Wellness

Concepts and Applications

Sixth Edition

David J. Anspaugh, PED, EdD, CHES
TRI-STATE UNIVERSITY

Michael H. Hamrick, EdD, CHES, FAAHE
THE UNIVERSITY OF MEMPHIS

Frank D. Rosato, EdD
THE UNIVERSITY OF MEMPHIS

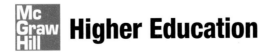 **Higher Education**

Boston   Burr Ridge, IL   Dubuque, IA   Madison, WI   New York   San Francisco   St. Louis
Bangkok   Bogotá   Caracas   Kuala Lumpur   Lisbon   London   Madrid   Mexico City
Milan   Montreal   New Delhi   Santiago   Seoul   Singapore   Sydney   Taipei   Toronto

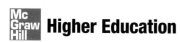

Higher Education

WELLNESS: CONCEPTS AND APPLICATIONS
SIXTH EDITION

Published by McGraw-Hill, a business unit of The McGraw-Hill Companies, Inc., 1221 Avenue of the Americas, New York, NY, 10020. Copyright © 2006, 2003, 2000, 1997, 1994, 1991 by The McGraw-Hill Companies, Inc. All rights reserved. No part of this publication may be reproduced or distributed in any form or by any means, or stored in a database or retrieval system, without the prior written consent of The McGraw-Hill Companies, Inc., including, but not limited to, in any network or other electronic storage or transmission, or broadcast for distance learning.

Some ancillaries, including electronic and print components, may not be available to customers outside the United States.

This book is printed on acid-free paper.

1 2 3 4 5 6 7 8 9 0 QPD/QPD 0 9 8 7 6 5

ISBN 0-07-297270-X

Editor in Chief: *Emily Barrosse*
Publisher: *Bill Glass*
Sponsoring Editor: *Nicholas Barrett*
Director of Development: *Kathleen Engelberg*
Developmental Editor: *Lynda Huenefeld*
Executive Marketing Manager: *Pamela S. Cooper*
Managing Editor: *Jean Dal Porto*
Project Manager: *Jill Moline-Eccher*
Production Service: *Jan Nickels*
Art Director: *Jeanne Schreiber*
Designer: *Cassandra J. Chu*

Text Designer: *Matthew Baldwin and Amy Evans McClure*
Cover Designer: *Yvo Riezebos*
Photo Researcher: *Natalia Peschiera*
Art Editor: *Katherine McNab*
Cover Credit: *© John Kelly/The Image Bank/Getty Images*
Media Producer: *Lance Gerhart*
Senior Media Project Manager: *Ron Nelms*
Production Supervisor: *Janean A. Utley*
Composition: *10/12 Sabon by GTS— Los Angeles, CA Campus*
Printing: *45 # Lighthouse Matte HB 88 Recycled, Quebecor World Dubuque Inc.*

Credits: The credits section for this book begins on page 527 and is considered an extension of the copyright page.

Library of Congress Cataloging-in-Publication Data

Anspaugh, David J.
  Wellness : concepts and applications / David J. Anspaugh, Michael H. Hamrick, Frank D. Rosato. — 6th ed.
    p.   cm.
  Includes bibliographical references and index.
  ISBN 0–07–297270–X
  1. Health. 2. Self-care, Health. 3. Medicine, Preventive. I. Hamrick, Michael H. II. Rosato, Frank D. III. Title.

RA776 .A57   2003
613—dc21

                          2001052194
                          CIP

The Internet addresses listed in the text were accurate at the time of publication. The inclusion of a Web site does not indicate an endorsement by the authors or McGraw-Hill, and McGraw-Hill does not guarantee the accuracy of the information presented at these sites.

www.mhhe.com

In Memoriam

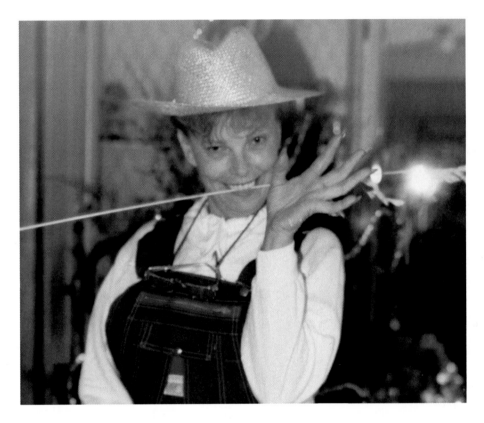

This edition is dedicated to the memory of Pat Rosato.
Pat courageously battled breast cancer for six and
a half years. She never lost her positive attitude, her
sense of humor, or her desire to help others
throughout the course of her illness.
She will be missed.

What's in This for You?

Are you looking for wellness and fitness information online? Working hard to get in shape? Trying to improve your grade? The great features in *Wellness: Concepts and Applications* will help you do all this and more! Let's take a look.

Online Learning Center Resources

Want to get a better grade? This box reminds you about the study aids and other resources available at McGraw-Hill's free Online Learning Center and describes some of the useful study tools you'll find there.

Chapter Key Terms

The opening page of each chapter lists the main terms for that chapter, helping you know which terms to pay close attention to as you study the chapter.

Chapter Objectives

The opening page of each chapter also lists the objectives for that chapter to help you understand what concepts you should know by the conclusion of the chapter. This will help you in test preparation.

Goals for Behavior Change

The opening page of each chapter contains a list of behavior change goals specific to that chapter to help you as you strive to achieve a better state of wellness.

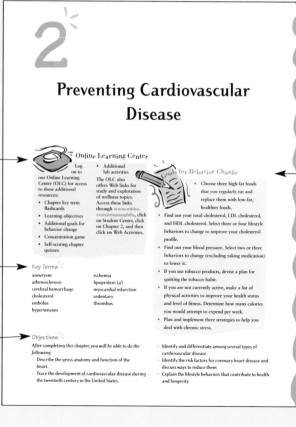

2

Preventing Cardiovascular Disease

Online Learning Center

Log on to our Online Learning Center (OLC) for access to these additional resources:
- Chapter key term flashcards
- Learning objectives
- Additional goals for behavior change
- Concentration game
- Self-scoring chapter quizzes

- Additional lab activities

The OLC also offers Web links for study and exploration of wellness topics. Access these links through www.mhhe.com/anspaugh6e, click on Student Center, click on Chapter 2, and then click on Web Activities.

Key Terms

aneurysm
atherosclerosis
cerebral hemorrhage
cholesterol
embolus
hypertension

ischemia
lipoprotein (a)
myocardial infarction
sedentary
thrombus

Objectives

After completing this chapter, you will be able to do the following:
- Describe the gross anatomy and function of the heart.
- Trace the development of cardiovascular disease during the twentieth century in the United States.

- Identify and differentiate among several types of cardiovascular disease.
- Identify the risk factors for coronary heart disease and discuss ways to reduce them.
- Explain the lifestyle behaviors that contribute to health and longevity.

Goals for Behavior Change

- Choose three high-fat foods that you regularly eat and replace them with low-fat, healthier foods.
- Find out your total cholesterol, LDL cholesterol, and HDL cholesterol. Select three or four lifestyle behaviors to change to improve your cholesterol profile.
- Find out your blood pressure. Select two or three behaviors to change (excluding taking medication) to lower it.
- If you use tobacco products, devise a plan for quitting the tobacco habit.
- If you are not currently active, make a list of physical activities to improve your health status and level of fitness. Determine how many calories you would attempt to expend per week.
- Plan and implement three strategies to help you deal with chronic stress.

Table 2-2 Risk Profile—Lipid and Lipoprotein Concentrations

Total Cholesterol	Category of Risk
< 200 mg/dL.*	Desirable
200–239 mg/dL	Borderline
≥ 240 mg/dL**	High

LDL Cholesterol	Category of Risk
<100 mg/dL	Optimal
100–129 mg/dL	Near optimal/above optimal
130–159 mg/dL	Borderline high
160–189 mg/dL	High
≥ 190 mg/dL	Very high

HDL Cholesterol	Category of Risk
≤ 40 mg/dL.***	Increased risk
≥ 60 mg/dL	Heart-protective

Triglycerides	Category of Risk
<150 mg/dL	Normal
150–199 mg/dL	Borderline high
200–499 mg/dL	High
≥ 500 mg/dL	Very high

SOURCE: Adapted from Revised cholesterol guidelines. 2001. *Harvard Heart Letter* 11 (July): 6–7.

* < is less than

** ≥ is equal to or greater than

*** ≤ is equal to or less than

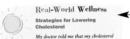 **Real-World Wellness**

Strategies for Lowering Cholesterol

My doctor told me that my cholesterol level is too high. How can I lower it to reduce my risk of having a heart attack or stroke?

First, establish a realistic goal, such as about how much you think you can lower your cholesterol. Second, identify the lifestyle changes that can lower cholesterol. Third, attempt to do all of the following that apply to you:

- Reduce your fat consumption to less than 30 percent of total calories (25 percent would be better).
- Reduce your saturated fat and trans fats consumption to less than 10 percent of total calories (8 percent would be better).
- Reduce your dietary cholesterol to less than 300 mg/day (less than 200 mg/day would be better).
- Lose weight if you are overweight.
- Stop smoking cigarettes and/or stop using other tobacco products.
- Increase your consumption of soluble fiber, found in fruits, vegetables, and grains.
- Do aerobic exercise at least three times per week for at least 30 minutes each time.

If these strategies fail to normalize your cholesterol level in six months, you may have to consider taking cholesterol-lowering drugs.

some common foods that contain cholesterol and saturated fat.

A number of population studies during the last 20 years have indicated a positive relationship between serum cholesterol (the level of cholesterol circulating in the blood) and the development of coronary heart disease. The National Heart, Lung, and Blood Institute reviewed this evidence and concluded that high circulating levels of serum cholesterol cause heart disease.

Values of serum cholesterol above 200 milligrams per deciliter (mg/dL) of blood are higher than the average risk. Table 2-2 shows the values of risk associated with total cholesterol (TC), LDL and HDL cholesterol (to be discussed shortly), and another serum lipid (blood fat), the triglycerides.

An important collaborative study involving 12 research centers throughout the United States provided clinical evidence implicating cholesterol as a culprit in coronary heart disease.[11] Half of a group of 3,806 subjects was given a cholesterol-lowering drug, and the other half was given a placebo. The subjects were followed for approximately 7.4 years, at which time the data indicated

that the drug group reduced their cholesterol levels by 13 percent, suffered 19 percent fewer heart attacks, and experienced 24 percent fewer fatal heart attacks. The incidence of coronary bypass surgery and angina were also significantly reduced. The researchers concluded that each 1 percent reduction in cholesterol level results in a 2 percent reduction in the risk for coronary heart disease.

A later follow-up of this study indicated that the reduction in coronary heart disease is probably closer to 3 percent for every 1 percent that cholesterol is lowered.[12] The strategies for lowering cholesterol in the blood are presented in Real-World Wellness: Strategies for Lowering Cholesterol.

The Cholesterol Carriers. The amount of cholesterol circulating in the blood accounts for only part of the total cholesterol in the body. Unlike sugar and salt, cholesterol does not dissolve in the blood, so it is transported by protein packages, which facilitate its solubility. These transporters are the lipoproteins manufactured by the body. They include the chylomicrons, very low-density lipoprotein (VLDL), intermediate-density lipoprotein

---

Real-World Wellness

These question-and-answer boxes show you how to put wellness concepts into practice. Helpful tips give practical advice for initiating behavior change and staying motivated to follow a wellness lifestyle.

Nurturing Your Spirituality

These boxes cover such topics as living well with cancer, making decisions about sex, and enjoying healthy pleasure, showing how wellness goes beyond just the physical dimension.

 Nurturing Your Spirituality

Can Spirituality Improve Your Physical Health?

It's all in your mind. Or is it in your body? Or both? The interconnections between mind and body are the bases for many types of alternative health practices. Spirituality is believing in a source of value that transcends the boundaries of the self but also nurtures the self. Mind-body medicine builds on spirituality, encouraging methods for improving the body by altering the mind. The National Institutes of Health (NIH) suggests the following spiritual practices:

- *Psychotherapy* focuses on the mental and emotional health of the patient and has been proven to reduce the amount of time required to recover from an illness.
- *Support groups* give patients the consolation that others have endured similar health challenges and survived, instilling hope.
- *Meditation*, formerly associated solely with religious practice, is a self-governed exercise for relaxation. Regular practice of meditation is recommended for reducing blood pressure and anxiety and increasing quality of life and longevity.
- *Imagery* includes use of all the senses to encourage attitude change, behavior, or physiological responses. Uses of imagery include pain control in cancer patients and increased immunity in elderly patients.
- *Hypnosis* is an ancient practice molded to fit modern needs. Today physicians, dentists, psychologists, and other mental health professionals use hypnosis to help people overcome addictions, control pain, and deal with phobias.

- *Biofeedback* provides patients with a picture of what is occurring physiologically in their bodies and an understanding of how trial-and-error adjustments of mental processes can affect these physiological behaviors. This technique is used in treatment for a wide variety of disorders, such as epilepsy, respiratory diseases, migraines, vascular disorders, and hypertension.
- *Yoga* is a disciplined practice of altering mental and physiological processes previously thought to be outside an individual's control. These alterations, performed on a regular basis, can reduce anxiety, lower blood pressure, treat arthritis, and increase the efficiency of the heart.
- *Dance therapy* uses body movement for therapeutic purposes. It is proven effective for achieving such goals as improving self-concept and self-esteem, minimizing fears, reducing body tension, improving circulatory and respiratory functions, promoting healing, and reducing depression.
- *Music therapy* puts to good use the power of music on the psyche. Do you ever listen to music to make you feel better? So do stroke, Parkinson's, brain-injury, cancer, anxiety, cerebral palsy, and burn patients.
- *Art therapy* uses self-expression through art to enhance healing. Art therapy is used with patients being treated for burns, emotional problems, chemical addictions, and sexual abuse.
- *Prayer and mental healing* involves communication with some form of higher power. A wide variety of healing techniques fall within this category. Examples are being physically touched by a religious healer and experiencing healing through personal prayer or attendance at church. Studies link regular church attendance with reduced chance of dying from stroke or heart disease, lower blood pressure, lower suicide rates, and reduced depression.

Researchers concluded that adults, young and old, should stay connected either to other people, a pet, or a favorite hobby.[5]

Physical

The physical component of wellness involves the ability to carry out daily tasks, develop cardiorespiratory and muscular fitness, maintain adequate nutrition and a healthy body fat level, and avoid abusing alcohol and other drugs or using tobacco products. In general, physical health is an investment in positive lifestyle habits. Separate chapters in this text are devoted to many of these physical dimensions of wellness.

Emotional

Emotional wellness is the ability to control stress and to express emotions appropriately and comfortably. It is the ability to recognize and accept feelings and not be defeated by setbacks and failures. Achieving emotional wellness allows you to cope with life's ups and downs effectively.

Many studies report on the connection between wellness and emotional health. Anger, for example, is a powerful emotion that has been linked to heart attacks. In a recent six-year study of 12,986 men and women, 256 participants had heart attacks. Individuals who were more prone to anger were almost three

Just the Facts

Special material in these boxes will encourage you to delve into a particular topic or more closely examine an important health issue.

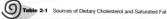

Just the Facts

Guidelines for Fat and Cholesterol

The National Cholesterol Education Program through the auspices of the National Heart, Lung, and Blood Institute released its newest recommendations for detecting and lowering high cholesterol in adults in May 2001. This revision represents the first major change since 1993. The following are some selected highlights recommended by a panel of 27 experts:

1. Physicians are strongly encouraged to pay more attention to the "metabolic syndrome," representative of a significant risk for heart disease. This syndrome is a combination of excessive abdominal fat, high blood pressure, high blood glucose, elevated triglycerides, and low HDL cholesterol.
2. HDL cholesterol is considered a major risk if it is below 40 mg/dL, instead of the previous 35 mg/dL.

3. Dietary intake of cholesterol should be less than 200 mg/day for those at high risk and less than 300 mg/day for all others.
4. There should be more aggressive treatment of triglycerides.
5. Less than 10 percent of calories should come from saturated fat and trans fats together.
6. Dietary fat may be increased to 35 percent of the total daily calories instead of the previous 30 percent, provided that the majority of these come from monounsaturated and polyunsaturated sources.
7. The new recommendations strongly urge the necessity of attaining and maintaining normal body weight, as well as consistent participation in physical activity.

Table 2-1 Sources of Dietary Cholesterol and Saturated Fat

	Cholesterol (mg)*	Saturated Fat (g)**		Cholesterol (mg)*	Saturated Fat (g)**
Meats (3 oz.)			**Seafood (3 oz.)**		
Beef liver	372	2.5	Squid	153	.4
Veal	86	4.0	Oily fish	59	1.2
Pork	80	3.2	Lean fish	59	.3
Lean beef	56	2.4	Shrimp (6 large)	48	.2
Chicken (dark meat)	82	2.7	Clams (6 large)	36	.3
Chicken (white meat)	76	1.3	Lobster	46.4	.08
Egg	215	1.7			
			Other Items of Interest		
Dairy Products (1 Cup; Cheese, 1 oz.)			Pork brains (3 oz.)	2,169	1.8
Ice cream	59	8.9	Beef kidney (3 oz.)	683	3.8
Whole milk	33	5.1	Beef hot dog (1)	75	9.9
Butter (1 tsp.)	31	7.1	Prime ribs of beef (3 oz.)	66.5	5.3
Yogurt (low-fat)	11	1.8	Doughnut	36	4.0
Cheddar	30	6.0	Milk chocolate	0	16.3
American	27	5.6	Green or yellow vegetable or fruit	0	Trace
Camembert	20	4.3	Peanut butter (1 tbsp.)	0	1.5
Parmesan	8	2.0	Angel food cake	0	1.96
			Skim milk (1 cup)	4	.3
Oils (1 tbsp.)			Cheese pizza (3 oz.)	6	.8
Coconut	0	11.8	Buttermilk (1 cup)	9	1.3
Palm	0	6.7	Ice milk, soft (1 cup)	13	2.9
Olive	0	1.8	Turkey, white meat (3 oz.)	59	.9
Corn	0	1.7			
Safflower	0	1.2			

* There are 1,000 mg in a gram.

** There are 28 g in an ounce and 454 g in a pound.

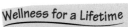

Wellness for a Lifetime

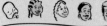

Childhood Origins of Heart Disease

Behavior patterns established during childhood that increase the likelihood of coronary heart disease often persist into adulthood. A physically inactive child is likely to become a physically inactive adult.[13] Only 50 percent of young people in the United States (ages 12 to 21 years) regularly participate in vigorous physical activity, and one-fourth report no physical activity at all.[14,15] Physical inactivity is a primary contributor to the unprecedented explosion of overweight and obesity among children in the United States. The percentage of overweight adolescents today has tripled since 1980, and this trend shows no signs of abating or reversing in the near future.[16] Approximately 30.3 percent of 6- to 11-year-old children are overweight and 15.3 percent are obese; 30.4 percent of adolescents are overweight, while 15.5 percent are obese.[17] One of the serious consequences of early obesity has been the emergence of Type 2 diabetes—a disease with life-threatening complications that in the recent past occurred almost exclusively in middle-aged adults—which is currently occurring among American adolescents. The two major reasons for this trend are (1) overweight/obesity and (2) physical inactivity.[17] The American Diabetic Association and the American Academy of Pediatrics recommend that at-risk children be screened with a blood test every two years starting at the age of 10.[18] An estimated 1.7 million Americans became regular cigarette smokers in 1998. More than half were younger than 18 years of age.[4] Smoking is a major risk for many diseases that tend to track into adulthood.

Leading health authorities presented a list of 10 high-priority public health concerns in *Healthy People 2010*. Topping the list was the need for Americans, young and old, to become more physically active. The second concern was the unprecedented number of overweight and obese people in the United States.[19]

In a recent study using sophisticated measuring techniques, children 9 to 11 years old whose cholesterol was higher than normal had blood vessels stiffer than expected for their young age. Arterial dilation was less than normal in these children, while resistance to blood flow was greater than normal in response to the heart's contractions.[20]

Obese children show blood vessel abnormalities that can lead to premature heart disease later in life.[21]

Cardiovascular disease is the third leading cause of death for children under the age of 15, and approximately 197,000 cardiovascular procedures were performed on youngsters 15 years of age and younger in the year 2001.[4]

Attempts to prevent heart disease need to begin in childhood. Knowledgeable parents can serve as role models who practice, rather than just talk about, healthy behaviors. Active parents should be the strongest influence, but they are not the only influence. Schools need to offer quality physical education programs throughout the 12 years of precollege education, and communities should offer opportunities and provide facilities for active participation in games and recreational play.

Autopsy studies of American combat battle casualties, whose average age was 22 years, in the Korean and Vietnam wars showed obstructions in the coronary arteries. These obstructions are caused by **atherosclerosis**, a slow, progressive disease of the arteries that can originate in childhood.[11] It is characterized by the deposition of plaque beneath the lining of the artery (figure 2-4). Plaque consists of fatty substances, cholesterol, blood platelets, fibrin, calcium, and cellular debris. The atherosclerotic process is responsible for 80 percent of the coronary heart disease deaths in the United States. The current theory of the development of atherosclerosis is explained in the section dealing with cholesterol as a risk factor.

Between 3 and 4 million people have silent **ischemia** or silent heart attacks.[12] These people typically do not experience chest pain or chest discomfort, nor do they have arm, neck, or jaw pain.[22] Those most likely to experience

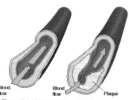

Figure 2-4 Progressive Narrowing of a Normal Coronary Artery (Atherosclerosis)

Blood flow   Blood flow   Plaque

Wellness for a Lifetime

These boxes address wellness concepts throughout the life span by looking at issues such as childhood origins of heart disease, alcohol and other drug use among young women, and strength training for older adults.

Wellness on the Web

These behavior change activities take you to quizzes, questions, and self-assessments on the text's Online Learning Center. Completing these activities will help you assess your current practices and design a more wellness-oriented lifestyle.

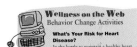

Online Learning Center

www.mhhe.com/anspaugh6e

The text's Online Learning Center (OLC) provides a wide variety of helpful studying tools—including interactive quizzes, key term flashcards, online labs, daily news feeds, and additional activities.

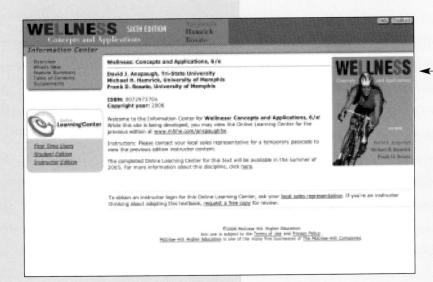

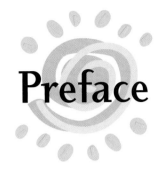

Preface

ellness: Concepts and Applications assumes that health is not a destination but a journey. Wellness is not a static condition but a continual balancing of the different dimensions of human needs—spiritual, social, emotional, intellectual, physical, occupational, and environmental. Because each of us is responsible for our growth in these areas, this edition continues to strive to emphasize the importance of self-responsibility. And because we know that knowledge alone stimulates change for very few people, the reader will be challenged to be actively involved in the learning process by constantly assessing how the information presented affects lifestyle from a personal perspective.

Wellness: Concepts and Applications is neither a fitness book nor a personal health text. Instead, this text is designed to help students gain knowledge and understanding in a variety of areas, with the goal of using that information to make behavior changes that will have a positive impact on their lives. In many cases, these changes are necessary if people are to develop the skills, attitudes, beliefs, and habits that will ultimately result in the highest possible level of health and wellness.

Audience

When the fitness and wellness concept appears in university courses and programs, it is usually a scaled-down model of the traditional personal health course or an upscale version of physical fitness courses. In some cases, it is a hybrid of personal health and fitness courses, with emphasis on self-participation in the medical marketplace. *Wellness: Concepts and Applications* is a hybrid because the physical components of wellness are blended with its many other components. The primary objectives of this text are to present cognitive health and wellness information appropriate for today's college students and to offer suggestions for their application. These suggestions relate to lifestyle behaviors over which people can exert some control. The emphasis is on self-responsibility, and this theme is implemented through a strong self-analysis and assessment component.

Approach

Important features unique to *Wellness: Concepts and Applications* distinguish it from other texts.

Balanced approach: Unlike other approaches that emphasize only physical fitness as a route to wellness, *Wellness: Concepts and Applications* provides a balanced presentation of the health benefits of exercise, diet, and cardiovascular wellness, along with the management of lifestyle change and consumer responsibility to achieve lifetime wellness.

Complete lifestyle decision-making information: Along with Goals for Behavior Change, Real-World Wellness boxes, Wellness on the Web Behavior Change Activities, and Assessment Activities that help apply the content, coverage of substance use, sexually transmitted diseases, cancer, and chronic health conditions is provided to enable and encourage responsible student decision making.

Consumer orientation: Chapter 15, "Becoming a Responsible Health Care Consumer," offers information to help students become wise consumers.

Interdisciplinary author team: Two health educators and a fitness educator currently teaching wellness courses have combined their expertise to provide the most balanced presentation possible.

Full color: A full-color format is used in the photographs, line drawings, and design of the text to increase visual appeal and to enhance the teaching-learning process.

Highlights of This Edition

Every chapter of *Wellness: Concepts and Applications* has been carefully updated. New tables, figures, references, and issues found in this edition are highlighted here.

Online Learning Center

In every chapter, the chapter-opening page contains an Online Learning Center box directing the reader to additional online information and study resources for that chapter.

Wellness on the Web: Behavior Change Activities

The text includes activities in every chapter that take students to online quizzes, questions, and self-assessment activities. This feature has been completely revised from the previous edition, with the reader being directed to the Online Learning Center at www.mhhe.com/anspaugh6e to complete the activities. This ensures that the links will be active when the reader tries to access them.

Just the Facts

Special material in newly written Just the Facts boxes encourages students to delve into a particular topic or closely examine an important health issue.

Wellness for a Lifetime

New content appears in the Wellness for a Lifetime features throughout the textbook.

New or Expanded Topics

We are committed to making this textbook the most up-to-date wellness text available. Following is a sampling of topics that are either completely new to this edition or covered in greater depth than in the previous edition:

Chapter 1: Wellness and Fitness for Life

- New and updated figures and tables
- New Just the Facts boxes on laughter as medicine, how communities can promote wellness, and selected health disparities by race, ethnicity, level of education, and gender
- Updated statistics on causes of death in the United States

Chapter 2: Preventing Cardiovascular Disease

- New and updated figures and tables
- New information regarding coronary heart disease
- New information on the relationship between high resting heart rates and sudden death
- New section on unhealthy lifestyle habit involvement in heart attacks
- New guidelines for the prevention and treatment of high blood pressure
- Information on the DASH diet

Chapter 3: Increasing Cardiorespiratory Endurance

- New and updated figures and tables
- New information on the Institute of Medicine's exercise recommendation
- New information on the importance of warming up before exercise

Chapter 4: Building Muscular Strength and Endurance

- New and updated figures and tables
- New information on establishing 1RM
- New Wellness for a Lifetime box on resistive training for American youth
- ACSM's revised resistance training guidelines for average healthy adults
- New information on vitamins, ginseng, and chromium
- New sections on co-enzyme Q10 (ubiquinone), conjugated linoleic acid (CLA), androstenedione ("andro"), and human growth hormone (hGH)

Chapter 5: Improving Flexibility

- New and updated figures and tables
- Expanded definition of *flexibility*
- New Just the Facts box about neck pain

Chapter 6: Forming a Plan for Good Nutrition

- New and updated figures and tables
- New information on low-carb, net carb, and carbohydrate loading
- New information on RDAs, DRIs, and DVs
- New information on enhanced foods
- New dietary recommendations regarding carbohydrate, protein, and fat intake
- New Just the Facts boxes on estimating calorie sources, low carbs vs. net carbs, vitamin D, water intake, enhanced foods, and the Food Guide Pyramid
- Updated nutrient information of selected legumes
- Updated information on trans fat
- New guidelines on water intake
- Updated discussion on dietary fiber
- New discussion on Glycemic Index and Glycemic Load

Chapter 7: Understanding Body Composition

- New and updated figures and tables
- Revised Wellness for a Lifetime box about body composition of children and adolescents
- New section on Dual-Energy X-Ray Absorptiometry (DEXA)

Chapter 8: Achieving a Healthy Weight

- New and updated figures and tables
- New Nurturing Your Spirituality box on body image and weight loss
- New Just the Facts boxes on the difference between overweight and obesity, weight maintenance, low-carbohydrate diets, ephedra, cutting back of calories, and walking
- New information on the Framingham Heart Study and obesity studies at Johns Hopkins
- New Nurturing Your Spirituality box titled "Obesity: Nature vs. Nurture"
- New section on portion sizes and volume eating
- Enhanced section on low-carbohydrate diets
- Expanded section on diet drugs
- New information on the National Academy of Sciences recommendations for time spent in physical activity

Chapter 9: Coping with and Managing Stress

- New and updated figures and tables
- Updated information on the autonomic nervous system
- New information on a study involving cancer patients with malignant melanoma
- New Real-World Wellness boxes about sleep and stress reduction and how to use a to-do list
- New section about tai chi
- New section on spirituality

Chapter 10: Taking Charge of Your Personal Safety

- New and updated figures and tables
- New Just the Facts boxes with U.S. crime clock statistics, on post-9/11 safe air travel, and on disasters
- Expanded section on relationship violence
- New section on violence in dating

Chapter 11: Taking Responsibility for Drug Use

- New and updated figures and tables
- New section on what causes addiction
- New Just the Facts boxes on products containing caffeine and 12-step programs
- New section on how to protect oneself from being a victim of club drugs

Chapter 12: Preventing Sexually Transmitted Diseases

- New and updated figures and tables
- New section on the treatment of HIV and AIDS
- New table on drugs approved to treat HIV infections

Chapter 13: Reducing Your Risk for Cancer

- New and updated figures and tables
- New section on antiangiogenesis therapy

- New section on bone marrow and peripheral blood stem cell transplants

Chapter 14: Managing Common Conditions

- New and updated figures and tables
- New section on pre-diabetes
- New section on gestational diabetes
- New Just the Facts box about advances in treating diabetes
- New information on the FDA's approval of alendronate, raloxifene, and resedronate
- New information on the relationship between asthma and immune malfunction
- New information on the treatment of migraines

Chapter 15: Becoming a Responsible Health Care Consumer

- New and updated figures and tables
- New information on relative and absolute risks
- New guidelines for determining whether information found on the Internet can be trusted
- Additional information on when it is wise to seek health care
- New Real-World Wellness box about when to seek treatment for a fever
- New data on common reasons for hospitalization and average length of stay
- New Just the Facts box on grading hospitals
- Revised tips on patient-physician communication
- New information on pharmacist consultations
- New information on sigmoidoscopy and colonoscopy procedures
- New section on direct-access testing (DAT)

Successful Pedagogical Features

Wellness: Concepts and Applications continues to use a variety of learning aids to enhance student comprehension.

Key Terms: The most important terms for student retention have been set in boldface type in the text for easy identification.

Chapter Objectives: These are introduced at the beginning of each chapter. They help the student identify the chapter's key topics. Accomplishing the objectives indicates fulfillment of the chapter's intent.

Goals for Behavior Change: These are listed at the beginning of each chapter, giving students objectives that help them apply what they learn in the text. They reinforce the concept of self-responsibility on which the text is based.

Nurturing Your Spirituality: These boxes cover such topics as living well with cancer, making decisions about sex, and enjoying healthy pleasure, showing students that wellness goes beyond the physical dimension.

Wellness on the Web: These are activities that take students to quizzes, questions, and self-assessments on the text's Online Learning Center. Completing these activities will help students assess their current practices and design a more wellness-oriented lifestyle.

Wellness for a Lifetime: These boxes address wellness concepts throughout the life span by looking at issues such as childhood origins of heart disease, alcohol and other drug use among young women, and strength training for older adults.

Real-World Wellness: These question-and-answer boxes show students how to put wellness concepts into practice. Helpful tips give students practical advice for initiating behavior change and staying motivated to follow a wellness lifestyle.

Just the Facts: Special material in these boxes encourages students to delve into a particular topic or closely examine an important health issue.

Chapter Summaries: These identify the main parts of the chapter and reinforce the chapter objectives.

Review Questions: Questions are provided to help students review and analyze material for overall understanding.

References: Accurate and current documentation is given at the end of the chapters.

Suggested Readings: Additional current resources are provided for students to obtain further information.

Assessment Activities: Each chapter concludes with at least two Assessment Activities to help students apply the content learned in the chapter to their decision making. The text is perforated for easy removal of the Assessment Activities.

Appendix: In the Food Composition Table, more than 1,200 common foods and fast foods are analyzed. This comprehensive table helps students complete Assessment Activities in Chapter 6.

Glossary: A comprehensive glossary is provided at the end of the text that includes all key terms, as well as additional terms, used in the text.

Technology: The Key to Teaching and Learning

Just a quick glance through the pages of *Wellness: Concepts and Applications* will show that technology is woven through every chapter. Similarly, the ancillary package that accompanies the text emphasizes technology while acknowledging the merit of the printed ancillaries. Together, the text and its ancillaries offer the ideal approach to teaching and learning—one that integrates the best tools that technology has to offer, challenging both instructors and students to reach higher.

Supplemental Instructor Materials

An extensive ancillary package is available to qualified adopters to enhance the teaching-learning process. We have made a concerted effort to produce supplements of extraordinary utility and quality. This package has been carefully planned and developed to help instructors derive the greatest benefit from the text. We encourage instructors to examine them carefully. Many of the products can be packaged with the text at a discounted price. Beyond the following brief descriptions, additional information about these ancillaries is available from your McGraw-Hill sales representative.

Instructor's Resource CD-ROM ISBN 0-07-297271-8

This interactive CD-ROM combines all the elements of the Course Integrator Guide with the electronic instructor resources offered with the text. The resources on the CD-ROM include the Course Integrator Guide, PowerPoint slides, Image Set, downloadable Test Bank, and Computerized Test Bank:

- *Course Integrator Guide:* This manual includes all of the features of a useful instructor's manual, including learning objectives, suggested lecture outlines, suggested activities, media resources, and Web links. It also integrates the text with all the wellness resources McGraw-Hill offers, such as the Online Learning Center (OLC), the image bank, and the PowerPoint presentations. The guide also includes references to relevant print and broadcast media.
- *PowerPoint Presentations:* A complete PowerPoint lecture for the course is included in the instructor's portion of the Online Learning Center, as well as on the Instructor's Resource CD-ROM. This presentation, ready to use in class, was prepared by a professional in the wellness field. It corresponds to the content in each chapter of *Wellness: Concepts and Applications*, making it easier for instructors to teach and ensuring that students can follow lectures point by point. Instructors can modify the presentation as much as they like to meet the needs of their course.
- *Image Set:* The Image Set is a bank of images for use in the classroom and in the accompanying PowerPoint presentation. The Image Set includes all of the figures from the text.
- *Test Bank:* This downloadable manual includes more than 2,000 questions, including multiple choice, true/false, and short essay. The questions have been entered into the computerized test bank.
- *EZ Test Computerized Test Bank:* McGraw-Hill's EZ Test is a flexible and easy-to-use electronic

testing program. The program allows instructors to create tests from book-specific items. It accommodates a wide range of question types, and instructors can add their own questions. Multiple versions of the test can be created, and any test can be exported for use with course management systems, such as WebCT, BlackBoard, or PageOut. The program is available for Windows and Macintosh environments.

Course Management Systems

www.mhhe.com/support

Now instructors can combine their McGraw-Hill Online Learning Center with today's most popular course management systems and/or McGraw-Hill's PageOut. The McGraw-Hill Online Learning Center has also been converted into a cartridge that can be used in most course management systems. Our Instructor Advantage program offers customers toll-free telephone support and unlimited e-mail support. Instructors who use 500 or more copies of a McGraw-Hill textbook can enroll in our Instructor Advantage Plus program, which provides on-campus, hands-on training from a platform specialist. We have also built an interactive support site accessible to anyone with an Internet connection. Located at www.mhhe.com/support, instructors can ask questions of the prebuilt database or e-mail a McGraw-Hill specialist. Instructors can consult their McGraw-Hill sales representative to learn what other course management systems are easily used with McGraw-Hill online materials.

Quia™

The Online Wellness Lab Manual and Workbook, developed in collaboration with Quia™, offers an electronic version of labs, assessments, and quizzes compiled from the text and its main supplements. This new online supplement offers the student such benefits as interactive labs and assessments, self-scoring quizzes, and instant feedback. The instructor benefits from a grade book that automatically scores, tracks, and records students' results and provides the opportunity to review individual and class performance. Instructors also have the ability to customize activities and features for their course by using Quia's™ activity templates. Instructors who want to find out more about this new online supplement and how they can package it with their textbooks can contact their McGraw-Hill sales representative.

Online Learning Center (OLC)

www.mhhe.com/anspaugh6e

This Web site offers resources to students and instructors. It includes downloadable ancillaries, Web links,

student quizzing, additional information on topics of interest, and much more.

Resources for the instructor include

- Downloadable PowerPoint presentation
- Lecture outlines
- Interactive links
- Links to professional resources

Resources for the student include

- Flashcards of chapter key terms
- Interactive activities
- Self-grading quizzes

PageOut®: The Course Web Site Development Center

www.pageout.net

PageOut® enables instructors to develop a Web site for their course. The site includes

- A course home page
- An instructor home page
- A syllabus (interactive and customizable, including quizzing, instructor notes, and links to the Online Learning Center)
- Web links
- Discussions (multiple discussion areas per class)
- An online grade book
- Student Web pages
- Design templates

This program is now available to registered adopters of McGraw-Hill textbooks. Instructors can contact their sales representative for assistance.

Video Library

Instructors can choose from the McGraw-Hill videotape library, which contains many quality videotapes, including selected Films for Humanities and all videos from the award-winning series *Health Living: Road to Wellness*. Digitized video clips are also available.

NutritionCalc Plus

NutritionCalc Plus can be used to analyze and monitor personal dietary needs and health goals. The database includes thousands of ethnic foods, supplements, fast foods, and convenience foods. Individual foods can be added to the food list. The database also includes the latest DRI values for essential nutrients, vitamins, and minerals. A wide variety of reports and graphs are generated based on the user's personal profile and intake analysis. An easy-to-use interface and the reliability of the database make NutritionCalc Plus the best source for nutrition analysis software.

Testwell by the National Wellness Institute

This is a self-scoring, pencil-and-paper wellness assessment developed by the National Wellness Institute in Stevens Point, Wisconsin, and distributed exclusively by McGraw-Hill Publishers. It adds flexibility to any wellness course by allowing adopters to offer preassessments and postassessments at the beginning, end, or any time during the course.

Diet and Fitness Log by McGraw-Hill

This logbook helps students track their diet and exercise programs. It serves as a diary to help students log their behaviors. Each log offers a brief introduction, followed by an evaluation section, in which they can assess their improvements and setbacks. It can be packaged with the textbook for an additional $1.00.

Acknowledgments

We wish to thank the following people for modeling for the photos:

Scott T. Belzer

Shonteh Henderson

Holly Ruth Henry

Chad Kirksick

Stacy Lancaster

Christopher Rasmussen

We wish to thank the reviewers, whose contributions have added significantly to the text. To the following, a grateful acknowledgment of their expertise and assistance:

For the Sixth Edition

John McIntosh
Northwest-Shoals Community College

Dick Newman
Presbyterian College

Karen Reynolds
Jefferson David Community College

Tim Rickabaugh
Defiance College

Christine Standefer
University of Maine–Presque Isle

Robert Walker
John Brown University

Daniel Williams
College of Southern Maryland

David J. Anspaugh

Michael H. Hamrick

Frank D. Rosato

Brief Contents

Contents

Wellness and Fitness for Life

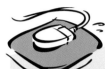 Online Learning Center

Log on to our Online Learning Center (OLC) for access to these additional resources:

- Chapter key term flashcards
- Learning objectives
- Additional goals for behavior change
- Concentration game
- Self-scoring chapter quizzes

- Additional lab activities

The OLC also offers Web links for study and exploration of wellness topics. Access these links through **www.mhhe.com/anspaugh6e**, click on Student Center, click on Chapter 1, and then click on Web Activities.

Goals for Behavior Change

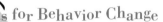

- Implement four new health-promoting behaviors.
- Increase physical activity to improve overall wellness.
- Choose and implement three countering strategies.
- Formulate a self-help plan for lifestyle change.
- Identify and discuss the main wellness challenges for Americans.
- Identify obvious and subtle factors that help shape behavior.
- Discuss some of the underlying assumptions of lifestyle change.
- Identify and describe the six stages of change.
- Describe strategies that can be useful in designing and implementing an action plan for change.

Key Terms

contracting
countering
health-behavior gap
health disparities
Leading Health Indicators (LHIs)
lifestyle diseases
locus of control

psychosomatic diseases
risk factors
self-efficacy
self-help
shaping up
transtheoretical model of behavior change
wellness

Objectives

After completing this chapter, you will be able to do the following:

- Discuss the wellness approach to healthy living.
- Identify benefits of living a wellness lifestyle.
- Describe the dimensions of wellness.

- Cite evidence of the relationship between physical health problems and social, emotional, and spiritual stressors.
- Identify health disparities that exist in the United States.
- Compare and contrast the major influences on the health of Americans today with those of Americans of the past.

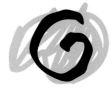

ood health is one of our most cherished possessions, one that is often taken for granted until it is lost. Some people convincingly argue that everything else in life is secondary to good health. For many, it is not difficult to recall instances when life's goals seemed unimportant because of sudden illness or a long-term debilitating health crisis.

Fortunately, the prospects of good health for Americans have never been better. The extent to which good health is realized is contingent on many factors. Chief among these factors are our actions and the choices we make. We can make choices that will promote health and well-being, prevent or delay the premature onset of many chronic illnesses, and improve our quality of life (see Real-World Wellness: Benefits of Living a Wellness Lifestyle). Staying healthy is not just a matter of common sense. Rather, it is a lifelong process that requires self-awareness, introspection, reflection, inquiry, accurate information, and action. This process relies on the concept of wellness and implies that each of us has the opportunity and the obligation to assume responsibility for factors that are under our control and to shape our health destiny. The wellness approach represents a formidable challenge because the processes leading to today's serious health threats are insidious, often originate in childhood or adolescence, flourish throughout adulthood, and finally culminate in full-blown disease in middle age or later. Lifestyle interventions initiated late in life produce limited success, but begun early in life they have maximum effect.

Components of Wellness

Wellness is defined as a lifelong process that at any given time produces a positive state of personal well-being; of feeling good about yourself; of optimal physical, psychological, and social functioning; and the control and minimization of both internal and external risk factors for both diseases and negative health conditions.[1] Wellness is a process rather than a goal. It implies a choice, a way of life. It means integrating the body, mind, and spirit. It symbolizes acceptance of yourself. It suggests that what you believe, feel, and do have an influence on your health. However, it does not imply that we make the best choice in every situation.

Consider the brief profiles of David, Susan, Carlos, and Maria. How would you rate each of them in terms of health and wellness?

David is physically active, places a high priority on his social life, barely makes passing grades in school, and engages in binge drinking almost every weekend. Susan is a perfectionist and her grades reflect it. To her, a *B* means failure. She spends an inordinate amount of time studying, regularly

Real-World Wellness

Benefits of Living a Wellness Lifestyle

I am a full-time student, work 20 plus hours a week, and help with family responsibilities. At the same time, I'm trying to maintain my academic scholarship. There just isn't enough time in the day to be concerned about health and wellness. What am I to gain from a wellness lifestyle?

A wellness lifestyle offers the following benefits:

- Increases energy level and productivity at work and school
- Decreases absenteeism from school and work
- Decreases recovery time after illness or injury
- Supplies the body with proper nutrients
- Improves awareness of personal needs and the ways to meet them
- Expands and develops intellectual abilities
- Increases the ability to communicate emotions to others and to act assertively rather than aggressively or passively
- Promotes the attitude that life's difficulties are challenges and opportunities rather than overwhelming threats
- Acts from an internal locus of control
- Increases ability to cope with stress and resist depression
- Improves the cardiorespiratory system
- Increases muscle tone, strength, flexibility, and endurance
- Improves physical appearance
- Helps prevent or delay the premature onset of some forms of chronic disease
- Regulates and improves overall body function
- Promotes self-confidence
- Delays the aging process
- Promotes social awareness and the ability to reach out to, understand, and care about others

skips meals, has no physical activity outlet, and rarely socializes. Her family tells her to "get a life." She needs the entire weekend to recover from the stress of academics. Carlos runs 3 miles every day, works out with weights three times a week, eats a balanced diet almost every day, has a close circle of friends, refuses to use his seat belt when driving, and smokes an average of two packs of cigarettes daily. Maria is a worrier. She makes good grades but is rarely

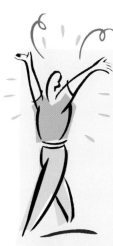

Nurturing Your Spirituality

Can Spirituality Improve Your Physical Health?

It's all in your mind. Or is it in your body? Or both? The interconnections between mind and body are the bases for many types of alternative health practices. Spirituality is believing in a source of value that transcends the boundaries of the self but also nurtures the self. Mind-body medicine builds on spirituality, encouraging methods for improving the body by altering the mind. The National Institutes of Health (NIH) suggests the following spiritual practices:

- *Psychotherapy* focuses on the mental and emotional health of the patient and has been proven to reduce the amount of time required to recover from an illness.

- *Support groups* give patients the consolation that others have endured similar health challenges and survived, instilling hope.

- *Meditation,* formerly associated solely with religious practice, is a self-governed exercise for relaxation. Regular practice of meditation is recommended for reducing blood pressure and anxiety and increasing quality of life and longevity.

- *Imagery* includes use of all the senses to encourage attitude change, behavior, or physiological responses. Uses of imagery include pain control in cancer patients and increased immunity in elderly patients.

- *Hypnosis* is an ancient practice molded to fit modern needs. Today physicians, dentists, psychologists, and other mental health professionals use hypnosis to help people overcome addictions, control pain, and deal with phobias.

- *Biofeedback* provides patients with a picture of what is occurring physiologically in their bodies and an understanding of how trial-and-error adjustments of mental processes can affect these physiological behaviors. This technique is used in treatment for a wide variety of disorders, such as epilepsy, respiratory diseases, migraines, vascular disorders, and hypertension.

- *Yoga* is a disciplined practice of altering mental and physiological processes previously thought to be outside an individual's control. These alterations, performed on a regular basis, can reduce anxiety, lower blood pressure, treat arthritis, and increase the efficiency of the heart.

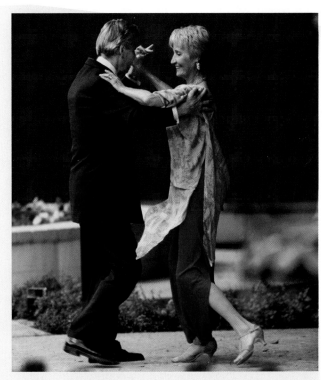

Enjoyable physical activity improves wellness inside and out.

- *Dance therapy* uses body movement for therapeutic purposes. It is proven effective for achieving such goals as improving self-concept and self-esteem, minimizing fears, reducing body tension, improving circulatory and respiratory functions, promoting healing, and reducing depression.

- *Music therapy* puts to good use the power of music on the psyche. Do you ever listen to music to make you feel better? So do stroke, Parkinson's, brain-injury, cancer, anxiety, cerebral palsy, and burn patients.

- *Art therapy* uses self-expression through art to enhance healing. Art therapy is used with patients being treated for burns, emotional problems, chemical addictions, and sexual abuse.

- *Prayer and mental healing* involves communication with some form of higher power. A wide variety of healing techniques fall within this category. Examples are being physically touched by a religious healer and experiencing healing through personal prayer or attendance at church. Studies link regular church attendance with reduced chance of dying from stroke or heart disease, lower blood pressure, lower suicide rates, and reduced depression.

In a recent six-year study of 12,986 men and women, 256 participants had heart attacks. Individuals who were more prone to anger were almost three times more likely to have a heart attack than those who were less prone to anger.[6,7] Examples of anger tendencies include being quick tempered, flying off the handle, saying nasty things when upset, and reacting aggressively and furiously when annoyed. Researchers suggested that a history of anger is as strong a risk factor for heart attacks as is smoking and hypertension.[8] They concluded that people with a penchant for high levels of anger should consider anger management therapy.

Many other health problems are rooted in emotional stressors. Health conditions ranging from hives to cancer may have as their origin a breakdown in the body's immune system caused by the body's response to emotional stressors. These stressors, by disrupting the body's delicate balance of powerful hormones, may serve as the triggering mechanism for myriad health problems. The growing acceptance of stress-coping techniques, like those presented in Chapter 9 of this text, is evidence of the trend toward nonphysical strategies for preventing and treating many health problems.

Intellectual

The intellectual component of wellness involves the ability to learn and use information effectively for personal, family, and career development. Intellectual wellness means striving for continued growth and learning to deal with new challenges effectively. It means acting on accepted principles of wellness and assuming responsibility for eliminating the discrepancy between knowledge and behavior, often referred to as the **health-behavior gap.** For example, people know that they should wear their seat belts and that they should not smoke, yet many people do not buckle up and continue to use tobacco products. For wellness to occur, people must internalize information and act on it.

An intellectually well person understands and applies the concepts of locus of control and self-efficacy. **Locus of control** refers to a person's view or attitude about his or her role in wellness and illness. A person's locus of control may be either internal or external. When people view problems concerning their health or other parts of their lives as generally out of their control (when they view themselves as being at the mercy of other people, places, and events), they have an external locus of control. On the other hand, people who have an internal locus of control view their own behaviors as having significant effects, feel that they are at least partially the masters of their fate, and recognize that they can change the course of their health. People with an internal locus of control are more likely to succeed in wellness activities, because they assume the necessary responsibility for their actions.

Just the Facts

Laughter as Medicine

If it is true that powerful negative emotions, such as anger, have a deleterious effect on health, might it also be true that powerful positive emotions, such as humor and laughter, are good for health? Research has long associated anger and hostility with increased heart disease risk. Recent studies now suggest that laughter may be heart-protective. Researchers at The University of Maryland found that people with heart disease were 40 percent less likely to laugh in uncomfortable situations and were less likely to recognize humor, compared with people of the same age without heart disease.

The health-protective mechanism of laughter is not clearly understood. Several possible explanations include

1. Laughter decreases the secretion of serum cortisol, a stress hormone related to several diseases, including heart disease.
2. Laughing releases chemicals, such as nitrous oxide (also known as laughing gas), that relaxes blood vessels.
3. Laughter increases blood levels of immunoglobulin A, an antibody that fights bacterial and viral infections.
4. Laughter may boost disease-fighting T-cells and natural killer cells, which are depressed during and after stressful experiences.
5. A hearty laugh involves the contraction and relaxation of muscles in the face, shoulders, abdomen, and diaphragm and may have a palliative effect on pain associated with arthritis.
6. Laughing changes the normal breathing pattern, ventilation, and circulation. Oxygen levels improve and help people with compromised breathing.
7. Laughter promotes fun and a sense of enjoyment with friends and family.
8. Laughter can improve your mood and help take your mind off your troubles. It is difficult to laugh and worry at the same time.

SOURCE: Consumers Union. 2001. Taking humor seriously. *Consumer Reports on Health* 13(10):7.

Locus of control serves as a simple but powerful yardstick of the relationship among attitudes, health perceptions, and wellness. People who appear optimistic about their health and believe they can have a direct influence on their well-being recover faster from surgery, have less heart disease, have better mental health, enjoy a higher quality of life, report more vitality and less pain, and live longer than people who have a pessimistic outlook.[9,10] Assessment Activity 1-2 at the end of this chapter will help you determine whether you have an internal or external locus of control.

Another influence on intellectual wellness is self-efficacy. **Self-efficacy** refers to a person's belief in his or her ability to accomplish a specific task or behavior. Perhaps the most important influence on the achievement of a wellness goal is the perception that it can be accomplished. Although the support of others is a source of encouragement, success is likely to require generating a personal sense of competence. Self-efficacy is not earned, inherited, or acquired; it is something you bestow on yourself.

For high-level wellness to be achieved, people must see themselves as successful and believe that they can accomplish a task. Although locus of control establishes an attitude toward one's role in achieving wellness, self-efficacy establishes behavior. Self-efficacy links knowing what to do and accomplishing the task. Together, an internal locus of control and a strong sense of self-efficacy are powerful tools in promoting wellness and coping with illness.

Occupational

Occupational wellness is the ability to achieve a balance between work and leisure time. Attitudes about work, school, career, and career goals greatly affect work or school performance and interactions with others. Striving for occupational wellness adds focus to your life and allows you to find personal satisfaction in your life through work.

Occupational wellness does not come without its challenges. Changes in careers and jobs are common and are associated with psychosocial stress. Such stress may affect health, either through neuroendocrine pathways or through increases in high-risk behaviors. For example, an unstable employment history and shorter duration of current job are linked with a greater prevalence of smoking and greater alcohol consumption.[11] Careers of today demand increased levels of flexibility and mobility. A person's level of wellness is a key factor in carving out and maintaining a successful career path. Finding work is easier for healthy persons; also, people who need to find work repeatedly are likely to drop out of the workforce if their health deteriorates.[11]

Environmental

Environmental wellness is the ability to promote health measures that improve the standard of living and quality of life in the community, including laws and agencies that safeguard the physical environment.

To illustrate the impact of environment on wellness, consider the differences in mortality (incidence of deaths) and morbidity (incidence of sickness) between earlier times and today. At the beginning of the twentieth century, the average life span of Americans was 47 years. Today it is 77.4 years,[12] an all-time high. In 1900, communicable, or infectious, diseases (diseases that can be transmitted from one person to another) were the major causes of death. Influenza, pneumonia, tuberculosis, smallpox, polio, diphtheria, and dysentery were often fatal and were greatly feared. Only 50 percent of children were expected to reach their fifth birthday. Environmental conditions were appalling; water was dirty and food was often unsafe for consumption. People generally had little control over their health, and prospects for a long life were greatly influenced by fate and circumstance. By comparison, children born today have a 99 percent rate of survival to their fifth birthday. Governmental agencies at the federal, state, and local levels now assume responsibility for protecting health and preventing infectious diseases. Vaccinations have eradicated many dreaded diseases. The world food supply has improved. Adult literacy has increased. Mind-boggling advancements in medical technology have given rise to diagnostic and surgical procedures far beyond the wildest imaginations of early-twentieth-century physicians. Still, even with all of the discoveries of modern medicine, the greatest improvement in the health of Americans is due to a much more basic element of the environment: safe water. No other factor, not even vaccinations or antibiotics, has had as significant an impact on mortality reduction and population growth as safe water.[13]

Today, environmental influences include more than safe water, food, and air. Subtle influences, such as the socioeconomic factors of income, housing, poverty, and education, play a crucial role in the health status of various population groups. As a rule, the less education you have and the less money you earn, the shorter your life expectancy and the greater your chances of getting many diseases.[14] People with lower socioeconomic status are less likely to work and, when they do, they are more likely to be exposed to unhealthy conditions. They do not have health care coverage, are underweight or overweight, are smokers, have high blood pressure and diabetes, or do not participate in leisure activities, compared with their peers who enjoy a higher socioeconomic status. Regardless of socioeconomic status and education level, people can safeguard their health by making healthy lifestyle choices. But even more can be done through policies and environments that support healthy behaviors and promote quality of life for entire communities.[15] (See Just the Facts: Communities Can Promote Wellness on page 8.)

ᔋᔋ Just the Facts ᔋᔋ

Communities Can Promote Wellness

Communities can create environments and policies that promote health and wellness. Examples include

- Enhanced 9-1-1 emergency medical transport services

- Fire stations and pharmacies that offer free blood pressure checks

- Health fairs where free cholesterol and diabetes screenings are available

- Walking and bicycle trails

- No smoking policies

- Smoking cessation services

- Health and wellness programs at schools and work sites and in faith- and community-based settings

- Availability of a full range of quality health services

- Programs that focus on eliminating racial, ethnic, and socioeconomic-based health disparities

- Accessible grocery stores stocked with fresh, affordable fruits and vegetables

SOURCES: Marks, J. S. 2003. We're living longer, but what about our quality of life? *Chronic Disease: Notes and Reports* 16(1):2–16; U.S. Department of Health and Human Services. 2003. *The power of prevention.* Washington, DC: U.S. Government Printing Office.

Health disparities are differences in the incidence, prevalence, mortality, and burden of diseases and other adverse health conditions that exist among specific population groups in the United States.[16] The National Institutes of Health has identified six focus areas in which racial and ethnic minorities experience serious disparities in health access and outcomes:

1. Infant mortality
2. Cancer screening and management
3. Cardiovascular disease
4. Diabetes
5. HIV infection/AIDS
6. Immunizations

These areas were selected for emphasis because they reflect areas of disparity known to affect multiple racial and ethnic minority groups at all life states (see Just the Facts: Selected Health Disparities by Race, Ethnicity, Level of Education, and Gender). Research on health disparities related to socioeconomic status will be addressed later in this text.

An important assumption of the wellness approach to living is that good health is best achieved by balancing each of the seven components. The body, mind, and spirit are inseparably linked. When they work together in a fully unified, integrated biological system, the body can ward off or overcome many diseases. When any of these components breaks down, wellness is threatened. Although the association between disease and physical causes (such as pathogens) is obvious, some people are reluctant to accept the association between illness and its mental, social, and spiritual aspects.

Nonphysical causes of illness are intangible and difficult to assess. Many people experience poor health because of guilt, anger, hostility, poor interpersonal skills, loneliness, anxiety, and depression. Any of these factors can interfere with the body's immune system and lay the foundation for the disease process. Medical records are replete with examples of **psychosomatic diseases,** in which physical (soma) symptoms are caused by mental and emotional (psycho) stressors. Such symptoms are just as real as if caused by disease-producing germs. Every disease involves interplay among the components of wellness. Fortunately, after a long-standing obsession with medical technology, many health care providers are beginning to focus on treating the whole person, and more people are demanding more than test-tube medical care.

Assessment Activity 1-1 at the end of this chapter provides an assessment of various aspects of wellness.

The Wellness Challenge

The most serious health problems of today are largely caused by the way people live and are referred to as **lifestyle diseases.** Lifestyle accounts for about two-thirds of life expectancy.[17] The leading causes of death in the United States among all age groups are heart disease, cancer, and stroke; they account for 58 percent of all deaths (Table 1-1 on page 10).[12] These are chronic diseases that are often caused by behaviors established early in life. *Chronic diseases* are health conditions that often begin gradually, have multiple causes, and usually persist for an indefinite time. Heart disease, diabetes, arthritis, and hypertension are examples of chronic illnesses. By contrast, *acute illnesses* come on suddenly, often have identifiable causes, are usually treatable, and often disappear in a short time. Appendicitis, pneumonia, and influenza are examples of acute illnesses.

Diseases are not the only causes of death. Accidents, homicide, and suicide are the leading killers of Americans between the ages of 15 and 24. Most (75 percent) accidental deaths among this age group involve motor vehicle accidents, many of which are alcohol-related. For young adults 25 to 44 years old, accidents, cancer, heart disease, suicide, human immunodeficiency virus (HIV) infection, and homicide are the leading causes of death.

Just the Facts

Selected Health Disparities by Race, Ethnicity, Level of Education, and Gender

The gap in life expectancy according to race, ethnicity, and gender has narrowed during the past 10 years. Still, disparities persist. Some racial and gender disparities in mortality are not as large as reported in 2000, while others are wider. Consider the following disparities by race and ethnicity, level of education, and gender:

Race/Ethnicity

1. Infant mortality rates have declined for all racial and ethnic groups. Still, disparities exist. The infant mortality rate is highest for infants of non-Hispanic black mothers and lowest for infants of mothers of Chinese origin.
2. Life expectancy at birth increased more for the black than for the white population. Still, life expectancy at birth is seven years longer for the white than for the black population.
3. Overall mortality is 31 percent higher for black Americans than for white Americans. Death rates for the black population exceed those for the white population by 40 percent for stroke, 29 percent for heart disease, 25 percent for cancer, and nearly 800 percent for HIV disease.
4. Homicide is the leading cause of death for young black males 15–24 years of age and the second leading cause of death for young Hispanic males. Homicide rates for young black and Hispanic males remain substantially higher than for young non-Hispanic white males.
5. HIV death rates are much higher for Hispanic and black males than for non-Hispanic white males 25–44 years of age.
6. Motor vehicle–related injury and suicide rates for young American Indian males are about 45 percent higher than the rates for young white males.
7. Overall mortality is almost 40 percent lower for Asian males than for white males. Death rates for cancer and heart disease for Asian males are 38–41 percent lower than corresponding rates for white males. The death rate for stroke is 3 percent lower for Asian males than for their white counterparts.

Level of Education

1. Infant mortality is inversely related to the mother's level of education. The less educated the mother, the higher the infant mortality rate.
2. Death rates for persons 25–64 years of age with fewer than 12 years of education is nearly three times the rate for persons with 13 or more years of education.

Gender

1. Life expectancy gains at birth are two years for males and one year for females.
2. Mortality from lung cancer is declining for men and increasing for women.
3. Mortality from chronic lower respiratory diseases is stable for men, while it is increasing for women.
4. The five-year survival rate for black females diagnosed with breast cancer is 15 percentage points lower than the survival rate for white females.

SOURCE: National Center for Health Statistics. 2003. *Health, United States, 2003.* Hyattsville, MD: U.S. Department of Health and Human Services.

For too many Americans these conditions reflect the dangers of negative lifestyle choices. Despite this, much of Americans' health-related anxiety involves exotic diseases. The current fear that some sort of strangely mutated disease will soon pose the greatest threat to life on Earth ironically coincides with a reduction in attention to chronic diseases that do kill in large numbers. The fear of bizarre pathogens leading to runaway deaths in the United States has been fueled primarily by newspaper headlines, fictional books, and movies. Five recent headlines serve as examples:

- "Mad cow disease spreads to U.S."
- "Anthrax kills postal workers"
- "West Nile Virus spreads to 37 states"
- "SARS shuts down travel to China"
- "Bioterrorism alert: botulism threatens the food supply"

Although the appearance of bioterrorism is possible and the spread of new viruses in a global community is a genuine concern, the real threats to Americans are mundane and are less likely to be featured as the lead stories in the evening news. As scary as some exotic diseases sound, the chances of getting them are remote, especially when comparing them with the chance of getting illnesses that people can take practical steps to avoid.[18]

Healthy lifestyles that involve diet, physical activity, and personal health habits offer the most potential for preventing health problems or delaying them until much later in life. More specifically, the following 10 health issues have been identified in the landmark document *Healthy People 2010*[19] as priority areas. These priority areas are referred to as **Leading Health Indicators (LHIs)** and are discussed in detail in this text. The LHIs are

Table 1-1 Ten Leading Causes of Death in 1900 and Today*

Rank	All Ages, 1900**	%	All Ages, Today***	%	15–24 Years, Today***	%	25–44 Years, Today***	%
1	Pneumonia and influenza	12	Heart disease	28	Accidents	46	Accidents	21
2	Tuberculosis	11	Cancer	23	Assault (homicide)	15	Cancer	15
3	Diarrhea and enteritis	8	Stroke	7	Intentional self-harm (suicide)	12	Heart disease	12
4	Heart disease	8	Chronic respiratory disease	5	Cancer	5	Intentional self-harm (suicide)	9
5	Stroke	6	Accidents	4	Heart disease	3	HIV disease	6
6	Nephritis	5	Diabetes mellitus	3	Congenital problems	1	Assault (homicide)	6
7	Accidents	4	Influenza and pneumonia	3	HIV disease	1	Liver disease and cirrhosis	3
8	Cancer	4	Alzheimer's disease	2	Chronic respiratory disease	1	Stroke	2
9	Diphtheria	2	Nephritis	2	Stroke	0.5	Diabetes mellitus	2
10	Meningitis	2	Septicemia	1	Diabetes mellitus	0.5	Influenza and pneumonia	1
	All other causes	38	All other causes	22	All other causes	15	All other causes	23

* Percentage mortality: i.e., percentage of all deaths in that year.

** Novartis Nutrition and McGraw-Hill. 2000. *Obesity: A modern epidemic. Innovations: Nutrition updates and applications.* New York: McGraw-Hill.

*** Kochanek, K. D., and B. L. Smith. 2004. Deaths: Preliminary data for 2002. *National Vital Statistics Reports.* Vol. 52, no. 13. Hyattsville, MD: National Center for Health Statistics.

1. Physical activity
   - Vigorous physical activity in adolescents *[30 min/day]*
   - Moderate physical activity in adults
2. Overweight and obesity
   - Overweight and obesity in children and adolescents
   - Obesity in adults
3. Tobacco use
   - Cigarette smoking by adolescents
   - Cigarette smoking by adults
4. Substance abuse
   - Alcohol and illicit drug use by adolescents
   - Illicit drug use by adults
   - Binge drinking by adults
5. Responsible sexual behavior
   - Responsible adolescent sexual behavior
   - Condom use by adults
6. Mental health
   - Treatment for adults with recognized depression
7. Injury and violence
   - Deaths from motor vehicle crashes
   - Homicides
8. Environmental quality
   - Ozone pollution exposure
   - Exposure to environmental tobacco smoke
9. Immunization
   - Fully immunized children aged 19 to 35 months
   - Flu and pneumococcal vaccination in high-risk adults
10. Access to health care
    - Persons with health insurance
    - Source of ongoing care
    - Early prenatal care

The risk factor most strongly associated with preventable death and chronic disease is cigarette smoking.[20] In studies that try to pinpoint the cause of death, tobacco use is responsible for 435,000 deaths or 18.1 percent of all deaths (see Figure 1-3).[21]

For the smoker, his or her primary wellness challenge is to stop smoking; if that proves impossible, significant reduction in the frequency and duration of smoking will attenuate some of the risk factors that threaten health. Second in importance to the smoker and first in importance to the nonsmoker as a wellness challenge are improvements in the diet and an increase in physical activity. This is the most formidable challenge for Americans of all ages because more people are overweight or obese (59 percent) than are poor (14 percent), are smokers (19 percent) or are heavy drinkers (6 percent).[22] Obesity is epidemic and its prevalence underscores the importance of physically

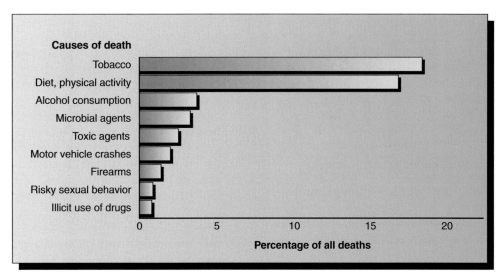

Figure 1-3 Underlying Causes of Death in the United States[21]

SOURCE: Mokdad A. H., J. S. Marks, D. F. Stroup, and J. L. Gerberding. 2004. Actual causes of death in the United States, 2000. *Journal of the American Medical Association* 291(10): 1238–45.

active lifestyles, weight control, and improvements in eating habits as health priorities for most Americans. Almost two-thirds of adults do not engage in any leisure-time periods of vigorous physical activity lasting 10 minutes or more per week.[23] Experts predict that obesity will soon be the leading cause of death and disease in the United States. However, there is a new development (see This Just In on page 21 for an update).

Americans' propensity for sedentary lifestyles comes at a time when evidence of the benefits of an active lifestyle is compelling. Physically active people outlive those who are inactive, and physical activity enhances the quality of life for people of all ages. Regular physical activity lessens the risk for heart disease, diabetes, colon cancer, high blood pressure, osteoporosis, arthritis, and obesity. It also improves symptoms associated with mental health, such as depression and anxiety.[20] Although the benefits of exercise are dose-related, moderate amounts of physical activity improve health and reduce the incidence of premature death (see Wellness for a Lifetime: Tips for Staying Physically Active on page 12). For people who are inactive, even small increases in physical activity are associated with measurable health benefits. The benefit of physical activity is the underlying theme of this text and, ideally, will serve as an impetus for you to establish an active lifestyle.

Achieving Lifestyle Change: A Self-Help Approach

A fundamental assumption underlying lifestyle-change programs is that behavior is a learned response. For example, we are not born with a taste for some foods and a dislike for others. And using seat belts is not a function

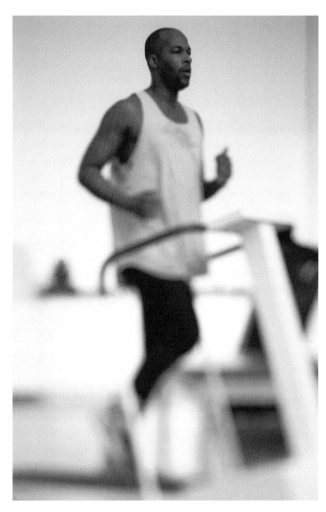

Running is a challenging activity that builds cardiorespiratory endurance.

Wellness for a Lifetime

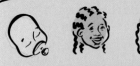

Tips for Staying Physically Active

Sedentary lifestyles are the most formidable wellness challenge for Americans of all ages. More people are at risk for premature death and/or morbidity due to physical inactivity than to any of the other risk factors. For years, medical experts have advised regular exercise to improve fitness and health, to prevent disease and disability, even to lengthen life. Unfortunately, most people starting an exercise program drop out, usually within the first six months. About one-fourth of Americans succeed in making exercise a regular part of their lives. How do they do it? What are they doing right? What are the basic principles of their success stories? Here are some tips from leading exercise experts who practice what they preach.

1. Team up. People who exercise regularly often team up with at least one other person. It might be a roommate, spouse, neighbor, or friend. It might be a workout at the fitness club with a half-dozen friends; it might be a midday break to shoot baskets; it might be an early morning walk with a member of the family.
2. Use exercise as a pick-me-up. Tired from the demands of work, many people resist expending energy on exercise. However, many experts do the opposite by turning to exercise as a source of energy. For them, exercise is a tranquilizer; it makes them more productive at work and home, it refreshes and relaxes them, and it helps them sleep.
3. Get a jump on the day. Many people are more consistent in their exercise routines when they exercise early. Quoting one expert, "You can't plan how your day is going to end, but you can plan how it will start."
4. Break up your workout. Exercise recommendations call for 30 minutes of moderate exercise most days of the week. But it doesn't have to be in one shot. Short bursts scattered throughout the day count, too. Look for opportunities to add exercise to your daily regimen. For example, use the stairs instead of the elevator; park farther away and walk briskly to class; or, when shopping, grab the first parking space (which is usually farther away); if you're waiting for someone, walk while you wait.
5. Seek variety. Engage in a variety of activities. If you work inside all day, you might exercise outside. Try seasonal activities. Catch the evening news while working out on a treadmill. Remember, if you enjoy your workout, you are more likely to continue working out.
6. Revel in your success. The more you make exercise feel like an accomplishment rather than a chore, the more you'll look forward to each session. One lifelong jogger logs his mileage because it boosts his lifetime record. A walker wears a pedometer, so he can monitor his progress as he attempts to walk at least 10,000 steps each day.

SOURCE: Consumers Union. 1999. Success stories: How the experts stay active. *Consumer Reports on Health* 11(4):8–9.

of heredity. Like most other behaviors, health behaviors are learned responses to both obvious and subtle influences. This learning begins at birth and continues throughout life. This is as true for behaviors that promote wellness as for behaviors that diminish it.

Examples of obvious influences that help shape behavior include parents and family, role models, advertising, and social norms. In many instances, these influences are combined to form a single powerful influence on behavior, such as exemplified by an advertisement for cigarettes using "ideal" masculine or feminine models, depending on the brand of cigarettes and the target population. Advertisers are successful not only at marketing products but also at influencing people to think they need those products.

Subtle forces also shape behavior. A good example is *subliminal advertising,* a technique in which messages, words, and symbols are embedded, or hidden, in the pictures, sounds, or words used in advertisements. Theoretically these messages, though not directly observable, can be perceived by the subconscious mind in such a way as to influence behavior.

Much of our behavior is also motivated by psychological needs. An infant whose main source of attention and stimulation comes during feeding time may learn to associate food with the deeper psychological needs of love and affection. A parent who consistently uses food to appease an unhappy child may be inadvertently establishing a preoccupation with food that will endure far beyond childhood.

Sometimes, behavior is motivated in response to force or coercion. *Reactance motivation,* a theory of behavior that has been associated with drinking among college students, suggests that telling people to abstain completely from doing something often produces the opposite reaction. For many people, it isn't difficult to recall instances in their lives in which they behaved a certain way primarily because they were told that they could not or should not behave that way. Coercion, in particular, leads to the arousal of reactance, which in turn tends to reduce compliance.

These examples help explain the myriad complex forces that contribute to behavior and illustrate why successful lifestyle change is so difficult to achieve. The hope and promise of any lifestyle-change program is that, while easier said than done, bad habits can be unlearned and new habits can be learned.

A Self-Help Plan

A **self-help** approach assumes that individuals can manage their lifestyle changes and can learn to control those features in the environment that are detrimental to health. In other words, expensive, long-term, professional help is not a prerequisite for everyone trying to make a lifestyle change. The self-help approach puts you in control of your health, requires your involvement, and permits you to determine what to do and how and when to do it. However, to be successful, this approach requires considerable time and thought devoted to planning. Successful lifestyle change is almost impossible to achieve without a plan.

The self-help approach that follows is based on the **transtheoretical model of behavior change**.[24] This model of lifestyle change is presented in six stages (Figure 1-4), as described next, along with recommended strategies. In applying this model of change, it is helpful to remember several important assumptions:

1. Each of the six stages is well defined and entails a series of tasks that need to be completed before moving to the next stage.
2. A linear progression through the stages of change, although possible, is rare. Most people lapse at some point, and it is possible to get stuck at one stage. However, the important thing is to formulate a plan and act on it. Even if a relapse takes you back temporarily to an earlier stage, you are more likely to succeed than a person who never tried at all.[25]
3. A key to successful change is knowing what stage you are in for the health issue or behavior at hand. Behavioral research reveals that people who try to accomplish changes they are not ready for set themselves up for failure. Similarly, too much time spent on a task already mastered—such as understanding

Stage	1. Precontemplation	2. Contemplation	3. Preparation	4. Action	5. Maintenance	6. Termination
Characteristic	Lack of awareness Denial	Awareness of the need to change Thinking about changing	Planning to change within a month Thinking about the future	Engaging in strategies Commitment to change	Greater difficulty than action stage Duration from six months to a lifetime	Problem behavior no longer an issue
Goal	Feedback on need to change Consciousness raising	More consciousness raising Emotional arousal	Public affirmation of change Development of a plan	Application of strategies Changes in environment Forming of or joining of support groups Establishment of rewards Countering	Application of same strategies as in action stage	Exit from cycle of change
Stage	1. Precontemplation	2. Contemplation	3. Preparation	4. Action	5. Maintenance	6. Termination

Figure 1-4   Stages, Characteristics, and Goals of Lifestyle Change

your problem—may result in an indefinite delay in taking action.

4. Although nearly all change begins with precontemplation, only the most successful ends in termination. But you cannot skip stages. Most people who succeed follow the same road for every problem. However, you may be at different stages of change for different problems.

5. Successful behavior change does not typically happen all at once; it takes time.

Precontemplation stage

In the precontemplation stage, individuals have no intention of changing in the near future. Precontemplators may be unaware of the health risks associated with their behaviors. Or they may feel a situation is hopeless; maybe they've tried to change before without success. They often use denial and defensiveness to keep from going forward. They feel safe in precontemplation because they can't fail there. A recent study on alcohol abuse among college freshmen and sophomores illustrates the tendency toward denial. Researchers found that 70 percent of freshmen and sophomores participating in the study were in the precontemplation stage. Less than 10 percent were aware of their problem-drinking behavior and in the preparation stage for stopping alcohol abuse.[26]

Strategies. Consciousness raising is a key strategy. If less than 10 percent of alcohol abusers are aware of their problem, for example, there should be little surprise that many problem-drinking intervention programs fail. Sometimes awareness comes from a visit to the doctor, a health-threatening diagnosis, a headline news story, or feedback from others. One way to encourage consciousness raising is to take an inventory of personal health habits and practices. A good way to start is to make a list of your health-promoting behaviors, practices you engage in to maintain or improve your level of wellness (see Just the Facts: Examples of Health-Promoting Behaviors). Make another list of health-inhibiting behaviors, practices that may be detrimental to your health (see Assessment Activity 1-3). If your lists are specific and identify behaviors that relate to wellness in its broadest sense (that is, the physical, social, emotional, and psychological aspects of health), comparing the two should give you insight into and information about your lifestyle.

Detailed, comprehensive lifestyle questionnaires, such as in Assessment Activity 1-1, can provide even more information about specific health practices and behavioral tendencies that can be targeted for change. Many of these questionnaires are similar to those you

Just the Facts

Examples of Health-Promoting Behaviors

- I avoid the extremes of too much or too little exercise.
- I get an adequate amount of sleep.
- I avoid adding sugar and salt to my food.
- I include 15 to 20 g of fiber in my diet each day.
- I plan my diet to ensure consumption of an adequate amount of vitamins and minerals.
- I brush and floss my teeth after eating.
- I avoid driving under the influence of alcohol or other drugs.
- I drive within the speed limit.
- I wear my seat belt whenever traveling in an automobile.
- I avoid the use of tobacco.
- I consume fewer than two alcoholic drinks per day.
- I know the instructions provided with any drug I take.
- I do my part to promote a clean and safe environment.
- I feel positive and enthusiastic about my life.
- I can express my feelings of anger.
- I can say no without feeling guilty.
- I engage in activities that promote a feeling of relaxation.
- I am able to develop close, intimate relationships.
- I am interested in the views of others.
- I am satisfied with my study habits.
- I am satisfied with my spiritual life.
- I am tolerant of the values and beliefs of others.

might complete for your physician. Regardless of the tool you use, remember that the goal is to learn more about yourself.

Contemplation stage

Contemplators have a sense of awareness of a problem behavior and begin thinking seriously about changing it. However, it is easy to get stuck in the contemplation stage for years. Perhaps making a change requires more effort than someone is willing to expend or the rewards or pleasures of the current behavior seem to outweigh the benefits of change. Traps[27] include the search for absolute certainty (nothing in life is guaranteed); waiting for the magic moment (you need to make the moment);

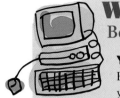

Wellness on the Web
Behavior Change Activities

Your Wellness Profile

How much do you really know about your family's health history and the resulting risks to your own personal health? The knowledge of your family's health history should influence the lifestyle choices you make every day. Go to the Online Learning Center at www.mhhe.com/anspaugh6e, select Student Center, then Chapter 1, then Wellness on the Web, then Activity 1 and answer several questions about your own health history.

Is there a history of heart disease or other cardiovascular problems in your family?

Have either of your parents suffered a heart attack before the age of 60?

Is there a history of cancer in your family?

Is there a history of stroke in your family?

Is there a history of diabetes in your family?

Is there a history of high blood pressure in your family?

The Health-Behavior Gap

The discrepancy between knowing what behavior is good for your health and actually doing it is called the health-behavior gap. The key to striving for high-level wellness is motivation, since no single principle or incident can provide the stimulus necessary to institute change and maintain positive lifestyle habits.

It is also important to recognize the links among your physical, spiritual, emotional, social, and intellectual health. What are some of the changes you can make in your own life to shrink the ever-widening health-behavior gap? Go to the Online Learning Center at www.mhhe.com/anspaugh6e, select Student Center, then Chapter 1, then Wellness on the Web, then Activity 2 and answer the questions found there regarding your own wellness.

Do you think of yourself as a confident person?

Do you have high self-esteem?

Do you make time in your schedule for relaxation?

Do you read for your own enjoyment?

Do you engage in activities that keep your body and mind active?

Do the people you surround yourself with serve as positive health role models?

Do the people in your life support you in your quest for a healthier lifestyle?

and wishful thinking (hoping for different results without changing your behavior).

Strategies. Contemplators need more consciousness raising. Reading, studying, and enrolling in courses are good ways to promote an awareness of the potential problems associated with certain behaviors. (One goal of this text, for example, is to increase your consciousness of habits and practices that promote wellness and of risk factors that may threaten your health.) Getting involved in activities that expose you to information about various aspects of health and wellness allows you to focus on the negatives of your current health practices and to imagine the consequences down the line if your behavior doesn't change.

Cognitive dissonance, the internal conflict that occurs when people feel that their behavior is inconsistent with their intentions or values (such as exhibited by a smoking parent who doesn't want his or her child to smoke), helps in this stage. Also, *emotional arousal,* sometimes accomplished by watching a movie or news story on the subject in question (such as about the sudden death of a child caused by drunken driving), spurs someone to action. Social strategies also help. For example, a problem drinker might attend an Alcoholics Anonymous meeting as a way of experiencing social support for behaving differently.

Preparation stage

Most people in the preparation stage are planning to take action within a month. They think more about the future than about the past, more about the pros of a new behavior than about the cons of the old one. Many people motivate themselves by making their intended change public rather than keeping it to themselves. This stage involves developing a plan customized to a person's unique circumstances and personality.

Most people make three serious mistakes when starting a lifestyle change. First, they expect miracles and set unrealistic goals. Setting goals that are too ambitious often guarantees failure. For many people, the fear of failure easily discourages future efforts at a lifestyle change.

Second, people oversimplify the complexities associated with lifestyle change and view it as a willpower issue. The strategy of choice for these people is "cold turkey," which involves picking a day for the change and, through determination and willpower, refraining from the target behavior. Experts disagree on the effectiveness of this strategy for changing many health behaviors, arguing that, while it may work for some because it forces them to adopt new habits, it inflates the "hold" over people by assigning it more power than it

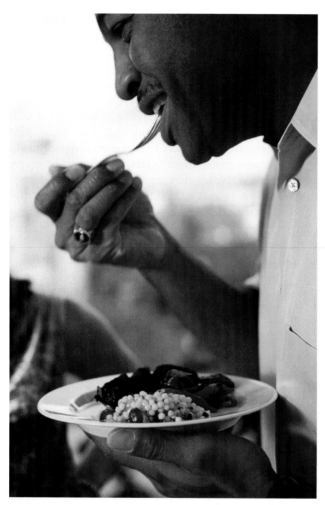

Behavior change, such as following a healthier diet, should be viewed as a lifetime goal, not a temporary fix.

deserves.[28] A dieter, for example, who decides to cold-turkey his consumption of high-fat, gourmet-style ice cream may actually encourage an obsession with this forbidden food. In this approach, little learning takes place, with the possible exception that willpower by itself is usually insufficient to cause a permanent change in behavior.

Third, people often view lifestyle change as a temporary goal rather than as a lifetime change. Perhaps more than anything else, this attitude accounts for the high *recidivism* (the tendency to revert to the original behavior) rate of many programs. One of the best examples is weight-loss programs. In weight-loss programs, for example, people typically set a goal, diet until they reach their goal, revert to their original eating habits, and invariably regain the lost weight. The proper way is to change eating habits, so that they will endure for a lifetime. When people try to change some aspect of behavior, they have to deny themselves something that feels comfortable or that provides enjoyment or pleasure.

Denial often triggers a preoccupation that worsens the health behavior being changed. This is the reason dieters often become more interested in food during a diet (see Real-World Wellness: Are You Ready for a Lifestyle Change?).

No single strategy for lifestyle change is right for everyone. The key is to get involved in planning your personal program and to use your imagination to create the most suitable plan.

Strategies. In this stage, a firm, detailed plan is developed that involves (1) assessing behavior and (2) setting specific, realistic goals.

Assess behavior. Behavior assessment, the collection of data on target behaviors, is the lifeline of any lifestyle-change plan. It involves the process of counting, recording, measuring, observing, and describing. Any behavior that can be qualified is assessed.

Real-World Wellness

Are You Ready for a Lifestyle Change?

I've started an exercise program four times during the past two years. Each effort resulted in failure. I don't want to start again until I know I'm ready. How will I know that I'm ready to begin a lifestyle-change program?

If you can answer yes to the following questions, you are ready to begin a lifestyle-change program:

- Do you view lifestyle change as a lifetime goal rather than as a temporary, short-term goal?
- Are you willing to get personally involved in planning a lifestyle-change program?
- Are you prepared for some disappointments?
- Are you willing to experiment with different ideas?
- Do you have the patience to accept success in small increments stretched over a long period?
- Are you willing to set modest, realistic goals?
- Are you willing to establish some time benchmarks for success?
- Are you willing to make some changes in the way you live?
- Are you willing to tell others about your goals?
- Can you accept a relapse as a temporary setback rather than as a full-blown failure?
- Are you willing to formulate a plan that makes provisions for countering, avoidance, contracting, shaping up, reminders, and support?

Assessment tools provide objective data regarding behavioral patterns, health changes, and/or results. They may be daily logs, journals, and diaries or medical diagnostic tools (e.g., blood pressure machine). Data should be collected long enough to note trends, usually for a minimum of one to two weeks. Often, people are surprised at what they learn about themselves. In a study of 235 nonexercising adults, participants were asked to record how much time they spend sitting or lying down. They were shocked when they found they were sleeping 8 hours a day and spending 15 of the remaining 16 hours sitting down.[29]

Sometimes a behavior assessment will prompt a change in behavior without any other action. In most lifestyle-change programs, a plan of action is not started until it is clear that assessment alone will not be enough to alter the behavior completely. For example, some people attach an electronic pedometer to their waistband to count the number of steps taken each day. The average sedentary person usually takes about 3,000 steps a day (2,000 steps equals a mile).[30] For some people the first step is the only step required. Counting serves as a sufficient intervention to behavior improvement. Several studies have shown that people who engage in self-assessment activities do better than people who don't, even if they don't write down everything. It's not so much that you write it down, but the act of recording that seems to make a difference, perhaps because it forces you to face your actions.[31]

The assessment phase also provides clues to a person's commitment to making a change in lifestyle. A thorough, detailed log is a good sign that a person has the motivation to carry out the plan.

When the assessment phase is finished, there should be sufficient information to form a behavioral profile, state specific goals, and customize an intervention program that matches goals and strategies to a person's unique circumstances and personality.

Set specific, realistic goals. Setting specific goals means setting goals that focus on concrete, observable, measurable behaviors. A behavioral goal to overcome shyness is different from a goal that requires someone to initiate a conversation with a different person each day for the next week. If goals are specific, you know precisely what you are trying to accomplish and where, when, and how often. By using specific goals, you get instant feedback on your progress. Another way to increase specificity is to establish a timetable for achieving goals. A timetable adds structure to the plan and provides a way to evaluate progress.

Realistic behavioral goals are reasonable and relate to personal circumstances. Setting realistic goals also means forming them in the context of correct information. For example, an informed dieter knows that setting a goal to lose 10 pounds in a week is not reasonable. A more achievable goal is 1 to 2 pounds.

When setting goals, starting off small is best. Setting a modest goal initially facilitates some degree of success, which increases confidence. For complex lifestyle changes, behavioral psychologists recommend breaking down an ambitious, long-range goal into a set of intermediate goals, beginning with the easier ones and then moving gradually to more difficult ones. Goals should be structured in moderation. Extreme goals promote the erroneous attitude that lifestyle change is temporary. They create a strong sense of denial, encourage preoccupation with target behaviors, and invariably lead to failure. Exceptions include cigarette smoking, alcoholism, and other drug dependence, for which abstinence is still the primary treatment.

Action stage

In the action stage, a person overtly makes changes in behavior, experiences, or environment. This is the busiest stage of change. It's also the stage most visible to others. New behaviors, such as exercising, not smoking, or actively changing a dietary pattern, can be observed.

Strategies. People in the action stage implement their plan for change. In doing so, they apply their sense of commitment to the change. Rewards and incentives are important elements of this stage. **Countering,** or behavior substitution, in which a new behavior is substituted for the undesirable one, is the most common and one of the most powerful strategies available to people trying to make a change. When this technique is applied, the goal is to think of a behavior incompatible with the one being altered. Examples include chewing gum to suppress the urge to smoke, substituting diet colas for sweetened colas, and going for a walk instead of watching television. Some effective countering techniques are summarized in Just the Facts: Countering Strategies on page 18.

Making changes in the environment is another key element of the action stage. Avoidance, or the elimination of the circumstances associated with an undesirable behavior, is a fundamental technique of the control process. A smoker cannot smoke if there are no cigarettes, an ice cream binge is not possible if there is no ice cream parlor, and loud music cannot interfere with studying if the radio is put away.

Avoidance is not limited to objects. It may also include jobs, school, and even people. If taking 18 hours of coursework while working 20 hours per week is compromising your academics, you may feel justified in dropping several courses or withdrawing from school if a reduction in your workload isn't possible. By the same token, it may be necessary to associate less often with people who contribute to a problem behavior.

～～Just the Facts～～

Countering Strategies

The following are some countering strategies you can use to replace problem behaviors:

- Exercising
- Cooking
- Playing a musical instrument
- Relaxing (see Chapter 9)
- Cleaning
- Doing crossword puzzles
- Walking
- Reading a book
- Calling a friend
- Going to a movie
- Keeping busy
- Learning to be more assertive
- Learning a new skill
- Joining a fitness club
- Organizing
- Playing a game
- Surfing the Internet
- Learning to use new software
- Watching a favorite television show
- Practicing thought stopping (counterthinking) by substituting positive thoughts for negative ones

The use of reminders is also a key element of an action plan. These may be in the form of a daily planner, a calendar, clocks, sticky notes, signs on a door, or a to-do list. During times when behavior change is not an issue, the list might read "call home, library, 2:00–4:00 p.m.; racquetball, 4:30–5:30; dinner date, 6:00–8:30; study time, 9:00–11:00." If you are working on an action plan for lifestyle change, adding action goals is a natural extension. If, for example, you are working on social skills, you might add "initiate a conversation with a classmate" or "eat lunch with someone different." A positive benefit of reminders, in addition to their reinforcement of positive behaviors, is the satisfaction that results from checking something off a list.

Contracting is another common action strategy. Written contracts tend to be more powerful than spoken ones. They usually include a statement of long-range and intermediate health goals; target dates for completion of each goal; intervention strategies; and rewards and incentives, such as "I will deposit $5 in my new car savings account for every day that I attend all of my classes between now and the end of the semester." These contracts are not legal documents, so simplicity and creativity are in order.

Shaping up is an another essential part of lifestyle change. It requires a person to allow him- or herself opportunities to practice desired behaviors, usually in small increments. The saying "Behavior begets behavior" is the essence of shaping up. This is also true for harmful behaviors. For example, cigarette smokers rarely enjoy their first cigarette; they learn to enjoy smoking by smoking. The same is true for most beer drinkers. Typically, shaping up occurs gradually until it becomes fully integrated into one's behavioral repertoire.

The acquisition of positive health behaviors occurs the same way. A step-by-step approach, with reinforcement following each successive movement, promotes success. In overcoming a fear of flying, a person might first visit the airport; the next step might be to tour an airplane; next the person may take a seat, fasten up, and visualize flying. Each step brings the person closer to flying, each step is reinforced, and any feelings of anxiety are countered with relaxation. People forget that problem behaviors are formed cumulatively and reflect many years of conditioning. It is only reasonable to expect that acquiring a preference for a new behavior will also require considerable time, thought, and reinforcement.

Another good strategy in an action plan is the formation of a support group, which may include a roommate, family, friends, classmates, or someone who can identify with the lifestyle goal. Dieting may be easier and more tolerable when done with a friend. Two people may accomplish their goals more effectively than either can alone. For example, two roommates may be more successful at maintaining their exercise regimen together than separately. Involving someone else in the process of change makes it easier to stick to your action plan, provides a source of encouragement, and holds you accountable for your goals. Social factors, such as the involvement of a support group, companion, or buddy system, are keys to success for health behavior improvement, particularly in the area of exercise and physical activity.[32]

Maintenance stage

The goal in the maintenance stage is to retain the gains made during the action and other stages and to try hard to prevent a relapse. Change never ends with action. Although people tend to view maintenance as a static stage, it is actually a continuation of the action stage and can last six months to a lifetime. Programs that promise easy change usually fail to acknowledge that maintenance is a long, ongoing process. This is why trendy, extreme programs, such as many diet programs, have a high recidivism rate. People may achieve their weight-loss goal, but they cannot maintain their strategy for losing weight for life. When this happens, a person may erroneously view the action plan as a temporary strategy. This is the opposite of maintenance and lifestyle change.

Most people experience a relapse and return to the precontemplation or contemplation stage of change, maybe several times, before eventually succeeding in maintaining the change. People move through the change process at different paces, and relapse is a part of behavior change. Learn from any relapse instead of reacting to it by giving up. It is important to remember that the real test of a program's success is not how many people reach their goals but how many people successfully maintain that goal for at least two years.

Strategies. Strategies used in the action plan should be continued in maintenance. Provisions for avoidance, reminders, contracting, countering, shaping up, and support groups apply during maintenance, just as they do during the action stage.

Termination stage

The termination stage is the ultimate goal for people trying to make a lifestyle change. In this stage, the problem behavior is no longer tempting. A person becomes confident that his or her problem behavior will never return; it becomes a nonissue. The cycle of change is exited.

Strategies. Some experts believe that termination is impossible, that the most anyone can hope for is a lifetime of maintenance. The key strategy is to be aware of early warning signs of relapse, such as overconfidence, that can recycle the problem behavior.

Regardless of the results, maintaining the proper perspective about success and failure is important. Many people have the attitude that they either completely succeed or completely fail. This way of thinking can be devastating to a person's motivation. When goals are not fully realized, the proper attitude is to view the shortcoming as justification for making adjustments in the program. The goals may have been too general or unrealistic. The intervention strategies may have lacked relevance. Look at relapse as a learning tool. Reshaping goals, setting a more realistic schedule, changing the rewards and penalties, or formulating different intervention strategies may be necessary.

Above all, you should maintain a healthy perspective about yourself and not burden yourself with guilt if you fall short of your goals. What seems important now becomes insignificant when viewed within a broader context. You may consider how significant this event is likely to be to you two years from now. Doing this helps establish the right perspective on your progress. More important than total success are the answers to the following questions: What did you learn from this experience? What did you learn about yourself? What can you do differently? Lifestyle change is a lifelong project that requires insight, skillful planning, and plenty of practice.

Summary

- Wellness is a lifelong process that requires self-awareness, introspection, reflection, inquiry, accurate information, and action. It means assuming attitudes and engaging in behaviors that promote health and well-being.
- Health is a constantly changing state of being that moves along a continuum from optimal health to premature death and is affected by an individual's attitudes and activities.
- Lifestyle diseases represent the major threat to the health and quality of life of Americans.
- Wellness requires the consistent balancing of spiritual, social, physical, emotional, intellectual, occupational, and environmental dimensions.
- An internal locus of control is the attitude that a person is in control of his or her life. An internal locus of control is consistent with the principles of wellness. An external locus of control is the belief that factors affecting health are outside one's control.
- *Self-efficacy* refers to the beliefs people have in their ability to accomplish specific tasks or behaviors. A strong sense of self-efficacy is consistent with the principles of wellness.

- The mind, body, and spirit are inseparably linked. A breakdown in any one of these can threaten health and wellness.
- Psychosomatic diseases occur when physical symptoms are caused by psychological, social, spiritual, or emotional stressors.
- *Healthy People 2010* has as one of its goals the elimination of health disparities that exist among population groups.
- Lifestyle diseases are those caused by the way people live. The major lifestyle diseases are heart disease, cancer, and stroke. Together these account for almost two-thirds of deaths among Americans.
- Chronic diseases are those that persist for an indefinite time.
- Accidents are the leading cause of death among Americans between 15 and 44 years of age.
- The risk factor most strongly associated with premature death and chronic disease in the United States is cigarette smoking.
- Experts predict that obesity will be the leading cause of death and disease by 2005.
- An increase in physical activity is the most formidable challenge for Americans of all ages. More people are

overweight or obese (59 percent) than are poor (14 percent), are smokers (19 percent) or are heavy drinkers (6 percent).
- Lifestyle change is one of the most pervasive human endeavors.
- A fundamental belief in lifestyle-change programs is that health behavior is a learned response and therefore can be changed.

- Health behavior is influenced by many complex forces, including family, role models, social pressure, advertising, and psychological needs.
- The six stages of change are precontemplation, contemplation, preparation, action, maintenance, and termination.
- Action strategies include countering, avoidance, reminders, contracting, shaping up, and support groups.

Review Questions

1. How are the health problems of today different from those of 50 years ago? Of 100 years ago?
2. This book suggests that wellness is a process rather than a goal. What does this mean? What are the implications of this statement?
3. What are the components of wellness? How are they similar? Dissimilar?
4. Define *psychosomatic diseases*. Cite four examples of psychosomatic conditions.
5. Cite some data that confirm the relationship between physical health problems and the spiritual, social, and emotional dimensions of wellness.
6. What are the differences between an internal locus of control and an external locus of control? Which of the two is more consistent with the principles of wellness?
7. Define the concept of self-efficacy. What is the relationship between the concepts of locus of control and self-efficacy?
8. How does the impact of environmental improvements compare with advancements in medical technology in increasing health and longevity among Americans?
9. To what does the term *health disparities* refer? Give three examples.
10. How do the leading causes of mortality today compare with those of 100 years ago? How do the leading causes of mortality among all Americans compare with those of young adults between the ages of 25 and 44?

11. To what does the term *Leading Health Indicator* refer? Identify 10 Leading Health Indicators.
12. What do medical experts consider the risk factor most strongly associated with premature death and chronic disease?
13. This book suggests that the most formidable wellness challenge for Americans of all ages is overcoming a sedentary lifestyle. What is the rationale for identifying physical activity as more important than diet or cigarette smoking?
14. Identify and briefly describe the six stages of change as presented in the transtheoretical model of behavior change.
15. What are some common mistakes people make in trying to modify some aspect of their health behavior?
16. What is a major reason for the high recidivism rate in many lifestyle-change programs?
17. If a college student wants to use countering strategies as a way to cope with compulsive eating, what can he or she do or use?
18. Your roommate wants to improve his or her study habits. Identify for your roommate four strategies that apply the techniques recommended in the action stage of lifestyle change.
19. Give an example of a specific and realistic lifestyle goal.
20. Identify three strategies experts recommend for staying physically active.

References

1. Wellness Program SUNY at Stony Brook. 2001. Wellness is . . . (http://naples.cc.sunysb.edu/pres/wellness.nst/pages/definition).
2. Hawks, S. 2004. Spiritual wellness, holistic health, and the practice of health education. *American Journal of Health Education* 35(1):14.
3. Harvard Medical School. 2002. Sending prayers: Does it help? *Harvard Health Letter* 27(7):7.
4. Mayo Clinic. 1999. Staying connected: Close ties promote health. *Mayo Clinic Health letter* 17(11):7.
5. New England Journal of Medicine. 2000. Exercising away depression. *HealthNews* 7(5):7.
6. Ahmad, K. 2000. Anger and hostility linked to coronary heart disease. *Lancet* 355(9215):1621.

7. Tufts University. 2000. The mind and the heart: They really are connected. *Tufts University Health and Nutrition Letter* 18(6):1, 4.
8. Harvard Medical School. 2000. Anger and heart disease risk. *Harvard Heart Letter* 10(11):1.
9. Tufts University. 2003. Optimistic people live longer. *Tufts University Health and Nutrition Letter* 20(11):4.
10. Consumers Union. 2004. Happier and healthier? *Consumer Reports on Health* 16(3):1, 4.
11. Metcalf, C., G. D. Smith, J. A. C. Sterne, P. Heslop, J. Macleod, and C. Hart. 2001. Individual employment histories and subsequent cause specific hospital admissions and mortality: A prospective study of a cohort of male and female workers with

21 years follow up. *Journal of Epidemiology and Community Health* 55(7):503.
12. Kochanek, K. D., and B. L. Smith. 2004. Deaths: Preliminary data for 2002. *National vital statistics reports*. Vol. 52, no. 13. Hyattsville, MD: National Center for Health Statistics.
13. Knox, R. 1998. Longevity reshaping the globe. *The Commercial Appeal* 159(132):2.
14. Harvard Medical School. 2003. The latino paradox. *Harvard Health Letter* 28(8):3.
15. Marks, J. S. 2003. We're living longer, but what about our quality of life? *Chronic Disease: Notes and Reports* 16(1):2–16.
16. National Institutes of Health. 2004. Addressing health disparities; the NIH pro-

gram of action (http://healthdisparities.
nih.gov/whatare.html).

17. Environmental Nutrition. 2002. Lifestyle, not genes, offers best hope of living healthier, longer. *Environmental Nutrition* 25(4):1, 4.

18. Tufts University. 2001. Is mad-cow disease a threat in the U.S.? *Tufts University Health and Nutrition Letter* 18(12):1, 6.

19. U.S. Department of Health and Human Services. 2000. *Healthy people 2010. Understanding and improving health.* 2d ed. Washington, DC: U.S. Government Printing Office.

20. National Center for Health Statistics. 2003. *Health, United States, 2003.* Hyattsville, MD: U.S. Department of Health and Human Services.

21. Mokdad, A. H., J. S. Marks, D. F. Stroup, and J. L. Gerberding. 2004. Actual causes of death in the United States, 2000. *Journal of the American Medical Association* 291(10):1238–45.

22. Environmental Nutrition. 2001. Overweight tops even smoking as health risk. *Environmental Nutrition* 24(7):1.

23. Lucas, J. W., J. S. Schiller, and V. E. Benson. 2004. *Summary health statistics for U.S. adults: National health interview survey, 2001.* National Center for Health Statistics. *Vital Health Stat* 10(218).

24. Prochaska, J., J. C. Norcross, and C. C. DiClemente. 1994. *Changing for good.* New York: William Morrow and Company.

25. Tufts University. 2003. New Year's resolution can start any day you want. *Tufts University Health and Nutrition Letter* 21(1):8.

26. Prochaska, J. M., J. O. Prochaska, F. C. Cohen, S. O. Gomes, R. G. Laforge, and A. L. Eastwood. 2004. The transtheoretical model of change for multi-level

interventions for alcohol abuse on campus. *Journal of Alcohol and Drug Education* 48(13):34–51.

27. Prochaska, J. 1996. "Just do it" isn't enough: Change comes in stages. *Tufts University Diet and Nutrition Letter* 14(7):4–6.

28. Tufts University. 2002. Is sugar really addictive? *Tufts University Health and Nutrition Letter* 20(8):5.

29. Consumers Union. 1999. Workouts that work. *Consumer Reports* 64(2): 31–34.

30. Consumers Union. 2000. Try a movement motivator. *Consumer Report on Health* 12(10):3.

31. Environmental Nutrition. 1999. Combat holiday overeating: Nag yourself. *Environmental Nutrition* 22(11):3.

32. De Bourdeaudhuij, I. and J. Sallis. 2002. Getting adults to exercise by modifying psychosocial variables. *Physical Activity Today* 8(3):3.

Suggested Readings

Giller, C.A. 2004. *Port in the storm: How to make a medical decision and live to tell about it.* Washington, DC: Lifeline Press. This book assumes that making a medical decision requires both technical information and human considerations. Dr. Cole Giller leads patients through six steps of the medical decision-making process to help them make choices that are best for them, in keeping with their beliefs, values, and priorities. The book includes tips and real-life stories demonstrating the best use of doctors, how to decipher medical information, and how to make a decision that is consistent with personal needs, values, personality, and lifestyle.

National Center for Health Statistics. 2003. *Health, United States, 2003.* Hyattsville, MD: U.S. Government Printing Office. This book serves as a major reference on health trends and statistics. Charts, tables, and figures present current data on health risk factors, mortality, health care resources, chronic diseases, life expectancy, and much more. Data are complied by the National Center for Health Statistics and Centers for Disease Control and Prevention.

Svec, C. 2001. *After any diagnosis: How to take action against your illness using the best and most current medical information available.* New York: Three Rivers Press.

Medical writer Carol Svec presents a "how to" guide for becoming an active patient in working with medical providers to determine the best options when faced with a diagnosis of a chronic or an acute life-threatening illness. This book provides advice on communicating with physicians; finding current books and articles about a specific disease; distinguishing between good and bad Internet sites; sorting through contradictory information on various health topics; researching doctors, hospitals, and support groups; and interpreting medical information.

☆ This Just In

There is an update on the death rate from the combination of physical inactivity and obesity that was referred to on page 11 of this chapter and page 54 of Chapter 2. It appears that the study sponsored by the U.S. Centers for Disease Control and Prevention, which was published in the March 10, 2004 edition of the *Journal of the American Medical Association,* overestimated the number of deaths attributed to physical inactivity and obesity. A statistical error occurred in the study that overestimated these deaths by as much as 80,000. Prior to the discovery of this error, the authors projected that deaths from physical inactivity and obesity would surpass the number of deaths associated with tobacco usage sometime in mid-2005. While physical inactivity and obesity will probably overtake tobacco usage as the leading cause of death, it probably will not occur for a few more years.

SOURCE: Mokdad, A. H., et al. 2005. Actual causes of death in the United States, 2000. *Journal of the American Medical Association* 293(3): 293–294.

Name _____ Date _____ Section _____

Assessment Activity 1-3

Assessing Your Health Behaviors

Before planning a lifestyle-change program, you should take an inventory of your health behaviors. This reveals important information about your lifestyle and should also help identify areas in need of improvement.

Directions: In this assessment, you are asked to make two lists. In the left column, list the things you do to maintain or improve your level of health. These are your

health-promoting behaviors. In the right column, list the things you do that may be detrimental to your health. These are your health-inhibiting behaviors. Try to be specific. Include the things that affect your mental, emotional, social, spiritual, and physical health. If you have a difficult time thinking of specific activities, you can refer to Assessment Activity 1-1.

Health-Promoting Behaviors	**Health-Inhibiting Behaviors**
1. _____	1. _____
2. _____	2. _____
3. _____	3. _____
4. _____	4. _____
5. _____	5. _____
6. _____	6. _____
7. _____	7. _____
8. _____	8. _____
9. _____	9. _____
10. _____	10. _____
11. _____	11. _____
12. _____	12. _____
13. _____	13. _____
14. _____	14. _____
15. _____	15. _____

Which health-inhibiting behavior would you be willing to change right now? _____

_____

2

Preventing Cardiovascular Disease

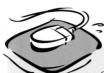

Online Learning Center

Log on to our Online Learning Center (OLC) for access to these additional resources:

- Chapter key term flashcards
- Learning objectives
- Additional goals for behavior change
- Concentration game
- Self-scoring chapter quizzes

- Additional lab activities

The OLC also offers Web links for study and exploration of wellness topics. Access these links through **www.mhhe. com/anspaugh6e**, click on Student Center, click on Chapter 2, and then click on Web Activities.

Key Terms

aneurysm
atherosclerosis
cerebral hemorrhage
cholesterol
embolus
hypertension

ischemia
lipoprotein (a)
myocardial infarction
sedentary
thrombus

Objectives

After completing this chapter, you will be able to do the following:

- Describe the gross anatomy and function of the heart.
- Trace the development of cardiovascular disease during the twentieth century in the United States.

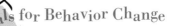

Goals for Behavior Change

- Choose three high-fat foods that you regularly eat and replace them with low-fat, healthier foods.
- Find out your total cholesterol, LDL cholesterol, and HDL cholesterol. Select three or four lifestyle behaviors to change to improve your cholesterol profile.
- Find out your blood pressure. Select two or three behaviors to change (excluding taking medication) to lower it.
- If you use tobacco products, devise a plan for quitting the tobacco habit.
- If you are not currently active, make a list of physical activities to improve your health status and level of fitness. Determine how many calories you would attempt to expend per week.
- Plan and implement three strategies to help you deal with chronic stress.

- Identify and differentiate among several types of cardiovascular disease.
- Identify the risk factors for coronary heart disease and discuss ways to reduce them.
- Explain the lifestyle behaviors that contribute to health and longevity.

ardiovascular disease encompasses a group of diseases that affect the heart and blood vessels. Cardiovascular disease—the leading cause of death in the United States—accounts for 38.5 percent of deaths.[1] About 25 percent of Americans (approximately 64.4 million people) have one or more forms of heart or blood vessel disease.

The most prevalent form of heart disease, coronary heart disease (CHD), also referred to as ischemic heart disease or coronary artery disease, kills more Americans than all other forms of heart disease combined. Approximately 340,000 people die annually of CHD, either in a hospital emergency room or before reaching the hospital. These deaths are usually the result of cardiac arrest (the heart stops beating due to interference of its electrical impulse).[1]

Coronary heart disease is but one of many types of heart disease, but it produces about half of all heart disease deaths in people under the age of 75. It is the leading cause of death for both men and women, although the development of CHD in women lags behind men about 10 years. With advancing age, however, the mortality rate between the sexes begins to equalize.[1]

The death rate from heart disease in the United States has been steadily declining for the last 50 years. The decline in death rate from heart disease has been largely responsible for the improvement in life expectancy. According to the Centers for Disease Control and Prevention, the average life expectancy (the number of years that a newborn can expect to live) has risen to 77.4 years.[2] If all major forms of cardiovascular disease were eliminated, life expectancy would increase by about 7 years.[1] One of the greatest public health successes of the twentieth century has been the decline in the death rate from cardiovascular disease—a 60 percent decline since the 1950s.[3]

Research has convincingly shown that following a heart-healthy lifestyle can significantly lower the risk for heart disease, and it has been a major contributor to the decline in heart disease mortality.[4] The medical profession, through the development and use of sophisticated diagnostic procedures and vastly improved after-the-fact treatments, has equally contributed to the downward trend in the death rate from cardiovascular disease.

Circulation

Circulation is better understood if you are familiar with the basic anatomy and function of the heart. The heart consists of cardiac muscle and weighs between 8 and 10 ounces. It is about the size of a fist and lies in the center of the chest. The heart is divided into two halves, or pumps, by a wall (the septum), and each half is subdivided into an upper chamber (the atrium) and a lower chamber (the ventricle). The right heart, or pulmonary pump, receives deoxygenated blood from the tissues and

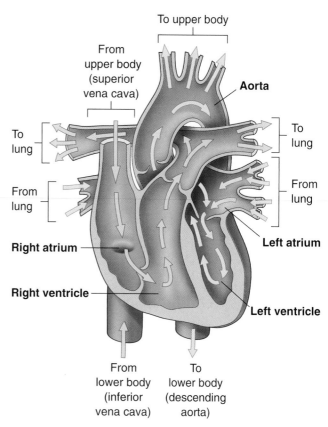

Figure 2-1 Circulatory System

pumps it to the lungs, so that carbon dioxide can be exchanged for a fresh supply of oxygen. From the lungs, the oxygen-rich blood is sent to the left heart, or systemic pump, so that the oxygenated blood can be pumped to all the tissues of the body. Both pumps work simultaneously. The systemic pump carries the heavier workload of the two and thus has a more muscular ventricular wall. Figure 2-1 illustrates the circulatory system.

The arteries carry oxygenated blood away from the heart, while the veins carry deoxygenated blood to the heart. There are two exceptions, one in the arterial system and one in the venous system. First, the pulmonary artery carries *deoxygenated* blood from the right heart to the lungs to exchange carbon dioxide for a fresh supply of oxygen. Second, the pulmonary vein carries *fully oxygenated* blood from the lungs to the left heart for distribution throughout the body.

The primary function of circulation is to provide a constant supply of blood and nutrients to the cells while removing their waste products. Under ordinary circumstances, the interruption of blood flow for as little as four to six minutes can result in irreversible brain damage due to oxygen deprivation.

The average heart beats 70 to 80 times per minute at rest. Endurance athletes often have resting heart rates in the 30- and 40-beat range, whereas some overweight and sedentary smokers have resting heart rates in the 90s.[5] The low heart rates of endurance athletes reflect physiological adaptations to training that represent normal values for this group. The Framingham Heart Disease Study showed that a rapid resting heart rate increased the risk for death from heart attack. Mortality increased progressively with higher resting heart rates, especially among men.[6] Men with resting heart rates greater than 75 beats per minute were 3.5 times more likely to die suddenly, compared with men whose heart rate was below 60. There are three plausible factors supporting the relationship between high resting heart rate and sudden death. First, medical researchers discovered that at least half of all heart attacks occur when atherosclerotic plaque is unstable. Unstable plaque has a thin, fibrous cap and is more likely to rupture than stable plaque. Blood rushing over unstable plaque threatens to rip off the fibrous cap. This situation is made more threatening by a high resting heart rate because more waves of blood rush over the cap in a given amount of time.[6] Second, a high resting heart rate is indicative of an inefficient heart that has less time between beats (the diastolic phase of the heart cycle) to deliver blood, oxygen, and nutrients to the myocardium (heart muscle). Third, a high resting heart rate could be an indicator of poor health habits, such as lack of exercise or diabetes, or could be the result of undiagnosed weakened heart muscle.

The heart is self-regulating; it contains its own conduction system fully capable of establishing and maintaining the heartbeat without outside neural stimulation. The heart's beating rate and rhythm are established by the sinoatrial node (SA node, or pacemaker), located in the right atrium, as shown in Figure 2-2. The atria contract, forcing blood into the ventricles as the electrical impulse travels from the SA node to the atrioventricular node (AV node), located between the right atrium and right ventricle. The electrical impulse pauses for one-tenth of a second at the AV node to allow the ventricles to fill with blood and then resumes down the system and spreads throughout the ventricular walls. The ventricles contract during this time, ejecting blood from these chambers.

Blood that enters the chambers of the heart does not directly nourish the heart muscle because there are no direct circulatory routes from the heart's chambers into its muscular walls. Instead, blood must first be ejected from the heart to the aorta (the largest artery in the body) and then to the coronary arteries that supply the myocardium (heart muscle) with blood and oxygen. The majority of blood is received by the myocardium during diastole (between beats) because the blood vessels dilate during this time, increasing their capacity to accept and deliver blood.

Coronary circulation is illustrated in Figure 2-3. The left coronary artery supplies a major portion of the myocardium with blood, whereas the right coronary artery serves less of it. Both vessels divide and subdivide downstream and eventually culminate in a dense network of capillaries (the smallest blood vessels in the body). Blood supply to the myocardium is so important that every muscle fiber is supplied by at least one capillary. The coronary veins return deoxygenated blood to the right atrium, so that it can enter pulmonary circulation. The veins bring deoxygenated blood from all tissues back to the right atrium.

Blood plasma is a clear, yellowish fluid that carries approximately 100 chemicals. Plasma represents 55 percent

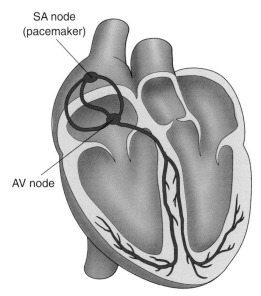

Figure 2-2 Electrical Conduction System of the Heart

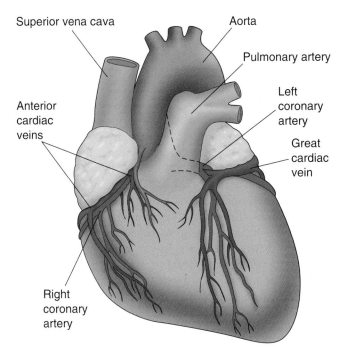

Figure 2-3 Coronary Circulation

of the blood content. The remaining 45 percent consists of blood solids—the erythrocytes (red blood cells), the leukocytes (white blood cells), and the blood platelets. The red blood cells are the most abundant of the blood solids, composing about 99 percent of the total. These cells carry oxygen and carbon dioxide attached to hemoglobin, an iron-rich protein pigment and a main component of red blood cells. The white blood cells are an important part of the body's defense system against invading microorganisms and other foreign substances. The blood platelets are involved in the complex processes that lead to the formation of clots for repairing damaged blood vessels.

Cardiovascular Disease: A Twentieth-Century Phenomenon

Cardiovascular disease, a relatively rare event 100 years ago, reached epidemic proportions during the middle of the twentieth century. The term *angina pectoris* (chest pain) was introduced into the medical literature by William Heberden, a British physician, in the latter part of the eighteenth century, but he was unable to offer any treatment for this strange malady. It was not until 1910 that physicians made the connection between recurrent episodes of angina pectoris and heart disease. Chest pain and other manifestations of a heart attack were not identified with obstructions of the coronary arteries until the early 1900s. An American physician gave the first accurate description of the events associated with a heart attack in 1912. The illness he described, which afflicted a 55-year-old man with no previous evidence of disease, is now a common occurrence in American life. The man died three days after the onset of symptoms. A postmortem examination of the heart revealed that a clot had occluded, or blocked, one of the major coronary arteries. In 1912, this was a medical rarity.

Coronary heart disease is responsible for the majority of heart attack deaths, but other forms of heart disease contribute to disability and death. Congenital heart defects, which exist at birth, affect approximately 36,000 newborns annually. Approximately 6,300 of these infants die from their defects.[1] The most common type of birth defect is abnormalities in the development of the heart. Heart defects affect nearly 1 percent of all newborns, and 10 times as many occur in spontaneously aborted pregnancies.[7] Rheumatic heart disease, caused by a streptococcal infection of the throat or ear, is virtually 100 percent preventable. Antibiotic treatment during the infection stage arrests the processes that could lead to rheumatic heart disease. Congestive heart failure occurs when the heart muscle is so damaged that it can no longer contract with sufficient force to pump blood throughout the body. The leading causes of congestive heart failure are poorly controlled or uncontrolled long-standing hypertension, a history of heart attacks, or both. Approximately 5 million Americans have congestive heart failure and about 52,800 die annually of this condition.

Coronary Heart Disease

Coronary heart disease is a disease of the arteries that supply the heart with blood and nutrients. A diagnosis of coronary artery disease is made if any artery is narrowed by 60 percent. A heart attack, or **myocardial infarction** (death of heart muscle tissue), occurs when an obstruction or a spasm disrupts or blocks blood flow to a portion of the heart muscle. The amount of heart muscle damage is determined by the location of the obstruction or spasm and the speed with which medical intervention is begun. Heart attacks of any magnitude produce irreversible injury and myocardial tissue death. It usually takes five to six weeks to form a fibrous scar around dead cardiac tissue. This area of dead tissue can no longer contribute to the pumping of blood, resulting in a less efficient heart. Massive heart attacks that cause extensive muscle damage result in death.

Although most heart attacks occur after the age of 65, the dysfunctions leading to them often begin before adolescence. These processes occur most often without symptoms and often go undetected until, without warning, a heart attack occurs. The attack is sudden, but the circumstances leading to it develop over many years. There is considerable evidence that the silent phase of coronary heart disease begins as early as childhood.[8,9]

Risk factors are genetic predispositions, lifestyle behaviors, and environmental influences that increase one's susceptibility to disease. Elevated blood pressure and blood fats (cholesterol and triglycerides) that occur during adulthood can often be traced back to childhood. See Wellness for a Lifetime: Childhood Origins of Heart Disease for more information about this connection.

The ongoing Framingham Study, which began in 1949, identified the risk factors connected with heart disease.[10] Cigarette smoking, high blood pressure, elevated cholesterol levels, diabetes, obesity, stress, physical inactivity, age, gender, and family history were found to be highly related to heart attack and stroke. As the risks were discovered, the realization evolved that heart disease is not the inevitable consequence of aging or bad luck but a preventable, acquired disease. After a few years, researchers realized that preventive efforts should begin in childhood.

Autopsy studies of 18-year-olds who died in accidents have shown a positive relationship between blood cholesterol levels and the prevalence of fatty streaks on the walls of the coronary arteries and aorta. The evidence indicates that the average cholesterol level in children in overfed, underexercised societies, such as the United States, is too high.

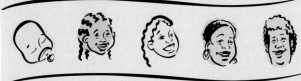

Wellness for a Lifetime

Childhood Origins of Heart Disease

Behavior patterns established during childhood that increase the likelihood of coronary heart disease often persist into adulthood. A physically inactive child is likely to become a physically inactive adult.[13] Only 50 percent of young people in the United States (ages 12 to 21 years) regularly participate in vigorous physical activity, and one-fourth report no physical activity at all.[14,15] Physical inactivity is a primary contributor to the unprecedented explosion of overweight and obesity among children in the United States. The percentage of overweight adolescents today has tripled since 1980, and this trend shows no signs of abating or reversing in the near future.[16] Approximately 30.3 percent of 6- to 11-year-old children are overweight and 15.3 percent are obese; 30.4 percent of adolescents are overweight, while 15.5 percent are obese.[17] One of the serious consequences of early obesity has been the emergence of Type 2 diabetes—a disease with life-threatening complications that in the recent past occurred almost exclusively in middle-aged adults—which is currently occurring among American adolescents. The two major reasons for this trend are (1) overweight/obesity and (2) physical inactivity.[17] The American Diabetic Association and the American Academy of Pediatrics recommend that at-risk children be screened with a blood test every two years starting at the age of 10.[18] An estimated 1.7 million Americans became regular cigarette smokers in 1998. More than half were younger than 18 years of age.[1] Smoking is a major risk for many diseases that tend to track into adulthood.

Leading health authorities presented a list of 10 high-priority public health concerns in *Healthy People 2010*. Topping the list was the need for Americans, young and old, to become more physically active. The second concern was the unprecedented number of overweight and obese people in the United States.[19]

In a recent study using sophisticated measuring techniques, children 9 to 11 years old whose cholesterol was higher than normal had blood vessels stiffer than expected for their young age. Arterial dilation was less than normal in these children, while resistance to blood flow was greater than normal in response to the heart's contractions.[20]

Obese children show blood vessel abnormalities that can lead to premature heart disease later in life.[21]

Cardiovascular disease is the third leading cause of death for children under the age of 15, and approximately 197,000 cardiovascular procedures were performed on youngsters 15 years of age and younger in the year 2001.[1]

Attempts to prevent heart disease need to begin in childhood. Knowledgeable parents can serve as role models who practice, rather than just talk about, healthy behaviors. Active parents should be the strongest influence, but they are not the only influence. Schools need to offer quality physical education programs throughout the 12 years of precollege education, and communities should offer opportunities and provide facilities for active participation in games and recreational play.

Autopsy studies of American combat battle casualties, whose average age was 22 years, in the Korean and Vietnam wars showed obstructions in the coronary arteries. These obstructions are caused by **atherosclerosis**, a slow, progressive disease of the arteries that can originate in childhood.[11] It is characterized by the deposition of plaque beneath the lining of the artery (Figure 2-4). Plaque consists of fatty substances, cholesterol, blood platelets, fibrin, calcium, and cellular debris. The atherosclerotic process is responsible for 80 percent of the coronary heart disease deaths in the United States. The current theory of the development of atherosclerosis is explained in the section dealing with cholesterol as a risk factor.

Between 3 and 4 million people have silent **ischemia** or silent heart attacks.[12] These people typically do not experience chest pain or chest discomfort, nor do they have arm, neck, or jaw pain.[22] Those most likely to experience

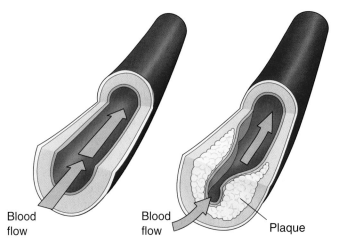

Blood flow   Blood flow   Plaque

Figure 2-4 Progressive Narrowing of a Normal Coronary Artery (Atherosclerosis)

Heart Attack: The Warning Signs

The Warning Signs

- Uncomfortable pressure, fullness, a squeezing sensation as if a band were being tightened around the chest, pain in the center of the chest lasting longer than 10 minutes
- Pain that spreads to the shoulders, arms, or neck
- The preceding warning signs accompanied by dizziness, fainting, sweating, nausea, and shortness of breath

What to Do If These Signs Appear

If you have chest discomfort lasting more than 10 minutes,

- Do not deny what may be occurring.
- Call emergency services first; if they cannot respond then have a friend or family member drive you to the nearest hospital that has 24-hour emergency cardiac care.
- Know in advance which hospitals have emergency cardiac care.
- Prominently display in your home the telephone number of the emergency rescue service and carry a copy with you.

a silent heart attack are older people, diabetics, females, those who have had a prior stroke or heart failure, non-whites, and those who are under chronic stress or who are lonely, angry, and negative most of the time.[12] The absence of chest pain, a hallmark of heart attacks, can more than double the risk of dying, probably because these people wait longer before seeking medical treatment. Three to four million Americans experience cardiac ischemia without knowing it. Ischemia (reduced blood flow) occurs as the result of arterial disease or arterial spasms that restrict blood flow to any part of the body, including the heart.[1] Silent ischemia can initiate heart attacks without prior warning. However, the typical heart attack is obvious, and the symptoms are pronounced. See Just the Facts: Heart Attack: The Warning Signs.

Stroke (Brain Attack)

The majority of strokes (cerebrovascular accidents, or brain attacks) follow the same sequence of events that results in coronary heart disease. A stroke is essentially the result of diseased blood vessels that supply the brain. It shares the same risk factors as coronary heart disease, and it takes years to develop.

Strokes are caused by a **thrombus** (a clot that forms and occludes an artery supplying the brain) or an **embolus** (a clot that forms elsewhere in the body

and fragments, dislodges, and is transported to one of the cerebral blood vessels that is too small for its passage). **Cerebral hemorrhage** (the bursting of a blood vessel in the brain caused by trauma, arterial brittleness, or aneurysm) is also a cause of stroke. An **aneurysm** is a weak spot in an artery that forms a balloonlike pouch, which can rupture. It may be a congenital defect or the result of uncontrolled or poorly controlled hypertension.

Between 70 and 80 percent of all strokes are due to a thrombus or an embolus. Brain cells once supplied by these blood vessels die and do not regenerate. As a result, the functional losses that occur (e.g., paralysis on one side of the body, difficulty speaking) cannot be fully recovered. That brain cells die also means that treatment will not be very effective. Many stroke victims are unable to return to a normal lifestyle unless the stroke was mild, in which case a full recovery is possible.

Strokes caused by hemorrhages result in a 50 percent mortality rate. Victims die from the pressure imposed by blood leaking into the brain. Those who survive this type of stroke are likely to recover more of their normal functions than are those whose strokes were caused by a blood clot. The blood that spills in and on the brain during a hemorrhagic stroke produces pressure, which gradually abates as the blood is absorbed by the body. Function is regained as the pressure relents.

On many occasions a stroke is preceded by warning signs and signals days, weeks, or months before a major stroke. These must be recognized and then acted on, so that prompt medical and lifestyle interventions can be instituted to prevent or delay a stroke.

Preventing a stroke is similar to preventing coronary heart disease. Both involve blood pressure and cholesterol control, smoking cessation, weight management, exercise, and proper nutrition. See Just the Facts: Stroke: The Warning Signs, which identifies the major warning signs.

Stroke: The Warning Signs

The American Heart Association suggests that people be familiar with the following warning signs:

- Temporary loss of speech or difficulty in speaking or understanding speech
- Unexplained dizziness, unsteadiness, or sudden falls
- Temporary dimness or loss of vision, particularly in one eye
- Sudden, temporary weakness or numbness of the face, arm, and leg on one side of the body
- Occurrence of a series of minor strokes, or transient ischemic attacks (TIAs)

Risk Factors for Heart Disease

The major risk factors for heart disease are increasing age, male gender, heredity, and race.[1] While these risk factors cannot be changed, their impact on heart disease can be reduced by a heart-healthy lifestyle. Tobacco smoke, high blood cholesterol, high blood pressure, physical inactivity, obesity and overweight, and diabetes mellitus are major risk factors that can be modified by a heart-healthy lifestyle and medication if needed. Other contributing risk factors include an individual's response to stress, hormonal factors, birth control pills, and excessive alcohol consumption. See Figure 2-5 (page 40) for the major risk factors.

These risk factors account for the majority of cardiovascular disease in the United States. However, there are many other factors that can be involved, some backed by a sound and growing body of evidence. These include high serum homocysteine, lipoprotein (a), high blood fibrinogen, and high blood insulin levels. Other possible risk factors, supported by inconclusive evidence, include short stature, baldness, ear lobe creases, and high serum uric acid level. A few of the more important of these risk factors are covered later in this chapter.

Major Risk Factors That Cannot Be Changed

Age

Cardiovascular disease is the leading cause of death and disability among the elderly because atherosclerotic disease is usually more advanced late in life. Approximately 55 percent of heart attacks occur in people 65 years of age or older. This age group accounts for more than 80 percent of fatal heart attacks.[1]

Male Gender

Until recently, the incidence of coronary heart disease among women was largely unexplored. Men have been the primary subjects in coronary heart disease and risk factor studies because of the high incidence of both among men. However, coronary heart disease is also the leading cause of death and disability among women, accounting for almost 250,000 deaths annually.[1] Women have less heart disease than men, particularly before menopause. See Wellness for a Lifetime: Women and Coronary Disease: Pre- and Postmenopause.

An alarming trend is the increased incidence of heart attacks in premenopausal women who have been smoking cigarettes long enough for it to affect their health, especially when combined with oral contraceptive use.

Heredity and Race

According to the American Heart Association, "a tendency toward heart disease or atherosclerosis appears to

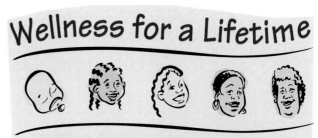

Women and Coronary Heart Disease: Pre- and Postmenopause

Heart attacks are relatively rare among premenopausal women because of the production and presence of estrogen (the female sex hormone responsible for the development of secondary sexual characteristics and the various phases of the menstrual cycle and essential for bone formation). Estrogen is also protective in that it lowers LDL cholesterol (the harmful form), raises HDL cholesterol (the protective form), and may increase blood flow to the heart.

During and after menopause, the production of estrogen decreases and eventually stops, and the protection from heart disease diminishes. Women tend to develop coronary heart disease about 10 years later than men. At age 65, the risk for men and women equalizes.[24]

A survey of women conducted by the American Heart Association indicated that most respondents perceived breast cancer as their greatest threat to health, even though heart disease kills and disables more women. Breast cancer killed 40,800 women in 2003, while approximately 500,000 women died from cardiovascular disease.[25] Heart attack symptoms—such as nausea; shortness of breath; fatigue; and jaw, shoulder, and back pain—tend to be far less dramatic in women. Such nonspecific symptoms may induce women to delay seeking medical treatment long enough to render angioplasty or blood-thinning drugs ineffective.

Because women are typically older than men when they develop heart disease, they usually have comorbid conditions, such as diabetes or high blood pressure. These complications interfere with postheart-attack healing processes.

Women should not take hormone replacement treatment for heart protection. This was standard treatment just a few years ago. But the results of two large placebo-controlled, randomized studies showed that hormone replacement therapy did not prevent heart disease; in fact, those subjects who were in the hormone replacement group had a higher incidence of heart attacks and strokes than the subjects who were taking a placebo.[26]

Risk factors that cannot be changed

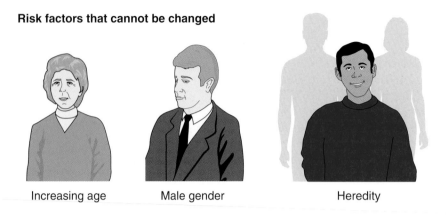

Increasing age   Male gender   Heredity

Risk factors that can be changed

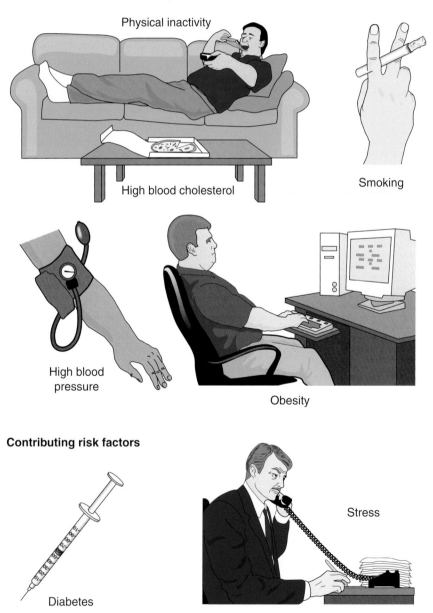

Physical inactivity

High blood cholesterol

Smoking

High blood pressure

Obesity

Contributing risk factors

Stress

Diabetes

Figure 2-5   Cardiovascular Disease Risk Factors

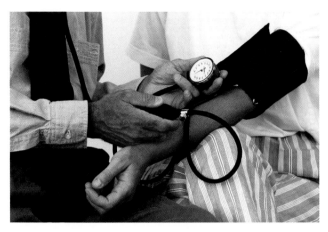

Keeping your blood pressure under control helps keep your heart healthy.

be hereditary, so children of parents with cardiovascular disease are more likely to develop it themselves."[1] A history of first-degree male relatives (father, grandfather, and brothers) who have coronary heart disease or who died of coronary heart disease before the age of 55 or first-degree female relatives (mother, grandmother, and sisters) who have coronary heart disease or who died of coronary heart disease before the age of 65 indicates a strong familial tendency.[23] If the family history is positive, the modifiable risk factors must be controlled. Some minority groups have a higher rate of heart disease than would be expected. For example, African Americans have a high incidence of hypertension. One in three African-American adults is hypertensive, compared with one in four adults in the general public. They also experience higher rates of morbidity (illness) and mortality (death) from consequences of hypertension, such as strokes and kidney failure.[27] Other minority groups— Mexican Americans, Native Americans, Native Hawaiians, and some Asian Americans—have high rates of heart disease primarily due to rampant obesity and one of its major consequences, diabetes.[1]

Although age, male gender, heredity, and race are major risks not under our direct control, we can modify their effects by living a wellness lifestyle. Abstaining from tobacco products; exercising regularly; controlling blood pressure, cholesterol, and body weight; managing stress; and maintaining a social support system can lessen the impact of these unchangeable risk factors.

Major Risk Factors That Can Be Changed

A well-designed study, whose results were reported in 2003, showed that approximately 90 percent of all coronary heart disease victims had one or more of the following risk factors: cholesterol abnormalities, high blood pressure, cigarette smoking/tobacco use, physical inactivity, obesity, and diabetes.[28] The data examined in this investigation came from three major heart disease studies that featured thousands of subjects. The authors of the current study stated that the evidence gathered in the three previous studies convincingly challenges the frequently made claim that only 50 percent of heart attacks occur to those with known risk factors. The facts indicate quite the opposite. The data showed that 90 percent of all heart attack victims had one or more of the five risk factors. Heart attacks don't occur unless there are reasons for their occurrence.

Cholesterol

Cholesterol is a steroid that is an essential structural component of neural tissue; it is used in the construction of cell walls and for the manufacture of hormones and bile (for the digestion and absorption of fats). A certain amount of cholesterol is required for good health, but high levels in the blood are associated with heart attacks and strokes.

The National Heart, Lung, and Blood Institute suggests that Americans reduce cholesterol consumption to less than 200 milligrams per day (200 mg/day) for those at high risk for cardiovascular disease and less than 300 mg/day for all other Americans.[29] Fat intake may be increased to a maximum of 35 percent of the total calories consumed, but saturated fat plus trans fats should be reduced to no more than 10 percent of the total calories. (See Just the Facts: Guidelines for Fat and Cholesterol on page 42.) Many authorities are convinced that limiting total fat and saturated fat is more important than being overly restrictive of cholesterol.

Americans should consume no more than 7 to 10 percent of their total calories in the form of saturated fat and trans fatty acids.[30] Monounsaturated fats should make up half of the total fat intake, with the remainder of fat intake consisting of polyunsaturated fats. Monounsaturates and polyunsaturates are heart-healthy fats, while saturates and trans fats are very harmful.

Today the average daily consumption of cholesterol is 331 mg/day by males and 231 mg/day by females. The average consumption of total fat is approximately 33 percent of total calories; 13 percent is saturated fat, 3 percent is trans fats, and the remainder consists of monounsaturated and polyunsaturated fats.[29]

Cholesterol is consumed in the diet (exogenous, or dietary cholesterol), but it is also manufactured by the body from saturated fats (endogenous). Cholesterol synthesis in the body would occur even if a cholesterol-free diet were consumed. The liver manufactures about 80 percent of endogenous cholesterol, with the remainder being synthesized in the intestinal and arterial walls.

The liver alone produces enough cholesterol to meet the body's needs. Therefore, consuming cholesterol is not necessary to maintain health. Table 2-1 on page 42 lists

~~~~~~~~~~~~~~~~Just the Facts~~~~~~~~~~~~~~~~

Guidelines for Fat and Cholesterol

The National Cholesterol Education Program through the auspices of the National Heart, Lung, and Blood Institute released its newest recommendations for detecting and lowering high cholesterol in adults in May 2001. This revision represents the first major change since 1993. The following are some selected highlights recommended by a panel of 27 experts:

1. Physicians are strongly encouraged to pay more attention to the "metabolic syndrome," representative of a significant risk for heart disease. This syndrome is a combination of excessive abdominal fat, high blood pressure, high blood glucose, elevated triglycerides, and low HDL cholesterol.
2. HDL cholesterol is considered a major risk if it is below 40 mg/dL, instead of the previous 35 mg/dL.

3. Dietary intake of cholesterol should be less than 200 mg/day for those at high risk and less than 300 mg/day for all others.
4. There should be more aggressive treatment of triglycerides.
5. Less than 10 percent of calories should come from saturated fat and trans fats together.
6. Dietary fat may be increased to 35 percent of the total daily calories instead of the previous 30 percent, provided that the majority of these come from monounsaturated and polyunsaturated sources.
7. The new recommendations strongly urge the necessity of attaining and maintaining normal body weight, as well as consistent participation in physical activity.

Table 2-1 Sources of Dietary Cholesterol and Saturated Fat

	Cholesterol (mg)*	Saturated Fat (g)**		Cholesterol (mg)*	Saturated Fat (g)**
Meats (3 oz.)			**Seafood (3 oz.)**		
Beef liver	372	2.5	Squid	153	.4
Veal	86	4.0	Oily fish	59	1.2
Pork	80	3.2	Lean fish	59	.3
Lean beef	56	2.4	Shrimp (6 large)	48	.2
Chicken (dark meat)	82	2.7	Clams (6 large)	36	.3
Chicken (white meat)	76	1.3	Lobster	46.4	.08
Egg	215	1.7	**Other Items of Interest**		
Dairy Products (1 Cup; Cheese, 1 oz.)			Pork brains (3 oz.)	2,169	1.8
Ice cream	59	8.9	Beef kidney (3 oz.)	683	3.8
Whole milk	33	5.1	Beef hot dog (1)	75	9.9
Butter (1 tsp.)	31	7.1	Prime ribs of beef (3 oz.)	66.5	5.3
Yogurt (low-fat)	11	1.8	Doughnut	36	4.0
Cheddar	30	6.0	Milk chocolate	0	16.3
American	27	5.6	Green or yellow vegetable or fruit	0	Trace
Camembert	20	4.3	Peanut butter (1 tbsp.)	0	1.5
Parmesan	8	2.0	Angel food cake	0	1.96
Oils (1 tbsp.)			Skim milk (1 cup)	4	.3
			Cheese pizza (3 oz.)	6	.8
Coconut	0	11.8	Buttermilk (1 cup)	9	1.3
Palm	0	6.7	Ice milk, soft (1 cup)	13	2.9
Olive	0	1.8	Turkey, white meat (3 oz.)	59	.9
Corn	0	1.7			
Safflower	0	1.2			

* There are 1,000 mg in a gram.

** There are 28 g in an ounce and 454 g in a pound.

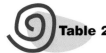

Table 2-2 Risk Profile—Lipid and Lipoprotein Concentrations

Total Cholesterol	Category of Risk
< 200 mg/dL*	Desirable
200–239 mg/dL	Borderline
≥ 240 mg/dL**	High

LDL Cholesterol	Category of Risk
<100 mg/dL	Optimal
100–129 mg/dL	Near optimal/above optimal
130–159 mg/dL	Borderline high
160–189 mg/dL	High
≥ 190 mg/dL	Very high

HDL Cholesterol	Category of Risk
≤ 40 mg/dL***	Increased risk
≥ 60 mg/dL	Heart-protective

Triglycerides	Category of Risk
<150 mg/dL	Normal
150–199 mg/dL	Borderline high
200–499 mg/dL	High
≥ 500 mg/dL	Very high

SOURCE: Adapted from Revised cholesterol guidelines. 2001. *Harvard Heart Letter* 11 (July): 6–7.

* < is less than

** ≥ is equal to or greater than

*** ≤ is equal to or less than

Real-World Wellness

Strategies for Lowering Cholesterol

My doctor told me that my cholesterol level is too high. How can I lower it to reduce my risk of having a heart attack or stroke?

First, establish a realistic goal, such as about how much you think you can lower your cholesterol. Second, identify the lifestyle changes that can lower cholesterol. Third, attempt to do all of the following that apply to you:

- Reduce your fat consumption to less than 30 percent of total calories (25 percent would be better).
- Reduce your saturated fat and trans fats consumption to less than 10 percent of total calories (8 percent would be better).
- Reduce your dietary cholesterol to less than 300 mg/day (less than 200 mg/day would be better).
- Lose weight if you are overweight.
- Stop smoking cigarettes and/or stop using other tobacco products.
- Increase your consumption of soluble fiber, found in fruits, vegetables, and grains.
- Do aerobic exercise at least three times per week for at least 30 minutes each time.

If these strategies fail to normalize your cholesterol level in six months, you may have to consider taking cholesterol-lowering drugs.

some common foods that contain cholesterol and saturated fat.

A number of population studies during the last 20 years have indicated a positive relationship between serum cholesterol (the level of cholesterol circulating in the blood) and the development of coronary heart disease. The National Heart, Lung, and Blood Institute reviewed this evidence and concluded that high circulating levels of serum cholesterol cause heart disease.

Values of serum cholesterol above 200 milligrams per deciliter (mg/dL) of blood are higher than the average risk. Table 2-2 shows the values of risk associated with total cholesterol (TC), LDL and HDL cholesterol (to be discussed shortly), and another serum lipid (blood fat), the triglycerides.

An important collaborative study involving 12 research centers throughout the United States provided clinical evidence implicating cholesterol as a culprit in coronary heart disease.[31] Half of a group of 3,806 subjects was given a cholesterol-lowering drug, and the other half was given a placebo. The subjects were followed for approximately 7.4 years, at which time the data indicated that the drug group reduced their cholesterol levels by 13 percent, suffered 19 percent fewer heart attacks, and experienced 24 percent fewer fatal heart attacks. The incidence of coronary bypass surgery and angina were also significantly reduced. The researchers concluded that each 1 percent reduction in cholesterol level results in a 2 percent reduction in the risk for coronary heart disease.

A later follow-up of this study indicated that the reduction in coronary heart disease is probably closer to 3 percent for every 1 percent that cholesterol is lowered.[32] The strategies for lowering cholesterol in the blood are presented in Real-World Wellness: Strategies for Lowering Cholesterol.

The Cholesterol Carriers. The amount of cholesterol circulating in the blood accounts for only part of the total cholesterol in the body. Unlike sugar and salt, cholesterol does not dissolve in the blood, so it is transported by protein packages, which facilitate its solubility. These transporters are the lipoproteins manufactured by the body. They include the chylomicrons, very low-density lipoprotein (VLDL), intermediate-density lipoprotein

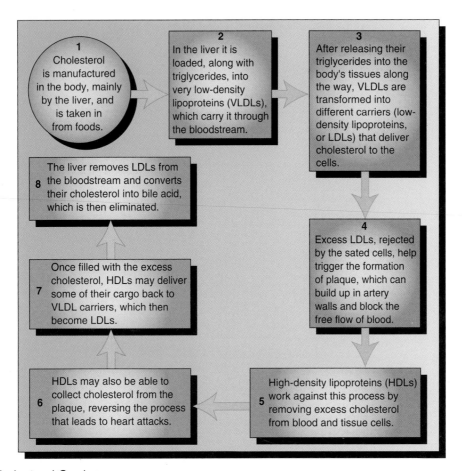

Figure 2-6 Cholesterol Carriers

(IDL), low-density lipoprotein (LDL), and high-density lipoprotein (HDL). Dietary cholesterol enters the body from the digestive system attached to the chylomicrons. The chylomicrons shrink as they give up their cholesterol to the cells of the body. The fragments that remain are removed by the liver and used to manufacture and secrete VLDLs, triglyceride-rich lipoproteins. The triglycerides represent 95 percent of the stored fats in the body. The VLDLs are degraded as their cargo of triglycerides is either used by the cells for energy or stored in adipose cells (fat cells). The VLDL remnants may be removed by the liver or converted to LDLs (Figure 2-6).

LDLs are the primary transporters of cholesterol—they carry 60 to 80 percent of the body's cholesterol—and the most capable of producing atherosclerosis. Michael S. Brown and Joseph L. Goldstein won a 1985 Nobel Prize in medicine and physiology for discovering that the liver and the cells of the body have receptor sites that bind LDLs, removing them from circulation. The liver contains 50 to 75 percent of these sites; the remainder are in other cells of the body. When LDL concentrations are excessive, the liver sites become saturated, and further removal of them from the blood is significantly impeded. As a result, plasma levels of cholesterol rise, leading to the formation and development of atherosclerotic plaque.

The development of atherosclerosis in the coronary arteries is complex. Since the early 1990s, the medical community has been seriously investigating the connection between disease and inflammation. Inflammation represents the body's major mechanism of defense against infection. Atherosclerosis—responsible for 80 percent of coronary disease—is a chronic inflammatory disease. The initial event in the atherosclerotic process is an injury (lesion) that occurs to the inner lining of the arteries. Such injuries occur because of prolonged exposure to tobacco smoke, high blood pressure, elevated LDL cholesterol, diabetes mellitus, high amounts of serum homocysteine, and viral and bacterial infections.[8] These injuries, which occur at multiple sites, allow LDL cholesterol to infiltrate under the artery lining, where they become oxidized (come in contact with oxygen). Oxidized LDLs become toxic. Oxidized LDLs resemble an infection, which triggers the immune system to initiate defensive actions. This is the connection between atherosclerosis and inflammation.[33] Monocytes from the immune system enter the artery wall and act as macrophages (long-lived cells that ingest foreign substances) to engulf and destroy oxidized LDLs.[6] The fat-filled macrophages become bloated with oxidized LDLs; in this state, they actually contribute to the formation of plaque. Plaque

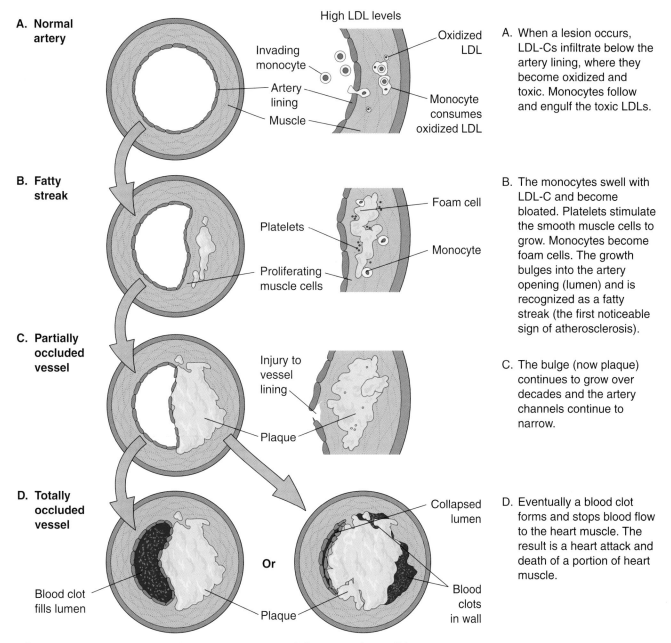

Figure 2-7 Progression of Atherosclerosis and Coronary Artery Disease

grows steadily over many years. The process initiates and maintains a low-grade inflammatory response by the body. Chronic inflammation damages the cells lining the arteries and can cause an acute heart attack by destabilizing plaque. Destabilized plaque has a thin fibrous cap which is likely to rupture causing a blood clot that can block blood flow in an artery resulting in a heart attack. Inflammation also contributes to the growth of the fibrous cap that seals over the plaque.

Cigarette smoke, lack of regular exercise, high blood pressure, cholesterol abnormalities, excessive body weight, an unhealthy diet, and a rapid heart rate result in continued inflammation and the growth of

plaque. Many plaques are unstable, meaning that they have a thin fibrous cap. These plaques are under constant threat of rupturing at any time. When a break in the cap occurs, plaque spews out through the opening, triggering further inflammatory responses by the body, which result in the formation of a blood clot. Often the clot is large enough to block the entire opening of the artery, the culmination of which is the stoppage of blood flow and oxygen to a portion of the heart muscle. This is a heart attack. See Figure 2-7 for an illustration of this process.

Physicians can test for chronic low-grade inflammation of the type that might be indicative of coronary heart disease. This is a simple blood test called high sensitivity C-reactive protein (hs CRP) test. This test has become a useful biomarker for assessing cardiovascular disease and in several studies it predicted future heart attacks more accurately than LDL cholesterol.[34] C-reactive protein is produced by the liver in response to an increase in the blood of Interleukin 6 (IL-6), which is the principal initiator of the inflammatory response. People who are overweight or obese or who have metabolic syndrome may spontaneously secrete sufficient IL-6 to mimic low-grade systemic inflammation, complete with an elevation of inflammatory proteins such as C-reactive protein.[35] Interleukin 6 increases with age. CRP levels of 3.0 milligrams per liter of blood (3 mg/L) or higher can triple the risk of having heart disease. The risk is higher for females than males. People whose CRP is less than 0.5 mg/L rarely have heart attacks.

Heart attacks are less likely to occur when LDL values are below 100 mg/dL. A national panel of experts has developed guidelines for safe and unsafe levels of LDL, and these appear in table 2-2. A high circulating level of LDL cholesterol is positively related to cardiovascular disease. Weight loss, a diet low in saturated fat and total fat, exercise, and medication (if needed) will lower LDL levels in the blood.

HDLs are involved in reverse transport; they accept cholesterol from the blood and tissues and transfer it to the liver, where it can be degraded and disposed of in the feces. This is a major route for removal of cholesterol. HDLs protect the arteries from atherosclerosis by clearing cholesterol from the blood. Cardiovascular health depends greatly on low levels of total cholesterol and LDLs and a high level of HDLs. Cigarette smoking, diabetes, elevated triglyceride levels, and anabolic steroids lower HDL, whereas physical exercise, weight loss, and moderate alcohol consumption raise it.

Moderate alcohol consumption (no more than two drinks per day for males and no more than one drink per day for females) increases HDL cholesterol. However, recent evidence has shown that three to four alcoholic drinks per week is sufficient to modestly raise HDL cholesterol. Caution should be exercised regarding alcohol intake because the health hazards associated with it far outweigh its few advantages. Alcohol consumption, even in moderate amounts, is not an acceptable way to raise HDL unless prescribed by a physician who is well aware of the patient's health and family history. An alcoholic drink is defined as a 5-ounce glass of wine, a 12-ounce beer, or 1½ ounces of 80-proof spirits. However, alcohol is a depressant that impairs judgment and removes inhibitions, so that people under its influence behave in ways they ordinarily would not while sober. Excessive alcohol intake is three drinks or more per day. Health is compromised at consumption levels above two drinks per day. The risks increase for heart disease, high

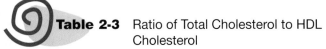

Table 2-3 Ratio of Total Cholesterol to HDL Cholesterol

Risk	Men	Women
Very low (one-half average)	< 3.4	< 3.3
Low risk	4.0	3.8
Average risk	5.0	4.5
Moderate risk (two times average)	9.5	7.0
High risk (three times average)	> 23	> 11

blood pressure, cirrhosis of the liver, breast cancer, and osteoporosis; also, the immune system weakens, red blood cell production slows down, and the brain is adversely affected. (See Chapter 10 for a more complete discussion of the effects of alcohol.)

Table 2-2 presents the current guidelines for HDL cholesterol levels in the blood. The higher the HDL, the greater the protection from cardiovascular disease. The average value for men is 46 mg/dL, and for women it is 56 mg/dL.[5] This biological difference in HDL levels between genders partly explains the lower incidence of heart disease in premenopausal women as compared with men. After menopause, HDL levels in women begin to decrease, as does their protection provided by this subfraction of cholesterol. The ratio between total cholesterol (TC) and HDL (TC/HDL) should also be considered when the risk is interpreted. This ratio is determined by dividing TC by HDL (Table 2-3).[5]

Another blood fat, the serum triglycerides, is involved in the development and progression of atherosclerosis. Normal serum triglycerides range from 50 mg/dL to 150 mg/dL. Table 2-2 identifies the risk associated with various serum triglyceride levels.

High serum triglycerides usually coexist with low HDL cholesterol, a proven risk factor for cardiovascular disease. Teasing out the independent effect of serum triglyceride levels has been difficult. But recent evidence has shown that high levels are a modest independent risk factor for heart disease and a reliable predictor when coupled with low HDL cholesterol.[36] Serum triglycerides greater than 190 mg/dL increase blood viscosity (blood thickness), resulting in sluggish blood flow. Viscous blood is more difficult to circulate, so oxygen and nutrients are not delivered as efficiently to the body's tissues, and these include the heart muscle.[8]

Table 2-2 shows the relative risk posed by high serum triglycerides. Levels below 150 mg/dL are in the normal category, but evidence suggests that an optimal level is below 100 mg/dL.[29]

A number of studies have shown that sedentary people with high triglycerides can reduce serum triglycerides substantially when they participate in moderately intense aerobic exercise for 45 minutes 4 days per week.[37]

Physically fit people metabolize serum triglycerides more effectively than do sedentary people and are able to clear these triglycerides from the blood more rapidly after a high-fat meal.[29] Fatty acids, stored in the body as triglycerides, are the primary type of fat used by muscle cells for energy.[38] This is the reason that exercise significantly lowers the triglyceride level in the body.

Other strategies for lowering serum triglycerides include weight loss; reductions in dietary sugar, fat, and alcohol; and the substitution of fish for meat a couple of times during the week. Increasing fish consumption, as long as it is not fried, lowers the dietary intake of calories and saturated fat and increases the intake of omega-3 fatty acids, which tend to lower serum triglycerides.

Blood pressure

Blood pressure, recorded in millimeters of mercury (mmHg), is the force exerted against the walls of the arteries as blood travels through the circulatory system. Pressure is created when the heart contracts and pumps blood into the arteries. The arterioles (smallest arteries) offer resistance to blood flow, and if the resistance is persistently high, the pressure rises and remains high. The medical term for high blood pressure is **hypertension.**

Hypertension is a silent disease that has no characteristic signs or symptoms, so blood pressure should be checked periodically. Blood pressure can be measured quickly with a sphygmomanometer. A cuff is wrapped around the upper arm and inflated with enough air to compress the artery, temporarily stopping blood flow. A stethoscope is placed on the artery below the cuff, so that the sound of blood coursing through the artery can be heard when the air in the cuff is released. The first sound represents the systolic pressure (the maximum pressure of blood flow when the heart contracts), and the last sound heard is the diastolic pressure (the minimum pressure of blood flow between heartbeats).

The guidelines for prevention and treatment of high blood pressure were revised in 2003 for the first time since 1997. The new guidelines were developed by a panel of experts under the direction of the National Heart, Lung, and Blood Institute.[39] The panel established a new category of blood pressure called "prehypertension." This category includes blood pressures ranging from 120/80 to 139/89. Fifty-eight million American adults have hypertension and 46 million are prehypertensive.[40] The blood pressures in the new category were considered normal under the old guidelines. The upgrade was made because a growing body of evidence showed that a blood pressure of 135/85 doubles the risk of having a heart attack or stroke when compared with a reading of 115/75.[41] The risk for death from heart disease or stroke begins to increase at

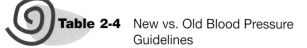

Table 2-4 New vs. Old Blood Pressure Guidelines

Category	Now (2003)	Before (1997)
No hypertension	Less than $\frac{120}{80}$	Less than $\frac{140}{90}$
Prehypertension	$\frac{120}{80}$ to $\frac{139}{89}$	———
Hypertension	$\frac{140}{90}$ or higher	$\frac{140}{90}$ or higher

SOURCE: Editors. July 2003. Why it pays to lower even "normal" blood pressure. *Heart Advisor* 6(7):2.

115/75 and doubles for each 20 mmHg systolic or every 10 mmHg diastolic. See Table 2-4 for the new versus the old guidelines.

Table 2-4 represents the latest thinking among medical researchers about the stages of blood pressure values. The higher the blood pressure, the greater the risk. The lower the blood pressure, the better. However, blood pressure can be too low if it causes symptoms such as lightheadedness or fainting. Recent evidence indicates that an increase in systolic blood pressure (SBP) accompanied by a decrease in the diastolic blood pressure (DBP) doubles the risk of dying from cardiovascular disease.[23] This combination seems to be more dangerous than when both pressures increase. The DBP decreases when the large arteries stiffen.

The difference between the SBP and DBP is called the "pulse pressure" (SBD minus DBP).[42] The SBP increases because age and poor lifestyle habits cause the arteries to lose their resilience. At the same time, the DBP decreases because the stiff arteries aren't as responsive to blood flow between heartbeats. A pulse pressure of 60 mmHg or more is associated with the development and progression of atherosclerosis.

Approximately 58 million American adults have high blood pressure, and 46,700 people die of its complications annually.[1] The cause of high blood pressure is not known in 90 to 95 percent of the cases. This is referred to as *essential hypertension. Essential* is a medical term that means "of unknown origin or cause." Essential hypertension cannot be cured, but it can be treated and controlled. The other 5 to 10 percent of the cases of hypertension have a specific cause. If the cause can be determined and eliminated, blood pressure will return to normal.

The heart is adversely affected by uncontrolled or undiagnosed hypertension of long duration. Pumping blood for years against high resistance in the arteries increases the workload of the heart, and it becomes enlarged in response to the strain. The heart receives inadequate rest because the resistance to blood flow is consistently high, and this produces overly stretched muscle fibers. They progressively lose the ability to rebound. The result is that they contract less forcefully. At this point the heart loses its efficiency and weakens. If intervention does not occur early, congestive heart failure is inevitable. Hypertension also damages the arteries and accelerates atherosclerosis.

Hypertension is the most important risk factor for brain attacks (strokes) as well as a major risk for heart disease. More than 700,000 brain attacks occur every year.[1] Certain segments of the population are at higher risk, such as African Americans, who are more likely to suffer a stroke or experience kidney damage than are white, Latino, or Asian Americans.[43]

Treatment for Hypertension. Treatment for hypertension may include all or some of the following: weight loss; salt and alcohol restriction; adequate intake of calcium, potassium, and magnesium; voluntary relaxation techniques; exercise; and medication. Excess body weight increases the work of the heart because it must meet the nutrient demands of the extra tissue.

High salt intake increases the blood pressure in those who are salt sensitive. Estimates indicate that at least 30 percent of Americans are salt sensitive, but the actual number is probably higher. Salt is an acquired taste that can be modified. Curbing salt consumption while blood pressure is still normal cannot hurt and it may help.[44]

Salt consists of sodium and chloride. Sodium, which makes up 40 percent of salt, is the culprit involved in raising blood pressure. According to the Institute of Medicine, Americans on average consume too much salt. The median intake for males is 7.8 to 11.8 grams per day (g/day), and for females it is 5.8 to 7.8 g/day.[45] The recommended consumption is 3.8 g/day and the most salt that anyone should consume is 5.8 g/day.

The average consumption of sodium is 3.5 to 5.0 g/day, compared with the recommendation, which is less than 2.4 g/day.[45] Reducing sodium consumption can lower the systolic blood pressure by 3 to 6 mmHg.

The diet, Dietary Approaches to Stop Hypertension (DASH), was specifically developed to lower blood pressure.[44] The diet emphasizes fruits, vegetables, low-fat dairy products, and low sodium intake. This diet has reduced systolic pressure by 10 to 12 mmHg. According to nutrition experts, the effectiveness of the diet is due to its rich content of calcium, potassium, and magnesium.

The daily potassium requirement has been increased to 4.7 g/day,[46] the calcium requirement is 1,200–1,500 mg/day,[46] and the magnesium requirement is 320 mg/day.[47]

Yoga, meditation, hypnotherapy, biofeedback, and other relaxation techniques can lower the pressure of hypertensive people. They can also reduce the pressure of normotensive people (those with normal blood pressure).[48] Meditating hypertensive people lowered their systolic pressure by 11 points and their diastolic pressure by 6 points more than did people in a control group counseled on the importance of losing excess weight, exercising regularly, cutting salt consumption, and drinking less alcohol.[112]

Many people drink alcohol because it relaxes them, but the ingestion of more than 2 ounces of alcohol per day raises blood pressure in some people. The same precautions regarding the use of alcohol and HDL cholesterol apply for hypertension.

The American College of Sports Medicine (ACSM) has developed a position paper on the relationship between exercise and hypertension.[40] Some of the more important conclusions follow:

1. Endurance exercises lower blood pressure by 5 to 7 mmHg. This is a significant reduction because small decrements in systolic blood pressure, as little as 2 mmHg, reduce the risk for stroke by 14 percent and coronary heart disease by 9 percent; a 2 mmHg decrease in diastolic blood pressure reduces the risk for stroke by 17 percent and coronary heart disease by 6 percent.
2. Blood pressure is reduced for up to 22 hours after a single bout of endurance exercise, with the greatest decreases occurring in those with the highest baseline blood pressures.
3. Moderate-intensity endurance exercise (40 to 60 percent of the heart rate reserve—explained in Chapter 3) will lower blood pressure.
4. The recommended exercise prescription for lowering blood pressure is as follows:
   (a) Frequency: on most, preferably all days of the week
   (b) Intensity: moderate
   (c) Time: 30 minutes or more
   (d) Type: endurance exercise supplemented with resistance training

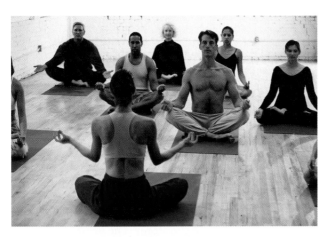

Stress-relieving activities, such as meditation, soothe the spirit and may even lower your risk for heart disease and other chronic illnesses. How do you manage stress?

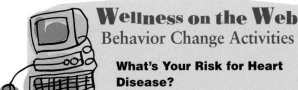

Wellness on the Web
Behavior Change Activities

What's Your Risk for Heart Disease?

In the battle to maintain a healthy heart, you have a powerful ally. The American Heart Association (AHA) is dedicated to educating and informing you on how to fight heart disease and stroke. Go to the OLC at www.mhhe.com/anspaugh6e, select Chapter 2, click on Wellness on the Web, and complete Activity 1. This assessment will show you what factors place you at greater risk for heart disease and allow you to take charge of your health by making more healthful lifestyle choices. Complete the 16 items and then click on the Submit button for your results. Which of your risk factors cannot be changed? Which can you change?

What Questions Should I Ask My Physician?

Often we tend to think of doctors as all-knowing gurus who can tell us everything we need to know to live a healthy life. The fact is, your relationship with your physician is a partnership—for best results, you need to know what to ask when you visit your doctor. The American Heart Association reminds you that, after making healthful lifestyle changes, your second-best friend in the fight against heart disease and stroke is your doctor. For help in formulating questions for this vital partner in your health care, go to the OLC at www.mhhe.com/anspaugh6e, select Chapter 2, click on Wellness on the Web, and read Activity 2. Help your physician help you live a healthier life!

Several mechanisms have been proposed to explain how endurance exercise can lower blood pressure. Endurance exercise

1. Lowers the blood levels of the catecholamines (epinephrine, norepinephrine, and dopamine), which are vasoconstrictors that increase resistance to blood flow
2. Lowers total peripheral resistance to blood flow by dilating blood vessels
3. Lowers body weight; evidence suggests that systolic blood pressure is lowered by 5 to 22 mmHg for every 22 excess pounds lost[49]
4. Improves cellular sensitivity to insulin, which encourages the kidneys to excrete sodium

Medications that control blood pressure have been developed. However, they have side effects, including weakness, leg cramps, stuffy nose, occasional diarrhea, heartburn, drowsiness, anemia, depression, headaches, joint pain, dizziness, impotence, and skin rash. The side effects are unique to the drugs being used to control blood pressure. Despite these side effects, many people find it easier to take the medicine than to make the difficult lifestyle changes that lower blood pressure. However, the effort to control blood pressure with medication should not negate the importance of controlling the lifestyle factors that contribute to hypertension. Medicine and lifestyle efforts are not mutually exclusive—each contributes to blood pressure management.

Cigarette smoking/tobacco use

Many medical authorities consider cigarette smoking the most harmful of the preventable risk factors associated with chronic illness and premature death.[50] More than 48 million adults in the United States currently smoke (approximately 23 percent of adults).[51] About 443,000 smokers died of smoking-related diseases each year between 1995 and 1999. Twenty-four percent of these deaths were cardiovascular-related.[1] In 1987, lung cancer became the leading cause of cancer death among women, replacing breast cancer. In 2002, 66,000 women died of lung cancer, compared with 40,000 who died of breast cancer.[52]

Harmful Products in Cigarettes. Nicotine; carbon monoxide; and other poisonous gases, tars, and chemical additives for taste and flavor are the hazardous products in cigarettes. Carbon monoxide and nicotine have a devastating effect on the heart and blood vessels. Nicotine is an addictive stimulant that increases the resting heart rate, blood pressure, and metabolism. For this reason, it should be reclassified as a drug and placed under the jurisdiction of the Food and Drug Administration (FDA).

A brief summary of nicotine's effects on the cardiovascular system is found in Just the Facts: Nicotine (page 50). Carbon monoxide, a poisonous gas that is a by-product of the combustion of tobacco products, displaces oxygen in the blood because hemoglobin has a greater affinity for it than for oxygen. The diminished oxygen-carrying capacity of the blood is partly responsible for the shortness of breath that smokers experience with mild physical exertion.

Cigarettes and other tobacco products are not regulated by the FDA because tobacco is not classified as a food or drug. The tobacco industry is under no mandate to disclose the nature and type of chemicals added to tobacco products. Some of these additives are harmful. The public has a right to know, but the tobacco industry has successfully resisted attempts by governmental agencies and consumer groups to force disclosure.

The harmful effects of cigarette smoking are insidious and take time to appear. The medical profession

～～Just the Facts～～

Nicotine

Nicotine is a powerful stimulant that

- Increases LDL and lowers HDL levels
- Causes the platelets to aggregate, increasing the probability of arterial spasms
- Increases the oxygen requirement of cardiac muscle
- Constricts blood vessels
- Produces cardiac dysrhythmias (irregular heartbeat)
- Is a causative agent in the 30 percent of coronary heart disease deaths related to smoking
- Increases the viscosity of the blood

measures the damage from smoking in pack years. Smoking one pack of cigarettes per day for 15 years is equal to 15 pack years (15 years × 1 pack per day = 15 pack years). Two packs per day for 15 years is equal to 30 pack years (15 × 2 = 30). Medical problems become evident after 25 to 30 pack years.

The Challenge of Quitting. To quit the tobacco habit, you have to simultaneously break the addiction to nicotine and the psychological dependence on smoking.[53] This involves changing behavior and effectively dealing with the social and situational stimuli that promote the desire to smoke. One-third of current cigarette smokers attempt to stop smoking every year but less than 10 percent of them succeed.[54] Most quitters make 4 to 10 unsuccessful attempts and try several stop smoking methods before finally succeeding. Quitting the smoking habit is a formidable challenge. However, 50 percent of active smokers have managed to stop smoking in the last 50 years. While exceedingly difficult, it can be done if one finds the right motivation. Since 1964, more men than women have quit, more whites than African Americans, and more non-Hispanics than Hispanics. More elderly people and more educated people also have higher quit rates.[55]

Complicating the effort to quit, particularly among young women, is the fear of gaining weight. Approximately 65 percent of those who quit do gain weight, but the physiological adaptations that occur may account for only a 10-pound weight gain. The physiological mechanisms responsible are probably associated with a slowing of metabolism, a slight increase in appetite, and slower transit time of food in the digestive system, so that more is absorbed by the body. Weight gain beyond 10 pounds is probably caused by altered eating patterns rather than physiology. Food smells and

tastes better when a person is not smoking. Food may substitute for a cigarette, especially during social activities. It may provide some of the oral gratification previously obtained from smoking, and it may relieve tension. Weight gain can be avoided by eating sensibly and exercising moderately and frequently; however, for best results, these new lifestyle habits need to be established before one attempts to quit smoking. It is very difficult to establish major lifestyle habits while attempting to quit another major habit.

Cigarette smoking increases the risk for many chronic diseases because of the direct effects of nicotine, carbon monoxide (CO), tars, and more than 4,000 chemicals that are inhaled with every puff.[56] Several studies have shown that smokers have higher blood levels of CRP, fibrinogen, and homocysteine than nonsmokers.[57] Fibrinogen and CRP are both involved with inflammation. Fibrinogen and homocysteine are risk factors that are covered later in this chapter. Both of these are components in the formation of blood clots.[58] Elevations of these three factors appear to be important mechanisms by which smoking promotes atherosclerotic disease.

Smoking encourages the accumulation of visceral fat (abdominal fat), which, from a health perspective, is the most harmful way to store fat. Visceral fat can be determined by a circumferential measurement of the waist. Evidence indicates that a waist circumference of 35 inches or more for females and 40 inches or more for males predisposes one to coronary heart disease, stroke, diabetes, and some forms of cancer.[59] Visceral fat also leads to a constellation of risk factors, collectively referred to as metabolic syndrome (also known as syndrome X or insulin-resistance syndrome). Metabolic syndrome begins with abdominal fat, which leads to insulin resistance, high blood pressure, low HDLs, high triglycerides, and elevated inflammatory proteins that substantially increase the risk for diabetes and cardiovascular disease.[60] An estimated 20 to 25 percent of Americans have metabolic syndrome.

Passive Smoking and Smokeless Tobacco. Involuntary, or passive, smoking (inhaling the smoke of others) is associated with premature disease and death. Estimates indicate that 53,000 nonsmokers who are regularly exposed to environmental smoke die annually from smoking-related causes.[61] The majority of these (35,000) die from ischemic heart disease, and 3,000 die from lung cancer. There is a dose-response effect. The more the nonsmoker is exposed to environmental smoke, the greater his or her risk for premature morbidity (illness) and mortality (death).

Children of smoking parents are more likely to experience a higher incidence of influenza, colds, bronchitis, asthma, and pneumonia. The impact of passive smoking on them can last a lifetime and ranges from delayed physical and intellectual development to the hazards associated with prolonged exposure to carcinogenic substances.

An alarming trend is the escalating sale of smokeless tobacco products. Chewing tobacco and dipping snuff have become popular among high school and college men. The World Health Organization (WHO) has described the growing use of smokeless tobacco as a new threat to society. Nicotine is an addictive drug regardless of the method of delivery, and its effects are similar whether it is inhaled, as in smoking, or absorbed through the tissues of the oral cavity, as in dipping and chewing. The incidence of oral cancer may be 50 times higher among long-term users of smokeless tobacco products than among nonusers.[62] Smokeless tobacco is addictive and deadly, and its use is rising among adolescent males.

Cigar sales in the country had been flat for 25 years until 1994, when sales began to increase as the result of a marketing campaign by the magazine *Cigar Aficionado*, cigar invitation-only dinners, and celebrity endorsements of cigar smoking, characterizing it as sophisticated and glamorous. Cigar smoking is no longer looked upon as the sole dominion of males; many women have taken up the habit. Cigar sales increased from 3.4 billion in 1993 to 5.1 billion in 1997.[40]

Cigars were not specifically included in the 1984 law that required tobacco companies to place labels on packages of cigarettes warning that they are hazardous to health. As a result, cigars carry no such warning label. This does not mean that cigar smoking is not harmful to health. See Just the Facts: Cigar Smoking: A Hazard to Health for the facts on cigar smoking.

Some benefits of quitting the cigarette smoking habit. There are many benefits to quitting the tobacco habit. Some occur within 20 minutes; others may take years. Following are a few of the benefits that occur after smoking the last cigarette.[56]

1. Blood pressure and heart rate decrease, and the temperature of hands and feet returns to normal in 20 minutes.
2. The risk for a sudden heart attack decreases in the first 24 hours.
3. Circulation improves and lung function increases up to 30 percent within two weeks to three months of quitting.
4. The risk for coronary heart disease declines by 50 percent after one year.
5. Lung cancer risk decreases by 50 percent after five years and coronary heart disease risk recovers to that of a never-smoker after five years.
6. Lung cancer death rate is similar to that of a never-smoker after 10 years.

∿ Just the Facts ∿

Cigar Smoking: A Hazard to Health

A common assumption is that cigar smoking is not as hazardous as cigarette smoking because people usually don't inhale cigar smoke. The facts regarding the dangers of cigar smoking are

- Nicotine reaches the brain by being absorbed through the lining of the mouth rather than from the lungs, but the effect is the same. See Just the Facts: Nicotine for a summary of nicotine's harmful effects on the heart and blood vessels.

- Cigars have larger quantities of nicotine, carbon monoxide, hydrogen cyanide, and other chemicals than cigarettes.[64]

- Nicotine is more easily absorbed by the cells lining the mouth and nose because cigar smoke is more acidic than cigarette smoke.[64]

- Cigars have been exempted from displaying disease warning labels but this will change soon. In June 2000, the Federal Trade Commission announced a settlement with seven of the largest U.S. cigar companies requiring health warning labels on cigar products.[65] Warning labels on cigars may appear as early as 2005.

Physical inactivity

Physical inactivity has been officially recognized as a major risk factor for cardiovascular disease by the American Heart Association.[1] The upgrading of physical inactivity, which appeared in the AHA's 1993 report, reflects the importance of participating in physical activities regularly. The AHA made the upgrade because the weight of the evidence that has been accumulating in the last few decades shows that exercise produces many important health benefits. This is good news for those who have been physically active, and it may motivate some **sedentary** people to become active. People who do not engage in 30 minutes of moderately intense physical activity on most days of the week are considered to be sedentary.

Physical inactivity (hypokinesis) is debilitating to the human body. A couple of weeks of bed rest or chair rest produce muscle atrophy, bone demineralization, and decreases in aerobic capacity and maximum breathing capacity. The human body was constructed for and thrives on physical exertion. The rapid deterioration of the human body from physical inactivity was exemplified in the 1966 Dallas Bed Rest study and follow-up 30 years later in 1996.[63] In 1966, five healthy 20-year-old males volunteered to remain in bed for three weeks for the cause of science. Those three weeks resulted in significant losses in muscle size and strength, a large decrease in maximal oxygen consumption, substantial losses in breathing capacity, and loss of bone mineral density. Bed rest was followed by eight weeks of vigorous aerobic exercise training, which completely reversed the declines experienced during the bed rest phase of the study.

The atrophy that bed rest produced in the young, healthy volunteers had an influence on the way cardiologists began to treat heart attack patients. The new philosophy emphasized rehabilitation and exercise instead of extended bed rest.

Thirty years later, the five subjects, then age 50, returned to the lab for follow-up testing. They had gained an average of 50 pounds, their body fat had doubled, and they exercised irregularly, if at all. In spite of these negative physical changes, as well as 30 years of aging, their cardiorespiratory endurance was higher at age 50 than it was at age 20 after three weeks of bed rest. The men then consented to participate in a six-month training program featuring jogging, brisk walking, and stationary cycling. At the end of the training program, the men became almost as physically fit as they were after eight weeks of training in 1966. In other words, the training program almost completely reversed a 30-year decline in fitness. Many experts have been proclaiming that the closest thing to a fountain of youth is exercise. According to the results of the Dallas Bed Rest study, exercising like a 20-year-old can make you almost as fit as one.

Two major reviews have shown that physical inactivity poses a significant risk of developing heart disease. In one review, the researchers critiqued 43 studies and concluded that physical inactivity increased the risk for coronary heart disease by 1.5 to 2.4 times.[66] The risk associated with physical inactivity is similar to that of the other major risk factors. According to the Centers for Disease Control and Prevention, the need for regular exercise by the general public should be promoted as vigorously as efforts to control blood pressure, lower cholesterol, and stop smoking. A later review by another team of researchers concluded that inactive people have a 90 percent greater risk of developing coronary heart disease than do active people.[67] With few exceptions, the results of later studies are consistent with the results of these two reviews. Some of the more recent studies have indicated a dose-response relationship between level of physical activity and cardiovascular disease.[68] This means that (1) men at high risk who regularly participate in light- to moderate-intensity physical activity expending about 1,500 calories per week will likely lower their risk for coronary heart disease by about 25 to 50 percent, and (2) men who engage regularly in more intense physical activity (above the moderate level) lower their risk for coronary heart disease by 60 to 70 percent and experience greater longevity.

Several studies examined the effect on coronary heart disease of level of physical fitness rather than of total numbers of calories expended per week in physical activity. These studies corroborated the results of the calorie expenditure studies that physically fit people are less inclined to develop coronary heart disease than are unfit people.[69] A later study indicated that people in the lowest 20th percentile of physical fitness had a significantly higher risk for coronary heart disease than those whose fitness level was in the top 20th percentile and their CRP and fibrinogen levels were also significantly higher.[70] In another study, subjects who performed below the 20th percentile on a maximal graded treadmill test were three to six times more likely to develop diabetes, hypertension, and metabolic syndrome than subjects who performed at or above the 60th percentile on the same test.[71] Physical fitness is protective because it increases the pliability of the blood vessels, it increases the efficiency of the heart, and it has an ameliorating effect on hypertension, diabetes, and dyslipidemias (cholesterol and triglycerides).

In summary, people actively engaged in leisure-time or occupational physical activity as well as those who participate in physical activities for the purpose of developing fitness are at a lower risk for death from cardiovascular disease and all-cause mortality. Major studies have supported the view that people who regularly engage in physical activities of moderate intensity have significantly fewer heart attacks and experience fewer deaths from all causes than do people who exercise little or not at all. Moderate activity was described as the equivalent of walking 1 to 2 miles per day for a total of 5 to 10 miles per week at a speed of 3 to 4 MPH. The greatest health benefits were gained by those who expended 1,500 to 2,000 calories per week (15 to 20 miles of walking) in physical activity. A total of 17,000 men were followed for more than 30 years. Those who regularly walked, climbed stairs, or participated in sports activities decreased their risk from all causes of mortality. Those who expended a minimum of 500 calories per week (5 miles of walking or its equivalent) to a maximum of 3,500 calories per week (35 miles of walking or its equivalent) experienced a progressive increase in longevity.

Investigators at the Cooper Institute for Aerobics Research[72] studied the relationship between physical fitness and mortality from all causes. The uniqueness of this study was twofold: first, the researchers measured the physical fitness levels of all subjects by treadmill testing; second, more than 3,000 of the 13,344 subjects were women. Because of their lower risk for cardiovascular disease, women have essentially been neglected as subjects in heart disease studies. The results of this study indicated that a low physical fitness level increased the risk for both men and women for death from cardiovascular disease, cancer, and all other forms of disease. The difference in all-cause mortality was greatest between those in the moderately fit category and those in the low-fit category. The difference between the moderately fit and the highly fit was insignificant. Physical inactivity increases the risk for coronary heart disease at a rate that is comparable to that observed for high blood pressure, high blood cholesterol, and cigarette smoking.[73]

A study using only women as subjects investigated the physical fitness benefits versus the health benefits of three levels of walking intensity.[74] One group walked at 5 MPH, a second group walked at 4 MPH, and a third group walked at 3 MPH. The results showed that physical fitness improved on a predictable dose-response basis. The fastest walkers improved the most and the slowest walkers improved the least, but the cardiovascular risk was reduced equally among the three groups. Low-level exercise was as effective as the highest level in promoting cardiovascular health. Exercise for health does not have to be as strenuous as exercise for physical fitness.

Graded treadmill tests of males hooked to an electrocardiograph have been used effectively as a diagnostic test for coronary heart disease. The effectiveness of this test for women has been less than desirable because women have too many false positive tests (the test shows they have heart disease, when in reality they do not).[75] However, graded maximal treadmill tests for women are more effective in predicting future heart disease when physicians assess fitness level and recovery heart rate.[76,77] Women who had higher fitness levels and faster recovery heart rates posttest had the lowest risk of dying from coronary heart disease during several years of follow-up.

Evidence also suggests that physical fitness is an important factor in the cardiovascular health of males.[78] Lower exercise capacity is a reliable predictor of mortality among normal men and men with existing cardiovascular disease.

The American College of Sports Medicine and the Centers for Disease Control and Prevention reacted to the results of these studies by jointly issuing a recommendation for exercise for Americans. The guideline states that "every U.S. adult should accumulate 30 minutes or more of moderate intensity physical activity on most, preferably all, days of the week."[79] This is a minimum guideline for exercise and was not intended to replace previous recommendations regarding more vigorous exercise for the purpose of improving physical fitness. Instead, the recommendation is directed at the 28 percent of American adults who report that they are completely inactive and another 42 percent who are not at least moderately active for the recommended 30 minutes per day, five or more days per week.[80] The entire 70 percent are considered sedentary because the definition of sedentary is anyone who does not get at least 30 minutes

of physical activity on most days of the week. Health professionals hope that the recommendation will motivate physically inactive and underactive Americans to participate in a more active lifestyle.

The term *physical activity* refers to any physical movement that results in energy expenditure. Physical activity includes but is not limited to walking, climbing stairs, mowing the lawn (using a riding mower does not count), raking leaves without a blower, mopping and vacuuming floors, washing and waxing the car (by hand), dancing, and playing with children and grandchildren. Moderate-intensity physical activity can be achieved by walking 3 to 4 MPH or through any other activity that burns as many calories as walking at those speeds.

People who consistently exercise above the moderate level not only receive the health benefits but also develop a higher level of physical fitness. Those who exercise in accordance with the guidelines gain about the same health benefits as those who are more physically active, but they will not attain the same degree of physical fitness. That 70 percent of the population inclined to ignore the advice to exercise regularly can become part of the estimated 435,000 premature deaths per year attributed to a sedentary lifestyle and a poor diet.[80]

The health and longevity returns from exercise and a physically active lifestyle are significant. Estimates indicate that longevity is increased by 1 minute for every minute spent walking and by 2 minutes for every minute spent jogging.[81] The potential for improving the health status of Americans through appropriate lifestyle behaviors is evident from estimates indicating that the leading determinants related to all-cause mortality have dramatically shifted from infectious diseases in 1900 to the chronic diseases that are considerably influenced by modifiable lifestyle and behavioral factors, such as smoking, obesity, and sedentary death syndrome in 2000.[82,83] Sedentary death syndrome includes "weak skeletal muscles, low bone density, hyperglycemia (high blood sugar), glucosuria (excessive sugar in the urine), low HDL, obesity, low physical endurance, and resting tachycardia (rapid heart rate)." This cluster makes up the sedentary death syndrome. Sedentary death syndrome is one of the top three causes of mortality, and it directly contributes to obesity, the second leading cause of death.

Obesity

Obesity strains the heart and coexists with many of the modifiable risk factors that promote cardiovascular disease. Obese people who have no other risk factors are still more likely to develop heart disease or stroke. Obesity continues to rise precipitously in the United States. Sixty-five percent of adults (people over 18 years of age) are overweight or obese.[84] *Overweight* is defined as carrying excess weight for one's height regardless of body composition. *Obesity* is defined as carrying an excess of body fat regardless of height.[85] The trend in the last couple of decades is that the number of overweight/obese, physically inactive Americans is continuing to rise and by mid-2005 will surpass smoking as the leading cause of preventable death.[86] (However, there is a new development. See This Just In in Chapter 1 for an update.) More alarming is the increase in the number of people who are 100 pounds overweight (this is extreme, or morbid, obesity). There are four times as many people in this category today than 15 years ago and five times as many people who are 150 pounds overweight than 15 years ago.[87] The rate of illness and death from obesity increases in proportion to the amount of excess weight. Obesity is a chronic, severe condition that can also worsen other medical conditions and disabilities. Not only is obesity associated with an increased risk for heart disease, but the manner in which fat is distributed in the body might also accentuate the risk.[85] Fat that accumulates in the upper half of the body (referred to as *visceral* or *central abdominal obesity*) is likely to be accompanied by high triglycerides, low HDL cholesterol, insulin resistance, and hypertension. This cluster of factors is called metabolic syndrome X, and it is associated with a significant increase in the likelihood of developing cardiovascular disease.

Cardiovascular disease is the leading cause of death in children 3–15 years of age.[1] In one study, the number of overweight students with high blood pressure was more than double that of normal-weight students.[88] In another study, overweight children were more likely to have metabolic syndrome, compared with normal-weight children.[89] The increase in overweight/obesity in young adulthood is increasing the prevalence of diabetes in this age group.[90] Children and adolescents need treatment to reduce these risks to prevent them from tracking into adulthood.

Obese people can lower their risk with a modest weight loss of 5 to 10 percent. This is a realistic, attainable goal. But the risk remains lower only if the loss of weight is maintained. Approximately 95 percent of people who lose weight regain it in a few years. Although calorie restriction is the primary method for losing weight, regular exercise is the most effective method for maintaining the loss. Diet and exercise are not mutually exclusive; instead, they complement each other, and both are important players in weight management.

Diabetes mellitus

Diabetes mellitus is a metabolic disorder in which the body cannot make use of sugar (glucose) as a fuel. The hormone insulin must be produced and secreted into the bloodstream, so that blood sugar can be transported into the cells. The cells have receptor sites, to which insulin attaches, making the cell amenable to the entrance of sugar.

In Type 1 diabetes, no insulin is produced, so it must be injected daily. Type 1, insulin-dependent diabetes mellitus (IDDM), usually occurs early in life. Type 2, or noninsulin-dependent diabetes mellitus (NIDDM), usually occurs in middle-aged, overweight, sedentary adults. However, more cases of Type 2 diabetes are showing up in children and adolescents, attributed to increasing overweight and decreasing physical activity in these groups.[91] Excessive weight is a factor because it increases cellular resistance to insulin, so that more insulin than normal is required to effect the passage of sugar from the blood to the cells. In contrast, exercise decreases insulin resistance, making cellular membranes more permeable to sugar. About 90 percent of diabetes mellitus is of the Type 2 variety. Data indicate that at least 75 percent of new cases of Type 2 diabetes can be prevented through regular exercise and the maintenance of normal weight.[92] An estimated 18 million Americans have diabetes—about 17 million of them have Type 2 diabetes; the remainder have Type 1 diabetes. About 16 million other Americans have prediabetes, in which their blood glucose levels are higher than normal but they are not yet diabetic.[93] This category was developed to alert physicians that the complications of diabetes begin at the prediabetic level and treatment needs to begin at this level.

Diabetes mellitus has numerous long-range complications. These primarily involve degenerative disorders of the blood vessels and nerves. Diabetics who die prematurely are usually the victims of cardiovascular lesions and accelerated atherosclerosis. The incidence of heart attacks and strokes is higher among diabetics than nondiabetics. Diabetes increases the risk for coronary artery disease by two to three times the normal rate in men and three to seven times the normal rate in women.[50] In fact, diabetes is such a potent risk factor for coronary heart disease that, by itself, it is the risk-equivalent of having had a previous heart attack.[94]

The arteries supplying the kidneys, eyes, and legs are particularly susceptible to atherosclerosis. Kidney failure is one of the long-term complications of diabetes. Diabetes is also the leading cause of blindness in U.S. adults. Impaired delivery of blood to the legs may lead to gangrene, necessitating the amputation of the affected tissues. In addition to circulatory problems, degenerative lesions in the nervous system may result, leading to multiple diseases that result in dysfunction of the brain, spinal cord, and peripheral nerves.[95] Unfortunately, medical science has been unable to identify the biological mechanisms responsible for these long-term vascular and neural complications. However, these complications can be mitigated by leading a balanced, well-regulated life, thereby keeping diabetes under control. Control includes dietary manipulation, exercise, weight control, rest, and medication if needed.

The landmark Physician's Health Study was the first major effort to show that exercise reduces the risk of developing Type 2 diabetes. The physicians participating in the study who exercised vigorously five or more times per week had a 42 percent greater reduction in the incidence of Type 2 diabetes than did those who exercised less than one time per week. The reduction in risk was particularly pronounced among those at greatest risk: the obese. The researchers concluded that at least 24 percent of cases of Type 2 diabetes were related to sedentary living. Even high-risk men (those who were overweight and had a parental history of diabetes) benefited from regular exercise. Every 500 calories burned per week in leisure-time physical activity reduced the risk for Type 2 diabetes by 6 percent.[96]

Data collected from more than 70,000 women subjects ages 40 to 65 years indicated that those who participated in moderate exercise on a regular basis lowered their risk of developing Type 2 diabetes, compared with women who did not exercise regularly.[97] Accumulating evidence shows that the effect of exercise on Type 2 diabetes prevention applies to both men and women.

Stress

Stress is difficult to define and quantify. Authorities agree that distress, or chronic stress, produces a complex array of physiological changes in the body. Together, these physiological events are called the *fight or flight response*. The hormones released by the body during these events produce the stress response. This includes (1) increases in heart rate, breathing rate, and blood pressure; (2) the tendency for blood platelets to aggregate (clump together); (3) blood sugar rushing to the muscles to provide more energy; and (4) the activation of the immune system. The stress response represents a significant strain on the body.

Stressors (events or situations that cause stress) may be acute or chronic. Acute stressors are situational and temporary. Taking a midterm exam and making an oral presentation are examples of events that provoke acute stress. When such an event is over, the body returns, within a short time, to its prior state of balance and harmony. However, chronic stress (characterized by prolonged elevations of stress hormones and a general feeling of uneasiness that permeates one's life) presents a much more serious problem. Constant worry about work, finances, or relationships and persistent feelings of anger and isolation are examples of chronic stress. Is chronic stress a causative agent in the development of chronic diseases in general and heart disease specifically?

See Nurturing Your Spirituality: Can Stress and Depression Make You Sick? on page 56.

Preventing and Reversing Heart Disease

Preventing heart disease is much preferred to treating it after the fact. Prevention includes regular exercise, maintenance of optimal body weight, sound nutritional practices, abstinence from tobacco products, nonuse of alcohol (or use in moderation), and abstinence from drugs. Dealing with stress in constructive ways, removing oneself as much as possible from destructive and disease-producing environmental conditions, and having periodic medical examinations are other aspects of prevention. It is much better physically, psychologically, and economically to make the effort to enhance health now than to reject or ignore health-promotion principles and treat disease later. It is never too late to change behavior. Even patients with coronary artery disease can benefit from lifestyle changes.

Until recently, medical thinking indicated that established atherosclerotic plaques in the coronary arteries were there to stay. Progression of the disease seemed inevitable unless medical corrective procedures were employed. But evidence has surfaced indicating that reversal of the disease is possible with appropriate lifestyle behaviors.

Dean Ornish showed that comprehensive behavior changes are required to reverse established coronary artery disease. Ornish devised a program that included a vegetarian diet in which only 6.8 percent of the calories came from fat; 4.4 hours of moderate aerobic exercise per week; stress management techniques consisting of stretching exercises, practicing of breathing techniques, meditation, progressive relaxation, and the use of imagery; smoking cessation; and attendance at regular group support meetings. The subjects in this study were evaluated against a control group who received "usual and customary" care.[99]

At the end of the first year, 82 percent of the subjects in the Ornish program showed regression of atherosclerosis, compared with only 10 percent of the usual care group. Over the following four years, the Ornish subjects showed further regression, whereas the usual care group experienced progression of atherosclerosis.[100]

Other investigators have examined the effect of less stringent interventions than those advocated by the Ornish program on the regression of atherosclerosis. These attempts have been less successful than the Ornish program but more successful than the usual care program.

The main criticism of the Ornish program was that lifelong compliance would be difficult. Twenty-nine percent of the study participants dropped out during the last four years of the program. It is not easy to permanently

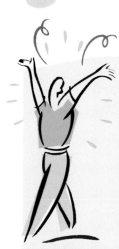

Nurturing Your Spirituality

Can Stress and Depression Make You Sick?

A convincing body of evidence suggests that chronic anger, anxiety, loneliness, or depression can be catastrophic for people with coronary artery disease.[96] At the same time, emerging evidence shows that the same mood states and feelings in healthy people may increase the likelihood of developing heart disease in the future.

Scientists are beginning to unravel the connection between mood states and heart disease. Consistently high levels of stress hormones circulating in the bloodstream suppress the immune system by interfering with the normal repair and maintenance functions of the body. This increases one's vulnerability to infections and disease.[97] Continuing high levels of cortisol and norepinephrine stimulate a prolonged fight or flight response, which can eventually lead to wear and tear on the heart and arteries. Frequent and prolonged periods of stress increase blood pressure, and that usually leads to injuries of the artery walls. These injuries are the first step in the development and ultimate progression of atherosclerosis.[6] Data indicate that exaggerated responses to stress may be a triggering mechanism for heart attack and stroke.

Depression can be a temporary or chronic mental disorder; it is characterized by feelings of sadness, loneliness, despair, low self-esteem, and self-reproach. Depression that occurs later in life increases the risk for coronary heart disease in two ways: (1) by reducing blood flow to the heart in those whose blood vessels are narrowed and (2) by causing heart rhythm disturbances.[96]

Scientists have much to learn about the relationship between the heart and mind. Physicians are beginning to acknowledge that depression is a significant factor in producing cardiovascular complications for those who already have heart disease. The good news is that depression is treatable. Mild depression responds to regular exercise and voluntary relaxation techniques, both of which reduce the production of stress hormones. On the other hand, severe depression requires psychological counseling and medication, plus regular exercise and relaxation training. Eighty percent of people with severe depression respond to treatment.

Regular exercise promotes relaxation, reduces the response to stress, enhances emotional well-being, and lowers cardiac reactivity (high heart rate, blood pressure, and resistance to blood flow). Cardiac reactivity occurs when modest stressors produce physiological responses by the heart and circulatory system that are out of proportion to the stressor. If these occur frequently, the development of atherosclerosis may well be the result.

Exercise acts as a safety valve that enables people to "let off steam" in a constructive way. Jogging, swimming, cycling, weight training, racquetball, and other physical activities focus our energies in worthwhile pursuits that rid the body of stress products that have accumulated. Exercise training, a physiological stressor, helps build tolerance to psychological and emotional stressors. In other words, the "physiological toughness" developed through exercise training enables us to cope more effectively with other types of stressors.[98]

Do stress and depression cause heart attacks? The answer is a qualified yes. We should have a more definitive answer after a few more years of research.

---

change bad habits, but the hard work associated with following a low-fat diet, exercising consistently at a moderately intense level, and giving up smoking can make people with coronary artery disease feel better and may allow them to avoid surgery.

Refer to Assessment Activity 2-1 at the end of this chapter. Respond to each of the risk questions about factors to determine your risk status.

Other Risk Factors

Iron-Enriched Blood

In 1992, a study completed in Finland found that men with high levels of iron (as measured by serum ferritin) also had a high probability of incurring heart problems.

Since then, a number of studies completed in the United States have failed to confirm the high iron–high heart disease connection. These American studies found the opposite. Women with high normal iron levels were found to have half the heart disease risk as women with low iron stores, and men in the high iron group were 20 percent less likely to die of heart disease than were men with the lowest levels.[101] The rationale is that low iron levels lead to a reduction in oxygen-carrying hemoglobin, so that less oxygen is transported to the tissues. It is possible that the decrease in oxygen transport to the cells, including the cells of the heart, is responsible for the heart problems that occur with greater frequency in those who are iron deficient.

Now that you are aware of the major risk factors for heart disease, refer to Assessment Activities 2-1 and 2-2 to test your risk and your knowledge. Be as accurate as

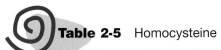 **Table 2-5** Homocysteine

Blood Level Micromoles/Liter	Risk
5–15	Normal
16–30	Moderate
31–100	Intermediate
> 100	Severe

> greater than

possible when providing the necessary information for Activity 2-1. Read the case study (Assessment 2-2) and respond to all of the questions.

Homocysteine

Homocysteine is a sulphur-containing amino acid produced as a normal by-product of methionine metabolism. Methionine is an essential amino acid that must be obtained through the diet.[102] Under normal conditions, homocysteine is either converted back to methionine or it splits into two harmless nonessential amino acids, which are easily flushed from the body through the urine. These conversions are accomplished by adequate intakes of folic acid, vitamin B_6, and vitamin B_{12}. Inadequate consumption of these three vitamins, folic acid in particular, results in a buildup of homocysteine in the blood. Homocysteine contributes to atherosclerosis because (1) it has a direct toxic effect, resulting in lesions that damage the cells lining the inside walls of the arteries; (2) it interferes with clotting factors; and (3) it oxidizes low-density lipoprotein (LDL).

Homocysteine is measured by drawing blood after a 12-hour fast. See Table 2-5 for a breakdown of the categories of risk.

Two major meta-analyses were reported in the *Journal of the American Medical Association*, indicating that elevated homocysteine may not be as dangerous a risk factor as earlier studies suggested. Meta-analysis is a procedure using statistics to interpret the results of many studies, often with conflicting conclusions, by treating the results of each investigation as a discrete bit of data. These two studies led to the conclusion that elevated homocysteine appears to be a modest risk factor at best for heart disease and stroke.[103] It is also unclear at this time whether lowering homocysteine actually reduces the incidence of heart attacks and strokes. Further research is needed in order to shed more light on this risk factor.

Lipoprotein (a)

Lipoprotein (a) is a molecule of bad LDL cholesterol with an extra protein attached.[104] A high level of Lp(a) may be harmful because it appears to interfere with the body's clot-busting system. However, cardiologists are not sure that elevated Lp(a) translates into an increase in heart attacks and strokes. The research is still equivocal on this point.[105] But high levels of Lp(a) circulating in the blood seem to be an independent predictor of stroke, death from vascular diseases, and death from any cause in elderly men, but not elderly women.[106]

Lp(a) values above 30 milligrams per deciliter (mg/dL) of blood are considered to be high and a very high value is above 50 mg/dL.[107] Lp(a) blood levels are determined primarily by one's genetic makeup, as opposed to lifestyle factors.[105]

Lp(a) is not routinely measured by physicians. It is likely to be measured when physicians need more information regarding the diagnosis of heart disease. For now, most physicians will continue to rely on the tried and true risk factors previously covered in this chapter.

High Sensitivity C-Reactive Protein (hs-CRP)

C-reactive protein (CRP), a biomarker for inflammation, was discovered 75 years ago. CRP is elevated in many diseases that have an inflammatory component, such as colorectal cancer, hypertension, rheumatoid arthritis, sepsis (blood poisoning), diabetes mellitus, and metabolic syndrome.[61] CRP is made by the liver in response to infection, inflammation, injury, or stress and elevations can be detected by a blood test. This test has been available for many years but it was not sensitive enough to detect low levels of inflammation that are indicative of atherosclerosis. The new and improved version, high sensitivity C-reactive protein (hs-CRP) can identify inflammation earlier and at lower levels than its predecessor. Atherosclerosis, the underlying cause of 80 percent of coronary heart disease, is a low-level inflammatory process. The newer, more sensitive test shows promise as a diagnostic tool for detecting atherosclerosis early, so that an intervention program can be developed and put in place early in the process.

While many major prospective studies in the United States and other countries have found CRP to be a strong, robust, independent risk factor for cardiovascular disease, others are questioning their results. A large European meta-analysis has provided data indicating that CRP is a relatively moderate predictor of future coronary heart disease and that it adds only marginally to the predictive value of the major risk factors.[108] On the other hand, many other studies have found that CRP is more predictive of heart disease than are high LDLs. More research is needed to resolve this issue.

Fibrinogin

An elevated fibrinogin level in the blood is positively correlated with heart disease and stroke. Fibrinogin adds to the viscosity (thickness or stickiness) of the blood and enhances the formation of blood clots.[50] High fibrinogin levels are more common in men than women, in smokers than nonsmokers, in those physically inactive than those who are active, and in those with high serum triglycerides than those with low levels.

Medical Contributions

Diagnostic Techniques

Diagnosing cardiovascular disease is becoming more sophisticated. Diagnosis begins with a medical examination and patient history. This procedure may be supplemented with a variety of tests, which may confirm or refute the physician's suspicions of the presence of cardiovascular disease. Graded exercise tests (GXTs) using a motor-driven treadmill with the patient hooked to an electrocardiogram (ECG) have gained popularity in the last 10 years or so. Such noninvasive tests use surface electrodes on the chest that are sensitive to the electrical actions of the heart. Mechanical abnormalities of the heart produce abnormal electrical impulses displayed on the ECG strip. These are read and interpreted by the physician.

The treadmill "road tests" the heart as it works progressively harder to meet the increasing oxygen requirement as the exercise protocol becomes more physically demanding. This test is more accurate for men than women. The gender difference in response to the treadmill test is not completely understood, but it is believed that women's breasts and extra fat tissue interfere with the reception of electrical impulses by the chest electrodes. But the treadmill test is still a useful tool in diagnosing potential heart problems for women if attention is shifted to a woman's physical fitness level and how quickly her heart rate recovers immediately after the test ends.[71,76]

In some cases, a thallium treadmill test is required because it is more sensitive; however, it is also much more expensive. This involves the injection of radioactive thallium during the final minute of the treadmill test. Thallium is accepted, or taken up, by normal heart muscle but not by ischemic heart muscle. The absorption or nonabsorption of thallium can be seen on a monitor. The thallium stress test increases diagnostic sensitivity to cardiovascular disease to approximately 90 percent.

Echocardiography is a safe, noninvasive technique that uses sound waves to determine the size of the heart, the thickness of the walls, and the function of the heart's valves. *Cardiac catheterization* is an invasive technique in which a slender tube is threaded from a blood vessel in an arm or a leg into the coronary arteries. A liquid contrast dye that can be seen on X-ray film is injected into the coronary arteries. X-ray films are taken throughout the procedure to locate where and how severely the coronary arteries are narrowed.

Medical Treatment

A variety of drugs are used in cardiovascular therapies. These drugs lower blood pressure and cholesterol level, minimize the likelihood of blood clotting, and dissolve clots during a heart attack.

Plain aspirin is proving to be an effective drug in the fight against heart disease. Low-dose (one-fourth of a regular aspirin) aspirin therapy consisting of a single daily dose for those who have heart disease reduces the risk of having another heart attack or dying from a subsequent attack. Low-dose aspirin therapy is more effective when supplemented with a "booster" dose of one whole aspirin on the first and fifteenth of each month. Also, regular aspirin use may prevent a first heart attack from occurring in apparently healthy people, but no one should take aspirin or any other drug without first consulting a physician. Aspirin is effective because it is an anti-inflammatory agent and atherosclerosis is an inflammatory disease.[109] Aspirin also plays a role in the prevention of blood clots that might form in arteries. Additionally, there is growing evidence that aspirin may help reduce the risk for colorectal, esophageal, stomach, prostate, and ovarian cancer because it may inhibit the chemical pathways that fuel tumor growth.

Surgical techniques have also affected the treatment of cardiovascular disease. *Coronary artery bypass graft (CABG) surgery* is designed to shunt blood around an area of blockage by removing a leg vein and sewing one end of a leg vein into the aorta and the other end into a coronary artery below the blockage, thereby restoring blood flow to the heart muscle (Figure 2-8). The internal mammary arteries also are used for bypass grafts. Many authorities consider these to be the ideal grafts. There are two internal mammary arteries, but the one in the left side of the chest is preferable because it is nearer to the coronary arteries. Many surgeons would rather not use both arteries in the same patient because the diminished flow of blood to the chest impairs healing of the surgical wound. Also, fashioning bypass grafts out of these arteries is time-consuming precision surgery, and there are only two of them and they don't reach all parts of the heart. The

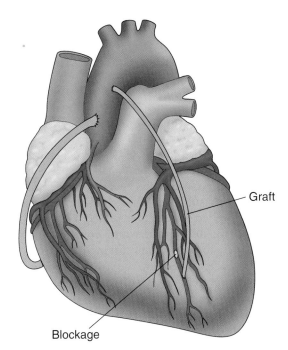

Figure 2-8 Coronary Artery Bypass Graft

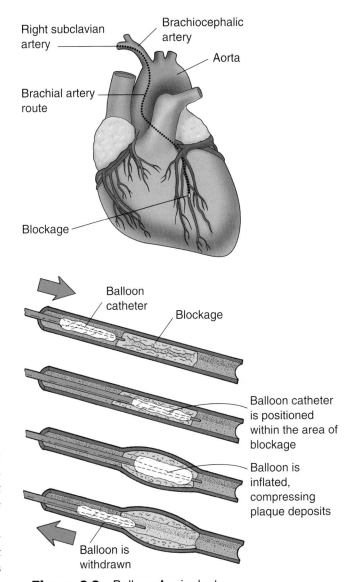

Figure 2-9 Balloon Angioplasty

advantage is that 95 percent of them remain open 20 to 30 years after surgery.

In 2001, 516,000 CABG surgical procedures were performed, at an average cost of $60,853 each.[1] This procedure requires the surgical team to place the patient on a heart-lung machine, which pumps blood to the body's tissues while the heart is stopped for repairs. Postsurgical complications, primarily temporary short-term memory loss, may occur. Research indicates that this loss probably occurs because the heart-lung bypass machine produces microemboli (tiny blood clots), which flow to the brain and reduce its oxygen supply.

A new off-pump procedure has been developed that does not require stoppage of the heart while the surgeon sews the bypass grafts. This procedure is accomplished laparoscopically—that is, long, slender surgical instruments are inserted through several small incisions. While there are fewer complications and a shorter rehabilitation with off-pump procedures, long-term survival versus on-pump procedures are yet to be fully determined.[110]

Balloon angioplasty uses a catheter with a doughnut-shaped balloon at the tip. The catheter is positioned at the narrow point in the artery, and the balloon is inflated, which cracks and compresses the plaque, stretches the artery wall, and widens the blood vessel to allow greater blood flow (Figure 2-9). An estimated 571,000 of these procedures were performed in 2001, at an average cost of $28,858 each.[1] Laser angioplasty uses heat to burn away plaque if the catheter can be maneu-

vered into the correct position. This technology appears to be useful for patients with certain types of atherosclerotic narrowings or blockages. Coronary atherectomy, one of the newest techniques, uses a specially tipped catheter equipped with a high-speed rotary cutting blade to shave off plaque.

Catheterization techniques are also used to implant a coronary stent in a diseased artery. The stent is a flexible, metallic tube that functions as a scaffold to support the walls of diseased arteries, thus maintaining an open passage for blood flow (Figure 2-10, page 60). Stents are positioned in such arteries by a catheter. When correctly positioned, a balloon inside the stent is inflated, causing the stent to expand. This action stretches the artery. Then the balloon is withdrawn, leaving the expanded stent behind to keep the blood vessel open. The problem

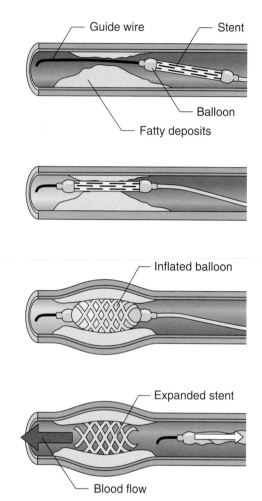

- Guide wire
- Stent
- Balloon
- Fatty deposits

- Inflated balloon

- Expanded stent

- Blood flow

Figure 2-10 Coronary Stent

stents coated with drugs that stop prolific muscle cell growth have been developed. These drug-eluting stents show great promise in averting restenosis (renarrowing of the artery), compared with stents without the drug. Two large studies have shown no restenosis at the 6- and 12-month marks after the procedure.[111]

Artificial valves have been developed to replace defective heart valves, and these work well. In the summer of 2001, the first successful self-contained mechanical heart was implanted in the chest of a male patient whose life expectancy was literally being measured in days. This device is considered experimental and its long-term success rate has yet to be demonstrated. However, it is a technological giant step forward, compared with its predecessors, and with modifications it seems to have great potential for extending the lives of people whose hearts are so severely damaged that conventional medical treatments are ineffective.

Mechanical devices (left ventricular assist devices) have been used to aid the failing hearts of patients awaiting donor hearts. These devices take over the burden of pumping blood throughout the body and may keep patients alive for several months or more.

Heart transplants have prolonged many lives. The outlook for patients has improved considerably because of the development and use of medicines to suppress the immune system in such patients and because of refinements in the prevention and early detection of the body's attempts to reject donor hearts. As a result, about 86 percent live longer than one year, 77 percent survive for three years, and the five-year survival rate is 71 percent.[1] In 1968, 23 heart transplants were performed; in 2002, 2,154 were performed.

Candidates for transplants are those whose hearts are irreversibly damaged with disease that does not respond to conventional treatment. Without a new heart, these people will die. The main problems associated with heart transplantation are insufficient numbers of donors, the difficulty of procuring compatible donor hearts, and the constant threat of organ rejection by the recipient.

with this procedure is the damage that occurs to the fragile inner lining of the artery during the placement of the stent. The body's response to this injury is inflammation, accompanied by rampant cell growth, which is needed to heal the wound. Cell growth occurs around and into the stent, narrowing the artery and reducing blood flow. In order to circumvent this occurrence,

Summary

- Approximately 1.5 million heart attacks occur each year, and 500,000 of these result in death.
- The heart is two pumps in one: the pulmonary pump, which sends deoxygenated blood to the lungs, and the systemic pump, which sends oxygenated blood to all tissues of the body.
- Blood plasma is a clear, yellowish fluid that makes up about 55 percent of the blood. The remaining 45 percent consists of blood solids—red blood cells, white blood cells, and blood platelets.

- Strokes are caused by a thrombus, an embolus, or a hemorrhage.
- Coronary heart disease is a disease of the coronary blood vessels that take nourishment and oxygen to the heart.
- Many of the risk factors for heart disease originate in childhood.
- The treatment of heart disease includes the development of appropriate lifestyle habits and medical intervention.
- The major risk factors that cannot be changed are age, male gender, and heredity.

- The major risk factors that can be changed are elevated cholesterol levels, hypertension, cigarette smoking, physical inactivity, and obesity.
- The other contributing risk factors are diabetes mellitus and stress.
- Cholesterol is a steroid that is essential for many body functions, but too much circulating in the blood creates a risk for cardiovascular disease.
- Low-density lipoproteins are associated with the development of atherosclerotic plaque.
- High-density lipoproteins protect the arteries from the formation of plaque.
- Blood pressure is the force exerted against the walls of the arteries as blood is pumped from the heart and travels through the circulatory system.
- *Hypertension* is the medical term for high blood pressure.
- Cigarette smoking may be the most potent of the risk factors associated with chronic illness and premature death.

- Involuntary, or passive, smoking is associated with premature disease and death.
- Obesity is a major risk factor that often coexists with many of the other risk factors for cardiovascular disease.
- Diabetes mellitus must be controlled to reduce the accompanying cardiovascular complications.
- Regular exercise significantly reduces the risk for Type 2 diabetes mellitus.
- Stress predisposes a person to illness and may hasten the disease process.
- Elevated levels of homocysteine and of Lp(a) in the blood are proving to be important risk factors for heart disease.
- Medical research has made a significant contribution to reducing the incidence of heart disease through the development of sophisticated technological advances in diagnosis and treatment.

Review Questions

1. Define *pulmonary pump* and *systemic pump* and discuss the function of each.
2. Describe the advent of heart disease in the United States.
3. Identify and describe the causes of stroke.
4. What is coronary heart disease? Discuss the available treatment options.
5. What are the risk factors for heart disease and how are they categorized by the AHA?
6. What is cholesterol? LDL? HDL?
7. What is the relationship between total cholesterol and HDL?
8. What is essential hypertension?
9. What ingredients in cigarettes increase the risk for cardiovascular disease? Describe their effect on the heart and blood vessels.
10. What is the risk associated with smokeless tobacco products?
11. Defend the proposition that a moderate level of exercise improves health and increases longevity.
12. What are the cardiovascular complications of diabetes mellitus?
13. How does stress contribute to cardiovascular disease?
14. Can heart disease be prevented or at least delayed? Identify the lifestyle behaviors that may be involved in the process.
15. Can atherosclerosis be reversed? Cite evidence to support your answer.
16. What contributions has the medical profession made to decreasing the death rate from heart disease?

References

1. American Heart Association. 2003. *Heart disease and stroke statistics—2004 update.* Dallas: American Heart Association.
2. Kochanek, K. D., and B. L. Smith. 11 February 2004. *National vital statistics reports deaths: Preliminary data for 2002.* Washington, DC: U.S. Department of Health and Human Services.
3. National Center for Health Statistics. 2001. *Health, United States 2001.* Hyattsville, MD: U.S. Government Printing Office.
4. Editors. *Heart Advisor.* 2004. Heart care counters multiple threats. *The Cleveland Clinic Heart Advisor* 7 (April): 1, 7.
5. Nieman, D. C. 2003. *Exercise testing and prescription.* Boston: McGraw-Hill.
6. Editors. *Harvard Heart Letter.* 2003. Keeping plaque in its place. *Harvard Heart Letter* 13 (January): 1–3.
7. Olson, E. N. 27 May 2004. A decade of discoveries in cardiac biology (www.medscape.com/viewarticle/477676).
8. Squires, R. W. 2001. Coronary artherosclerosis. In *ACSM resource manual.* 4th ed. Edited by J. L. Roitman. Philadelphia: Lippincott Williams and Wilkins.
9. McArdle, W. D., F. I. Katch, and V. L. Katch. 2000. *Essentials of exercise physiology.* Philadelphia: Lippincott Williams and Wilkins.
10. Kannell, W. B., et al. 1968. Epidemiology of acute myocardial infarction: The Framingham Study. *Medicine Today* 2:50.
11. U.S. Department of Health and Human Services. 1996. *Physical activity and health: A report of the surgeon general.* Atlanta: U.S. Department of Health and Human Services, Centers for Disease Control and Prevention, National Center for Chronic Disease Prevention and Health Promotion.

12. Waldstein, S. R., et al. 2004. Stress-induced blood pressure reactivity and silent cerebrovascular disease. *Stroke* 35:1294–98.

13. U.S. Department of Health and Human Services. July 2003. *Statistics related to overweight and obesity.* Washington, DC: U.S. Government Printing Office.

14. American Heart Association. 2003. Physical Inactivity. *Statistical fact sheet—Risk factors.* American Heart Association. Dallas, TX.

15. Aaron, D. J., et al. 2002. Longitudinal study of the number and choice of leisure time physical activities from mid to late adolescence. *Archives of Pediatric and Adolescent Medicine* 156:1075–80.

16. Pi-Sunyer, F. X. 11 March 2002. The role of weight loss in improving metabolic outcomes. *Medscape—Clinical Update* (www.medscape.com/viewprogram/1440-pnt).

17. Ogden, C. L., et al. 2003. Prevalence and trends in overweight among U.S. children and adolescents, 1999–2000. *Journal of the American Medical Association* 288 (29 August): 1728–32.

18. Tufts University. 2000. More kids are getting diabetes—and more should be screened for it. *Tufts University Health and Nutrition Letter* 18(2):2.

19. U.S. Department of Health and Human Services. 2000. *Healthy people 2010: Understanding and improving health*, Washington, DC: U.S. Department of Health and Human Services, U.S. Government Printing Office.

20. Porter, V. 2004. Even children have heart disease—Especially those who are overweight. *Medscape—Cardiology* (www.medscape.com/viewarticle/478258-print).

21. Diet, exercise improve blood vessels in obese kids. 14 April 2004. *Heart Center Online for Cardiologists and Their Patients* (www.heartcenteronline.com).

22. Harvard Medical School. 2000. Heart attacks without chest pain: The danger is greater. *Harvard Heart Letter* 11(1):5–6.

23. Margolis, S., and G. Gerstenblith. 2001. *Coronary heart disease.* Baltimore: The Johns Hopkins Medical Institutions.

24. Weil, A. 2003. Not me—Women and heart disease. *Dr. Andrew Weil's Self Healing*, December, 4–5.

25. Leitch, A. M. July 2004. Breast cancer overview. *Women's Surgery Group* (www.womenssurgerygroup.com/conditions/BreastCancer/overview.asp).

26. How to protect women's hearts. 2004. *Heart Advisor* 7 (July): 3.

27. Brookes, L. June 2004. More new guidelines, antihypertensive medications, and research on special populations. *Medscape—Cardiology* (www.medscape.com/viewarticle/480467).

28. Greenland, P., et al. 2003. Major risk factors as antecedents of fatal and nonfatal coronary heart disease events. *Journal of the American Medical Association* 290(7): 891–97.

29. Wardlaw, G., J. Hampl, and R. DiSilvestro. 2004. *Perspectives in nutrition.* 6th ed. St. Louis: McGraw-Hill.

30. Wilder, L. B., L. J. Cheskin, and S. Margolis. 2004. *The Johns Hopkins white paper: Nutrition and weight control for longevity.* New York: Medletter Associates.

31. Editors. 1984. The Lipid Research Clinics coronary primary prevention trial results. I. Reduction in incidence of coronary heart disease. *Journal of the American Medical Association* 251:351.

32. La Rosa, J. C., et al. 1990. The cholesterol facts: A summary of the evidence relating dietary facts, serum cholesterol, and coronary heart disease: A joint statement by the American Heart Association and the National Heart, Lung, and Blood Institute. *Circulation* 81:1721.

33. Cunningham, D. S. 2004. Quenching the flames of inflammation. *Life Extension* 10 (July): 27–34.

34. Pepys, M. B., and G. M. Hirschfield. 2003. C-reactive protein: A critical update. *Journal of Clinical Investigation* 111 (June): 1805–12.

35. Tall, A. R. 2004. C-reactive protein reassessed. *New England Journal of Medicine* 350 (April): 1450–52.

36. Harvard Medical School. 2000. Triglycerides and heart disease. *Harvard Heart Letter* 11(1): 1–4.

37. Thomas, T. R., and T. P. La Fontaine. 2001. Exercise nutritional strategies, and lipoproteins. In *ACSM resource manual.* 4th ed. Edited by J. L. Roitman. Philadelphia: Lippincott Williams and Wilkins.

38. Powers, S. K., and E. T. Howley. 2004. *Exercise physiology.* 5th ed. Boston: McGraw-Hill.

39. Editors. *Harvard Health Letter.* 2003. Blood pressure normal? Maybe now it isn't. *Harvard Heart Letter* 28 (July): 7.

40. Pescatello, L. S., et al. 2004. Position stand—exercise and hypertension. *Medicine and Science in Sports and Exercise*, March: 533–53.

41. Editors. 2003. Why it pays to lower even "normal" blood pressure. *Heart Advisor*, 6 (July): 2.

42. Harvard Medical School. 2001. A better way of measuring hypertension? *Harvard Health Letter* 26(4):3.

43. Editors. *Harvard Health Letter.* 2003. High blood pressure isn't color blind. *Harvard Heart Letter* 13 (June): 1.

44. Moser, M. 2004. Effective treatment of hypertension without medication: Is it possible? *Journal of Clinical Hypertension* 6(5):219–21.

45. Reuters Health Information. 2004. Institutes of Medicine advises on water, salt, potassium intake. *Medscape* (www.medscape.com/viewarticle/469001).

46. Editors. April 2004. New consumption guidelines issued for water, sodium, and potassium. *Tufts University Health and Nutrition Letter*, 22(2): i, 4–5.

47. Cataldo, C. B., L. K. De Bruyne, and E. N. Whitney. 2003. *Nutrition and diet therapy.* Belmont, CA: Thompson Wadsworth.

48. Sotile, W. M. 2001. Stress management. In *ACSM resource manual.* 4th ed. Edited by J. L. Roitman. Philadelphia: Lippincott Williams and Wilkins.

49. Editors. 2003. What was normal blood pressure is now considered too high. *Tufts University Health and Nutrition Letter* 21 (July): 4–5.

50. American Heart Association. 2001. *Heart and stroke facts.* Dallas: American Heart Association.

51. Editors. 2004. The smoking section. *University of California Berkeley Wellness Letter* 20 (June): 8.

52. American Cancer Society. 2002. *Cancer facts and figures.* Atlanta: American Cancer Society.

53. Editors. *Harvard Health Letter.* 2003. Let the butt stop here. *Harvard Heart Letter* 14 (October): 4.

54. Hales, D. 2001. *An invitation to fitness and wellness.* Belmont, CA: Wadsworth Thompson Learning.

55. U.S. Department of Health and Human Services. 2000. *Healthy people 2010 with understanding and improving*

health and objectives for improving health. 2 vols. Washington, DC: U.S. Government Printing Office.

56. Hart, J. A. July 2004. Medical encyclopedia: Smoking and smokeless tobacco. *Medline Plus* (www.nlm.nih.gov/medlineplus/ency/article/002032.htm).

57. Bridenbaker, M. 2002. Going up in smoke: What smokers need to know. *Medscape Cardiology* (www.medscape.com/viewarticle/457496).

58. Reuters Health Information. June 2003. Clot, inflammation factors higher in smokers. *Heart Center Online* (www.heartcenteronline.com).

59. Purnell, J. Q. June 2003. Obesity. *Medscape* (www.medscape.com/viewarticle/457926).

60. American Diabetes Association. April 2004. The metabolic syndrome (www.diabetes.org/utils/printthispage.jsp?).

61. Cunningham, D. S. 2004. Secondhand smoke raises heart disease risk. *Life Extension* 10 (July): 21.

62. Academy of General Dentistry. July 2004. Is tobacco safe? *General Dentistry* (www.media@agd.org).

63. Editors. *Harvard Health Letter.* 2002. Daily bed rest study. *Harvard Heart Letter* 12 (January): 6.

64. Editors. *Harvard Health Letter.* 2004. Inhaling not necessary for cigars to trouble arteries. *Harvard Heart Letter* 14 (June): 7.

65. Centers for Disease Control and Prevention. August 2004. Warning label fact sheet. *Tobacco Information and Prevention Source* (www.cdc.gov/tobacco/sgr_2000/factsheets/factsheet_labels.htm).

66. Powell, K. E. 1987. Physical activity and the incidence of coronary heart disease. *Annual Review of Public Health* 8:253.

67. Berlin, J. A., and G. A. Colditz. 1990. A meta-analysis of physical activity in the prevention of coronary heart disease. *American Journal of Epidemiology* 132:612.

68. Whaley, M. A., and L. A. Kaminsky. 2001. Epidemiology of physical activity, physical fitness, and selected chronic diseases. In *ACSM resource manual.* 4th ed. Edited by J. L. Roitman. Baltimore: Lippincott Williams and Wilkins.

69. Blair, S. N., et al. 1995. Changes in physical fitness and all-cause mortality: A prospective study of healthy and un-

healthy men. *Journal of the American Medical Association* 273:1093–98.

70. Geffken, D. F., et al. 2001. Association between physical activity and the markers of inflammation in a healthy elderly population. *American Journal of Epidemiology* 153:242–50.

71. Barclay, L., and D. Lie. January 2004. Fitness important for cardiovascular health. *Medscape Medical News* (www.medscape.com/viewarticle/466028).

72. Blair, S. N., et al. 1989. Physical fitness and all-cause mortality—Prospective study of healthy men and women. *Journal of the American Medical Association* 262:2395.

73. American Heart Association. 2003. Physical inactivity. *Statistical Fact Sheet—Risk Factors,* 1–3.

74. Duncan, J. J., et al. 1991. Women walking for health and fitness. *Journal of the American Medical Association* 266:3295–99.

75. ACSM. 2000. *ACSM's guidelines for exercise testing and prescription.* 6th ed. Philadelphia: Lippincott Williams and Wilkins.

76. Kerr, M. March 2004. Fitness most important factor in assessing cardiac mortality risk in women. *Medscape Medical News* (www.medscape.com/viewarticle/471289).

77. Editors. 2004. Simple test reveals future health. *Heart Advisor* 7 (March): 6.

78. Myer, J., et al. 2002. Exercise capacity and mortality among men referred for exercise testing. *New England Journal of Medicine* 346 (March): 793–801.

79. Pate, R. R., et al. 1995. Physical activity and public health. *Journal of the American Medical Association* 273:402.

80. President's Council on Physical Fitness Sports. July 2004. Physical activity and health. *Fact Sheet* (www.fitness.gov/physical_activity_fact_sheet.html).

81. Lee, I. M., and R. S. Paffenbarger. 2000. Associations of light, moderate, and vigorous intensity physical activity with longevity: The Harvard Alumni Health Study. *American Journal of Epidemiology* 151:293–99.

82. Booth, F. W. 2002. Costs and consequences of sedentary living: New battleground for an old enemy. *PCPFS Research Digest* 3 (March): 1–8.

83. Centers for Disease Control and Prevention. 9 March 2004. Physical inactivity and poor nutrition catching up to tobacco as actual causes of death.

Fact Sheet (www.cdc.gov/od/oc/media/pressrel/fs040409.htm).

84. Flegal, K., et al. 2002. Prevalence and trends in obesity among U.S. adults 1999–2000. *Journal of the American Medical Association* 288:1723–27.

85. Purnell, J. Q. June 2003. Obesity. *WebMD Scientific American Medicine—Medscape* (www.medscape.com/viewarticle/457926).

86. Mokdad, A. H., et al. 2004. Actual causes of death in the United States, 2000. *Journal of the American Medical Association* 291:1238–45.

87. Editors. 2003. Americans getting heavier still. *Tufts University Health and Nutrition Letter* 21 (December): 2.

88. Sorof, J. M., et al. 2004. Overweight, ethnicity, and the prevalence of hypertension in school-aged children. *Pediatrics* 113:475–82.

89. Weiss, R., et al. 2004. Obesity and the metabolic syndrome in children and adolescents. *New England Journal of Medicine* 350:2362–74.

90. Hillier, T. A., and K. L. Padula. 2004. Complications in young adults with early-onset Type 2 diabetes; losing the relative protection of youth. *Diabetes Care* 26:2999–3005.

91. U.S. Department of Health and Human Services. February 2003. *Small steps, big rewards: Prevent Type 2 diabetes.* NIH Publication NO. 03-5344. U.S. Department of Health and Human Services.

92. Editor. 1996. How to avoid adult onset diabetes. *Nutrition Action Health Letter* 23(7):3.

93. Liebman, B. 2004. The gathering storm. *Nutrition Action Letter* 31 (June): 1–7.

94. Editors. 2001. New advice for a healthy heart. *University of California, Berkeley Wellness Letter* 17 (August): 1–2.

95. Champaigne, B. 2001. Exercise and diabetes mellitus. In *ACSM resource manual.* 4th ed. Edited by J. L. Roitman. Philadelphia: Lippincott Williams and Wilkins.

96. Reuters Health Information. March 2004. Anger, hostility linked to rhythm disorder in men. *Heart Center Online* (www.heartcenteronline.com).

97. Effects of stress on the body. April 2003. *Heart Center Online* (www.heartcenteronline.com).

98. Sime, W. W., and K. Hellweg. 2001. Stress and coping. In *ACSM resource manual.* 4th ed. Edited by J. L.

Roitman. Philadelphia: Lippincott Williams and Wilkins.

99. Ornish, D., et al. 1990. Can lifestyle changes reverse coronary heart disease? *The Lancet* 336:129.

100. Ornish, D., et al. 1993. Can lifestyle changes reverse atherosclerosis? Four-year results of the lifestyle heart trial. *Circulation* 88 (suppl.): 2064.

101. Editors. 1997. Iron's link to heart disease. *HealthNews* 3(3):7.

102. Study investigates homocysteine levels following heart attack. September 2003. *Heart Center Online* (www.heartcenteronline.com).

103. Wilson, P. W. F. 2002. Homocysteine and coronary heart disease. *Journal of the American Medical Association* 288:2042–43.

104. Komaroff, A. L. 2004. By the way doctor. *Harvard Health Letter* 29 (July): 8.

105. Lee, T. H. 2004. Ask the doctor. *Harvard Health Letter* 12 (June): 8.

106. Ariyo, A. A., T. Chaw, and R. Tracy. 2003. Lp(a) lipoprotein, vascular disease, and mortality in the elderly. *New England Journal of Medicine* 349 (November): 2108–15.

107. Segal, M., ed. 2003. *Disease prevention and treatment.* Hollywood, FL: Life Extension Media.

108. Danesh, J., et al. 2004. C-reactive protein and other circulating markers of inflammation in the prediction of coronary heart disease. *New England Journal of Medicine* 350 (April): 1387–97.

109. Weil, A. 2004. The latest on aspirin therapy. *Dr. Andrew Weil's Self Healing,* June, 8.

110. Reuters Health Information. February 2004. Long-term survival after CABG may be less good with off-pump procedure. *Medscape,* (www.medscape.com/viewarticle/469504).

111. Peck, P. March 2004. Sirolimus-eluting stents effective in direct stenting, treatment of small vessels lesions. *Medscape* (www.medscape.com/viewarticle/471253).

112. Editors. January 1997. Meditation lowers blood pressure as well as drugs. *Tufts University Diet and Nutrition Letter* 14(11): 3.

Suggested Readings

Editors. *The Cleveland Clinic Heart Advisor.* 2004. How to beat genes that raise risks. *Heart Advisor* 7 (August): 1, 7.
The following five suggestions summarize the article:
1. Record your family's health history.
2. Focus on first-degree relatives: mother, father, siblings, and children.
3. Discuss your family history of heart disease with your family physician.
4. Ask your doctor if you should undergo testing.
5. Reduce all of the risk factors under your control through lifestyle behaviors.

Editors. 2004. Cholesterol: How low should you go? *University of California at Berkeley Wellness Letter* 20 (July): 2.
Is it possible to lower one's cholesterol too much? Experts have focused in on LDL cholesterol and total cholesterol, but as yet there is no agreement, since the body requires some cholesterol in order to function. The conclusion is that it is virtually impossible for healthy people to lower cholesterol and its subfractions to the point where it would be harmful to health.

Editors. 2004. Heart attack vs. sudden cardiac arrest: What's the difference? *Harvard Health Letter* 29 (August): 7.
A heart attack occurs when the heart's muscle cells are abruptly cut off from blood and oxygen because the coronary arteries have been clogged. Sudden cardiac arrest is when the heart suddenly stops beating. The most frequent cause is a problem in the electrical system that establishes and synchronizes the heartbeat.

Editors. 2004. No age limit for blood pressure control. *Harvard Heart Letter* 14 (August): 1.
The latest findings on blood pressure control from the Framingham Heart Disease Study are discussed. The conclusion was that high blood pressure exists among all age groups, but it is more prevalent and least controlled among the elderly. Only 25 percent of the elderly hypertensive women and 32 percent of the elderly hypertensive men have their blood pressure under control.

Editors. 2004. Treating Type 2 diabetes. *Health News* 10 (August): 4.
Early-stage Type 2 diabetes can be controlled by weight management, regular exercise, and a healthy diet. But if these lifestyle behaviors fail to control the disease, then drug therapy is required. The last half of this article deals with the advantages and disadvantages of several common drugs and the importance of matching the drug to the individual diabetic.

3

Increasing Cardiorespiratory Endurance

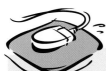 Online Learning Center

Log on to our Online Learning Center (OLC) for access to these additional resources:

- Chapter key term flashcards
- Learning objectives
- Additional goals for behavior change
- Concentration game
- Self-scoring chapter quizzes

- Additional lab activities

The OLC also offers Web links for study and exploration of wellness topics. Access these links through **www.mhhe. com/anspaugh6e**, click on Student Center, click on Chapter 3, and then click on Web Activities.

Key Terms

aerobic
aerobic capacity
cardiorespiratory
  endurance
cross-training

health-related fitness
hyperthermia
hypothermia
performance-related
  fitness

Objectives

After completing this chapter, you will be able to do the following:

- Identify and define the health-related components of physical fitness.
- Discuss the principles of conditioning.
- Calculate your target heart rate for exercise by two methods.

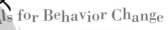 Goals for Behavior Change

- List three physical activities you normally do every week (exclusive of structured, planned exercise) and find and implement ways of making them more challenging.
- If you do not exercise regularly, list several factors that will motivate you to begin a cardiorespiratory endurance program. Begin a simple walking or other exercise program with these factors in mind.
- If you are physically active, list the main factors that will encourage you to improve the frequency, intensity, or duration of your activity. To help you stay motivated, post this list in a place where you will see it every day.
- Choose a piece of home exercise equipment that seems well suited to your exercise preferences and goals.

- Identify and discuss the health benefits of consistent participation in exercise.
- Describe the problems associated with exercise in hot and cold weather.

echnology has affected the lives of Americans by increasing productivity while reducing and in some cases eliminating the amount of physical work for the labor force. Therefore, physical fitness for most of the population can no longer be attained on the job, and leisure hours represent the only time for its development. Dozens of physical activities, exercise regimens, sports, games, and household and other physical chores that may contribute to health enhancement and fitness development are available. These activities are sufficiently different from each other, running the gamut from low- to high-skill requirement, so that almost anyone can find one or two enjoyable, fun, and challenging activities. This chapter focuses on the principles and concepts that have evolved for developing cardiorespiratory endurance for the purposes of health enhancement and physical fitness.

Components of Physical Fitness

According to the American College of Sports Medicine (ACSM), *physical fitness* is defined "as a set of attributes that people have or achieve that relates to the ability to perform physical activity."[1] *Physical activity* is an umbrella term defined "as bodily movement that is produced by the contraction of skeletal muscle and that substantially increases energy expenditure."[1] *Exercise* is a subset of physical activity. It is defined "as planned, structured, and repetitive bodily movement done to improve or maintain one or more components of physical fitness."[1]

Physical activity includes exercise and all other types of human movements, such as mowing the lawn, raking leaves, vacuuming the floors, climbing stairs, washing the car by hand, chopping wood, and shoveling snow.[2] These activities, many of which are daily chores, may improve physical fitness for some unfit sedentary people, but when engaged in regularly, are health-enhancing for most people. Health improvement can be attained with regular participation in lower-intensity physical activities, whereas higher-intensity physical activities that sustain an exercise target heart rate are necessary for improving physical fitness. In addition to the development of a higher level of physical fitness, the extra effort involved in more vigorous exercise includes a significant bonus. Greater exercise intensity lowers the risk for heart disease, more so than lower-intensity levels.[3,4]

Most physical fitness experts have accepted the concept of performance-related and health-related fitness. **Performance-related fitness,** or sports fitness, consists of the following components: speed, power, balance, coordination, agility, and reaction time. These are essential for sports performance, but they may or may not contribute significantly to those activities performed for

Just the Facts

What's the Difference?

Components of Fitness	Activities
Health-Related	*Health-Related*
• Cardiorespiratory endurance	• Walking
• Muscular strength	• Running
• Muscular endurance	• Jogging
• Flexibility	• Cycling
• Body composition	• Hiking
	• Swimming
Performance-Related	• Rope jumping
• Speed	• Weight training
• Power	• Cross-country skiing
• Balance	
• Coordination	*Performance-Related*
• Agility	• Racquetball
• Reaction time	• Handball
	• Squash
	• Tennis
	• Badminton
	• Soccer
	• Softball
	• Basketball
	• Football
	• Water polo

health enhancement (see Just the Facts: What's the Difference?).

Speed is velocity, or the ability to move rapidly. *Power* is the product of force and velocity and the rate at which work is performed. *Balance,* or equilibrium, is the ability to maintain a desired body position, either statically or dynamically. *Coordination* is the harmonious integration of the body parts to produce smooth, fluid motion. *Agility* is the ability to change direction rapidly. *Reaction time* is the time required (usually measured in hundredths of a second) to respond to a stimulus.

The components of **health-related fitness** are cardiorespiratory endurance, muscular strength, muscular endurance, flexibility, and body composition. In this text the exercise emphasis is on health-related fitness.

Performance-related and health-related fitness, although different, clearly are not mutually exclusive. For example, competitive athletes require an abundance of the performance-related components of fitness, but the natures of their sports may also require the simultaneous development of the health-related components. Athletes who play racquetball, tennis, basketball, soccer, and handball are some that fall within this category. Conversely, the same sports are appropriate for health and fitness enthusiasts who prefer to achieve their goals through friendly competition.

However, the development and maintenance of health-related fitness do not necessarily depend on athletic ability or activities high in the performance components. Fitness for health purposes can be achieved with minimal psychomotor ability through activities such as walking, jogging, cycling, hiking, backpacking, orienteering, swimming, rope jumping, and weight training. These are self-paced activities; that is, the exerciser selects a relatively comfortable pace that can be sustained for a minimum of 10 minutes. No competing opponent pushes the exerciser beyond his or her physiological limits.

Remember the adage "No pain, no gain"? Trying to comply with it has done more harm than good to sedentary people attempting to become physically active. The health benefits of exercise begin to occur when exercise is somewhat uncomfortable but not painful. Only the most dedicated health enthusiasts and competitors can face exercise that constantly produces pain. Although exercise for health enhancement should stress cardiorespiratory development, the other components of fitness should not be neglected. Flexibility exercises can be a part of warm-up and cooldown procedures. Flexibility exercises may be performed three to five times per week, and the best results occur during the cooldown period following the cardiorespiratory workout.[5,6] Stretching is most effective at this time because muscle temperature is elevated. Warm muscles respond well to stretching, and the likelihood of muscle injury is decreased. Resistance/strength training plays an important role and should be an integral part of a well-rounded fitness program.

As with all components of wellness, developing and sustaining an exercise program are the responsibilities of each individual. This text provides convincing evidence of the need for regular exercise and provides guidelines for initiating a sound program or reinforcement for those currently exercising.

Cardiorespiratory Endurance

Cardiorespiratory endurance is the ability to take in, deliver, and extract oxygen for physical work—that is, the ability to persevere at a physical task at a given intensity level.[7] Cardiorespiratory endurance improves with regular participation in aerobic activities, such as speed walking, jogging, cycling, swimming, cross-country skiing, and many others. The term **aerobic** means "with oxygen," but when applied to exercise, it refers to activities in which oxygen demand can be met continuously during performance.[8] Aerobic performance depends on a continuous and sufficient supply of oxygen to burn the carbohydrates and fats needed to fuel such activities. In other words, someone performing aerobically has the capacity to sustain the intensity or the energy requirement for longer than a couple of minutes,[8] a phenomenon known as *steady state*. Steady state can be achieved only during aerobic exercise, and it represents a level of exertion that feels relatively comfortable to the exerciser. It is also referred to as a *pay as you go system,* in that the oxygen cost of an activity is paid in full by the body during the activity. Steady state oxygen consumption can be maintained for an average of 10 to 60 minutes during submaximal continuous exercise. This may not apply for exercise during hot and humid weather. The stress of exercising during these conditions causes a steady upward drift in oxygen consumption.[8]

Cardiorespiratory endurance is also referred to as **aerobic capacity,** or maximum oxygen consumption (VO_2 max). It is the most important component of physical fitness and is the foundation of total fitness.

The physiological changes that result from cardiorespiratory training are referred to as the *long-term,* or *chronic, effects of exercise.* The effects of training are measurable and predictable.

Heart Rate

A few months of aerobic training lowers the resting heart rate by 10 to 15 beats per minute (bpm).[9] It also lowers the heart rate for a given workload. For example, a slow jog may produce a heart rate of 165 beats per minute before training and 140 beats per minute after a few months of training. The trained heart is a stronger, more efficient pump capable of delivering the required blood and oxygen with fewer beats.

Stroke Volume

Stroke volume is the amount of blood that the heart can eject in one beat. Aerobic training increases the stroke volume by (1) increasing the size of the cavity of the ventricles, which results in more blood filling the heart, and (2) increasing the contractile strength of the ventricular wall, so contraction is more forceful and a greater amount of blood is ejected from the ventricles.[9] The increase in stroke volume, both at rest and during exercise, is one of the primary effects of endurance training and one of the major mechanisms responsible for improvement in aerobic fitness.

Cardiac Output

Cardiac output is the amount of blood ejected by the heart in one minute. Cardiac output (Q) is the product of heart rate (HR) and stroke volume (SV) ($Q = HR \times SV$). Cardiac output increases with aerobic training during maximal effort—it does not increase at rest or during submaximal exercise. Cardiac output does not change during rest or submaximal exercise because the lowered resting heart rate compensates for the increase in stroke volume. What does change is the manner in which cardiac output is achieved. This is illustrated by the following example: An untrained 25-year-old man has a resting heart rate of 72 bpm and a stroke volume of 70 mL of blood per beat. His cardiac output at rest is calculated as follows:

$$Q = HR \times SV$$
$$= 72 \times 70$$
$$= 5,040 \text{ mL (5.0 L)}$$

The same person after two years of aerobic training has the same cardiac output at rest, but it is achieved differently: The resting heart rate is now decreased to 55 bpm and the stroke volume is increased to 92 mL of blood per beat.

$$Q = 55 \times 92$$
$$= 5,040 \text{ mL (5.0 L)}$$

The average cardiac output at rest is 4 to 6 liters of blood per minute. During maximal exertion, cardiac output reaches values of 18 to 20 liters of blood per minute for the average person but may reach as much as 40 liters per minute for large, well-conditioned athletes—what an incredible piece of work by an organ that weighs less than a pound! To put this in perspective, imagine 40 1-liter cola bottles filled with blood. This is the amount that the hearts of some highly conditioned people can pump in one minute. Maximal cardiac output improves with training primarily because of the resulting increase in stroke volume.[9] Maximal heart rate is essentially unaffected by training; therefore, its influence on maximal cardiac output is relatively constant. However, maximal heart rate declines with age by about 1 bpm per year after age 20. Training cannot stop the decline; it can only slow the process.

Blood Volume

Aerobic training increases total blood volume, plasma volume (the liquid portion of the blood), and blood solids (the red blood cells, white blood cells, and blood platelets). The increase is greatest in plasma volume, so the blood becomes more liquid. The increase in the ratio of plasma volume to red blood cell volume is an adaptation to exercise that lowers the viscosity, or thickness and stickiness, of the blood. This change decreases the resistance to blood flow, allowing it to circulate more easily through the blood vessels.

Blood is automatically shunted by the body to areas of greatest need. At rest, a significant amount is sent to the digestive system and kidneys. During vigorous exercise, as much as 85 percent of the blood is sent to the working muscles, reducing the amount sent to the digestive and urinary systems.[1]

Heart Volume

The muscles of the body respond to exercise by growing larger and stronger. As a muscular pump, the heart's volume and weight increase with endurance training.[10] Training that lowers the resting heart rate stimulates greater filling of the ventricles, whose muscle fibers respond to the increased pool of blood by stretching. This produces a recoil effect in the muscle fibers, which results in a stronger contraction with more blood ejected per beat. Continued training causes the ventricles to enlarge and grow stronger, so the weight and the size of the heart increase. The hypertrophied (enlarged) heart is a normal response to endurance training that has no long-term detrimental effects. Although maintaining this effect for life is beneficial, several months of inactivity will reduce heart weight and size to pretraining levels. The atrophy (wasting away) associated with physical inactivity is inevitable.

Respiratory Responses

The chest muscles that support breathing improve in both strength and endurance with exercise.[8] Vital capacity, the amount of air that can be expired maximally following a maximal inspiration, increases slightly. A corresponding decrease occurs in "dead space" air, or residual volume, the amount of air remaining in the lungs after a maximal expiration.

Training substantially increases maximal pulmonary ventilation (the amount of air moved in and out of the lungs).[8] Before training, the lungs can ventilate approximately 110 liters of air per minute. Pulmonary ventilation increases to about 135 liters of air following a few months of training. Highly trained athletes commonly ventilate 180 to 200 liters of air per minute.

Blood flow to the lungs, particularly to the upper lobes, appears to increase after training. This results in a larger and more efficient surface for the exchange of oxygen and carbon dioxide.

Metabolic Responses

Aerobic endurance training improves aerobic capacity by 5 to 25 percent in previously untrained, healthy adults. The magnitude of improvement is primarily dependent on the initial level of physical fitness. The lower the fitness level, the greater the gain from aerobic training.[9] A gain of 15 to 20 percent in aerobic capacity is typical for an average person who trains at 75 percent of maximal oxygen intake (VO_2 max), three days per week, for 30 minutes per workout over a six-month training period. Two to three years of highly intense training of greater frequency and longer duration has resulted in increases in VO_2 max in excess of 40 percent.

The improvement in aerobic capacity is the result of several physiological adaptations that increase the body's production of energy. First, adenosine triphosphate (ATP), the actual unit of energy for muscular contraction, is produced in greater quantities. The mitochondria, specialized organelles responsible for manufacturing ATP, respond to training by increasing in size and number to increase their output. Second, oxidative enzymes within the mitochondria that accelerate the production of ATP increase in quantity. Third, cardiac output and blood perfusion of the muscles performing the work increase. Fourth, training facilitates and increases the extraction of oxygen by the exercising muscles. These are some of the major adaptations that combine to enhance aerobic endurance.[8]

Aerobic capacity (VO_2 max) is limited by heredity and is finite. Studies of identical and fraternal twins and studies that examined family groups (parents and children) have produced estimates of the role of genetics in the development of maximal cardiorespiratory endurance. Separating the influence of genetics from the influence of training is very complex. As a result, the estimates of the genetic predisposition for maximal cardiorespiratory endurance ranges from a low of 25 percent to a high of 93 percent. At this point, the majority of the evidence indicates that the genetic component is probably closer to 40 to 50 percent.[8,11,12] Whatever the actual percentage turns out to be, the consensus among exercise scientists is that the role of genetics represents a substantial potential for the development of maximal cardiorespiratory endurance. The sensitivity of the VO_2 max response to aerobic training is to a significant degree dependent on heredity. If those who inherit the genetic potential for endurance events also train diligently, they become capable of exceptionally high levels of performance. Diligent training with an average genetic potential results in average or slightly above-average performance. Only a select few inherit the ability to produce world-class endurance performances. The majority of people are in the average category, but all can achieve their aerobic *potential* with training. However, the expectation that regularity of training will produce a fitness payback that is proportional to the effort is logical, albeit inaccurate. The relationship between genetics and sensitivity to training is complicated by the fact that some people are "responders" (capable of making significant improvement from consistent training), while others are "nonresponders" (their improvement is minimal, even though they are exposed to the same training program). Therefore, two people who are the same age, height, weight, and gender who train together and are equally compliant may obtain results that are very different, based on their response to training. The sensitivity

to training is genetic, and evidence indicates that it is dependent on mitochondrial mass and mitochondrial DNA.[8] Evidence also indicates that the mother's genes are responsible for mitochondrial mass.[11]

Three methods for assessing your cardiorespiratory endurance are presented in the Assessment Activities. These include the Rockport Fitness Walking Test, the 1.5-Mile Run/Walk Test, and the 3-Minute Bench Step Test. Each is accompanied by norms, so you can compare your performance against the standards.

Aerobic capacity reaches a peak after six months to two years of steady endurance training. At this point, it levels off and remains unchanged for a number of years, even if training is intensified. However, aerobic performance continues to improve with harder training, because a higher percentage of the aerobic capacity can be maintained for a longer period. For example, six months of appropriate training may allow you to jog 3 miles at 60 percent of your aerobic capacity. Another year of harder training may allow you to run 3 miles at 85 percent of your capacity. Capacity has not changed during this time, but physiological adaptations have occurred that enable the body to function at progressively higher percentages of maximum capacity.

Aerobic capacity decreases with age. During adulthood, peak aerobic energy steadily declines by an average of about 1 percent per year between the ages of 25 and 75.[13] A significant portion of the decline is related to the lack of physical activity that accompanies aging: Those who are physically active throughout their lifetimes experience declines in aerobic capacity but not at the same rate as those who are inactive. See Wellness for a Lifetime: Exercise Is for Everyone on page 74 for more details about the impact of exercising on aging.

The effects of training persist as long as training continues. Training of moderate intensity may increase the VO_2 max by 10 to 20 percent. However, the VO_2 max returns to pretraining levels within a few months if training is discontinued.[10] Most of the decline occurs during the first month and slows down during the next 2 months. Fitness developed through years of continuous training can be lost in months if training is interrupted or discontinued. Highly conditioned athletes respond to detraining in a similar manner. In a study, subjects who suspended training for 84 days after 10 years of active participation experienced a significant decline in aerobic capacity after 3 weeks of inactivity. They returned to pretraining levels in most fitness parameters by the end of the study. The exceptions to complete reversal were muscle capillary density and mitochondrial enzymes, which remained 50 percent higher than levels measured in sedentary control subjects. This study indicated that the results of inactivity are variable and affect some systems more quickly than others. Physical decline cannot be prevented with physical inactivity.

Wellness for a Lifetime

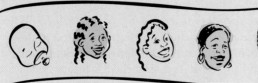

Exercise Is for Everyone

The ability of the body to take in, transport, and extract oxygen for physical work and exercise declines with age. On the average, aerobic capacity declines by about 8 to 10 percent every decade after the age of 25 in both males and females. One of the major sources of this decline in the United States is the decreasing level of physical activity that tends to accompany aging. This trend toward inactivity also results in a loss of muscle weight, an increase in fat weight, and a decrease in metabolic rate, all of which contribute to the decline in aerobic capacity. Although physiological aging does lower aerobic capacity, at least 50 percent of the decline is due to "disuse atrophy" caused by inactivity.[14]

Biological aging cannot be stopped. We cannot live forever. However, exercise comes as close to an antiaging pill as anything else available. Even older people who have been sedentary for decades can benefit from aerobic exercise and weight training.

The beneficial outcomes of regular exercise for older people include an increase in energy, a favorable change in body composition (loss of fat, gain of muscle), an increase in muscular strength and endurance, an increase in metabolism, and significant improvements in cardiovascular and musculoskeletal health.[7] All of these changes translate into a higher quality of life and longevity.

Physically fit 60- and 70-year-olds have the aerobic capacity of unfit 25-year-olds.[7] This means that physically fit elderly people have the energy to live independently during their later years. The ability to perform the daily chores of living and to participate in an active lifestyle with energy to spare develops confidence that contributes to the enjoyment of life.

Cardiorespiratory Endurance and Wellness

Most Americans believe that exercise is good for them, but the majority cannot explain how or why. This section provides some of the answers.

Consistent participation in exercise is necessary to improve health status. Sporadic exercise does not pro-

mote physical fitness or contribute to health enhancement. Infrequent participation increases the risk for sudden death during the time of exercise.[15] Physical inactivity is a major risk factor for coronary heart disease. The risk is approximately equal to that imposed by cigarette smoking, high blood pressure, and elevated serum cholesterol. Forty-two percent of American adults are marginally active—that is, they do not exercise a minimum of 30 minutes per day for at least 5 days per week.[16] Another 28 percent report that they are completely inactive. Therefore, 70 percent of the adult population is either inactive or not active enough for physical activity to improve their health. About 25 percent of 12- to 21-year-olds participate in light to moderate physical activity, such as walking and cycling nearly every day.[17] About 50 percent state that they regularly engage in vigorous physical activity. Approximately 25 percent report no vigorous physical activity and 14 percent report no physical activity at all. The number of physically inactive people exceeds the combined total of those who smoke, are hypertensive, and have high serum cholesterol.[15] Based on these numbers, promoting regular exercise for the general public should be an important priority of public health policy.

Coronary heart disease is rarely responsible for sudden cardiac death during or after exercise among people under the age of 30. Congenital heart defects or other cardiac abnormalities, such as faulty valves, enlarged hearts, heart muscle disease, and fatal cardiac arrhythmias are the usual culprits for this age group. Most exertional deaths occur among older Americans and are due to coronary heart disease and cardiomyopathy (wasting of cardiac muscle due to disease).[18] A study by Harvard medical researchers found that heavy physical exertion, such as shoveling snow, gardening, walking fast, jogging, playing softball, and playing tennis, can trigger a heart attack.[19] For the physically unfit, the risk of incurring a heart attack during and in the first hour after strenuous exertion increased by 107 times. The risk for physically fit people increased only 2.7 times. These data applied equally to men and women.

The danger attributed to physical exertion is greatly diminished in people who exercise regularly. The benefits they receive from physical training far outweigh the minimal risk associated with one bout of strenuous exercise. A similar study conducted at the same time in Germany found amazingly similar results.[20]

One and one-half million heart attacks occur every year in the United States. The Harvard researchers concluded that 75,000 of these are exertional and they usually occur after strenuous exercise. Most of these heart attacks occur among those who are physically inactive and at high risk.[19] See Just the Facts:

Just the Facts

Exercise-Related Problems

Many health, fitness, and cosmetic benefits occur to those who exercise on a regular basis. Although they are outweighed by the benefits, risks are associated with such behavior. Despite precautions, injuries occasionally occur. Beginning exercisers are particularly susceptible to injury because of their lack of knowledge about training coupled with their misguided attempts to achieve their goals too quickly. The following suggestions should result in safer workouts:

1. Dress according to the weather: shorts, T-shirt, mesh baseball-type cap in warm weather; layers of light clothing, hat, gloves, ear protection, and windbreaker in cold weather.
2. Wear appropriate shoes for the activity in which you participate: jogging shoes, walking shoes, aerobic shoes, or cross-trainers. In general, exercise shoes should be ½ to ¾ of an inch longer than your longest toe. There should also be room enough for the toes to spread out. The soles of most exercise shoes consist of three layers. The outer sole that contacts the floor or ground should be made of hard rubber. The next layer is the midsole, which protects the midfoot and toes. The last layer is made of a thick, spongy substance that absorbs most of the shock when the foot strikes the surface.
3. Warm up and cool down properly before and after exercise.
4. Exercise within your capacity—it should feel a little uncomfortable but not painful. According to the American College of Sports Medicine (ACSM), the initial stage of an exercise program should last a minimum of 4 weeks at a low intensity (50 to 60 percent of the maximal heart rate, or HR_{max}). Each exercise session should last for 15 to 20 minutes during the first week and increase to 25 to 30 minutes during the fourth week. At this point, the exerciser is ready to increase the intensity, frequency, and duration of each session.

5. While following these simple guidelines reduces the possibility of incurring pain or injury, beginning exercisers may experience, as a result of overuse, shin splints, side stitch, blisters, chafing, muscle cramps, muscle soreness, Achilles tendon injuries, and lower-back pain.
   a. Muscle soreness following exercise usually occurs among beginners who have yet to adapt to physical exertion or to those at any level of fitness who exceed their physical capabilities. Following the ACSM guidelines reduces exposure to muscle pain.
   b. Side stitches occur primarily among walkers and joggers. They consist of severe pain in the upper right quadrant of the abdomen. Side stitches may be caused by reduced blood flow to the diaphragm (a large, dome-shaped muscle that separates the abdominal cavity from the chest cavity), or they may be due to the collection of gas in the intestines. In either case, deep breathing and direct pressure applied with both hands at the site of the pain may provide relief. Sometimes, stopping the activity for a few minutes is required for the pain to subside.
   c. A common injury occurring among beginners is shin splints. Shin splints produce a burning pain that radiates along the inner surface of the large bones of the lower leg. These are nagging, painful injuries better prevented than treated. The causes of shin splints include training demands that exceed a person's capacity to perform. High-impact activities, such as jogging or aerobics to music; poor-quality exercise shoes; hard exercise surfaces; and walking or jogging on hilly surfaces are other contributing causes. Treatment includes applying ice, resting, wrapping or taping the affected shin, and placing heel lifts in the shoes.

Exercise-Related Problems for some tips on reducing the hazards associated with regular exercise. Some selected health benefits of regular exercise are listed in Table 3-1 on page 76. If these benefits could be distilled and sold in pill form, the American public would line up to pay any reasonable price to attain them, yet all of these benefits are readily available to anyone willing to commit the time and effort. While millions of people are exercising, 70 percent of the adult population is either inactive or marginally active.

Principles of Conditioning

Becoming familiar with the principles of exercise is necessary to maximize the results of a physical fitness program. Your objectives can be met through the appropriate manipulation of intensity, frequency, duration, overload, progression, and specificity. Setting of objectives, warm-up, cooldown, and careful selection of activity are important elements that add to the enjoyment and effectiveness of exercise.

Table 3-1 Health-Related Benefits Associated with Regular Aerobic Exercise

Reduces the Risk of Cardiovascular Disease

- Increases HDL cholesterol
- Decreases LDL cholesterol
- Favorably changes the ratios between total cholesterol and HDL-C and between LDL-C and HDL-C
- Decreases triglyceride levels
- Promotes relaxation; relieves stress and tension
- Decreases body fat and favorably changes body composition
- Reduces blood pressure, especially if it is high
- Makes blood platelets less sticky
- Decreases the incidence of cardiac dysrhythmias
- Increases myocardial efficiency
  1. Lowers resting heart rate
  2. Increases stroke volume
- Increases oxygen-carrying capacity of the blood
- Reduces the risk for colon cancer and breast cancer

Helps Control Diabetes

- Makes cells less resistant to insulin
- Reduces body fat

Develops Stronger Bones Less Susceptible to Injury

Promotes Joint Stability

- Increases muscular strength
- Increases strength of the ligaments, tendons, cartilage, and connective tissue

Contributes to Fewer Lower-Back Problems

Acts as a Stimulus for Other Lifestyle Changes

Improves Self-Concept

SOURCES: Tanasescu, M., et al. August 2002. Exercise type and intensity in relation to coronary heart disease in men. *Journal of the American Medical Association,* 288:1994–2000.

U.S. Department of Health and Human Services. August 2003. Physical activity fundamental to preventing disease (http://aspe.hhs.gov/health/reports/physicalactivity/).

National Center for Health Statistics. 2003. *Health, United States 2003,* Hyattsville, MD.

Davis, N. S. 2003. Exercise as a mode of treating diseases of the heart. *Journal of the American Medical Association,* 290:2614.

Intensity

Intensity refers to the degree of vigorousness of a single session of exercise. In 1995, the American College of Sports Medicine (ACSM) and the Centers for Disease Control and Prevention (CDC) developed and promoted the following recommendation for exercise: Every U.S. adult should accumulate 30 minutes or more of moderately intense physical activity on most and preferably all days of the week.[21] The recommendation refers to *physical activity* rather than *exercise.* This is an umbrella term that includes many types of physical exertion, including structured exercise. *Moderate intensity* refers to walking at a 3- to 4-mile-per-hour pace (15 to 20 minutes per mile) or engaging in any activity that burns a similar number of calories at a similar rate. The 30 minutes of activity can be split up into two or three bouts of 10 to 15 minutes each throughout the day. Table 3-2 provides a summary of the ACSM-CDC exercise principles and their application to the enhancement of health and physical fitness.

The recommendation for health enhancement is a minimum guideline designed to motivate and recruit the 70 percent of the population not physically active. It is not intended to lower the standard for those who currently

exercise at a higher level or whose primary goal is the development of physical fitness. Programs designed primarily to improve health may not improve or may minimally improve physical fitness. It takes higher-intensity exercise to significantly improve physical fitness. In fact, intensity is the most important principle for the development of physical fitness.[12] The higher the intensity, the greater the return. Those who exercise for physical fitness purposes also derive health benefits in a two-for-one deal. It takes a higher level of training to achieve both.

In September 2001, the Institute of Medicine (IOM), a private, nonprofit organization established by the U.S. Congress 150 years ago to advise the federal government on matters requiring technical and scientific expertise, issued an exercise recommendation of 60 minutes of brisk physical activity per day.[22] This recommendation was based on evidence indicating that successful maintenance of body weight occurs at this level of physical activity. *Brisk exercise* was defined as walking 4 miles per hour (a 15-minute-per-mile pace). The IOM also suggested that the cumulative effect of exercise is important for weight loss, so the 60 minutes does not have to be performed continuously—that is, it can be broken into segments scattered throughout the day. The caveat is that all segments

Table 3-2 Summary of Exercise Principles for the Development of Physical Fitness and Health

Exercise Principles	Exercise Goals	
	To Develop and Improve Level of Physical Fitness (1998 Guidelines)	To Develop and Improve Health Status (1995 Guidelines)
Intensity	• 55/65 to 90% of HR_{max} • 55 to 64% of HR_{max} for sedentary beginners • 40/50 to 85% of the cardiac reserve or • 40/50 to 85% of the VO_2 reserve*	• Moderate (walking 3 to 4 MPH)
Frequency	• 3–5 days per week	• Most, preferably all, days of the week
Duration (time)	• 20–60 minutes at 60 to 90% of HR_{max} • 200–300 calories per exercise session	• 30 minutes or more
Overload	• Should not exceed 10% of the previous workout	• NA**
Progression	• Based on physiological readiness • According to the schedule of overload	• NA
Specificity	• For competitors training for maximal performance	• NA

* The VO_2 reserve is VO_2 max minus VO_2 rest.

** Not applicable.

need to be performed at a brisk intensity level. The issuance of this recommendation produced some confusion on the part of the general public. The ACSM recommended 30 minutes per day; the IOM recommended 60 minutes per day. Which recommendation is correct? The answer is that they are both correct because the programs are designed to meet different goals. The ACSM recommendation is a starter program for the purpose of health enhancement for sedentary adults. Thirty minutes of physical activity per day will make only a minimum contribution to weight loss, hence the IOM recommendation of 60 minutes of exercise per day.

HR_{max} can be measured by a physical work capacity test on a treadmill or cycle ergometer. Because most people do not have access to such tests, HR_{max} can be estimated by subtracting age from 220. A 20-year-old person has an estimated HR_{max} of 200 beats per minute $(220 - 20 = 200)$. This formula predicts rather than measures HR_{max}; therefore, a measurement error of approximately plus or minus 10 to 12 beats per minute is associated with its use.

After the HR_{max} has been determined, the target for exercise may be calculated. The easiest method for determining the target zone for exercise is to use the percentage of HR_{max} recommended by ACSM (see the example that follows). The target zone for exercise provides the desirable heart rate for the development of physical fitness. For the 20-year-old person whose HR_{max} is 200 beats per minute, the target zone for exercise is calculated as follows:

$$\frac{\begin{array}{r} 200 \ (\text{estimated } HR_{max}) \\ \times \ 0.55 \ (55\% \text{ of } HR_{max}) \end{array}}{110 \ (\text{lower-limit target HR})}$$

$$\frac{\begin{array}{r} 200 \ (\text{estimated } HR_{max}) \\ \times \ 0.90 \ (90\% \text{ of } HR_{max}) \end{array}}{180 \ (\text{upper-limit target HR})}$$

This 20-year-old person should exercise at a heart rate range of 110 to 180 beats per minute, depending on objectives and level of fitness. A 20-year-old person who is sedentary, and possibly overweight, should exercise at the lowest percentage of HR_{max} (55 percent). A same-age subject who is at an average physical fitness level should exercise at 70 to 75 percent of the HR_{max}, and a 20-year-old person who is fit should exercise at 80 to 90 percent of the HR_{max}. The target for a person who has an average level of fitness is 140 to 150 beats per minute for exercise. The training effect occurs at heart rate levels below the maximum.

A slightly different emphasis was proposed by the ACSM concerning the prescription of exercise in the latest "position stand."[23] The suggestion was that exercise intensity should be monitored by the VO_2 Reserve

Table 3-3 Guidelines for Selecting Exercise Intensity Level

Fitness Level	Intensity Level (%)
Low	60
Fair	65
Average	70
Good	75
Excellent	80–90

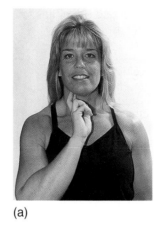
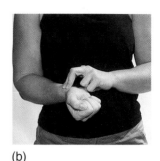

(a)   (b)

Figure 3-1 Sites for Taking a Pulse

The two sites for measuring pulse are (a) at the neck (carotid artery) and (b) at the wrist (radial artery).

(VO_2R) method. This approach is based on a given percentage of the VO_2R (the difference between VO_2 max and VO_2 rest). This is an excellent way to generate an exercise prescription, but it requires that an individual perform a maximal aerobic test on a treadmill or cycle ergometer. Realistically, most people don't opt for such testing, so this method will be used on a limited basis. But the good news is that the heart rate reserve method (the Karvonen formula) simulates the VO_2 Reserve without the measurements and it is much more applicable for the general public.

The Karvonen formula considers fitness level and resting heart rate. The training heart rate is calculated with this formula by using a percentage of the heart rate reserve (cardiac reserve), the difference between the HR_{max} and the resting heart rate. The best way to determine the resting heart rate for this method is to count your pulse rate for 15 seconds while in the sitting position immediately after waking in the morning. You should repeat this for four or five consecutive days and average the readings for a relatively accurate representation of your resting heart rate. Next, you should estimate your level of fitness based on your exercise habits and select a category from Table 3-3 to determine the appropriate exercise intensity level. If you cannot decide which category is the most appropriate, take one of the fitness tests at the end of this chapter. Your performance on these should place you in a category that reflects your physical fitness level.

The Karvonen formula is

$$THR = (MHR - RHR) \times TI\% + RHR$$

where THR is the training heart rate, or the heart rate that should be maintained during exercise; MHR is the maximum heart rate; RHR is the resting heart rate; and $TI\%$ is the training intensity (see table 3-3). Therefore, the exercise heart rate for a 25-year-old with a resting heart rate of 75 beats per minute and an average fitness level is calculated as follows:

$$\begin{array}{r} 220 \\ -25 \\ \hline 195\ (HR_{max}) \end{array}$$

$$\begin{aligned} THR &= (195 - 75) \times 0.70 + 75 \\ &= 120 \times 0.70 + 75 \\ &= 84 + 75 \\ &= 159 \end{aligned}$$

The training heart rate for this 25-year-old subject is 159 beats per minute. Assessment Activity 3-4 will enable you to determine your target heart rate for exercise.

Learning to take the pulse rate quickly and accurately is necessary to monitor exercise intensity by heart rate. Two of the most commonly used sites for taking the pulse rate are the radial artery on the thumb side of the wrist and the carotid artery at the side of the neck (Figure 3-1a and 3-1b). Use the first two fingers of your preferred hand to palpate (examine by touch or feel) the pulse. At the wrist, the pulse is located at the base of the thumb when the hand is held palm up. To find the carotid pulse, slide your fingers downward at the angle of the jaw below the earlobe to the side of the neck. You apply only enough pressure to feel the pulse, particularly at the carotid artery. Excessive pressure at this point stimulates specialized receptors that automatically slow the heart rate, leading to an underestimation of the rate achieved during exercise. The wrist is the preferred site for the palpation of the pulse rate. Palpate the carotid pulse if you cannot feel your pulse at the wrist.

Locate and count the pulse rate immediately after exercise stops. Count the beats for 10 seconds and multiply by 6 to get beats per minute. Regardless of which site you use, be consistent in its application. Some practice is required to locate the pulse quickly and count it accurately.

Another method for monitoring the intensity of exercise is to rate your subjective perception of the effort. On some days, exercise seems easier than normal, and on other days it may seem more difficult; therefore, it is important to adjust the intensity according to the perception of the effort. According to the ACSM, "the appropriate exercise intensity is one that is safe, is compatible with a long-term active lifestyle for that individual, and achieves the desired caloric output given the time constraints for the exercise session."[1]

The "Talk Test" is a simple subjective estimate that clearly demonstrates whether the individual is exercising too intensely. The intensity is excessive when the exerciser is unable to carry on a conversation without gasping for breath between each word or two. The remedy for such an occurrence is simple—*slow down the pace.*

Frequency

The *frequency* of exercise is the number of days of participation each week. The latest ACSM guidelines for improving physical fitness recommend that exercise be pursued three to five days per week for optimal results. Optimal results are the greatest gain for the time invested. Fewer than three days is an inadequate stimulus for developing fitness, and conversely, more than five days per week represents a point of diminishing returns from exercise and increases the likelihood of injury. Those who are exercising for health reasons and following the 1995 guidelines are advised to engage in physical activities on most, preferably all, days of the week.

You can overdo exercise—too much results in staleness or overtraining. The signs of overtraining include the following:

- Chronic fatigue and listlessness
- Inability to make further fitness gains or regression of the level of fitness
- Sudden loss of weight
- An increase of five beats per minute in the resting heart rate
- Loss of enthusiasm for working out
- Increase in the risk for injury
- Irritability, anger, and depression

Treatment requires that you cut back on training or stop completely for one to two weeks. When you resume exercise, it must be of lower intensity, frequency, and duration. You must rebuild and regain fitness gradually. Prevention is the best treatment for overtraining because people for whom exercise is a way of life are reluctant to discontinue training, even temporarily, for fear that they will lose their fitness edge. Convincing them that continuing to exercise is the worst possible action is extremely difficult.

Time (Duration)

Duration refers to the length of each exercise session. Intensity and duration are inversely related—the more intense the exercise, the shorter its duration. Some fitness

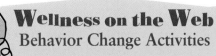

Wellness on the Web
Behavior Change Activities

Why Exercise?

How do experts define *physical fitness*? There's no general agreement, but most authorities endorse the concept of performance-related and health-related fitness. Like all aspects of wellness, you are responsible for developing an exercise program and sticking with it. Taking this step is much easier when you understand the importance of exercise as an integral part of a quality lifestyle. Stephen Seiler, PhD, is an endurance sport enthusiast and exercise physiologist who has a strong interest in the physiology of performance and in the role of exercise as "preventive medicine." To enhance your understanding of exercise physiology as it relates to wellness, read Dr. Seiler's articles at www.mhhe.com/anspaugh6e. Select Student Center, Chapter 3, Wellness on the Web, Activity 1. Scroll down the list of topics and read more about a specific area of exercise physiology as it relates to your wellness and fitness goals.

The Key to Your Heart

When we say someone is "heartless," we're speaking figuratively, not literally. From the moment we're conceived until we draw our last breath, our hearts work tirelessly to fuel the processes that give us life. In an average lifetime, the heart beats more than 2½ billion times without stopping to rest. Throughout history, this life-sustaining power has created an aura of mystery around the heart. Modern science has removed much of the mystery, but we continue to be fascinated and curious about this vital human organ. To explore the heart in detail, go to http://sln.fi.edu/biosci/biosci.html. In "The Heart: An Online Exploration," you'll discover the complexities of the heart's development and structure. You'll have the opportunity to follow the blood as it circulates through the blood vessels and the various body systems. Most important, you'll learn how to keep your heart healthy and how to monitor your heart's health.

experts employ the acronym "FIT Principle" as a means for people to remember the first three principles of exercise: F = frequency; I = intensity; and T = time/duration. Intensity is the most important consideration for the development of physical fitness. But reducing the intensity somewhat while increasing the frequency and duration is the safest and most beneficial method for novice exercisers to attain physical fitness and health enhancement. In 1990, the ACSM recommended 20 to 60 minutes of continuous or noncontinuous aerobic activity. The 1995 guidelines suggest the accumulation of 30 minutes or more of physical activity per day.[24]

Another way to monitor duration is to calculate the number of calories expended per exercise session. The ACSM recommends that, if you expend 300 calories per exercise session, you should exercise three times per week; if you expend only 200 calories per exercise session, you should exercise four times per week. These guidelines are sufficient for health benefits to accrue, but for fitness purposes, they should be viewed as a minimal level of exercise. There is a dose-response relationship between the amount of energy expended by exercising and all-cause mortality. The greater the dose, the greater the response and concomitantly the less the risk. One thousand calories expended per week will reduce all-cause mortality by 30 percent, and higher caloric expenditures further decrease the risk.[24, 25] (Table 8-5 in Chapter 8 discusses the way to determine how long you need to engage in the activities of your choice to achieve these goals.)

Progression, Overload, and Specificity

As people attain a level of fitness that meets their needs and when further improvement is not desired, the program switches from developing fitness to maintaining it. At this point, the principles of overload and progression may be set aside, but both are necessary for the improvement phase of fitness. *Overload* involves subjecting the body to unaccustomed stress. Challenging the body to periodically accept a slightly increased level of work forces it to adapt by attaining a higher level of fitness. Deciding when to impose each new challenge involves the principle of progression. The workload is increased only when the exerciser is ready to accept a new challenge. For aerobic exercise, target heart rate or perceived exertion may be used to establish criteria for scheduling the progression. For example, if you jog, swim, or cycle a certain distance, the exercise heart rate will decrease over time as your body adapts to training. When the exercise heart rate drops to a predetermined level or the effort required becomes comfortable, you should adjust the pace or distance to return to the original target zone. However, the new physical challenge should not exceed the current amount of exercise by more than 10 percent. This should ensure that the new workload is not excessive.

The principle of *specificity* of training suggests that the body adapts according to the specific type of stress placed on it. The muscles involved in any activity are the ones that adapt, and they do so in the specific way in which they are used. For example, jogging prepares one for jogging but is poor preparation for cycling. Cycling does not prepare one for swimming. Although these activities stress the cardiorespiratory system, they are sufficiently different in that there is little fitness carry-over among them.

The principle of specificity is particularly important for competitive athletes. Competitors attempt to maximize the returns from their training effort; therefore, runners must train by running, swimmers must swim, and cyclists must cycle. The focus is on maximal improvement in one activity, so that the body is trained in a specific manner. This locks athletes into regimented training programs, but noncompetitors who exercise for health and physical fitness reasons are not under such constraints. They can vary activities and prevent the boredom of participating in the same activity day after day, week after week. Cycling, jogging, swimming, racquetball, cross-country skiing, weight training, and other activities may be used in any combination or order for the development of physical fitness. This is the essence of **cross-training.** Not only does cross-training relieve boredom, but it may reduce the incidence of injury because it does not stress the same muscles in the same way during every workout.

Cross-training has many advantages and is an excellent technique for attaining the health benefits of exercise. Variety, the major attraction of cross-training, can also be a disadvantage, however. By participating in many different activities, you seldom become proficient in any one. However, if the objective is physical fitness or health enhancement, proficiency is incidental.

Identifying goals provides some direction for the activities selected and the way the principles of exercise are to be manipulated to increase the probability of success. Only one or two major goals should be selected, and these should be as specific as possible, so that an effective exercise program can be devised. Activities, objectives, and exercise principles must match.

When you have identified the objectives and know what you wish to achieve from an exercise program, identify the means for sustaining the program. The resolve to exercise is shakiest during the early stages of the program, usually because people push untrained bodies beyond their limits. This results in sore muscles, stiffness, and possible injury. Consequently, the dropout rate is highest in the beginning of any exercise program. The irony is that the greatest return for the effort is attained during this phase.[26] Some tips for sustaining that effort are presented in Just the Facts: Motivational Tips.

Other Exercise Considerations

Warming Up for Exercise

Warming up prepares the body for physical action. The process involves physical activities that gradually heat the muscles and elevate the heart rate. It is a transitional

~Just the Facts~

Motivational Tips

Follow these tips to stay motivated to exercise:

- Exercise with a friend. Make sure both of you have compatible goals and are similar in fitness level. Friends can help each other sustain a program, particularly during busy times when the temptation is high to push exercise out of an already crowded schedule.

- Exercise with a group. Exchange ideas and literature about exercise with group members.

- Elicit the support of friends and family. Their support is a powerful source of reinforcement.

- Associate with other exercisers. They represent an enthusiastic, positive, and informative group—and their values are contagious.

- Join an exercise class or a fitness club. This gives you a place to go and meet people who want to exercise.

- Keep a progress chart. This will give you an objective account of your improvement.

- Exercise to music. Music makes the effort appear easier.

- Set a definite time and place to exercise. This is particularly important during the early days of the program. Schedule exercise as you would any other activity of importance and then commit to the schedule.

- Participate in a variety of activities. Cross-training is excellent for the person who exercises for health or recreation.

- Do not become obsessive about exercise. Skipping exercise is not a good practice normally, but skipping is appropriate at times. Do not exercise when you are sick or overtired. Do not feel guilty about missing exercise for a day or two. Resume exercise as soon as you can.

stage that bridges the gap between rest and physical activity. For aerobic activities, the procedure involves physical movements that gradually raise muscle temperature, increase heart rate, and increase circulation. The intensity of the warm-up should be gradually increased over 5 to 10 minutes, ultimately reaching 50 percent of the planned exercise intensity.[27] Breaking out in a sweat is usually an indicator that the appropriate intensity has been achieved. The suggested warm-up for simple repetitive activities, such as jogging, cycling, and brisk walking, is to perform the specific activity at a lower intensity. For example, joggers should jog at a slower than exercise pace during the warm-up, gradually increasing the pace as the warm-up progresses. This procedure gradually warms up the muscles that are to be used during exercise

in the specific way in which they are to be used. Additionally, it reduces the oxygen deficit that normally occurs at the beginning of exercise. The oxygen deficit is the result of the body's inability to meet the oxygen demand of the exercise. It takes 2 to 3 minutes for the aerobic system to catch up and thus supply the oxygen needed to support the exercise. At this point, the exercise will feel more comfortable and can be maintained for a period of time. The oxygen deficit can be attenuated and possibly eliminated with a well-structured warm-up.

Increasing the heart rate gradually during the warm-up is most important. This allows the circulatory system to adjust to the load. If the heart rate elevates suddenly, circulation cannot adjust rapidly enough to meet the oxygen and nutrient demands of the heart muscle. The effects of this lag time are abolished in about two minutes, but increasing the heart rate quickly can be hazardous even during those two minutes, particularly for those with compromised circulation. Even a healthy heart may be affected when the gradual phase of warm-up has been eliminated. Abnormal electrocardiographic (ECG) responses were reported in several studies when the exercise sessions were not preceded by an active warm-up. Sudden strenuous physical exertion produced temporary left ventricular dysfunction and possible ventricular arrhythmias that were evident on the ECG.[10,28,29] However, another study failed to confirm the cardiovascular abnormalities cited in the previous studies.[30] The reason for the disparity in the results may very well be the difference in the assessment techniques used. In light of the equivocal nature of these data, a proper warm-up should precede exercise. The logic of this position has not been refuted.

Passive warm-up techniques, such as massage, sauna baths, steam baths, hot showers, hot towels, and heating pads, should not be used as substitutes for an active warm-up. These techniques may precede an active warm-up if a person feels stiff and sore from the previous workout.

Stretching exercises may be performed after the warm-up is completed. At this point, muscle temperature is elevated, so that stretching is more effective and muscle, tendon, and joint injuries are less likely to occur. Stretching is most effective during the cooldown following the workout because (1) muscles are heated and receptive to stretching and (2) muscles that have contracted repeatedly during exercise need to be stretched. Figures 5-1 through 5-8 in Chapter 5 illustrate some typical stretching exercises that may be used before and after the workout period.

Cooling Down from Exercise

The cooldown is as important as the warm-up. Cooldown should last 8 to 10 minutes and consist of two phases. The first phase involves approximately 5 minutes of walking or other light activities to prevent blood from pooling in the muscles that have been working. Light activity causes rhythmic contractions of the muscles, which in turn act as a stimulus to circulate blood from the muscles to the heart for redistribution throughout the body. This boost to circulation following exercise, often referred to as the *muscle pump*, is essential for recovery and shares some of the burden of circulation with the heart. The muscle pump effect does not occur if a period of inactivity follows exercise. An inactive cooldown forces the heart to work at a high rate to compensate for the reduced volume of blood returning to it because of blood pooling in the muscles. Exercisers run the risk of a hypotensive response (a sharp drop in blood pressure), which may result in dizziness and fainting. Also, elevated blood levels of catecholamines (epinephrine and norepinephrine) during the first couple of minutes of recovery may produce fatal heart arrhythmias.[31]

Light physical activity after exercise also speeds the removal of lactic acid that has accumulated in the muscles. *Lactic acid* is a fatiguing metabolite resulting from the incomplete breakdown of sugar. It is produced by exercise of high intensity or of long duration.

The second phase of cooldown should focus on the stretching exercises performed during the warm-up. Most participants find that stretching after exercise is more comfortable and more effective because the muscles are heated and more elastic.

Type of Activity

Many activities contribute to one or more components of health-related physical fitness. Activity selections should be based on objectives, skill level, availability of equipment, facilities, instruction, climate, and interest. Any rhythmic, continuous aerobic activity that uses large muscle groups and can be performed for an extended period is suitable for the attainment of health and fitness.

The President's Council on Physical Fitness and Sports (PCPFS) enlisted the aid of seven experts to evaluate 14 popular physical activities for their contribution to physical fitness and general well-being. Although this assessment occurred several years ago, the ratings are as valid today as when they were originally conceived. A summary of these appears in Table 3-4.

Selected sports have also been evaluated for their contribution to the health-related components of physical

 Table 3-4 Rating 14 Sports and Exercises

Exercise	Cardio-respiratory Endurance (Stamina)	Muscular Endurance	Muscular Strength	Flexibility	Balance	General Well-Being				Total
						Weight Control	Muscle Definition	Digestion	Sleep	
Jogging	21*	20	17	9	17	21	14	13	16	148
Bicycling	19	18	16	9	18	20	15	12	15	142
Swimming	21	20	14	15	12	15	14	13	16	140
Skating (ice or roller)	18	17	15	13	20	17	14	11	15	140
Handball/squash	19	18	15	16	17	19	11	13	12	140
Skiing—nordic	19	19	15	14	16	17	12	12	15	139
Skiing—alpine	16	18	15	14	21	15	14	9	12	134
Basketball	19	17	15	13	16	19	13	10	12	134
Tennis	16	16	14	14	16	16	13	12	11	128
Calisthenics	10	13	16	19	15	12	18	11	12	126
Walking	13	14	11	7	8	13	11	11	14	102
Golf**	8	8	9	9	8	6	6	7	6	67
Softball	6	8	7	9	7	7	5	8	7	64
Bowling	5	5	5	7	6	5	5	7	6	51

* The ratings are on a scale of 0 to 3; thus, a rating of 21 is the maximum score that can be achieved (a score by 3 of all 7 panelists). Ratings were made on the following basis: frequency, four times per week minimal; duration, 30 to 60 minutes per session.

** The rating was made on the basis of using a golf cart or caddy. If you walk the course and carry your clubs, the values improve.

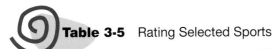

Table 3-5 Rating Selected Sports

Sport	Cardiorespiratory Endurance	Muscular Strength/Endurance		Flexibility	Body Composition
		Upper	Lower		
Badminton	M-H*	L	M-H	L	M-H
Football (touch)	L-M	L-M	M	L	L-M
Ice hockey	H	M	H	L	H
Racquetball	H	M	H	M	H
Rugby	H	M-H	H	M	H
Soccer	H	L	H	M	H
Volleyball	M	M	M	L-M	M
Wrestling	H	H	H	M-H	H

* *H,* high; *M,* medium; *L,* low. The values in this table are estimates that vary according to the skill and motivation of the participants.

fitness. These appear in Table 3-5. Lifetime sports (such as tennis, badminton, and racquetball) are more easily accessible than are team sports (such as volleyball, soccer, softball, and basketball) because fewer players are needed. Ideally, fitness should be developed and maintained primarily through self-paced activities (for example, jogging, cycling, walking, and swimming), but the challenge inherent in sports may be necessary to sustain motivation for some people. Lifetime sports are challenging and fun, and they offer variety. However, fitness attained from these activities depends on skill level and a willingness to exert maximal effort in competition. The orthopedic demands of these activities may be greater than a sedentary beginner can tolerate. Quick stops and starts, bursts of high-intensity activity, sudden changes of direction, and rapid twists and turns place a great deal of stress on the musculoskeletal system. The physically fit can handle the aerobic and musculoskeletal requirements of active sports, but attempting to "play yourself into shape" is a mistake. With knowledge of the principles of exercise, warm-up, cooldown, and the contributions of various physical activities to physical fitness, you can design an exercise program using Assessment Activity 3-5. See Real-World Wellness: Choosing Fitness Equipment for the Home on page 84 for helpful advice on exercising at home.

Environmental Conditions

People work and exercise in a variety of environmental conditions. Hot and cold weather produce unique problems for people who function outdoors. Their safety and comfort depend on their knowledge of the ways the body reacts to physical activity in different climatic conditions.

Heat is produced in the body as a by-product of metabolism. Physical activities significantly increase metabolism, generating more heat than normal. Heat must be dissipated efficiently, or it may build up, resulting in **hyperthermia,** abnormally high body temperature that can cause illness or even death. Human beings are homeotherms, which means that we function within a narrow range of internal body temperatures. Normal temperature ranges from 97° to 100° Fahrenheit (F). The average temperature is 98.6° F. Temperature control, or thermoregulation, represents a balance between heat produced by the body's metabolically active tissues plus heat gained from the environment compared to loss. The hypothalamus (a brain structure that maintains a constant internal environment) functions as a thermostat by decreasing heat production when the body temperature rises and increasing heat production when it falls. When heat is gained more rapidly than it is lost—such as during vigorous exercise—the temperature may rise to the point where heat stress illnesses may occur. Proteins that build body tissues and direct virtually all chemical processes can tolerate only small fluctuations in body temperature or they get too hot, change shape, and stop functioning.[32] At this juncture, heat stress illness may occur and may run the gamut from a relatively minor problem, heat syncope (loss of consciousness) to a major life-threatening medical emergency, heat stroke. *Heat exhaustion* is a serious condition but not an imminent threat to life. It is characterized by dizziness, fainting, rapid pulse, and cool skin. Treatment includes immediate cessation of activity. The victim should be moved to a cool, shady place; placed in a reclining position; and given cool fluids to drink.

Heat stroke is the most severe of the heat-induced illnesses. The symptoms include a high temperature (greater

Real-World Wellness

Choosing Fitness Equipment for the Home

I'm a working mother with two young children. My only chance to exercise is at home after the children have been put to bed. I'm most interested in purchasing a good piece of cardio equipment that will burn calories and increase my energy level. What advice can you give me for selecting such equipment?

Here are some helpful hints:

1. Some of the most effective cardio equipment includes motor-driven treadmills, stationary exercise bikes, stationary rowers, stair climbers, elliptical trainers, cross-country skiing machines, videotape aerobic workouts (with or without stepping benches), and jump ropes.

2. Selecting the right piece of equipment is important. Many well-intentioned home exercisers become bored with the equipment they purchase or find that it is not meeting their needs, so they quit exercising.

3. Try out a piece of equipment before buying it. Make sure it feels comfortable, is easy to use, and is the right size for you.

4. Give equipment the three-week test: Before making your purchase, borrow or rent the piece of equipment and use it three to five times per week for three weeks. At the end of three weeks, you should know whether you enjoy it well enough to use it regularly and whether it will meet your needs and goals. The best equipment in the world is useless unless you use it regularly.

5. Check the construction of equipment to make sure that it is sturdy. The machine should not rock or wobble, and it should perform smoothly.

6. Equipment made of lightweight sheet metal or with many plastic parts may not withstand regular use.

7. Do not buy the least expensive machine. Think of this purchase as a long-term investment. Usually a middle-of-the line product will do very well. These carry a 90-day warranty for parts, and the warranty may be extended to also include service.

8. Shop at a reputable sports equipment store that has a knowledgeable sales staff who can answer your questions and help you make the appropriate choice.

9. Make sure that the store will deliver and set up the equipment.

10. If marketing and promotional claims made for the equipment sound too good to be true, they probably are.

---

than 104° F) and dry skin caused by the cessation of sweating. These symptoms are accompanied by delirium, convulsions, or loss of consciousness. The early warning signs include chills, nausea, headache, and general weakness. Victims of heat stroke should be rushed immediately to the nearest hospital for treatment.

Mechanisms of Heat Loss

Heat is lost from the body by conduction, convection, radiation, and evaporation of sweat. Conduction, convection, and radiation are mechanisms responsible for heat loss *and* heat gain. These three depend on the difference between the temperature of the body and that of the environment. These mechanisms do not function alone to effect heat loss or gain.

Conduction occurs when direct physical contact is made between objects of which one is cooler than the other. The greater the difference in temperature between the objects, the greater the transfer of heat. An example is entering an air-conditioned room from outdoors on a summer day and sitting in a cool leather chair. Heat is lost through contact with the cooler chair, as well as the cooler air that is in contact with the skin. By the same token, sitting in a hot tub in which the temperature of the water is several degrees warmer than skin temperature results in the transfer of heat to the body rather than away from it.

Conductive heat loss occurs even more rapidly in water.[12] Water is not an insulator but a conductor. It absorbs 26 times more heat than does air at the same temperature. Air is an excellent insulator but a poor conductor. This is the reason that sitting at poolside is more comfortable than sitting in the pool, even if the temperatures of air and water are equal.

Heat loss or gain by *convection* occurs when a gas or water moves across the skin. Heat is transferred from the body to the environment more effectively if a breeze is blowing. Convective heat loss in water is increased when a person is swimming rather than floating because of the increased movement of the water across the body. The same principle applies to running outdoors because of the air flow over the body.

Humans, animals, and inanimate objects constantly transmit heat by electromagnetic waves to cooler objects in the environment. This heat loss through *radiation* occurs without physical contact between objects. Heat is transferred on a temperature gradient from warmer objects to cooler ones.

Heat loss by radiation is effective when the air temperature (ambient temperature) is well below skin temperature. This is one of the main reasons that outdoor exercise in cool weather is better tolerated than the same exercise in hot weather. Muscles fatigue more rapidly when exercise occurs in hot weather.[33] Exercise is more

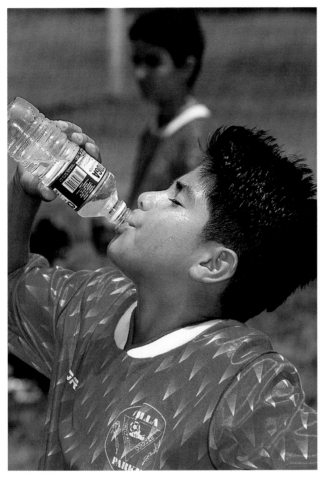

In hot, humid weather, drinking water and wearing loose clothing help prevent hyperthermia and heat stress illnesses.

difficult to sustain in hot weather because higher amounts of lactic acid are produced and greater amounts accumulate in the muscles, promoting fatigue and making muscle contraction more difficult.[34] Temperatures in the upper 80s and 90s often result in heat gain by radiation.

Evaporation of sweat is the main method of heat loss during exercise, and this process is most effective when the humidity is low. High humidity significantly impairs the evaporative process because the air is saturated and cannot accept much moisture. If both temperature and humidity are high, losing heat is difficult by any of these processes. Under these conditions, adjusting the intensity and duration of exercise or moving indoors, where the climate can be controlled, may be beneficial.

Heat loss by evaporation occurs only when the sweat on the surface of the skin is vaporized—that is, converted to a gas. The conversion of liquid to a gas at the skin level requires heat supplied by the body. As liquid sweat absorbs heat from the skin, it changes to a gaseous vapor carried away by the surrounding air, resulting in the removal of heat generated from exercise.

Small amounts of evaporative sweat remove large quantities of heat. For example, each pint of sweat that evaporates removes approximately 280 calories of heat. Beads of sweat that roll off the body do not contribute to the cooling process—only sweat that evaporates does.

Exercise in hot and humid conditions forces the body to divert more blood than usual from the working muscles to the skin in an effort to carry the heat accumulating in the deeper recesses to the outer shell. The result is that the exercising muscles are deprived of a full complement of blood and cannot work as long or as hard. Exercise is therefore more difficult in hot and humid weather.

Heat loss by evaporation is seriously impeded when a person wears nonporous garments, such as rubberized and plastic exercise suits. These garments encourage sweating, but their nonporous nature does not allow sweat to evaporate. This practice is dangerous because it may easily result in heat buildup and *dehydration* (excessive water loss), leading to heat stress illnesses. You should dress for hot-weather exercise by wearing shorts and a porous top. A mesh, baseball-type cap is optional. It is effective in blocking the absorption of radiant heat if you exercise in the middle of the day because the sun's rays are vertical. You do not need to wear a cap when exercising in the cooler times of the day or if the sun is not shining.

Guidelines for Exercise in the Heat

Guidelines for exercising in heat and humidity have been developed for road races, but these guidelines can be applied to any strenuous physical activity performed outdoors during warm weather. Ambient conditions are considered safe when the temperature is below 70° F and the humidity is below 60 percent. Caution should be used and people sensitive to heat and humidity should reconsider exercising when the temperature is greater than 80° F or the humidity is over 60 percent. People who are trained and heat acclimated can continue to exercise in these conditions, but they should be aware of the potential hazards and take precautions to prevent heat illness.

The keys to exercising without incident in hot weather are acclimating to the heat and maintaining the body's normal fluid level. Acclimation to heat is characterized by physiological adjustments that occur naturally from repeated exposure to exercise in the heat.[35] Acclimation includes the early onset of sweating, an increase in the rate of sweating, and the reduction of sodium in sweat. These adjustments result in less cardiovascular strain and a lower body temperature for a specific amount of exercise. The main consequence of dehydration (excessive fluid loss) is a reduction in blood volume. This results in sluggish circulation, which decreases the delivery of oxygen to the exercising muscles. Lowered blood volume results in less blood that can be sent to the skin to remove the heat generated by exercise. If too much of the blood volume is lost, sweating stops and the body temperature rises, leading to heat stress illness. Heat stress illness is a serious problem that can be avoided by following these guidelines designed to preserve the body's fluid level:

Estimating Water Loss

- Weigh yourself nude before and after exercise.
- Towel off sweat completely after exercise and then weigh yourself.
- Each pound of weight loss represents about 1 pint of fluid loss. Be sure to drink that and more after exercise. See Just the Facts: Fluid Consumption Before, During, and After Exercise.

Other Considerations

- Modify the exercise program by (1) working out during cooler times of day, (2) choosing shady routes where water is available, (3) slowing the pace or shortening the duration of exercise on particularly oppressive days, and (4) wearing light, loose, porous clothing to facilitate the evaporation of sweat.
- Never take salt tablets. They are stomach irritants, they attract fluid to the gut, they sometimes pass through the digestive system undissolved, and they may perforate the stomach lining.
- Exercise must be prolonged, produce profuse sweating, and occur over a number of consecutive days to reduce potassium stores. For the average bout of exercise, you do not need to worry about depleting potassium or make a special effort to replace it. The daily consumption of fresh fruits and vegetables, as suggested by the food pyramid, is all that is needed (see Chapter 6).
- Remember to use a sunscreen lotion when the weather is sunny or hazy. Be sure that the sunscreen you select has a sun-protection factor (SPF) of at least 15, and apply it liberally over exposed skin.

Guidelines for Exercise in the Cold

Problems related to exercise in cold weather include frostbite and **hypothermia** (abnormally low body temperature). *Frostbite* can lead to permanent damage or loss of a body part from gangrene. This can be prevented by adequately protecting exposed areas, such as fingers, nose, ears, facial skin, and toes. Gloves, preferably mittens or thick socks, should be worn to protect the fingers, hands, and wrists. Blood vessels in the scalp do not constrict effectively, so a significant amount of heat is lost if a head covering is not worn. A stocking-type hat is the best head covering because it can be

∿∿ Just the Facts ∿∿

Fluid Consumption Before, During, and After Exercise

The American College of Sports Medicine[36] has issued the following recommendations about fluid consumption:

1. Make a special effort to drink plenty of fluid every day, so that you will be fully hydrated prior to exercise.
2. For exercise lasting 60 minutes or less,
   - Drink a minimum of 1 pint (2 cups) of water about two hours prior to exercise.
   - Start drinking soon after exercise begins and continue drinking at regular intervals in an effort to replace the fluid lost from sweating.
   - Drink cool fluids (59° F to 72° F) flavored for palatability because cool fluids do not interfere with stomach emptying, they do not cause stomach cramping, and they absorb some of the body's internal heat.
3. For intense exercise lasting 60 minutes or more,
   - Drink fluids that contain a small amount of carbohydrates (sugar: glucose, sucrose; starch: maltodextrin) and sodium on a regular basis.
   - Regularly ingest carbohydrates to maintain blood glucose level and delay fatigue.
   - Ingest sodium in very small amounts (0.5 to 0.75 gram per liter of fluid) to enhance taste and promote fluid retention.
   - After the workout, continue drinking the same beverage until your thirst is satisfied and then drink some more.
4. Most exercisers are reluctant drinkers during workouts and do not drink enough to match the fluid they lose through sweating, but they should make a conscious effort to get enough fluid during exercise.
5. The general rule after exercise is to drink until you satisfy your thirst and then drink some more. The thirst mechanism of humans is a poor index of the body's need for fluid.
6. Water is an acceptable drink, but it may blunt the thirst drive before rehydration is complete. Therefore, find a tasty beverage that is noncarbonated, nonalcoholic, and caffeine-free to drink after exercise. Homemade lemonade, fruit juices cut in half with water to reduce the concentration of sugar, and commercial sports drinks fit the bill nicely.[7]

pulled down to protect the ears. In very cold or windy weather, use surgical or ski masks and scarves to keep facial skin warm and to moisten and warm inhaled air. All exposed or poorly protected flesh is vulnerable to frostbite when the temperature is low and the windchill high. Air temperature plus wind speed equals the windchill index. This value will help you know how to dress appropriately for outdoor exercise.

People often experience a hacking cough for a minute or two after physical exertion in cold weather. This is a normal response and should not cause alarm. Very cold, dry air may not be fully moistened when it is inhaled rapidly and in large volumes during exercise, so the lining of the throat dries out. When exercise is discontinued, the respiratory rate slows and the volume of inhaled air decreases, allowing enough time for the body to fully moisturize it. Coughing stops within a couple of minutes as the linings are remoistened.

Hypothermia is the most severe of the problems associated with outdoor activity in cold weather. Hypothermia occurs when body heat is lost faster than it can be produced. This can be a life-threatening situation. The adjustments made by the body to avoid excessive heat loss include shivering, nonshivering thermogenesis, and peripheral vasoconstriction. Shivering is the involuntary contraction of muscles. These contractions increase the body's heat production by four to five times that produced under normal resting conditions. Nonshivering thermogenesis raises body temperature through neural stimulation that increases metabolic rate. Peripheral vasoconstriction occurs from the neurally mediated contraction of smooth muscles located subcutaneously (beneath the skin). The contractions of these muscles constrict the small arteries beneath the skin, leading to decreased blood flow to the skin. This adjustment prevents unnecessary heat loss. However, hypothermia may still occur because these adjustments can be overcome by excessive exposure to cold.

Exercise in cold weather requires insulating layers of clothing to preserve normal body heat. Without this protection, body heat is quickly lost because of the large temperature gradient between the skin and environment. A layer or two of insulating clothing can be discarded if you get too hot.

Hypothermia can occur even if the air temperature is above freezing.[38] The rate of heat loss for any temperature is influenced by wind velocity. Wind velocity increases the amount of cold air molecules that come in contact with the skin. The more cold molecules, the more effective the heat loss. The speed of walking, jogging, or

Real-World Wellness

Exercising Safely in an Urban Environment

I live in a large city and like to jog outdoors in my neighborhood. How can I limit the risks associated with exercising in the heart of the city?

You can start by becoming familiar with the risks to avoid or lessen their impact. Some of the major hazards follow:

1. Traffic volume is one of the primary risks associated with jogging in a large city. This risk can be reduced by wearing reflective clothing, jogging during daylight hours, and jogging on the sidewalks rather than the streets. The best way to handle the problem is to find a nearby park or outdoor running track.

2. A second risk comes from air pollution, primarily carbon monoxide and ozone. The Centers for Disease Control and Prevention has identified outdoor exercisers as one group at high risk for the effects of ozone, carbon monoxide, and other air pollutants. Rapid, deep breathing during exercise results in inhaling more pollutants more deeply into the lungs. Some studies have shown that 30 minutes of jogging during heavy traffic conditions increased carbon monoxide levels in the blood to the equivalent of smoking half a pack of cigarettes.

Carbon monoxide interferes with the delivery of oxygen to the body's tissues and, when inhaled in high quantities, can cause illness and death. Carbon monoxide emissions from cars, trucks, and buses are most prevalent during rush hours, so avoid jogging on busy streets during these times.

Ozone causes lung inflammation and injury. The long-term effects of exercising in high ozone conditions are not known. Ozone tends to accumulate in the atmosphere after 10:00 a.m. It is heaviest during bright, sunny days because it is produced by the photochemical reaction of sunlight with hydrocarbons and nitrogen dioxide from motor vehicle exhaust.

Jogging before the rush hour begins will (1) help control your exposure to motor vehicle emissions and (2) allow you to exercise prior to the buildup of ozone in the atmosphere.

3. Joggers and other outdoor exercisers can be targets for crime. Carry no visible money or valuables, such as watches or jewelry. Carry an I.D. tag with your name and the telephone number of a family member or friend in case you are involved in an accident. Do not carry addresses, yours or your family's, in case you are mugged.

cycling into the wind must be added to the speed of the wind to properly evaluate the impact of windchill.

You should wear enough clothing to stay warm, but not so much as to induce profuse sweating. Knowing how much clothing to wear comes from experience exercising in various environmental conditions. Clothing that becomes wet with sweat loses its insulating qualities. It becomes a conductor of heat, moving heat from the body quickly and potentially endangering the exerciser.

If you exercise or work outdoors in cold weather, you may want to wear polypropylene undergarments.

Polypropylene is designed to whisk perspiration away from the skin, so that evaporative cooling does not rob heat from the body. You should wear a warm outer garment, preferably made of wool, over this material. If it is windy, wear a breathable windbreaker as the third, outer layer.

If you follow the guidelines for activity in hot and cold weather, you can usually participate comfortably all year long. Other hazards associated with outdoor exercise are discussed in Real-World Wellness: Exercising Safely in an Urban Environment on page 87.

Summary

- *Physical fitness* is defined in terms of performance-related and health-related fitness.
- Cardiorespiratory endurance is the most important component of health-related fitness.
- The long-term effects of physical training include modifications in heart rate, stroke volume, cardiac output, blood volume, heart volume, respiration, and metabolism.
- Aerobic capacity is finite, improves by 5 to 25 percent with training, and decreases with aging; this decrease is slower in those who are physically fit.
- The training effect is lost in stages if exercise is interrupted or discontinued.
- Exercise affects cholesterol levels, blood pressure, and triglyceride levels; may reduce the risks for diabetes mellitus and stress; and is an alternative method for quitting use of tobacco products.
- The principles of exercise can be manipulated to meet any exercise objective.
- Exercising by varying the activities per exercise session or during exercise sessions is cross-training.
- The heat generated by exercise is lost from the body by conduction, convection, radiation, and evaporation.
- Evaporation of sweat is the major mechanism for ridding the body of heat that develops during exercise.
- Hypothermia is the most severe problem associated with exercise in cold weather.

Review Questions

1. What are the physiological changes that occur from regular participation in aerobic exercise?
2. What are the health benefits that occur from regular participation in aerobic training?
3. Name and define the physiological changes that occur with exercise training.
4. Identify and define the principles of physical conditioning.
5. Define *cross-training* and give some examples.
6. Why should you warm up before exercise?
7. Identify and define the mechanisms of heat loss. Which of these is most important during exercise and why?
8. Describe fluid replacement before, during, and after exercise.

References

1. American College of Sports Medicine. 2000. *Guidelines for exercise testing and prescription.* 6th ed. Philadelphia: Lippincott Williams and Wilkins.
2. Editors. 2004. Exercise your right to health. *Harvard Heart Letter* 14 (July): 4–5.
3. Tanasescu, M., et al. 2002. Exercise type and intensity in relation to coronary heart disease in men. *Journal of the American Medical Association* 288:1994–2000.
4. Tomohiro, O., et al. 2003. Effects of exercise intensity on physical fitness and risk factors for coronary heart disease. *Obesity Research* 11:1131–39.
5. Malkin, M. 2004. Warming up, cooling down and stretching. *Fitness Management* 20 (January): 30–32.
6. Brehm, B. 2003. Stretching and flexibility: Changing ideas regarding benefits. *Fitness Management* 19 (February): 19.
7. Nieman, D. C. 2003. *Exercise testing and prescription.* New York: McGraw-Hill.
8. Powers, S. K., and E. T. Howley. 2004. *Exercise physiology.* New York: McGraw-Hill.
9. Franklin, B. A., and J. L. Roitman. 2001. Cardiorespiratory adaptation to exercise. In *ACSM's resource manual.* 4th ed. Edited by J. L. Roitman. Philadelphia: Lippincott Williams and Wilkins.
10. Coyle, E. F. 2001. Detraining and retention of adaptations induced by endurance training. In *ACSM's resource manual.* 4th ed. Edited by J. L. Roitman.

Philadelphia: Lippincott Williams and Wilkins.

11. Brooks, G. A., T. D. Fahey, T. White, and K. M. Baldwin. 2002. *Exercise physiology*. 3d ed. Mountain View, CA: Mayfield.

12. Wilmore, J. H., and D. L. Costill. 2004. *Physiology of sport and exercise*. Champaign, IL: Human Kinetics.

13. Williams, M. A. 2001. Human development and aging. In *ACSM's resource manual*. 4th ed. Edited by J. L. Roitman. Philadelphia: Lippincott Williams and Wilkins.

14. U.S. Department of Health and Human Services. 1996. *Physical activity and health: A report of the surgeon general*. Atlanta: U.S. Department of Health and Human Services, Centers for Disease Control and Prevention, National Center for Chronic Disease Prevention and Health Promotion.

15. Beckman, S. 2001. Emergency procedures and exercise safety. In *ACSM's resource manual*. 4th ed. Edited by J. L. Roitman. Philadelphia: Lippincott Williams and Wilkins.

16. President's Council on Physical Fitness and Sports. July 2004. Physical activity and health. *Fact Sheet* (http://fitness.gov/physical_activity_fact_sheet.html).

17. U.S. Department of Health and Human Services. July 2003. *Statistics related to overweight and obesity*. National Institutes of Health, NIH Publication No. 03-4158, July 2003.

18. Virmini, R., A. Burke, and A. Farb. 2001. Sudden cardiac death. *Cardiovascular Pathology* 10:211–18.

19. Mittleman, M. A., et al. 1993. Triggering of acute myocardial infarction by heavy physical exertion. *New England Journal of Medicine* 329(23):1677.

20. Willich, S. N., et al. 1993. Physical exertion as a trigger of acute myocardial infarction. *New England Journal of Medicine* 329(23):1684.

21. Pate, R. R., et al. 1995. Physical activity and public health. A recommendation from the Centers for Disease Control and Prevention and the American College of Sports Medicine. *Journal of the American College of Sports Medicine* 273:402.

22. Food and Nutrition Board, National Academy of Sciences. 2002. *Dietary reference intakes for energy, carbohydrates, fiber, fat, protein and amino acids*. National Academy Press.

23. American College of Sports Medicine. 1998. The recommended quantity and quality of exercise for developing and maintaining cardiorespiratory and muscular fitness, and flexibility in healthy adults. *Medicine and Science in Sports and Exercise* 30:975–91.

24. Rankimen, T., and C. Bouchard. 2002. Dose-response issues concerning the relations between regular physical activity and health. *PCPFS Research Digest* 3 (September): 1–8.

25. Lee, I. M., and P. J. Skerrett. 2001. Physical activity and all-cause mortality: What is the dose-response relation? *Medicine and Science in Sports and Exercise* 33:5459–71.

26. Brehm, B. A. 2002. Current issues in exercise adherence. *Fitness Management* 18 (March): 36, 38.

27. Holly, R. G., and J. D. Shaffrath. 2001. Cardiorespiratory endurance. In *ACSM's resource manual*. 4th ed. Edited by J. L. Roitman. Philadelphia: Lippincott Williams and Wilkins.

28. Foster, C., J. D. Anholm, and C. K. Hellman. 1981. Left ventricular function during sudden strenuous exercise. *Circulation* 63:592–96.

29. Foster, C., et al. 1982. Effects of warmup on left ventricular response to sudden strenuous exercise. *Journal of Applied Physiology* 53:380–83.

30. Chelser, R. M., et al. 1997. Cardiovascular response to sudden strenuous exercise: An exercise echocardiographic study. *Medicine and Science in Sports and Exercise* 29(10):1299–303.

31. Howley, E. T., and B. D. Franks. 2003. *Health fitness instructor's handbook*. 4th ed. Champaign, IL: Human Kinetics.

32. Editors. 2003. Don't let the heat beat your heart. *Harvard Heart Letter* 13 (June): 2–3.

33. Ftaiti, F., et al. 2001. Combined effect of heat stress, dehydration, and exercise on neuromuscular function in humans. *European Journal of Applied Physiology* 84:87–94.

34. Zuo, L., et al. 2000. Intra- and extracellular measurement of reactive oxygen species produced during heat stress in diaphragm muscle. *American Journal of Physiology* 279:C1058–66.

35. Bernard. T. E. 2001. Environmental considerations: Heat and cold. In *ACSM's resource manual*. 4th ed. Edited by J. L. Roitman. Philadelphia: Lippincott Williams and Wilkins.

36. American College of Sports Medicine. 1996. Position paper on exercise and fluid replacement. *Medicine and Science in Sports and Exercise* 28:1.

Suggested Readings

American Heart Association. 27 April 2004. Exercise is key to reversing obesity-related heart risk in children. *Journal Report*. (www.americanheart.org/presenter.jhtml?identifer=3020389).

This study found that the arteries of overweight children act like those of middle-aged smokers, increasing their risk for an early heart attack. But the damage can be reversed through diet and regular exercise.

Centers for Disease Control and Prevention. 9 March 2004. Physical inactivity and poor nutrition catching up to tobacco as actual cause of death. *Fact Sheet* (www.cdc.gov/od/oc/media/pressre/fs040309.htm).

This fact sheet presents statistics showing that poor diet and physical inactivity will soon surpass tobacco usage as the leading preventable cause of death in the United States.

Editors. 2004. But would you exercise to save someone else's life? *Tufts University Health and Nutrition Letter* 22 (May): 1–4.

This article discusses the many ways that people benefit from exercise while helping others. This usually involves walking for a worthy cause, such as breast cancer, diabetes, arthritis, and leukemia. These events help raise awareness about these diseases and raise money for research, treatment, services, and educational programs.

Editors. 2004. Can you be fat but fit? *University of California Berkeley Wellness Letter* 20 (July): 6.

Results of a study at the University of North Carolina showed that

1. People who were lean and fit had the lowest risk for premature death.
2. Those who were fat and unfit, especially women, had greater than 50 percent risk for premature death.
3. Those who were fat but fit reduced their excess risk by half.
4. For men, being fat but fit was much better than being lean and unfit.
5. For women, being fat but fit was equal to being lean and unfit.

Weil, A. 2004. Finding joy in movement. *Dr. Andrew Weil's Self Healing*, August 7. The ACSM guidelines for exercise for health enhancement are presented. For good health and an increase in energy level, Dr. Weil states that exercise is the closest thing to a "magic bullet." Some suggestions are given for starting and maintaining an exercise program.

20- to 29-year-old women

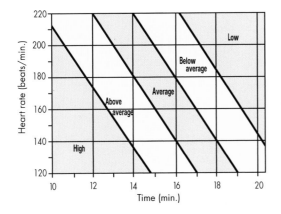

30- to 39-year-old women

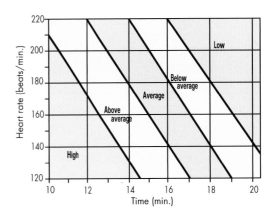

40- to 49-year-old women

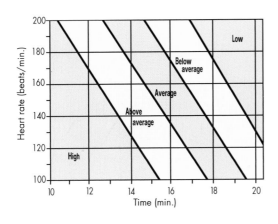

50- to 59-year-old women

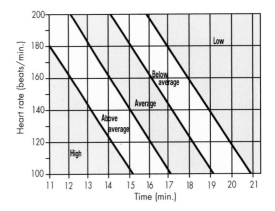

60-year-old and older women

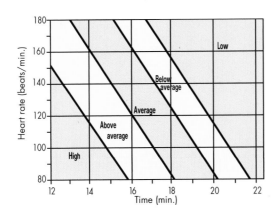

4

Building Muscular Strength and Endurance

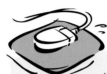 Online Learning Center

Log on to our Online Learning Center (OLC) for access to these additional resources:

- Chapter key term flashcards
- Learning objectives
- Additional goals for behavior change
- Concentration game
- Self-scoring chapter quizzes

- Additional lab activities

The OLC also offers Web links for study and exploration of wellness topics. Access these links through **www.mhhe. com/anspaugh6e**, click on Student Center, click on Chapter 4, and then click on Web Activities.

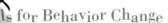 Goals for Behavior Change

- Begin a strength-training program or improve the one in which you already participate.
- Supply your close family members with at least five health-related reasons they should participate in resistance training.
- Identify the parts of your body where you would like to make the greatest physical change and explain why.
- Identify some of the tasks or sports that you perform daily, weekly, or monthly that would be easier to do if you increased your strength.

Key Terms

anaerobic
atrophy
circuit resistance
  training (CRT)
concentric contraction
eccentric contraction
hypertrophy

isokinetic
isometric
isotonic
muscular endurance
muscular strength
variable resistance

Objectives

After completing this chapter, you will be able to do the following:

- Explain the benefits of resistance training for older people.
- Define the different types of muscle contraction.
- Identify the various systems of dynamic and static exercise training.
- Describe the limitations of isometric exercise training.

- Explain the advantages and disadvantages of circuit resistance training.
- Define each of the principles of resistance training.
- Describe the short- and long-term effects of anabolic steroid use.
- Describe the health benefits of resistance training.
- Describe the progressive resistance technique that increases muscle endurance.

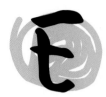vidence has been steadily mounting of the growing importance of muscular development for health enhancement, fitness, and aesthetic purposes. The muscular system improves through resistive forms of exercises, such as weight training and calisthenics. Resistive exercises complement aerobic forms of exercise, because each uniquely contributes to health, physical fitness, and personal appearance. Both types of exercise are required for a well-rounded conditioning program, and together they produce optimum results. However, best results are obtained by performing strength and endurance programs on separate days.[1]

Aerobic activities, which improve cardiorespiratory function and enhance health status in many ways, were presented in Chapter 3. Resistance exercises also contribute to physiological and psychological health. Many experts are convinced that resistance training is the only type of exercise capable of slowing, and possibly reversing, declines in muscle mass, bone density, and strength. Not long ago, these negative changes were considered to be the result of the aging process.[2] But today the evidence clearly indicates that a significant percentage of age-related losses are the result of *disuse atrophy.*[3] Disuse atrophy explains the loss of muscle mass and strength because of a sedentary lifestyle personified by low-level muscle stimulation well below the threshold for developing and maintaining muscle mass.[1]

The body contains more than 600 muscles, and 65 percent of these are located above the waist. All muscles, regardless of location, respond to the physiological law of use and disuse. "Use it or lose it" is an axiom that applies to all human beings during every phase of the life cycle. Americans tend to become more sedentary as they age. The declining stimulation results in a progressive shrinking and weakening of the muscles.

With few exceptions—notably cross-country skiing, rowing, and swimming—aerobic activities provide limited stimulation of upper body musculature. Sedentary living neglects the muscular system entirely and accelerates the loss of muscle tissue and body strength. The need for resistance training was illustrated in a study of runners during a 10-year period. Runners who did no resistance training suffered muscle **atrophy** in their upper bodies while maintaining muscle size in their legs.[4] Their arms, which received little stimulation from jogging, decreased in circumference.

Jogging is unable to stimulate the arms at or above the threshold needed for muscular development or maintenance, but the addition of resistive exercises can. This is an example of how the two types of training complement each other.

The Health Benefits of Resistance Training

Irrefutable evidence proves that strength training produces unique health benefits for people of all ages as well as for those with various types of infirmities. The American College of Sports Medicine, the American Heart Association, and the surgeon general's *Report on Physical Activity and Health* have all proclaimed and strongly supported the need for strength training for enhancing health and for improving quality of life. Strength training increases muscle mass and decreases the fat content of the body. The implications for weight loss and management are enormous, because muscle tissue is more metabolically active than is fat tissue. This means that the body burns more calories under any condition, including rest.[5]

An improvement in strength reduces the exerciser's heart rate and blood pressure while he or she is lifting weights. The practical application of these responses is that there is less stress on the heart when people lift or move moderately heavy objects in everyday life.[6] Heavy resistance training and circuit weight training have the potential to produce a high enough volume of work to improve cardiorespiratory endurance by as much as 5 to 10 percent.[7]

Resistance training increases the strength and endurance of the antigravity muscles, improving posture and producing less stress on the lower back.[2] Stronger, more stable joints are better able to withstand physical stress or trauma.

Strength training also enables one to perform the functions of daily life with less effort. Stronger muscles allow people to perform functional tasks that become more difficult as people age, such as getting in and out of a car, in and out of a bathtub, or up from an easy chair and climbing stairs. Dynamic forms of resistance training have a high degree of transferability to everyday activities.[8,9]

An increase in leg strength helps those who have osteoarthritis (wear-and-tear arthritis) because stronger muscles absorb a greater share of the physical stress at joints. In effect, stronger muscles spare the joint structures from some of the weight-bearing activity. Rheumatologists (physicians who specialize in the diagnosis and treatment of arthritic conditions) often recommend weight training to their patients because it alleviates symptoms and strengthens the muscles, tendons, and ligaments that surround the joints.[10]

An improvement in leg strength also leads to better balance and decreases the likelihood of falling, which reduces the chances that a fracture might occur.[6,8] Osteoporosis is a disease characterized by the deterioration of the skeletal system. Bone mineral content decreases, so that the bones become fragile and susceptible to fracture. Women are more prone to osteoporosis, but men are also affected as they age. People can protect the skeletal system

ᔕᔕᔕ Just the Facts ᔕᔕ

The Benefits of Resistance Training

Resistance training produces the following positive results:

• Increases muscle mass and decreases fat mass
• Increases strength and muscle endurance
• Increases basal metabolic rate (BMR)
• Develops the antigravity muscles (abdominal, lower back, hips, front and back of the thighs, both calves)
• Increases bone density (resulting in less risk for bone fracture)
• Decreases the risk for low-back pain
• Improves dynamic balance (resulting in less risk of falling)
• Improves mobility, such as that necessary for walking and stair-climbing
• Improves reaction time
• Contributes to more restful sleep
• Helps elevate the mood of mildly to moderately depressed people
• Improves body image, self-esteem, and self-confidence
• Improves the effectiveness of insulin in older adults
• Aids in weight loss and weight management
• May increase HDL cholesterol (the protective form)

by eating a nutritious diet and by participating regularly in weight-bearing and resistive exercise.[11] Resistive exercises are versatile, having the capacity to stress all of the joints and the bones that articulate with them, and they produce lateral forces that increase the thickness and density of bones, so they have the potential to prevent osteoporosis.[12]

The results brought about by resistance exercises allow people to live independently and with dignity as they age. Evidence indicates that Americans are living longer, and many will live with physical and functional limitations.[13] Illnesses occur with greater frequency and severity as we age, but much of the disability associated with aging is not due entirely to the aging process. Many authorities attribute at least 50 percent of these changes to disuse atrophy.[14] Our typically sedentary lifestyles, more prevalent among the aging population than among any other group of Americans, are responsible for a significant number of these illnesses. Those who stimulate their muscles regularly, regardless of their age, do not experience the type of physical deterioration observed in those who are physically inactive. Recent

research indicates that physical inactivity is responsible for the majority of age-related muscle loss.[10,15] The loss of muscle from aging and inactivity is referred to as sarcopenia, which literally means flesh or muscle loss.

Strength training also produces an impressive array of psychological and emotional benefits, which include improvements in self-esteem, self-confidence, and body image.[9,16,17] It helps improve the mood of mildly to moderately depressed individuals. Resistive exercise programs improve reaction time and may contribute to more restful sleep. Just the Facts: The Benefits of Resistance Training provides a summary of the positive outcomes that can be achieved through resistance training. Also see Wellness for a Lifetime: Strength Training for Older Adults (page 106).

Many cardiac patients participate in strength development exercise. Substantial benefits may be gained at minimal risk.[18] Improving upper and lower body strength allows cardiac patients to perform everyday lifting activities with less effort and greater movement efficiency. Also, strength training may have a positive impact on cardiorespiratory endurance, hypertension, blood fat levels, and psychological well-being, and it improves blood sugar and insulin control.[19]

Anaerobic Exercise

Strength development exercises are **anaerobic.** *Anaerobic* literally means "without oxygen," and when applied to exercise, it refers to high-intensity physical activities in which oxygen demand is above the level that can be supplied during performance. Short-term supplies of fuel stored in the muscles provide the energy for anaerobic activities. As a result, these can be sustained for only several seconds. Sprinting 100 yards, lifting a heavy weight, and running up two or three flights of stairs are some examples of anaerobic activities.

Muscular Strength

Muscular strength is the maximum force that a muscle or muscle group can exert in a single contraction. It is best developed by some form of progressive resistance exercise, such as weight training with free weights (barbells and dumbbells) or single or multistation machine weights.

Muscular strength is developed best through high-intensity exercise. Lifting heavier loads a few times to fatigue produces larger gains than does lifting lighter loads many times to fatigue. Weight trainers speak of the amount of work accomplished during the workout in terms of exercise repetitions and sets and in terms of the percentage of 1 repetition maximum (1 RM) for each exercise. A *repetition* is one complete lift of an exercise, beginning with the starting position, moving the weight through a full range of motion, and returning to the

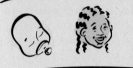

Wellness for a Lifetime

Strength Training for Older Adults

One of the realities of aging is muscle atrophy (decrease in size), resulting in a loss of strength, power, balance, and coordination. However, scientists have shown that a substantial amount of muscle loss is due to lack of appropriate physical activity rather than to the aging process. Engaging regularly in resistance exercises can build muscle, maintain muscle, and limit the loss of muscle tissue.

Inactive people can expect to lose approximately 50 percent of their muscle mass between 20 and 90 years of age.[20] This loss is accompanied by a 30 percent reduction in strength between 50 and 70 years of age. Data from the ongoing Framingham Study showed that 40 percent of female subjects 55 to 64 years of age, 45 percent of female subjects 65 to 74 years of age, and 65 percent of female subjects 74 to 85 years of age were unable to lift 10 pounds. The loss of muscle strength is most pronounced after age 70. Data show that muscle strength declines by approximately 15 percent per decade during the 60s and 70s and to 30 percent per decade thereafter.[21]

Because of this limitation, everyday functions taken for granted by the young become physical challenges, including opening bottle caps and jar lids, carrying groceries, and climbing stairs. If muscle atrophy progresses unabated, walking without assistance becomes difficult if not impossible, and the likelihood of falling increases.[22]

The good news is that the muscles of older people respond to training in much the same way as the muscles of young adults. Older people may make greater gains because of their initial level of debility (weakness). Studies have shown that the elderly can double or even triple their strength level in as little as three to four months of strength training.[20] Strength training also seems to have profound anabolic (muscle-building) effects in elderly people.

lifted 10 times but not 11. In other words, maximum fatigue occurs on repetition number 10, thereby preventing repetition number 11.

Do not attempt to establish 1 RM by lifting a maximum load for any exercise because untrained musculoskeletal systems are susceptible to injury. However, 1 RM can be safely predicted in a reasonably accurate fashion without having to attempt a maximum load.[23] The predicted 1 RM can be calculated by the selection of a weight that produces fatigue with fewer than 10 repetitions. For example, a subject can perform a maximum of 8 repetitions with 140 pounds in the bench press. From this data, what is this subject's predicted 1 RM for the bench press? The formula is as follows:

$$1\ RM = \frac{Weight\ lifted}{(1.0278 - .0278R^*)}$$

*R is the number of repetitions performed.

$$= \frac{140\ lbs.}{1.0278 - .0278\,(8)}$$

$$= \frac{140}{1.0278 - .2224}$$

$$= \frac{140}{.8054}$$

$$= 173.8,\ or\ 174,\ lbs.$$

Thus, 174 pounds is this subject's predicted 1 RM for the bench press exercise. One hundred forty pounds represents 80 percent of the 1 RM (140/174 = .80, or 80 percent). Eighty percent is more than a sufficient stimulus for developing strength and muscle hypertrophy (increase in muscle size). The American College of Sports Medicine suggests that beginners/intermediate participants should train with loads corresponding to 60 to 70 percent of 1 RM for 8 to 12 repetitions to fatigue. Our example subject with a predicted 1 RM of 174 pounds in the bench press would exercise with weights equal to 104 to 122 pounds.[22] Advanced weight trainers would select weights equal to 80 to 100 percent of 1 RM.

Children and adolescents (youth) should never lift maximum loads. In fact, resistive training for youth has been a controversial topic for decades. See Wellness for a Lifetime: Resistive Training for American Youth for a discussion of the efficacy and safety of resistance training for youth.

Muscle Contraction and Resistance Training

Muscle contraction is either static or dynamic. *Static contractions* occur when muscles exert force but do not move (shorten or lengthen). *Dynamic contractions* involve muscle contractions that are either *concentric*

starting position. Doing this 10 times in a continuous fashion is referred to as *10 repetitions,* or *10 reps,* and these 10 reps represent 1 *set* of that exercise. Repeating the entire sequence 2 more times completes *3 sets* of the exercise. One RM represents the heaviest load that can be lifted 1 time. Ten RM is a lighter load that can be

Wellness for a Lifetime

Resistive Training for American Youth

Evidence has been accumulating steadily over the last decade supporting resistive training for youth. The American Academy of Pediatrics, the American College of Sports Medicine, the American Orthopedic Society, and the National Strength and Conditioning Association strongly support resistive training for youth. The key elements of these programs are competent and skillful supervision and properly designed training programs.[24]

Resistive training is significantly different from competitive bodybuilding, Olympic-style weight lifting, and power lifting. The term *youth* refers to boys and girls who are prepubertal and postpubertal youngsters up to the age of 18.

The prevailing opinion, prior to the 1990s, among scientists, educators, and clinicians was that resistance training could not produce strength gains in prepubertal children. The reason given was that children were too young to produce testosterone, the hormone that is primarily responsible for increasing muscle size and strength. But recent studies featuring higher training volumes and longer workouts for children and adolescents have shown that gains in strength are not only possible but probable.[25]

Eight to 12 weeks of resistive training typically results in strength gains on the order of 30 to 50 percent. Percentage increases in strength among resistive-trained youth are similar to those made by resistive-trained adults.

Since children are deficient in testosterone, other mechanisms for developing strength become primary. Strength gains in children appear to be mediated by the nervous system. Neural adaptations to strength training include the recruitment of more motor units (one nerve and all of the muscle fibers that it innervates), motor unit coordination, and other factors. Learning contributes to performance as one's skill level on each exercise improves.

Muscle strength and endurance improve, but there are other benefits associated with resistive training, including an increase in bone mineral density, weight control, an improved cardiovascular risk profile, enhanced motor skills and sports performance, increased resistance to potential injuries from sports and recreational activities, and improved well-being.

Resistive training programs for youth should adhere to the following guidelines. They should (1) be developed and supervised by qualified professionals, (2) focus on proper technique instead of the amount of weight lifted, (3) gradually increase resistance as strength improves, (4) range from 6 to 15 repetitions per exercise, depending on age, needs, and goals, and (5) be varied to keep it fresh and challenging.

Resistance training is a safe and beneficial activity for youth of both sexes when the guidelines are followed.

(muscle shortening) or *eccentric* (muscle lengthening).[26] See Figure 4-1 for an illustration of each.

Some of the exercises commonly used to develop the major muscle groups of the body are shown in Figures 4-2 to 4-17. The anatomical charts in Figures 4-18 and 4-19 show the location of the muscles stressed in each exercise. These exercises are demonstrated on exercise machines and free weights, methods that are relatively equivalent and work the same muscle groups.

See Assessment Activity 4-1 for a method of determining your strength based on body weight and gender.

Static Training (Isometrics)

Isometric contractions (in which muscle length is constant) occur when muscles produce tension but do not shorten because the resistance is beyond the contractile force that can be generated by the exercising muscles. Examples of isometric contractions are pushing against a wall, pushing sideways or upward against a door jamb,

and loading a weight machine with poundage beyond one's capacity to lift. See Figure 4-20 for an illustration.

Optimal strength development from isometric contractions occurs with 5 to 10 sets of six-second contractions at 100 percent of maximum force.

Isometric exercises are effective for developing strength, but this approach has some important limitations. The most serious of these is a higher than expected rise in exercise arterial blood pressure and an increased workload on the heart throughout the entire contraction.[26] All-out straining isometric contractions should not be performed by people with heart and vascular disease. A second limitation is that strength developed isometrically is joint-angle specific. Maximum strength development occurs at the angle of contraction, with a training carryover of approximately 20° in either direction from that angle.[27] To develop strength throughout the muscle's range of motion, you must perform isometric contractions in at least three different points in the range of motion.

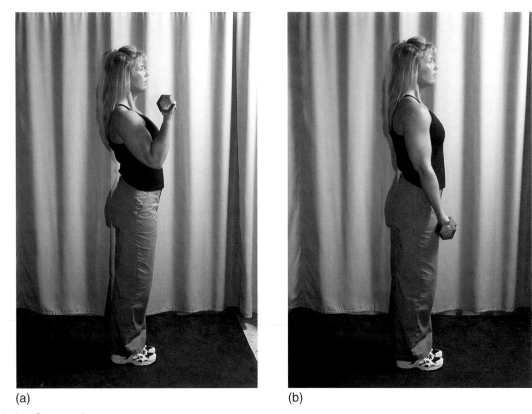

(a)   (b)

Figure 4-1 Contractions

The two types of contractions: (a) a concentric contraction; (b) an eccentric contraction.

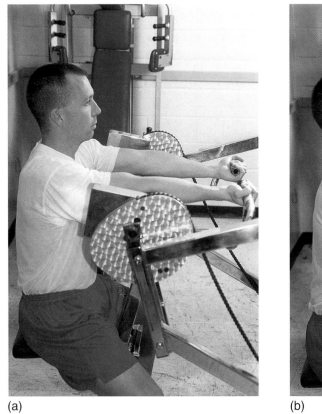
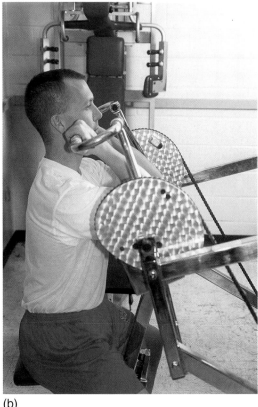

(a)   (b)

Figure 4-2 Biceps Curl

(a) Start with your arms extended, palms up. (b) Flex both arms, slowly move the weight through a full range of motion, and return to the starting position. The prime mover is the biceps brachii.

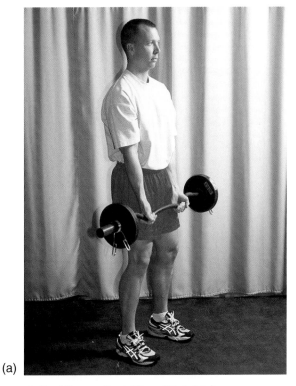
(a)

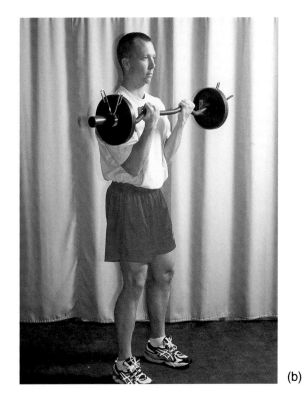
(b)

Figure 4-3 Biceps Curl (Free Weights)

(a) Start with the arms extended, palms facing forward. (b) Flex both arms and raise the weight through a full range of motion. The exercise above is performed in the standing position so the performer's knees are slightly bent to prevent excessive strain on the low back. The prime movers are the biceps muscles.

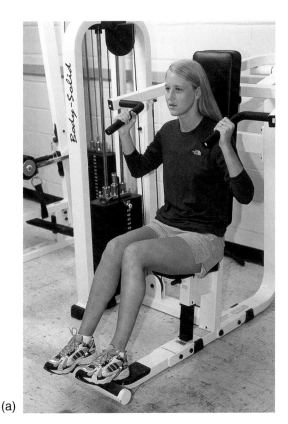
(a)

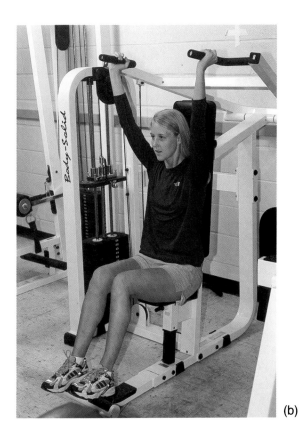
(b)

Figure 4-4 Overhead Press

(a) Sit upright with your hands approximately shoulder width apart. (b) Slowly press the bar upward until your arms are fully extended, and lower to the starting position. Avoid an excessive arch in your lower back. The prime movers are the triceps and deltoid muscles.

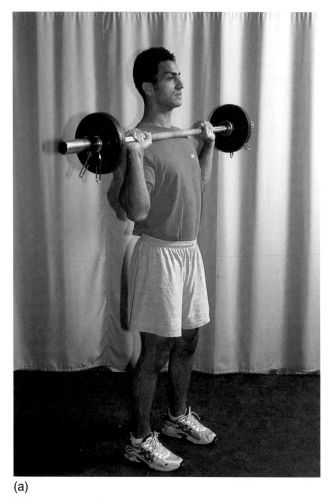

(a)

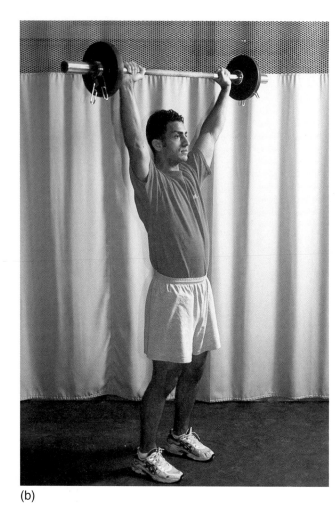

(b)

Figure 4-5 Overhead Press (Free Weights)

(a) Hold the bar at shoulder height. (b) Press the bar upward until the arms are fully extended and then lower the weight to the starting position. The knees are slightly bent throughout the movement to prevent excess strain on the low back. The prime movers are the triceps and deltoids.

Because muscles cannot overcome the resistance in isometric training, measuring improvement is difficult, constituting another limitation of this system. Improvements in strength can be measured if exercisers have access to specialized equipment, such as dynamometers and tensiometers, that record the amount of force applied. Motivation for exercise is difficult to sustain without feedback.

Research indicates that isometric exercise systems are as effective as dynamic exercise systems for developing strength. The question is not which system is better but which system best satisfies the intended use for the newly acquired strength. The transferability of strength to occupational and leisure pursuits is relevant.

Strength developed in the muscles is highly specific to the manner in which the muscles are trained. Muscles trained isometrically perform best when stressed isometrically; muscles trained dynamically perform best when stressed dynamically. There is some transfer of isometric training to everyday life. Carrying groceries, a baby, or

any object in a fixed position or pushing and pulling objects requires isometric strength, but most movements are dynamic, and transfer is more widely applicable from dynamic systems of training.

Dynamic Exercise

Dynamic exercises include **isotonic** (equal tension), variable resistance, free-weight, and **isokinetic** (equal speed) exercises.

Isotonic training

Isotonic muscle contractions occur when muscles shorten and move the bones to which they are attached, resulting in movement around the joints. Isotonic movements consist of concentric and eccentric muscle contractions. The **concentric contraction** occurs when a muscle shortens as it develops the tension to overcome an external resistance. The **eccentric contraction** occurs

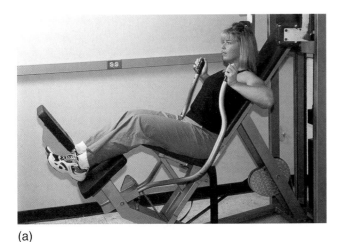
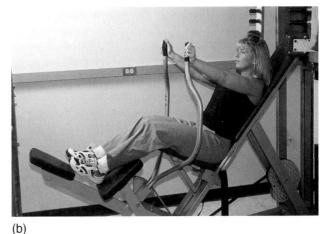

(a)   (b)

Figure 4-6 Bench Press

(a) Lie on your back with your knees bent and your feet flat on the bench to prevent arching your back. (b) Slowly press the bar forward, fully extending your arms, and return to the starting position. The prime movers are the pectoralis major, triceps, and deltoid muscles.

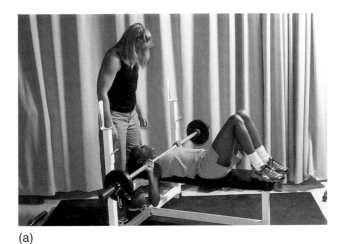
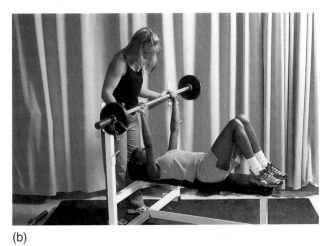

(a)   (b)

Figure 4-7 Bench Press (Free Weights)

(a) Lie on your back with knees bent and feet flat on the bench. (b) Press the bar overhead by completely extending your arms and return to the starting position. For safety, this exercise requires at least one spotter to assist the performer in returning the weight to the rack after the last repetition. The prime movers are the pectoralis major, triceps, and deltoids.

when the muscle lengthens and the weight (resistance) is slowly returned to the starting position. When muscles contract eccentrically, they are resisting the force of gravity as they lengthen, so that the weight is not allowed to free-fall. In general, muscles can produce about 30 to 40 percent more tension eccentrically than concentrically.[2,5,26] But no advantage exists for training programs that emphasize eccentric contractions. Research indicates that conventional isotonic programs develop as much strength and produce less of the delayed muscle soreness associated with eccentric contractions.

Isotonic exercises produce delayed muscle soreness 24 to 48 hours after a workout. Eccentric contractions cause microscopic damage to muscle fibers, their connective tissue, and the cell membranes.[1] Soreness occurs because the damaged tissues swell and apply pressure on the nerves. Delayed muscle soreness is more common among beginning exercisers, exercisers who attempt to overload too quickly, and those who change from one activity to another. Novice weight trainers should avoid intense exercise during the first 5 to 10 exercise sessions to minimize delayed onset muscle soreness and to allow time for the musculoskeletal system to adapt to the training stimulus. But delayed onset muscle soreness should not be completely avoided because the structural muscle damage that produces it and the subsequent healing process that occurs afterwards are necessary to maximize the training response.[5] In other words, beginners

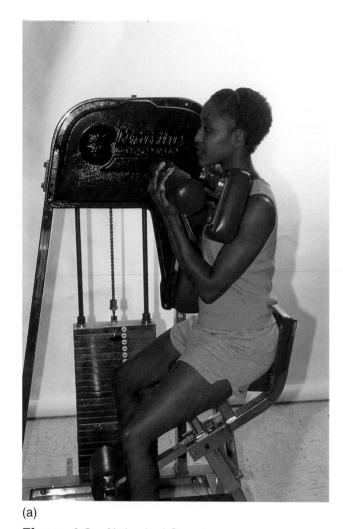

(a)

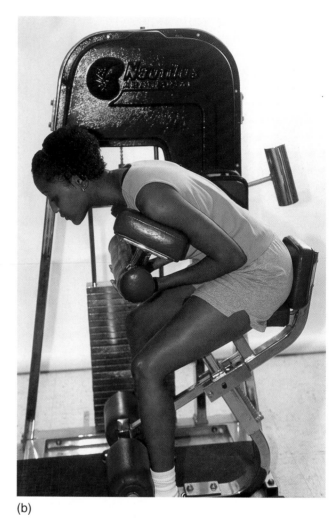

(b)

Figure 4-8 Abdominal Crunch

(a) Sit upright with your chest against the pads, hands folded across your stomach or lightly placed on the front pads. (b) Slowly press forward through a full range of motion, and return to the starting position. The prime mover is the rectus abdominis muscle.

should exercise hard enough to cause some muscle soreness the day following the workout.

Stretching exercises, light workouts, or complete rest may be required to alleviate muscle soreness. Prevention is the best treatment. Prevention involves allowing enough time to adjust to a new routine (at least one month), overloading the muscles in small increments (not trying to do too much too fast), and exercising within capacity. Because muscle soreness may last 48 hours, those who use isotonic exercise systems are advised to exercise no more than every other day. This schedule ensures that the next bout of exercise will occur after soreness has abated.

Variable resistance training

Variable resistance exercise equipment was developed because isotonic exercises do not maximally stress muscles throughout their full range of motion. The maximum weight lifted isotonically is limited to the weakest point in the musculoskeletal leverage system. The weight appears lighter at some points in the joint movement and heavier at others. In reality, the weight is constant and the human bony leverage system changes.

Variable resistance equipment is designed to provide maximum resistance through the full range of motion. Universal Gym equipment accomplishes this by altering the lifter's leverage. Decreasing the leverage increases the resistance at points in the movement where the muscles are strongest. Nautilus equipment uses a system of cams to decrease musculoskeletal leverage, which in turn increases lifting resistance. Variable resistance training challenges people to exert more force throughout the range of motion, which should result in greater returns. Whether variable resistance weight training is more effective than conventional weight training is yet to be resolved. Evidence indicates that it is as good and may be better, even though it varies the resistance imprecisely.[28]

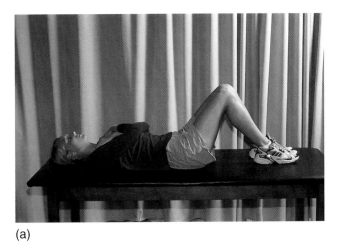
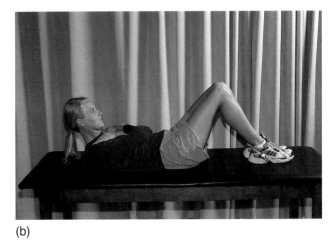

(a) (b)

Figure 4-9 Abdominal Crunch (Mat Exercise)

(a) Lie on your back (supine position), arms crossed over the chest, feet flat on the floor. (b) Lift your head and chest off the mat until your shoulder blades clear the mat. At this point, return to the starting position. The prime mover is the rectus abdominis.

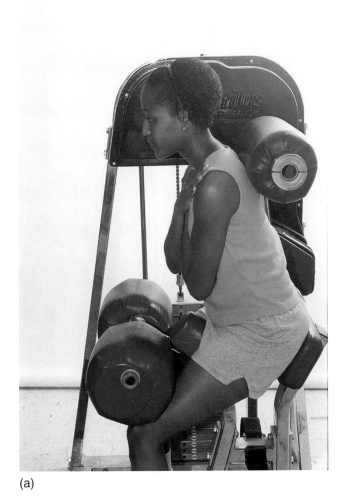
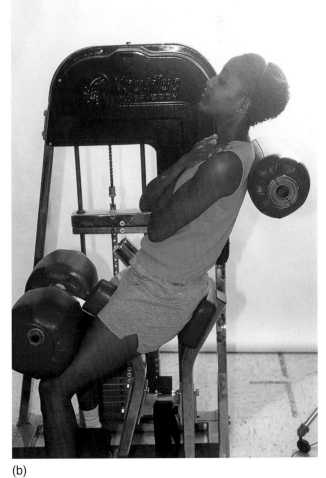

(a) (b)

Figure 4-10 Lower-Back Extension

(a) Place your thighs and back against the pads. (b) Slowly press backward until your back is fully extended, and return to the starting position. The prime movers are the erector spine and gluteus maximus muscles.

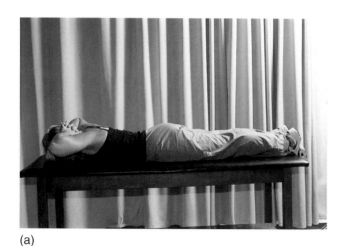
(a)

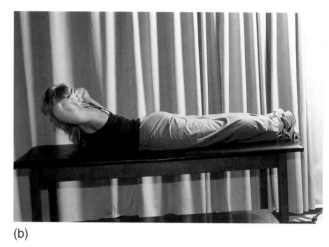
(b)

Figure 4-11 Back Extension (Mat Exercise)

(a) Lie face down (prone position) and clasp the hands together behind your head as shown. (b) Lift your upper torso off the mat. This should be uncomfortable but not painful. Do not hyperextend the spine. The prime movers are the erector spine and gluteus maximus.

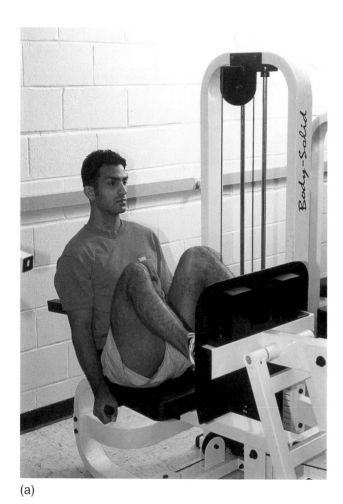
(a)

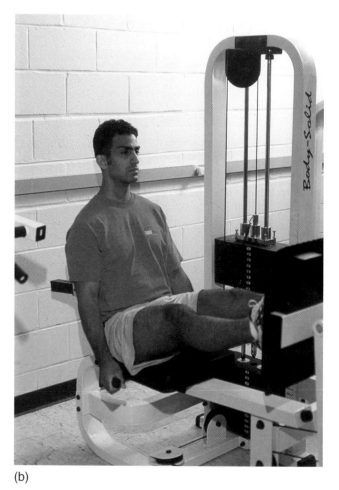
(b)

Figure 4-12 Leg Press

(a) Adjust the seat so that your legs are bent at approximately 90°. (b) Slowly extend your legs fully, and return to the starting position. The prime movers are the quadriceps and gluteus maximus muscles.

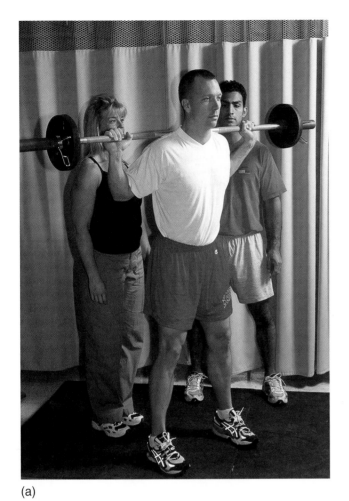
(a)

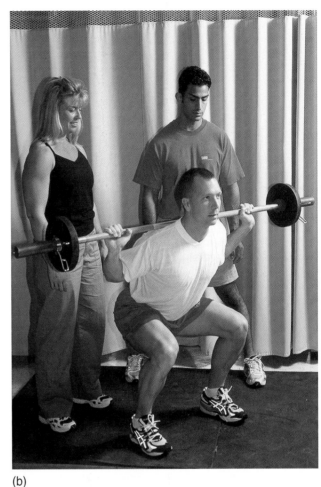
(b)

Figure 4-13 Half-Squat (Free Weights)

(a) Stand with the weight on your shoulders. (b) Squat down until your knees are bent at approximately 90° and return to the starting position. Keep your back straight throughout. There should be two spotters to place the weight on your shoulders at the start of the exercise and to remove it at the end. The prime movers are the quadriceps and gluteus maximus.

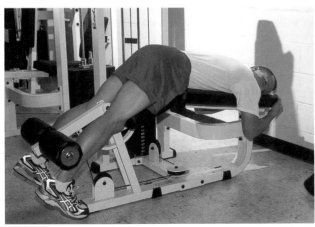
(a)

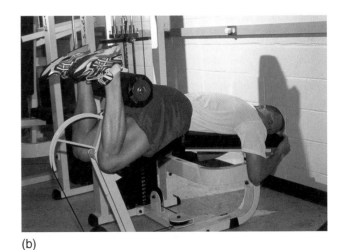
(b)

Figure 4-14 Hamstring Curl

(a) Lie face down with your lower legs under the pads. (b) Curl the weight approximately 90°, and return to the starting position. The prime mover is the hamstring muscle group.

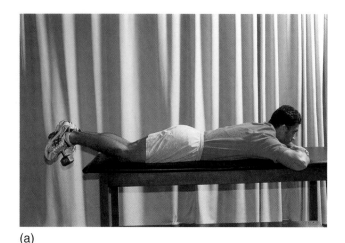
(a)

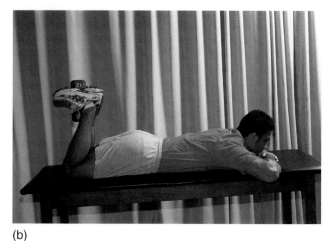
(b)

Figure 4-15 Hamstring Curl (Free Weights)

(a) Lie in the prone position holding a dumbbell between your feet as shown. (b) Bend your knees to raise the dumbbell to the vertical position and return to the starting position. Ankle weights can be substituted for a dumbbell. The prime mover is the hamstring muscle group.

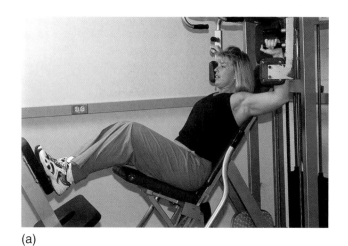
(a)

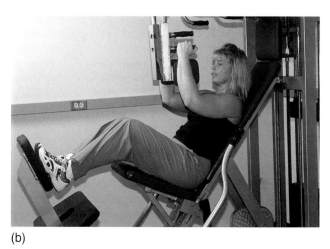
(b)

Figure 4-16 Chest Press

(a) Keep your upper arms parallel to the floor, bend your elbows at 90°, and place your hands on the handles. (b) Slowly push the bars until your elbows are pointing forward, and return to the starting position. The prime movers are the pectoralis major and deltoid muscles.

Free-weight training

Isotonic training with free weights continues to be an appropriate method of strength development. Free-weight training provides many advantages. For athletes, it yields some flexibility in strength development because the movements are not confined to a track. Exercises can be selected or improvised to simulate the movements required by specific sports, allowing the development of the muscles that will be used in competition. Concurrently, ancillary musculature that plays a supporting or stabilizing role for the major muscles is also stimulated and developed.

For noncompetitors, free weights have several advantages. The equipment is inexpensive and versatile. A starter set of free weights typically costs less than $150. Free weights do not require much space, so the workout can occur in the home.

The main limitation of free-weight exercise is that this system does not provide maximum resistance throughout the full range of motion. A second limitation is the need for one or two spotters to assist with exercises such as the bench press and half-squats.

Isokinetic training

Isokinetic resistance training involves dynamic movements performed on exercise devices that produce maximum resistance throughout the full range of motion. The movement speed is preselected by the exerciser

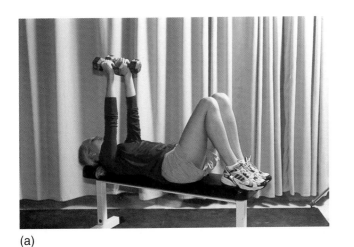
(a)

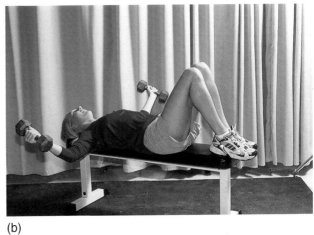
(b)

Figure 4-17 Lateral Supine Raises (Free Weights)

(a) Lie on your back, arms extended upward with a dumbbell in each hand. (b) Lower the weights laterally until the upper arms are parallel to the floor. Maintain a slight bend in the elbows throughout the movement. Then raise your arms in the same arc to the starting position. The prime movers are the pectoralis major and deltoids.

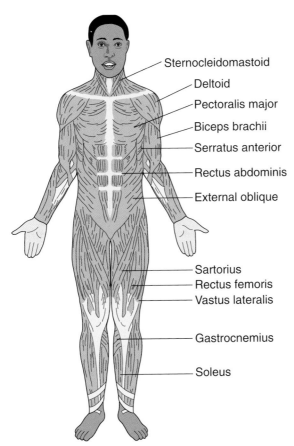

Sternocleidomastoid
Deltoid
Pectoralis major
Biceps brachii
Serratus anterior
Rectus abdominis
External oblique

Sartorius
Rectus femoris
Vastus lateralis

Gastrocnemius

Soleus

Figure 4-18 Selected Muscles of the Body—Front View

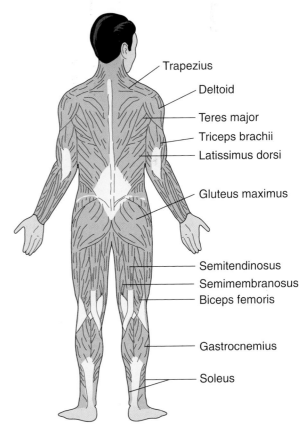

Trapezius
Deltoid
Teres major
Triceps brachii
Latissimus dorsi

Gluteus maximus

Semitendinosus
Semimembranosus
Biceps femoris

Gastrocnemius

Soleus

Figure 4-19 Selected Muscles of the Body—Rear View

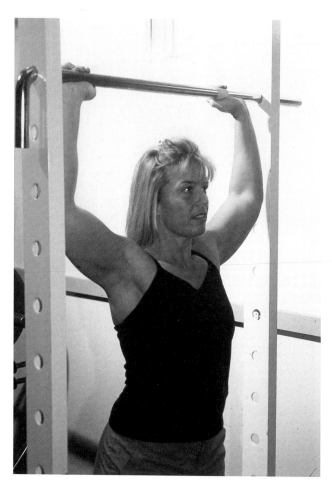

Figure 4-20 Isometric Contraction

An isometric contraction is a static contraction against an immovable object.

and remains constant throughout the movement. Isokinetic exercise theoretically improves on traditional and variable resistance dynamic systems.[29] Isokinetic devices adjust the resistance to accommodate the force applied by the exerciser. The greater the application of force, the greater the resistance to movement supplied by the device while the speed of movement is held at a constant rate. Maximum force applied through the full range of motion is countered with maximum resistance at all joint angles. This activates the greatest number of motor units and should produce greater gains in strength than other dynamic systems of exercise.

Historically, muscle fibers have been classified according to fiber type. The various fiber types and their respective percentages are influenced by genetics and exercise habits. The fiber composition of skeletal muscles has a significant influence on both endurance and power events. For more on muscle fiber types see Just the Facts: Muscle Fiber Types.

Circuit Resistance Training

Circuit resistance training (CRT) is effective for people who wish to develop several fitness dimensions simultaneously. Muscular strength and endurance, changes in body composition, and improvement in cardiorespiratory endurance can be attained together. Endurance is the application of repeated muscular force against a submaximal resistance.

A circuit usually consists of 8 to 15 exercise stations. The weight selected for each exercise station should equal 40 to 60 percent of 1 RM.[28,33] The exerciser does as many repetitions as possible for 15 to 30 seconds at each station. The rest interval between exercise stations should equal the exercise time spent at each station. The circuit is repeated two or three times for a total elapsed time of 30 to 50 minutes per workout. As fitness improves, overload can be applied by (1) increasing the amount of weight at each station, (2) increasing the amount of exercise time at each station (up to 30 seconds), (3) decreasing the amount of rest between stations, or (4) any combination of these.

The CRT system is challenging, versatile, and fun. Exercise stations can be rearranged, exercises that develop similar muscle groups can be substituted for each other, and the order in which the circuit is traversed can be changed. Because relatively light weights are used, the likelihood of injury is reduced. Circuits can be set up in small spaces. Machine weights are ideal for CRT because of the speed with which resistances can be changed, but free weights are adaptable to this system as well. The main limitation of CRT is that optimal gains in strength or cardiorespiratory endurance are difficult to achieve. Strength is most efficiently developed through lifting heavy weights combined with a substantial rest period between sets. Cardiorespiratory endurance can best be achieved through rhythmic and continuous activities, such as jogging, cycling, cross-country skiing, and rowing, performed for a minimum of 20 minutes per workout. An example of a circuit is presented in Just the Facts: Circuit Resistance Training.

Muscular Endurance

Muscular endurance is the application of repeated muscular force against a submaximal resistance. Inflating a tire with a bicycle pump, walking up five flights of stairs, lifting a weight 20 times, and doing 50 sit-ups are some examples of activities that develop muscular endurance. It is developed by many repetitions against resistances that are considerably less than maximum.

Research has shown that the greatest effect on muscle endurance occurs with submaximal loads that can be lifted 20 or more times.[33] Programs that emphasize low resistance and high repetitions produce limited improvement, if any, in *strength*. The primary stimulus of

~Just the Facts~

Muscle Fiber Types

In humans, muscles fall into one of two fiber types: slow-twitch, or Type I (also referred to as slow oxidative), and fast-twitch, which consists of two subtypes, Type IIa and Type IIb. The Type II fibers are called fast-glycolytic fibers because they contract rapidly without the involvement of oxygen.

Each fiber type can be identified by its speed of contraction, its contractile force, and its rate of fatigue. Type I fibers are aerobic, contract more slowly than Type II fibers, and are resistant to fatigue. They are slow to fatigue because of their rich supply of capillaries, myoglobin content, and number of mitochondria and mitochondrial oxidative enzymes.[30] The capillary density of these fibers allows for a greater exchange of oxygen between the blood and muscle fibers. Myoglobin, a compound similar to hemoglobin, accepts oxygen from the blood and shuttles it to muscle mitochondria, where it is used in conjunction with oxidative enzymes to break down foodstuffs to form adenosine triphosphate (ATP). As a result, Type I fibers are well equipped for endurance work. ATP is the actual unit of energy used for muscle contraction.

Fast-twitch fibers contract more forcefully and more rapidly but fatigue more quickly than Type I fibers. Their tendency to tire easily is due to a small number of mitochondria combined with very limited amounts of myoglobin.

Type IIa fibers are "intermediate fibers," or fast-oxidative glycolytic fibers, that are capable of using oxygen.

These fibers are adaptable to endurance training, and their oxidative capacity increases as a result. Endurance training converts Type IIb fibers to Type IIa fibers. However, the magnitude of change is approximately no more than a few percentage points.[31]

At this point, there appear to be no apparent age or sex differences in the distribution of muscle fiber type. The average male or female possesses 47 to 53 percent Type I fibers while endurance athletes range from 70 to 80 percent Type I fibers.[1] In contrast, power athletes have 70 to 75 percent Type II fibers.[1] The aging process results in a selective loss of Type II fibers, with most of the loss occurring from the Type IIb fibers.[32]

The ratio of slow-twitch to fast-twitch muscle fibers can be determined by examining under a powerful microscope muscle biopsies from selected sites in the body. The muscle composition of world-class aerobic athletes (distance runners, cyclists, cross-country skiers) is predominately slow-twitch, whereas the muscle composition of the world-class power or anaerobic event athletes (shot-putters, sprinters, power and Olympic weight lifters) is primarily fast-twitch. Knowing the ratio of fiber type could be important for these competitors, but it is relatively unimportant when one exercises for health reasons. Health enthusiasts can participate in a variety of activities with some degree of success and satisfaction regardless of fiber type.

~Just the Facts~

Circuit Resistance Training

The following is an example of a circuit. You should warm up before CRT and finish the workout with a cooldown.

Station 1	Leg presses or half-squats	15–30 secs.
Station 2	Bench presses	15–30 secs.
Station 3	Back hyperextensions	15–30 secs.
Station 4	Biceps curls	15–30 secs.
Station 5	Overhead presses	15–30 secs.
Station 6	Sit-ups or abdominal crunches	15–30 secs.
Station 7	Push-ups	15–30 secs.
Station 8	Lateral raises	15–30 secs.
Station 9	Hamstring curls	15–30 secs.
Station 10	Pull-ups	15–30 secs.

these programs is on the body's ability to supply blood and oxygen to the working muscles for them to contract on a repeated basis. Endurance exercises increase muscle capillarization and muscle myoglobin. An increase in muscle capillaries allows the muscles to accept more blood. The increase in oxygen carried by the capillaries is transferred to a greater quantity of myoglobin, which delivers it to the muscles. As with other types of isotonic resistance training programs, muscle endurance exercises should be performed no more than every other day.

Isometric, or static, muscle endurance is the ability to sustain, or hold, a submaximal contraction for a time.[2] Examples are carrying objects, such as groceries and other packages; pushing or pulling objects, such as a lawn mower; and carrying children.

Assessment Activity 4-2 presents a method of determining your muscular endurance. Assessment Activity 4-3 measures abdominal muscle endurance, and Assessment Activity 4-4 measures muscular strength and endurance with calisthenics.

Principles of Resistance Training

The principles of exercise—intensity, duration, frequency, overload, progression, and specificity—apply to resistance training as well as aerobic training. These principles were established over many years through research and experience. The current set of guidelines recommended for average healthy adults was published in 2002 by the American College of Sports Medicine (ACSM).[22]

Novice trainers should select loads (weights) that allow 8 to 12 repetitions maximum (RM). Intermediate and advanced trainers should use a wider loading range from 1 to 12 RM in a periodized fashion, gradually shifting emphasis to heavy loading (1 to 6 RM), with at least three minutes of rest between sets. Periodization is the introduction of variety into the resistance training program. Systematically adjusting the volume of work (repetitions and sets) and the intensity of work over a set period of time decreases the risk of incurring staleness. It also helps maintain motivation. Other recommendations advanced by the ACSM include the following:

1. Repetitions should be performed at a moderate speed—that is, one to two seconds for concentric contraction, one to two seconds for eccentric contractions.
2. Frequency of training should be two or three days per week for novice and intermediate weight trainers and four or five days per week for advanced weight trainers.
3. Weight training for muscle endurance should feature light to moderate loads (40 to 60 percent of 1 RM), more than 15 repetitions per set, and less than 90 seconds' rest between sets.

Intensity

Intensity refers to the amount of weight used for a given exercise. It is probably the most important variable in resistance training, and it is the most important stimulus associated with the development of strength and muscle endurance.[33]

The intensity level for resistance exercise varies according to the training system used. Optimal strength development through isometrics involves maximal contractions, 5 to 10 sets with a total contraction time of 30 to 60 seconds. Optimal strength development through dynamic systems of exercise should include 3 to 5 sets of 4 RM to 6 RM per set, with at least 3 minutes' rest between sets, and this should be performed three times per week. If muscle endurance is the primary goal, the workout should consist of 3 to 5 sets of 15 RM to 25 RM per set, with less than 90 seconds' rest between sets, performed three times per week. For bodybuilding or increasing muscle size, the recommended loading is 6 to

Wellness on the Web
Behavior Change Activities

How Much Do You Know About Muscle Strength and Endurance?

"Being buff" and "getting ripped" are key goals of many bodybuilders and other fitness enthusiasts. How important is muscle development for fitness, health, and aesthetic purposes? The body contains more than 600 muscles, and 65 percent of these are located above the waist. All muscles, regardless of location, respond to the physiological law of use and disuse. Americans tend to become more sedentary with age, and this decreased activity results in a progressive shrinking and weakening of the muscles. Go to the OLC at **www.mhhe.com/anspaugh6e**, select Student Center, Chapter 4, Wellness on the Web, Activity 1, to take a quiz on muscle strength and endurance. Answer the 12 multiple choice questions to test your current knowledge. How much did you know?

12 RM—that is, the weight selected should be light enough to allow a minimum of 6 repetitions but heavy enough not to exceed 12 repetitions.[22] There should be 1 to 2 minutes' rest between sets, and the exercises should be performed at a moderate speed. Multiple sets are needed to maximize muscle hypertrophy. Hypertrophy is an increase in muscle size.

There is a preferred order of exercise associated with resistance training. Large muscle multiple-joint exercises (half-squat, bench press, etc.) should precede small muscle exercises (biceps curl, triceps extension, etc.) because research has shown that, by first exercising the larger muscles the intensity of the workout can be increased.[22,33] The rationale supporting larger to smaller muscle groups is that exercises requiring the most muscle mass should be stressed while the exerciser is fresh. If the reverse order were followed, the smaller muscle groups would be fatigued, limiting their contribution to larger muscle exercises and thereby reducing the intensity of the workout.

Duration (Time)

The duration, or length, of each exercise session is dependent on the number of exercises, repetitions, and sets; the amount of rest between sets; and the time available to the performer. Conventional resistance programs (3 sets, 10 to 12 exercises, 8 to 12 reps) take about 50 minutes. Serious bodybuilding requires two to four hours in advanced weight training systems, six days per week. Availability of time and individual goals will dictate the length of the workout.

Frequency

Frequency refers to the number of training sessions per week. Dynamic resistance exercises (isotonic and isokinetic) should be performed every other day (seven training sessions every two weeks) or three times per week (six training sessions every two weeks). Near-maximum gains in strength for novice weight trainers occur with these exercise frequencies.

Isometrics can be performed every day because muscle soreness does not result. However, for physiological and psychological reasons, you should designate two to three days of rest throughout the week. Evidence indicates that alternate-day isometric training is 80 percent as effective as daily training.[28] However, daily training using maximal voluntary isometric contractions produces the best results.

Overload and Progression

The principle behind strength increase is straightforward—the muscles must be subjected periodically to greater resistance as they adapt to the previous resistance. This overload principle applies to all muscles, regardless of the system of training.

Overload may be applied by progressively increasing the amount of weight lifted or the number of repetitions performed or by decreasing rest time between sets. An increase in the number of repetitions leads to increases in muscle endurance, an increase in the amount of weight lifted leads to an increase in muscle strength, and a decrease in rest time increases muscular and aerobic endurance.

The principle of progression relates to the application of overload. It dictates how much and when an increase in resistance, reps, or sets or a decrease in rest time should occur. For example, the application of overload in a strength development program featuring 6 RM is accomplished by increasing the load when the exerciser can perform more than six reps on more than one occasion. The added weight reduces the number of reps that can be performed. Continued training improves strength and increases the number of reps. Once again, when the exerciser can perform more than six reps on more than one occasion, the weight is increased. This cycle is repeated for as long as strength development is the goal.

Specificity

The principle of specificity reflects the body's response to exercise. The type of training dictates the type of muscle development. Training programs that emphasize high resistance and low repetitions increase muscle strength and size. The gains are the result of muscle **hypertrophy,** an increase in the diameter of muscle fibers, and the recruitment of more motor units.

Training programs that emphasize low resistance and a high number of repetitions develop muscle endurance. The high volume of work increases the blood and oxygen supply to the muscles by increasing capillary density and muscle myoglobin concentration. Other adaptations are specific to the muscle actions involved, speed of muscular contraction, range of motion, muscle groups being trained, energy systems involved, and intensity and volume of training.[22]

The effectiveness of resistance training programs is based on the knowledgeable use of principles that guide such programs. However, other factors contribute to program effectiveness. These are found in Real-World Wellness: Other Important Considerations for Resistance Training (page 122).

Ergogenic Aids

Ergogenic aids are substances, techniques, or treatments that theoretically improve physical performance in addition to the effects of normal training. This discussion on ergogenic aids will be limited to a few of those reputed to accelerate muscle and strength development.

Many athletes and nonathletes take supplements of various types to accelerate muscle development. This short summary of a few of the many ergogenic aids suffices to show that some of these have performance-enhancing qualities, but many do not.

Protein Supplementation

The adult requirement for protein is 0.8 gram (g) per kilogram (1 kg = 2.2 lbs.) of body weight. Research has shown that resistance training may push this requirement to 1.6 to 1.8 g/kg of body weight.[34] Values such as these are easily obtained with the typical American diet, particularly for active people, who tend to consume more calories than does the average adult. Protein in excess of these values has resulted in no further gains in strength, power, or muscle size.[34]

Vitamins and Minerals

Physical performance is adversely affected by vitamin and mineral deficiencies. Those who have deficiencies can supplement their diets with the missing element or elements. However, the performance of well-nourished, physically active people is not improved through vitamin and mineral supplementation.

While vitamins do not furnish energy for muscle contraction, nor do they significantly contribute to body mass, they do provide functions that are crucial for normal energy metabolism, so it is important to obtain the daily requirement and then some. The antioxidant vitamins, such as C and E, may speed recovery from vigorous exercise. They also neutralize the free radicals (harmful

Real-World Wellness

Other Important Considerations for Resistance Training

In addition to the principles of resistance exercise, what factors should I consider to ensure the effectiveness and safety of my resistance training program?

Here are some other important factors for novice weight trainers:

- *Order of exercises.* Many people believe that large muscle exercises should precede small muscle exercises. This format allows one to train at a higher intensity level. Large muscle exercises, such as half-squats or leg presses, should be performed prior to hamstring curls; bench presses should precede triceps extensions. If small muscle group exercises precede large muscle exercises, fatigue (preexhaustion) is carried over to the large muscle exercises, which limits their effectiveness.

  Novice exercisers should not exercise the same muscles in consecutive exercises, because they are likely then to be less tolerant to the preexhaustion phenomenon that occurs from the buildup of lactic acid resulting from the previous exercise.

- *Rest intervals between sets.* The rest period depends on the goals of training. For example, if the goal is strength development, the rest period between sets should be 2 to 3 minutes. If bodybuilding is the goal, the rest period should be 1 minute or less. If circuit training is the system used, the rest period between exercises should be 15 to 30 seconds.

- *Speed of movement.* For the general public, speed of movement should be relatively slow and controlled. It should take 2 to 3 seconds for the concentric contraction and the same amount of time for the eccentric contraction.

- *Multiple sets versus single sets.* Although one set of each exercise performed two to three days per week increases strength, it is a minimal effort. Doing two to three sets three times per week is better.

- *Breathing patterns.* Most important, never hold your breath during physical exertion because this produces an extraordinary rise in blood pressure. Breathe rhythmically during exertion. The suggested pattern of breathing during weight training is to exhale during concentric contractions, while muscles are shortening, and to inhale during eccentric contractions, while muscles are lengthening and returning weights to starting positions.

- *Spotting.* Spotters are needed for certain exercises performed with free weights. These include multijoint exercises, in which weights must be returned to a rack on completion, and exercises during which weights need to be properly positioned. Half-squats and bench presses are examples of exercises requiring assistance.

- *Safety.* The chances of sustaining an injury from resistance training are relatively small, but as with all physical activities, the chance exists. Safety is enhanced by using correct lifting techniques, making use of spotters, breathing properly, maintaining equipment in good working order, and wearing proper exercise clothing.

- *Full range of motion.* To develop strength throughout the full range of motion, exercising muscles must produce force through complete flexion and extension. Be careful not to hyperextend or overextend, which can result in injury.

---

elements that may damage cells; they are the product of oxidation) that are produced during high-intensity exercise.[35] Vitamins C and E and other substances with antioxidant properties mop up and neutralize free radicals, but in the process become "used up" themselves. Free radicals are implicated in the aging process and diseases such as cancer, atherosclerosis, rheumatoid arthritis, and macular degeneration. Keeping them controlled is very important, and since vigorous exercise produces them, antioxidant supplementation is probably a good idea for very active people.

Creatine

Many, but not all, studies show that supplementing with creatine may enhance performance in short-term, high-intensity activities, such as resistance training. Creatine is a nitrogen-containing organic compound found in meat, poultry, and fish.[36] In addition to dietary crea-

tine, the body synthesizes creatine in the liver, kidneys, and pancreas from nonessential amino acids. A third source is supplemental creatine monohydrate, which comes in powder, tablet, and liquid form. Creatine monohydrate supplementation increases skeletal muscle creatine content for most people. It is particularly advantageous for strict vegetarians, who eat no animal flesh and have low dietary levels as a result. Creatine monohydrate supplementation promotes faster recovery from repetitive high-intensity exercises, so that users can perform a higher than normal volume of work.[37]

Evidence indicates that creatine supplementation is safe in the short term, but long-term data are lacking. It does not benefit the casual exerciser.

Ginseng

This herb has been used for centuries as a cure-all and an energizer. Theoretically, it improves physical performance by combating fatigue. In some animal studies, ginseng supplementation increased levels of free fatty acids in the blood while maintaining blood glucose level during exercise. Simultaneously, glycogen (stored sugar) values in the muscles were slightly higher.[38] This indicated that ginseng had a glycogen-sparing effect as the body selected the available fatty acids for fuel over glucose. Theoretically, this would improve endurance performance. However, studies with human subjects have not corroborated animal study results.

Chromium Picolinate

Chromium is a micromineral that contributes to carbohydrate and fat metabolism. Chromium may improve insulin's effectiveness in blood glucose regulation. Insulin has become an item of interest to those involved in sports and activities requiring muscle size, strength, and power because it decreases protein catabolism (breakdown of protein), increases protein synthesis (muscle building), and increases intramuscular availability of glucose.[39] When insulin is secreted into the blood, chromium is simultaneously released from the spleen, bones, and soft tissues. Chromium may facilitate the binding of insulin to cellular receptor sites, making it easier for the cells to receive glucose from the blood.

By itself, chromium is difficult to absorb. Chromium picolinate is a commercial preparation that is organic and somewhat more easily absorbed. Chromium deficiencies in the United States are rare.

The majority of available evidence to date indicates that chromium supplementation has little or no discernible effect on the development of muscle mass, fat loss, or exercise performance in humans.

Ubiquinone (Co-Q10)

Ubiquinone (Co-Q10) is a lipid found in the cell's mitochondria. It is an electron carrier that prevents oxidative damage to lipid tissues by donating electrons to free radicals (oxidants). Free radicals are rendered harmless when they receive an electron, so Co-Q10 functions as an antioxidant. Muscle concentrations of Co-Q10 decline with age, various disease states, and exercise.[35] As previously mentioned, physical activity generates free radicals, and physically active people should ensure an adequate intake of antioxidants through dietary and supplemental means, and this includes supplements of Co-Q10. Tissue concentrations were higher in physically active people but it did not seem to translate to improved aerobic performance in healthy people. However, there is evidence supporting improved physical performance on a treadmill in heart disease patients.[40]

Conjugated Linoleic Acid (CLA)

Conjugated linoleic acid (CLA) comes from the plant portion of the human diet. Animal studies indicate that CLA supplementation increases lean body mass; increases cellular responsiveness to growth factors, hormones, cellular messengers, and may deter catabolism (prevents the breakdown of muscle tissue).[39] Growth factors include strength training and various amino acids. The hormones include growth hormone, thyroid hormone, insulin, and sex hormones. The cellular messengers include chemical and neural transporters. However, human studies are scarce. One study showed a slight increase in arm girth and leg strength in a group receiving CLA versus a group receiving a placebo. Another study found improvement in bone mineral content and immune states in those subjects taking supplemental CLA. Obviously, more research is needed to evaluate the effectiveness as well as the safety of long-term use.

Androstenedione (Andro)

Androstenedione (andro) is a precursor hormone to the male hormone testosterone. It is manufactured in the adrenal glands, which sit atop the kidneys.[5] Proponents of andro claim that it burns fat, builds muscle, and slows aging. Studies in males of all ages have shown that andro did not increase testosterone level and did not contribute to muscle mass or strength gains in weight training subjects.[41] Half of the subjects received andro, while the other half were given a look-alike placebo. Strength gains and increases in muscle mass were equal in both groups, indicating that the gains made were solely the result of the weight training program. The conclusion at this time is that andro does not seem to be effective. Furthermore, the health effects of long-term use are unknown.

Human Growth Hormone (hGH)

Human growth hormone (hGH) is secreted by the pituitary gland, which historically was referred to as the body's master gland because it secretes a number of hormones that affect other glands and organs. But the consensus today is that the pituitary gland is controlled by the hypothalamus and functions more as a relay between the central nervous system and peripheral endocrine glands.

Human growth hormone, in the recent past, had to be extracted from human cadavers. It was in short supply and expensive. Now it is made in laboratories, it is still expensive, but limited supplies are no longer a problem. It is reputed to build skeletal mass, decrease fat mass, increase muscle mass, and shorten recovery from intense exercise.[2] Placebo-controlled studies do not support these claims in young, healthy, physically active subjects.

The major medical problem associated with human growth hormone usage in adults is the risk of developing

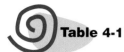

Table 4-1 Overview of Anabolic Steroid Effects

Effects Supported by Strong Evidence in Males and Females

Stunted growth when taken before puberty	Deepening of the voice (in women)
Coronary artery disease	Menstrual irregularities (in women)
Low HDL cholesterol	
Sterility, low sperm count (in men)	Development of facial and body hair (in women)
Liver tumors and liver disease	Decreased breast size (in women)
Death	Clitoris enlargement (in women)
Acne	
Water retention	Fetal damage (when taken during pregnancy)
Oily, thickened skin	
Male-pattern baldness (in women)	

Possible Effects in Males and Females

Diarrhea	Bone pains
Muscle cramps	Impotence (in men)
Breast development (in men)	Sexual problems
Aggressive behavior	High blood pressure
Headache	Kidney disease
Nausea	Depression

SOURCE: Adapted from Nieman, D. C. 2003. *Exercise testing and prescription.* New York: McGraw-Hill.

acromegaly. Acromegaly is a disorder that results in the growth and thickening of the bones of the brow, jaw, hands, and feet long after the skeleton's normal growth has ended. The internal organs also enlarge and the victim suffers muscle and joint weakness and ultimately heart disease. Cardiomyopathy is a serious disease of the heart that involves inflammation and reduced heart muscle function. It is the most frequent cause of death from human growth hormone usage; diabetes and hypertension are other reported side effects.

Anabolic-Androgenic Steroids

Anabolic-androgenic steroids are hormones. Their anabolic properties contribute to muscle enlargement, while their androgenic properties produce masculinizing effects. They build muscle mass and strength, and as a result, they improve, in some people's estimation, physical appearance and physical performance.

Anabolic steroid use by nonathletes is on the rise. This is particularly true for young men. A nationwide survey of 3,403 male high school seniors indicated that 6.6 percent of this group were current users or had pre-

viously been users of steroids and that 25 percent of the current users showed signs of dependency.[42] According to this report, the improvement in physical appearance reputed to occur with steroid use, accompanied by peer approval of those physical changes, functioned as a powerful reinforcer for continued use. Heavy steroid users were more likely than light users to take two or more steroids simultaneously and more apt to take these drugs by injection rather than in pill form. Injection as a method of delivery is highly characteristic of drugs that involve addiction. The steroid "hook" is insidious and powerful: 30 percent of the heavy users stated that they would not discontinue steroid use if steroids were proved to cause liver cancer, 31 percent would not stop if they were proved to cause heart attacks, and 39 percent would not stop if they were proved to cause infertility.[43]

Although definitive evidence of the long-term effects of steroid use is not available, the potential for long-term harm is certainly real. Predicting how and when the effects of steroids will be manifested is impossible because people respond differently to these drugs as a result of differences in body chemistry. The steroid effect is complicated further by the fact that black market preparations contain additives, and some preparations are contaminated. The potential for harm is readily discernible; 80 to 90 percent of steroids used are purchased through the black market. Table 4-1 presents some of the known and possible effects of steroid use.

Keeping a Daily Training Log

Beginning weight trainers should keep a daily log of their training activities. The advantages of keeping such a record far outweigh the minimal amount of bother, time, and effort required to make the entries during the workout. Each entry should be recorded during the rest period between sets.

The advantages of maintaining a daily training log include the following:

- You will always know which exercises you performed and the amount of weight used for each.
- You will always know the number of repetitions and sets that you performed of each exercise.
- The training log provides an objective account of your improvement. You can compare the amount of weight you are currently lifting with the amount at the beginning of your training.
- The training log provides an accurate history.
- The training log is a motivating device that provides objective feedback of performance improvement.

A sample training log is shown in Figure 4-21. A blank training log is given in Assessment Activity 4-5 for you to use to document your resistance training program. It will be helpful to make additional copies of this training log.

Name Cathy Smith   Starting date Jan. 1, 2005

Program objectives To gain strength and muscle definition

Exercise	Jan. 1			Jan. 3			Jan. 5			Jan. 7			Jan. 9			Jan. 11			Jan. 13		
	Resis. (lbs.)	Reps	Sets	Resis. (lbs.)	Reps	Sets	Resis. (lbs.)	Reps	Sets	Resis. (lbs.)	Reps	Sets	Resis. (lbs.)	Reps	Sets	Resis. (lbs.)	Reps	Sets	Resis. (lbs.)	Reps	Sets
1. Bench press	60	10	3																		
2. Biceps curl	25	10	3																		
3. Back extension	80	10	3																		
4. Leg press	150	10	3																		
5. Hamstring curl	30	10	3																		
6. Chest press	30	10	3																		
7. Abdominal crunch	—	25	3																		
8. Overhead press	35	10	3																		

Figure 4-21 Sample Training Log

Resistance (abbreviated as *Resis.*) refers to the amount of weight (in pounds) lifted or pressed. *Reps* (for *repetitions*) is the number of times the weight is lifted or pressed. *Sets* are the groups of reps.

Summary

- The physiological law of use and disuse applies to all human beings during all phases of the life cycle.
- The muscular systems of older adults are trainable and respond to resistance training with an increase in strength and muscle size.
- Muscular strength is the maximum force that a muscle or muscle group can exert in a single contraction.
- Dynamic exercises consist of concentric and eccentric muscle contractions.
- Isotonic exercises are dynamic in that muscles shorten and lengthen, producing movement around a joint.
- Variable resistance exercise equipment is designed to provide maximum resistance throughout the full range of motion.
- Circuit resistance training is a versatile system that allows a person to develop several fitness dimensions simultaneously.

- The principles of exercise—intensity, duration, frequency, overload, progression, and specificity—apply to resistance training. These can be manipulated to meet all muscle development objectives.
- Muscle fiber types are influenced by genetics and exercise habits.
- The suggested breathing pattern during resistive exercises is to exhale during the concentric contraction and inhale during the eccentric contraction.
- Many studies have shown that creatine supplementation may enhance performance in short-term, high-intensity activities.
- Anabolic steroids are performance-enhancing drugs that are harmful and illegal.
- Research in the last decade has shown that resistance training contributes to wellness in a variety of ways.
- Muscle endurance is the ability to apply repeated muscular force.

Review Questions

1. Define *muscular strength* and *muscular endurance*.
2. What are the differences among isometric, isotonic, isokinetic, and variable resistance exercises?
3. What are concentric and eccentric contractions?
4. What are the health benefits of participating in resistance exercise?

5. Name and define the principles of conditioning as they relate to resistance training.
6. What are the health consequences and physical performance benefits of steroid use?

References

1. Powers, S. K., and E. T. Howley. 2004. *Exercise physiology.* 5th ed. New York: McGraw-Hill.
2. Nieman, D. C. 2003. *Exercise testing and prescription.* 5th ed. New York: McGraw-Hill.
3. Dudley, G. A., and L. L. Ploutz-Snyder. 2001. Deconditioning and bed rest; musculoskeletal response. In *ACSM's resource manual.* 4th ed. Edited by J. L. Roitman. Philadelphia: Lippincott Williams and Wilkins.
4. American College of Sports Medicine. 1998. The recommended quantity and quality of exercise for developing and maintaining cardiorespiratory and muscular fitness and flexibility in healthy adults. *Medicine and Science in Sports and Exercise* 30(6):975.
5. Wilmore, J. H., and D. L. Costill. 2004. *Physiology of sport and exercise.* 3d ed. Champaign, IL: Human Kinetics.
6. Bryant, C. X., J. A. Peterson, and B. A. Franklin. 1998. Fountain of youth. *Fitness Management* 14(10):44.

7. Kraemer, W. J., J. S. Volek, and S. J. Fleck. 2001. Chronic musculoskeletal adaptations to resistance training. In *ACSM's resource manual.* 4th ed. Edited by J. L. Roitman. Philadelphia: Lippincott Williams and Wilkins.
8. Spain, C. G., and B. D. Franks. 2001. Healthy people 2010: Physical activity and fitness. *PCPFS Research Digest* 3(13):1–16.
9. Editors. 2004. Why everyone needs strength training. *University of California Berkeley Wellness Letter* 20 (May): 4–5.
10. Harvard University. 1998. Stay strong longer with weight training. *Harvard Health Letter* 23(12):1.
11. Kostuik, J. P., S. M. Jande Beur, and S. Margolis. 2004. *Back pain and osteoporosis.* Baltimore: Johns Hopkins Medicine.
12. Dawson-Hughes, B. 2003. Medical community far behind in preventing osteoporosis. *Tufts University Health and Nutrition Letter* 21 (October): 3.

13. Wagner, D. K., et al. 2001. Summary measures of population health: Addressing the first goal of healthy people 2010, improving health expectancy. *Statistical Notes* no. 22. Hyattsville, MD: National Center for Health Statistics.
14. U.S. Department of Health and Human Services. 1996. *Physical activity and health: A report of the surgeon general.* Atlanta, GA: U.S. Department of Health and Human Services, Centers for Disease and Prevention, National Center for Chronic Disease Prevention and Health Promotion.
15. Editors. 2003. Are you doing all you can to fight sarcopenia? *Tufts University Health and Nutrition Letter* 21 (March): 1, 4–5.
16. Bloomer, R. J. 2004. Resistance training and weight management. *Fitness Management* 20 (June): 32–35.
17. Brehm, B. A. 2003. Exercise and body image: A complex relationship. *Fitness Management* 19 (December): 22.

18. NSCA Position Statements. August 2004. Health aspects of resistance exercise and training. National Strength and Conditioning Association (www.nscalift.org/Publications/posstatements.shtml#Youth).

19. Editors. 2003. A big lift for your heart. *Harvard Heart Letter* 13 (February): 6.

20. American College of Sports Medicine. 1998. Exercise and physical activity for older adults. *Medicine and Science in Sports and Exercise* 30(6):992.

21. Williams, M. A. 2001. Human development and aging. In *ACSM's resource manual*. 4th ed. Edited by J. L. Roitman. Philadelphia: Lippincott Williams and Wilkins.

22. Kraemer, W. J., et al. 2002. Progression models in resistance training for healthy adults—ACSM position stand. *Medicine and Science in Sports and Exercise* 34(2):364–80.

23. Brzycki, M. 2004. What's a good formula for estimating a one-repetition maximum? *Fitness Management* 20 (July): 50.

24. Faigenbaum, A. D. 2003. Youth resistance training. *PCPFS Research Digest* 4 (September): 1–8.

25. Guy, J., and L. Micheli. 2001. Strength training for children and adolescents. *Journal of the American Academy of Orthopedic Surgeons* 9(1):29–36.

26. Bryant, C. X., J. A. Peterson, and J. E. Graves. 2001. Muscular strength and endurance. In *ACSM's resource manual*. 4th ed. Edited by J. L. Roitman. Philadelphia: Lippincott Williams and Wilkins.

27. Graves, J. E., M. L. Pollock, and C. X. Bryant. 2001. Assessment of muscular strength and endurance. In *ACSM's resource manual*. 4th ed. Edited by J. L. Roitman. Philadelphia: Lippincott Williams and Wilkins.

28. Fleck, S. J., and W. J. Kraemer. 1997. *Designing resistance training programs*. Champaign, IL: Human Kinetics.

29. American College of Sports Medicine. 2000. *ACSM guidelines for exercise testing and prescription*. 4th ed. Philadelphia: Lippincott Williams and Wilkins.

30. Brzycki, M. 2003. The role of muscle fibers in strength training. *Fitness Management* 19 (March): 48–51.

31. Rico-Sanz, J., et al. 2003. Familial resemblance for muscle phenotypes in the heritage family study. *Medicine and Science in Sports and Exercise* 35(8): 1360–66.

32. Carmeli, E., R. Coleman, and A. Reznick. 2002. The biochemistry of aging muscle. *Experimental Gerontology* 37:477–89.

33. Kraemer, W. J., and J. A. Bush. 2001. Factors affecting the acute neuromuscular responses to resistance exercise. In *ACSM's resource manual*. 4th ed. Edited by J. L. Roitman. Philadelphia: Lippincott Williams and Wilkins.

34. Batheja, A., and J. R. Stout. 2001. Food: The ultimate drug. In *Sport Supplements*. Edited by J. Antonio and J. R. Stout. Philadelphia: Lippincott Williams and Wilkins.

35. Lowery, L. M., M. Berardi, and T. Ziegenfuss. 2001. Antioxidant supplementation and exercise. In *Sport Supplements*. Edited by J. Antonio and J. R. Stout. Philadelphia: Lippincott Williams and Wilkins.

36. Williams, M. H., R. B. Kreider, and J. D. Branch. 2000. *Creatine: The power supplement*. Champaign, IL: Human Kinetics.

37. ACSM Consensus Statement. 2000. The physiological and health effects of oral creatine supplementation. *Medicine and Science in Sports and Exercise* 32:706–17.

38. Gammeren, D. V. 2001. Endurance performance. In *Sport Supplements*. Edited by J. Antonio and J. R. Stout. Philadelphia: Lippincott Williams and Wilkins.

39. Earnest, C. P., and C. Street. 2001. Skeletal muscle mass, strength, and speed. In *Sport Supplements*. Edited by J. Antonio and J. R. Stout. Philadelphia: Lippincott Williams and Wilkins.

40. Cataldo, C. B., L. K. De Bruyne, and E. N. Whitney. 2003. *Nutrition and diet therapy*. Belmont, CA: Thompson Wadsworth.

41. Earnest, C. P. 2001. Dietary androgen supplements. *Physician and Sportsmedicine* 29(5):63–70.

42. Yesalis, C. E., and M. S. Bahrke. 1995. Anabolic-androgenic steroids: Current issues. *Sports Medicine* 19:326–40.

43. Yesalis, C. E. 2000. *Anabolic steroids in sport and exercise*. 2nd ed. Champaign, IL: Human Kinetics.

Suggested Readings

Brehm, B. A. 2004. Menopause, weight gain, and physical activity. *Fitness Management* 20 (July): 22.

This article discusses the need for physical exercise for menopausal women. It emphasizes a well-balanced program consisting of cardiorespiratory, strength, and flexibility training. It discusses the benefits associated with such a program.

Editors. 2004. Why everyone needs strength training. *University of California Berkeley Wellness Letter* 20 (May): 4–5.

This article discusses the benefits versus the risks associated with strength training and offers tips on increasing the safety component. It provides a basic strength development program with good illustrations of 11 basic exercises.

Liebman, B. 2004. Give me strength. *Nutrition Action Healthletter* 31 (September): 1–7.

The information in this article comes from an interview with Miriam Nelson, PhD, from Tufts University. The article covers the need for weight training for diabetes, osteoporosis, fracture prevention, self-confidence, depression, arthritis, heart disease, and aging. It also provides tips on how to get started.

Mayo Clinic Health Information. August 2004. Strength training in women: Improve your muscle tone. *Mayo Clinic.Com* (www.cnn.com/HEALTH/library/HQ/01710.html).

This article discusses the need for strength training for women because it reduces body fat, it increases lean body mass, and the body will burn more calories more efficiently because the metabolic rate increases. Other benefits are discussed. Alternatives to lifting weights are also presented and discussed.

McGraw, J. J. 2004. Nutrition and children. *Fitness Management* 20 (March): 38–44.

This article discusses the problem of rising obesity among the nation's children. The solution includes healthy diets based on estimates of the caloric needs of children of various age groups. It discusses the role of aerobic exercise and resistive training and it provides guidelines for resistive training and tips for parental involvement.

University of Illinois. 2004. *Weight training guidelines and programs*. Urbana, IL: McKinley Health Center, University of Illinois.

This provides very good guidelines for weight training, including the order of exercises, intensity, rest periods, frequency, lifting techniques, warm-up, and cooldown. It also provides guidelines for meeting different program objectives, including endurance, health/fitness, strength, size, and power.

Name _____ Date _____ Section _____

Assessment Activity 4-1

Calculation of Strength (Selected Muscle Groups)

Directions: The calculation of strength by this method is expressed as the ratio of strength to body weight. The amount of weight accomplished for each lift is converted to a proportion of your body weight and is determined in the following manner:

1. Find your 1 RM for each of the following exercises: biceps curl (two arm), overhead press, bench press, half-squat or leg press, and hamstring curl.
2. Divide your 1 RM for each exercise by your body weight. For example, a 130-lb. woman performs a 1 RM bench press of 80 lbs. Her score is 80 ÷ 130 = 0.61. Look at the chart below for an interpretation of her score. Look under the Bench Press column

and note that her score of 0.61 is in the average category. In this example, the woman has the following results on the five lifts: biceps curl = 0.28 (fair), overhead press = 0.26 (fair), bench press = 0.61 (average), half-squat or leg press = 1.35 (good), and hamstring curl = 0.52 (good). These data are plotted in the first strength profile chart.

3. When you have computed a score for each of your lifts, turn to the strength profile charts. Plot your data in the blank chart provided.
4. Refer to figures 4-1 through 4-16 for a refresher on how to do these exercises.

Strength/Body Weight Ratio

Women

Biceps Curl	Overhead Press	Bench Press	Half-Squat or Leg Press	Hamstring Curl	Strength Category
0.45 and above	0.50 and above	0.85 and above	1.45 and above	0.55 and above	Excellent
0.38–0.44	0.42–0.49	0.70–0.84	1.30–1.44	0.50–0.54	Good
0.32–0.37	0.32–0.41	0.60–0.69	1.00–1.29	0.40–0.49	Average
0.25–0.31	0.25–0.31	0.50–0.59	0.80–0.99	0.30–0.39	Fair
0.24 and below	0.24 and below	0.49 and below	0.79 and below	0.29 and below	Poor

Men

Biceps Curl	Overhead Press	Bench Press	Half-Squat or Leg Press	Hamstring Curl	Strength Category
0.65 and above	1.0 and above	1.30 and above	1.85 and above	0.65 and above	Excellent
0.55–0.64	0.90–0.99	1.15–1.29	1.65–1.84	0.55–0.64	Good
0.45–0.54	0.75–0.89	1.00–1.14	1.30–1.64	0.45–0.54	Average
0.35–0.44	0.60–0.74	0.85–0.99	1.00–1.29	0.35–0.44	Fair
0.34 and below	0.59 and below	0.84 and below	Less than 1.0	0.34 and below	Poor

Strength Profile Charts

Example

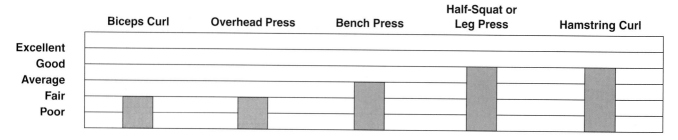

Your Data

	Biceps Curl	Overhead Press	Bench Press	Half-Squat or Leg Press	Hamstring Curl
Excellent					
Good					
Average					
Fair					
Poor					

Name _____ Date _____ Section _____

Assessment Activity 4-4

Assessing Muscular Strength and Endurance with Selected Calisthenic Exercises

Directions: The tests making up this assessment require minimal equipment and are easy to administer.

Chin-ups: Grasp an overhead horizontal bar, hands shoulder-width apart, palms facing your body. On the upstroke, your chin must go above the bar and your arms must extend fully on the downstroke. Your legs must remain extended throughout the exercise and should not be used to thrust your body upward (Figure 4-23).

Flexed-arm hang: Perform this exercise if you cannot do chin-ups. Have someone assist you to the exercise position with your chin above the bar, palms facing away from your body. A stopwatch is started as soon as you assume this position and is stopped if you tilt your head back to keep your chin above the bar, if your chin touches the bar, or if your chin drops below the bar. Record the time to the nearest whole second (Figure 4-24, page 136).

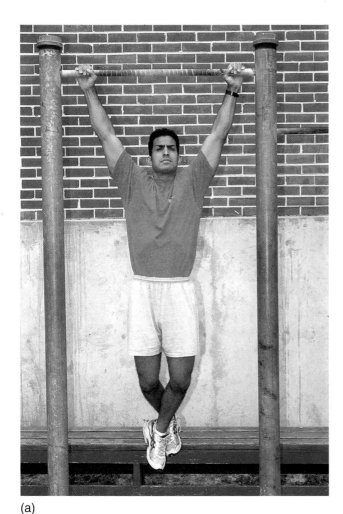

(a)

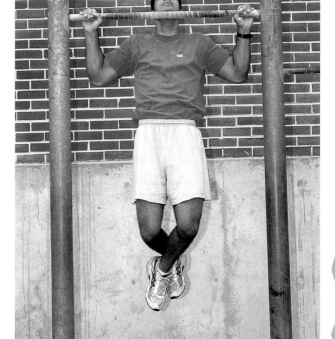

(b)

Figure 4-23 Chin-Ups

Push-ups: Assume a prone position (face down) with your arms extended, hands on the floor under your shoulders. Keep your back and legs straight and your feet together. The person counting the push-ups should place a fist under your chest. Bend your elbows, lowering your chest until contact is made with the counter's fist, and then return to the starting position by straightening your arms. Repeat as many times as possible without resting to a maximum score of 46 push-ups (Figure 4-25).

Modified push-ups: Perform this exercise if you cannot do the standard push-up. The modified version is performed in the same manner as the standard push-up, except that you support your body weight with your hands and knees. Do as many as you can without rest to a maximum of 24 (Figure 4-26).

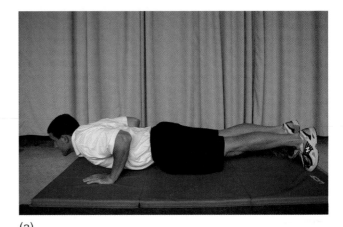

(a)

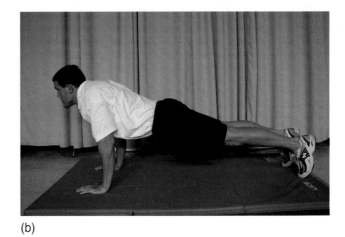

(b)

Figure 4-24 Flexed-Arm Hang

Figure 4-25 Push-Ups

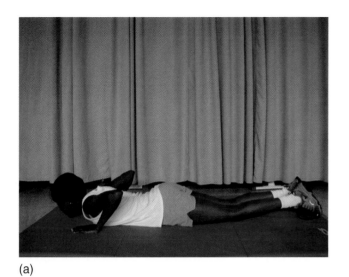

(a)

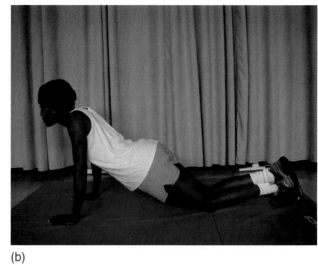

(b)

Figure 4-26 Modified Push-Ups

Muscular Strength and Endurance Standards

Chin-Ups	Flexed-Arm Hang (secs.)	Push-Ups	Modified Push-Ups	Strength Category
20 or more	30 or more	40 or more	24 or more	Excellent
15–19	24–29	32–39	14–23	Good
10–14	15–23	27–31	8–13	Average
6–9	9–14	20–26	2–7	Fair
5 or less	8 or less	19 or less	1 or less	Poor

Assessment Activity 4-5

Resistance Training Log

Directions: Keep a record of your resistance fitness activities on the form provided. Make copies of this form for repeated uses.

Daily Training Log

Name _____ Starting date _____

Program objectives _____

Exercise	Date: Resis.* (lbs.)	Reps	Sets	Date: Resis. (lbs.)	Reps	Sets	Date: Resis. (lbs.)	Reps	Sets	Date: Resis. (lbs.)	Reps	Sets	Date: Resis. (lbs.)	Reps	Sets

*Resis., resistance; reps, repetitions

5

Improving Flexibility

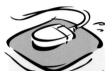

Online Learning Center

Log on to our Online Learning Center (OLC) for access to these additional resources:

- Chapter key term flashcards
- Learning objectives
- Additional goals for behavior change
- Concentration game
- Self-scoring chapter quizzes

- Additional lab activities

The OLC also offers Web links for study and exploration of wellness topics. Access these links through **www.mhhe. com/anspaugh6e**, click on Student Center, click on Chapter 5, and then click on Web Activities.

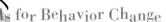

Goals for Behavior Change

- Begin participating regularly in a stretching program to improve flexibility.
- Identify some of the tasks or sports that you perform regularly for which being more flexible would be helpful.
- Practice correct lifting techniques when moving heavy objects.
- Modify your work or study area to lower the risk for neck and back pain.
- Try two safe ergogenic aids and analyze their effectiveness.

Key Terms

ballistic stretching
flexibility
goniometer
proprioceptive
  neuromuscular facilitation
  (PNF)

static stretching
stretch reflex

Objectives

After completing this chapter, you will be able to do the following:

- Define *flexibility*.
- Identify factors affecting flexibility.
- Distinguish among static, ballistic, and proprioceptive neuromuscular facilitation stretching.

- Assess and prescribe a personal flexibility program.
- Discuss the high incidence of neck pain, upper-back pain, and lower-back pain in the United States.
- Demonstrate proper lifting techniques for prevention of lower-back injury.

usculoskeletal conditioning includes exercises that increase muscle strength and endurance, and exercises that improve flexibility. This chapter examines the relationship between flexibility and wellness, identifies and illustrates safe and effective stretching exercises, discusses types of stretching and stretching techniques, and presents guidelines for developing a sound flexibility program.

Flexibility and Wellness

Flexibility programs are planned, deliberate, and regularly performed sets of exercises designed to progressively increase the range of motion of a joint or series of joints.[1,2] *Flexibility* may be defined and measured statically or dynamically. For the purpose of this text, it will be defined statically as the range of motion of a single joint or a series of joints.[3] The joints are surrounded by connective tissues consisting of muscles, tendons, and ligaments. The tendons connect muscles to bones and the ligaments connect bones to bones. These structures respond to stretching exercises, which result in the development of a greater range of motion (ROM). Athletes involved in sports that require greater than average flexibility devote much training time to improving this component of physical fitness. For instance, martial arts participants, ballet dancers, and gymnasts demonstrate an extraordinary range of motion well beyond the capacity of most people. Flexibility is an important component of health-related physical fitness but one that is often neglected even though it requires a minimal investment in time, effort, and equipment.

Factors that limit joint movement include (1) the bony structure of the joints (the skeleton is established by heredity, but it can be harmed by trauma, disease, calcium deposits, etc.); (2) the amount of tissue (muscle and fat) around and adjacent to the joint; (3) the elasticity of muscles, tendons, and ligaments; and (4) the skin (scar tissue from surgery or a laceration over a joint may limit movement). Other factors that influence flexibility are age, gender, and level and type of physical activity. Young people are more flexible than adults because tendons lose their elasticity with age. Preschool-age children are very flexible due to limited bony calcification—that is, the ends of the long bones have yet to ossify (the conversion of cartilage to bone). Peak flexibility occurs between 15 and 18 years of age and begins to decline by the mid-20s.[3] Inactivity may play a greater role than the aging process in the loss of flexibility because muscles and other soft tissues lose elasticity when not used. Also, aging is often accompanied by conditions, such as arthritis, that compromise range of motion. Active individuals are usually more flexible than inactive people.[4]

Women tend to be more flexible than men because the hormones that permit women's tissue to stretch during the childbirth process facilitate all body stretching.[2] The range of motion for most movements begins to decline in the mid-20s for men and women.[4] (Complete Assessment Activities 5-1 through 5-4 at the end of this chapter to determine your flexibility.)

Joint flexibility is important for several reasons. Inflexible muscles around the joints limit range of movement, eventually inhibiting activities of daily life. This phenomenon is most frequently seen in older people who have difficulty reaching down to tie their shoes or bending over to get a drink of water from a fountain. Lack of flexibility in the shoulders can affect the performance of normal daily activities, such as changing an overhead lightbulb or removing a can of vegetables from a cupboard.[3] Tight muscles may also contribute to joint deterioration by subjecting the bones to excessive pressure, causing pain and abnormalities in joint lubrication. Regular flexibility exercises can improve body posture. Flexibility exercises following aerobic activity reduce muscle soreness.[3]

According to the American College of Sports Medicine (ACSM), stretching exercises may prevent injuries.[5] The supporting data come primarily from observational studies, which are not as definitive as randomized, controlled clinical trials. Studies with larger samples and better controls indicate little relationship between stretching and the risk for injury. Even though scientific evidence does not strongly support flexibility training for injury prevention, sports medicine specialists advocate its use.[6] Based on the available evidence as well as experience, flexibility exercises help maintain a full range of joint motion. While this is true, people who are at the extremes of flexibility from inflexible to extremely

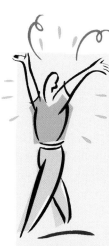

Nurturing Your Spirituality

The Ancient Arts of Tai Chi and Yoga

Medical health care training and delivery have been gradually adopting a more holistic view of treating patients. This holistic view recognizes the role of spirituality in the healing process. Johns Hopkins Medical School currently offers an elective course for its medical students on spirituality and healing.[10] The National Institutes of Health has awarded grants to a small number of medical schools to develop and promote courses on this subject.

At the same time that spirituality is making a medical comeback, Americans are searching for ways to alleviate stress, promote relaxation, and enhance health. Two physical arts that blend spirituality and health, tai chi and yoga, are gaining popularity.

Tai chi originated as a self-defense art, but it has evolved into a religious ritual, a relaxation technique, and an exercise program for people of all ages, including the elderly. Tai chi features slow, balanced, low-impact movements that may reduce stress and improve flexibility, balance, and strength.[11] It requires concentration, controlled breathing, and balance while body weight is shifted as a person transitions from one movement to another. It is often referred to as *movement meditation* because it promotes muscle relaxation through movement.[12]

The potential benefits of tai chi include the following:

- Improved flexibility
- Physical therapy, because it may assist in recovery from injury
- Improved balance and coordination
- Improved strength, particularly of the lower body (buttocks, thighs, and calves)
- Improved posture
- Increased ability to relax
- Possible slight reduction in the resting blood pressure

It takes years to become adept at tai chi, but several movements and positions can be learned with a few weeks of instruction.

Yoga originated in India about 6,000 years ago. There are several types, but hatha yoga seems to be most popular among Americans. Hatha yoga features a system of exercises that promote physical fitness and mental well-being.[13]

Yoga is a Sanskrit word that means "union." Its practitioners strive for total union in experience, a union of physical, mental, and spiritual states. Achieving this union results in a calm, relaxed, tranquil attitude.

Research indicates that yoga's meditative characteristics may prevent or at least decrease the severity of psychosomatic illness. Psychosomatic illnesses are mind-body maladies. They are caused by negative mental states and attitudes that produce changes in body physiology that result in disease. Some common psychosomatic diseases are tension headaches, ulcers, asthma, stress, essential hypertension, impotence, back pain, and menstrual problems.

Master practitioners can, at will, influence body responses controlled by the autonomic nervous system, such as breathing rate, heart rate, and blood pressure. But it takes years of practice to achieve this level of control.

The exercises and body positions featured in yoga promote mobility and flexibility, but some of these positions are potentially unsafe. It is important to learn from an experienced instructor to minimize mistakes.

Practiced regularly, yoga may lower resting blood pressure, relieve mild depression, and contribute to strength and balance. Anecdotal evidence (evidence that comes from personal reports) also indicates that practitioners experience more energy and feel calmer and more focused than nonpractitioners.[14]

---

flexible seem to be more susceptible to joint injury due to less stable joints.[7] Also, extreme flexibility appears to be detrimental to performance in running and weight lifting because tight muscles perform more efficiently in these activities.

Maintenance of flexibility is most important for the prevention of lower-back pain.[8] For example, a sedentary lifestyle characterized by sitting for long periods leads to a loss of flexibility and increases the likelihood of lower-back injury. Flexibility of the hamstring muscles (a group of muscles in the back of the thighs) and the lower-back muscles contributes to good posture. Posture is also improved by the development of strong abdominal muscles and the maintenance of normal body weight. Extra body weight, particularly that which accumulates around the abdominal area, throws the body out of balance and applies a forward force on the lower (lumbar) spinal area, which places extra stress on the lower back.[9]

The benefits of flexibility training are summarized in Just the Facts: Benefits of Flexibility Training. See also Nurturing Your Spirituality: The Ancient Arts of Tai Chi and Yoga.

Developing a Flexibility Program

Flexibility can be improved by exercises that promote the elasticity of the soft tissues. Figures 5-1 through 5-8 demonstrate exercises that can maintain and improve the flexibility of the major body sites. These 10-minute exercises can be done every day, both before and after exercise, and on days of rest from exercise.

When to Stretch

Stretching exercises can be included in the warm-up prior to exercise and in the cooldown following exercise and done on nonexercise days. Stretching prior to working out should occur only after the muscles have been warmed up with 5 to 10 minutes of such cardiovascular activities as brisk walking, slow jogging, stationary bike riding, or similar activity.[6,15] A gradual warm-up

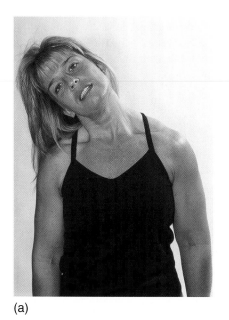
(a)

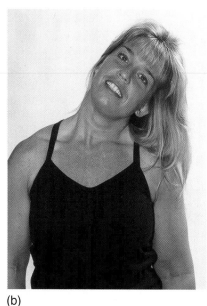
(b)

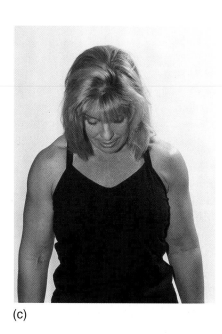
(c)

Figure 5-1 Neck Stretches

Slowly bend your neck from side to side and to the front. Do not do head circles, because these require hyperextension (excessive extension) of the cervical (neck) area of the spinal column, which produces potentially harmful compression of the intervertebral disks.

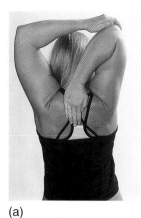
(a)

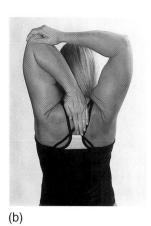
(b)

Figure 5-2 Shoulder Stretch

(a) Gently pull your right arm behind your head and hold for 15 to 30 seconds. (b) Repeat with the other arm.

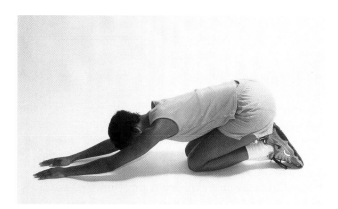

Figure 5-3 Chest and Shoulder Stretch

Stretch your arms to full extension with both palms on the floor and press your chest down to the floor. Hold 15 to 30 seconds and slowly release.

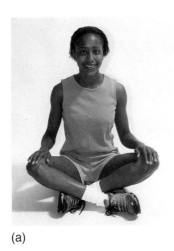
(a)

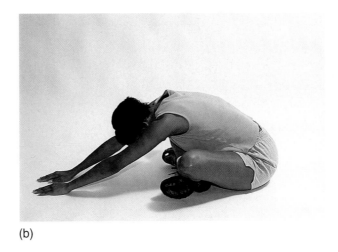
(b)

Figure 5-4 Back Stretch

(a) Cross your legs and lean forward, extending your arms to the front. (b) Hold for 15 to 30 seconds and slowly release.

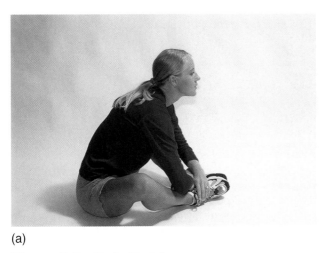
(a)

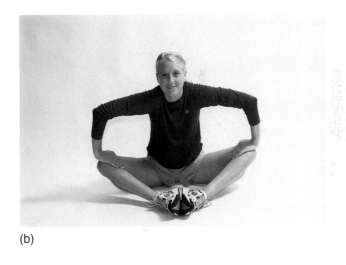
(b)

Figure 5-5 Groin Stretch

(a) Place the soles of your feet together and lean forward. Hold 15 to 30 seconds. (b) Variation: Push down gently on both knees and hold for 15 to 30 seconds.

increases heart rate slowly and raises the temperature of muscles, tendons, and ligaments by increasing blood flow to these structures. Stretching after a warm-up is safer and more productive than stretching before: Stretching cold muscles increases the probability of incurring a soft tissue injury.[16] Warm up prior to stretching for approximately 10 minutes on the days of rest between workouts.

The highest payback from stretching comes at the end of an aerobic or resistive workout. During this time, the muscles are thoroughly warmed and capable of stretching maximally and safely. Also, the muscles that have been contracting and shortening vigorously and continuously during the workout should be systematically stretched and lengthened after the workout. However, there is emerging evidence that stretching prior to exercise may

be counterproductive for activities that require strength. Stretching temporarily decreases muscle strength and as a result may produce a performance decrement.[3]

Types of Stretching

Muscles must contract for movement to occur. The contracting muscles are called *agonists* and are the prime movers. For an agonist to contract, shorten, and produce movement, a reciprocal lengthening of its *antagonist* must occur. For example, when the biceps muscle of the upper arm contracts, its opposite, the triceps muscle, must relax and lengthen. In this case, the biceps is the agonist and the triceps is the antagonist, but the triceps becomes the agonist for movements that require it to contract, making the

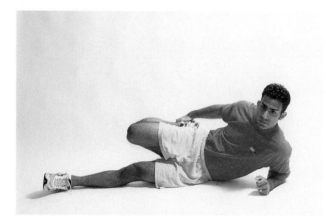

Figure 5-6   Quadriceps Stretch

Lie on your side as shown. Bend the knee of your top leg, grasp your ankle with your free hand, and slowly pull your heel toward your buttocks until you feel the stretch in the muscles in the front of your thigh. Hold 15 to 30 seconds, roll over to the other side, and repeat with your other leg.

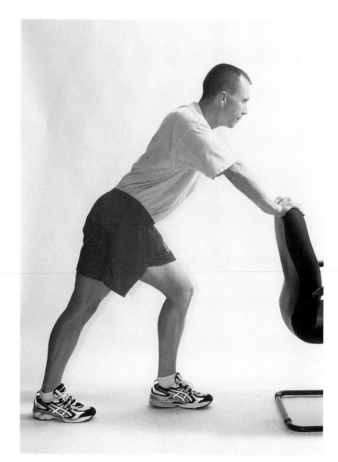

Figure 5-8   Calf and Achilles Tendon Stretch

Assume the position shown. Be sure the heel of your extended leg remains in contact with the floor and both feet are pointed straight ahead. Slowly move your hips forward until you feel the stretch in the calf of your extended leg. Hold 15 to 30 seconds and repeat with your other leg.

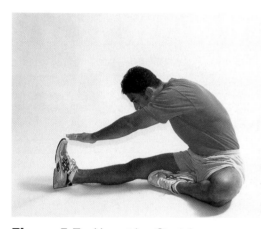

Figure 5-7   Hamstring Stretch

Place the sole of your left foot against the thigh of your extended right leg. Lean forward without bending the knee of your extended leg. Hold for 15 to 30 seconds and repeat with your other leg.

biceps the antagonist. Understanding these concepts is necessary to understanding stretching techniques.

Static stretching involves slowly moving to desired positions, holding them for 15 to 30 seconds, and then slowly releasing them. This method of stretching does not activate the **stretch reflex** (automatic or reflexive contraction of a muscle being stretched), so the muscle is essentially stretched without opposition.

The stretch reflex consists of two *proprioceptors*, sensory organs found in muscles, joints, and tendons that provide information regarding body movement and position. These proprioceptors are the muscle spindle and the Golgi tendon organ.[15] The muscle spindle is a receptor sensitive to changes in muscle length. The Golgi tendon organ is a receptor that is also sensitive to changes in muscle length but additionally responds to increases in muscle tension.[15]

Stretching the muscles also stretches their muscle spindles, which send volley sensory impulses, informing the brain that the muscles are being subjected to stretch. Impulses are sent back to the muscles, which cause them to contract reflexively, thus resisting the stretch. But if a muscle is stretched statically and the position is held for at least 6 seconds, the Golgi tendon organ responds to the change in length and tension by sending a volley of signals of its own to the brain via the spinal cord. Unlike the signals from the muscle spindle, those initiated by the Golgi tendon organ cause the antagonist muscle (the muscle being stretched) to relax reflexively. This protective mechanism allows the muscle to stretch through relaxation as the Golgi tendon organ nullifies or overrides the signals of the muscle spindle. Thus, stretching positions held for at least 6 seconds and preferably for 15 to

30 seconds allow muscles to lengthen and stretch with minimal chance of injury.

Static stretching should produce a feeling of mild discomfort but not pain. Static stretching (see Figures 5-1 to 5-8) results in little or no muscle soreness, has a low incidence of injury, requires little energy, and can be done alone. For these reasons, static stretching is the preferred system for increasing flexibility.

The following guidelines should be followed for safe and effective static stretching:[6]

- Warm up for a few minutes before stretching by walking, jogging slowly, doing light calisthenics, or doing a similar activity.
- Stretch to the point of mild discomfort.
- Do not stretch to the point of pain.
- Hold each stretch for 15 to 30 seconds minimum.
- Do not hold your breath during a stretch; breathe rhythmically and continuously.
- Move slowly from position to position.
- Perform each stretch at least four times.
- Stretch after the workout; this produces the greatest benefit because the muscles are warm and more amenable to stretching.
- Perform stretching exercises five or six times per week.

Deliberate attempts to improve flexibility should occur throughout the life cycle. See Wellness for a Lifetime: Flexibility Guidelines for Children and Older Adults for more specific information.

Proprioceptive neuromuscular facilitation (PNF) is another effective and acceptable stretching technique. It is more complex than most methods of stretching, but it is the most effective.[2,5,15] By combining slow, passive movements (the force for passive movement is supplied by a partner) with maximal voluntary isometric contractions, you can bypass the stretch reflex stimulation that accompanies changes in muscle and tendon length.

All variations of PNF stretching require a partner and some combination of passive stretching and isometric contractions. Two of the common PNF methods, contract-relax (CR) and slow reversal-hold-relax (SRHR), are presented in Figures 5-9 and 5-10 (page 148). For comparison, both figures exemplify stretching the hamstring group (muscles in the back of the thigh). The hamstrings are the antagonist muscle group, and the quadriceps muscles (muscles in the front of the thigh) are the agonists. For example, the CR method is performed as follows (Figure 5-9):

1. A partner gently pushes the upraised leg in the direction of arrow *A*. This movement passively stretches the antagonist (hamstrings).
2. The subject follows this with a six-second maximal contraction of the agonist (quadriceps).
3. This is followed by another passive stretch of the hamstrings.

Wellness for a Lifetime

Flexibility Guidelines for Children and Older Adults

Flexibility peaks from ages 15–18 for men and women and declines thereafter in people who are not actively engaged in physical activities that include planned exercises for the purpose of maintaining or increasing range of motion. Evidence indicates that flexibility can be increased in healthy older adults who participate in aerobic activities supplemented with stretching exercises.[4] Physical activities, such as walking and aerobic dance, coupled with stretching exercises increase the range of motion of older adults.

Recommendations for improving the flexibility of children are somewhat different. Because children are more flexible than adults, 5- to 9-year olds need less time devoted to flexibility exercises than do older adults.[17,18] However, some formal stretching is required, and activities such as tumbling and climbing are suggested. For older children, ages 10 through 12, the amount of time spent on improving flexibility should be greater than that of younger children but less than that of adults. Children, especially some boys, may begin to lose flexibility at this early age, so regular stretching exercises and physical activities, such as tumbling, that promote flexibility are recommended.

It is important to establish the habit of regularly stretching the muscles, tendons, and joints throughout one's lifetime. Stretching becomes even more important as we become older.

This is repeated twice, with a few seconds of rest between sequences.

The SRHR method is performed in the following manner (Figure 5-10):

1. A partner gently pushes the upraised leg in the direction of arrow *A*.
2. The subject then performs a six-second maximal voluntary isometric contraction (MVIC) of the antagonists (hamstrings) against resistance supplied by the partner.
3. The subject follows this with a six-second maximal contraction of the agonists (quadriceps).
4. This is followed by another passive stretch of the hamstrings.

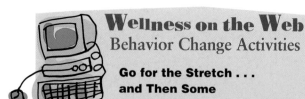

Wellness on the Web
Behavior Change Activities

**Go for the Stretch . . .
and Then Some**

Flexibility affects both your health and your wellness. If you think flexibility is related to the muscles only, then you are mistaken. While muscle flexibility is important, the ligaments that attach muscle to muscle and tendons that attach bone to bone are just as, if not more, important.

If you are not flexible, you have a higher risk for joint and muscle injury.

Each joint in the body must be tested for flexibility separately. To learn how to test your major joints for flexibility, go to **www.mhhe.com/anspaugh6e**. Click on Student Center, then Chapter 5, then Wellness on the Web, and then Activity 1.

Ready, Set, Stretch!

Flexibility is an important part of your exercise program, yet it's often a neglected part. How often have you gone through your routine and then decided to skip stretching because you're tired or ready to get home? Being flexible will help you function better throughout the day and make you feel good.

Keeping your muscles and ligaments flexible is important because tight muscles can cause chronic pain. For example, sitting all day can cause tight hip flexors and loose gluteal muscles. This muscular imbalance can make the joint weaker as parts of the bone surface bear more weight than they should. And what about your back? In many cases, back pain is caused by tight hamstrings, which cause the hips and pelvis to rotate back, flattening the lower back and causing back problems.

Other benefits of stretching include:

- Reduced potential for injury
- Improved performance
- Reduced soreness and lower-back pain
- Increased blood flow to the body
- Improved coordination

And it keeps you active and mobile as you age.

To learn more about stretching, and about some of the tools you can use in a stretching routine, go to www.mhhe.com/anspaugh6e, click on Student Center, then Chapter 5, then Wellness on the Web, and then Activity 2.

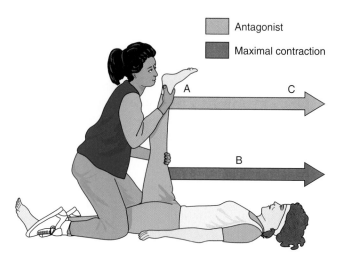

Figure 5-9 Contract-Relax (CR) Technique

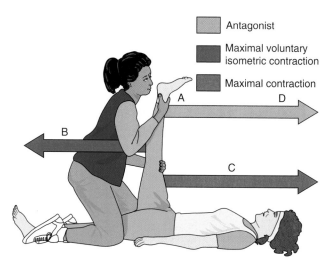

Figure 5-10 Slow Reversal-Hold-Relax (SRHR) Technique

This sequence is repeated twice, with a few seconds of rest between exercises.

Although PNF appears to be the most effective stretching method for enhancing flexibility, it has some limitations. It requires a partner; it produces more pain and muscle stiffness; it requires more time; and it increases the risk for injury, particularly when used by novices.[6]

Ballistic stretching uses dynamic movements or repetitive bouncing motions to stretch muscles. Each time a muscle is stretched in this manner, the muscle spindle (one of two receptors that make up the stretch reflex) located in that muscle is also stretched. It responds by sending a volley of signals to the central nervous system that order the muscle to contract, thus resisting the stretch. This not only is counterproductive—the muscle is forced to pull against itself—but also can lead to injury because the elastic limits of the muscle may be exceeded. Ballistic stretching is not recommended for flexibility development for the general public.[6] Many competitive athletes—performers participating in track and field, gymnastics, martial arts, dancing, and so on—use ballistic stretching to improve sport-specific flexibility.[19] Years of training using ballistic stretching enables these athletes to adapt and withstand the rigors of such training in relative safety.

Flexibility Assessment

Measuring flexibility is rather difficult, and several instruments have been developed for this purpose. Probably the most widely used device is the **goniometer.** This is a protractor-like device that measures the range of motion of a specific joint. This method is an accurate means of assessing flexibility.[20] However, for the average person, assessing flexibility by using a goniometer is not practical.

Several tests are suitable for measuring flexibility when more sophisticated means cannot be used. (The directions and norms for these tests are provided in the assessment activities.) You should warm up and follow the rules for general stretching before taking the assessments.

Preventing Back and Neck Pain

All people experience tense muscles and muscle soreness in various parts of the body on an occasional basis. The neck, shoulder, and back are particularly susceptible to the types of pressures that cause pain. Sedentary lifestyles contribute to back pain; unfortunately, 70 percent of Americans are sedentary or marginally active. Also contributing to neck and back pain are occupations that require workers to stand for long periods or to spend a significant amount of time sitting behind a desk, in front of a computer, or behind the wheel of an automobile. See Just the Facts: Neck Pain for more on neck pain. According to the Bureau of Labor Statistics, approximately 92,500 cases of occupational injuries and illnesses are due to repetitive motion. Typing or key entry; repetitive use of tools; and the repetitive placing, grasping, or moving of objects other than tools result in such injury.[24] Musculoskeletal problems are highly associated with these work-related physical tasks when the level of exposure is high. Performing unaccustomed physical work or engaging in unfamiliar sports also produces stress on the back and neck. Activities that require repetitive overhead reaching or extended sitting at a computer may produce pain and discomfort in the back, shoulders, and neck. The exercises in Figures 5-1 through 5-4, coupled with a few minutes of moving

Just the Facts

Neck Pain

There are more than 70 million visits to physicians and other health care professionals for neck and back pain every year.[21] Approximately 10 to 15 percent of the population experience neck pain at any given time.[22] Most cases are transitory annoyances that usually resolve themselves in about seven days. Normally, visiting a physician is unnecessary unless neck pain lasts longer than two weeks or is accompanied by any of the following signs and symptoms:

1. Severely restricted movement on turning the head left or right or an inability to touch the chin to the chest
2. Headaches, fever, weight loss
3. Pain that worsens at night
4. Rest and pain-killing medications provide no relief
5. Pain, numbness, or tingling sensations in the fingers, arms, or legs
6. Difficulty walking, clumsiness, or weakness
7. Problems with the bladder or bowels or sexual dysfunction

A study in Finland showed that endurance or resistance exercises for the neck alleviated neck pain.[23] The endurance exercises consisted of repeatedly lifting the head while lying face-up and then face-down. The resistive program used special elastic bands to exercise the neck muscles. Free weights were used to exercise the arms and shoulders. Also, all subjects regularly engaged in aerobic exercise. The subjects who participated in neck endurance and neck resistance exercises had less pain and disability at the end of one year than a control group who performed only aerobic exercises.

about, may prevent or alleviate pain in these areas of the body.

These problems can be significantly lessened if (1) employers ergonomically design the layout of workstations, job methods, tools, and materials to reduce exposure to the physical factors related to performing repetitive tasks and (2) employees become aerobically fit and engage in activities to promote muscle and joint flexibility.

The lower back consists of five lumbar bones, six shock-absorbing disks, the spinal cord, nerves, muscles, and ligaments. Lower-back pain affects 80 to 90 percent of American adults at some point in their lives.[22] It is one of the main reasons people visit their primary care physicians, even though 90 percent of people affected recover within a month.[22]

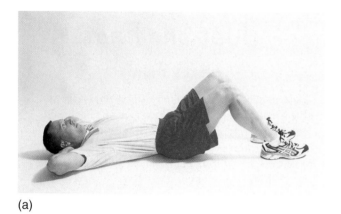

(a)

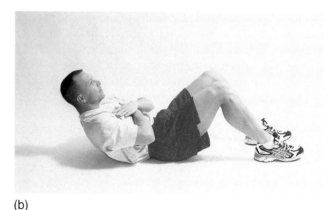

(b)

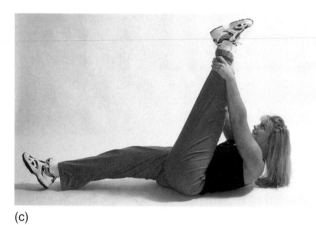

(c)

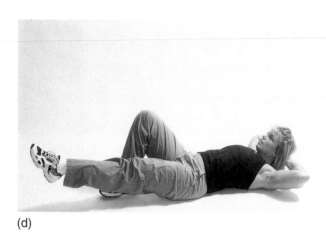

(d)

Figure 5-11   Maintaining a Healthy Back

(a) To develop the abdominal muscles, lie on your back in the position shown, and contract your abdominal muscles to force the lower back against the floor. Hold for 6 to 10 seconds. Relax and repeat 5 to 10 times.

(b) To develop the abdominal muscles, lie on your back, cross your arms over your chest, and raise your shoulder blades off the floor as shown. Return to the starting position. Repeat 5 times and work up to 25.

(c) To stretch the hamstrings, hips, and buttocks, raise one leg and extend the other. Reach up and grasp the upright leg below the calf. Alternate legs and work up to 20 repetitions with each.

(d) To develop lower abdominal muscles, keep one leg bent with that foot flat on the floor. Raise the extended leg about 6 inches off the floor, and return to the starting position. Do 10 reps and repeat with the other leg. Work up to 25 reps.

The high incidence of lower-back pain is caused by the following: excess body weight, weak abdominal muscles, weak and inflexible back muscles, weak and inflexible hamstring muscles, poor posture, cigarette smoking, the lifting of objects incorrectly, work- or sports-related injuries, and diseases such as osteoarthritis and osteoporosis.

Excess body weight stresses the lower back by pulling the spinal column forward. This causes an excessive amount of arch in the lower back, which results in poor alignment of the spine. As a result, obese people are more susceptible to lower-back problems than are normal-weight people.[25]

Weak abdominal muscles, weak and inflexible back muscles, and tight hamstring muscles distort upright posture and tilt the pelvis forward, which increases stress on the lower back.[25] Figure 5-11 illustrates exercises that stretch the lower back and develop the abdominal muscles.

Smokers have a higher incidence of lower-back pain than do nonsmokers. Smoking appears to increase degenerative changes in the spine. Smoking also prolongs lower-back pain and hampers the healing process by reducing the oxygen supply to the affected areas of the back. This occurs because the carbon monoxide in cigarette smoke attaches readily to hemoglobin, crowding out oxygen.

Figure 5-12 demonstrates correct and incorrect ways to lift a weight from the floor. Lifting correctly substantially lowers the risk of sustaining a lower-back injury. See Just the Facts: Tips for Preventing and Treating Back and Neck Pain.

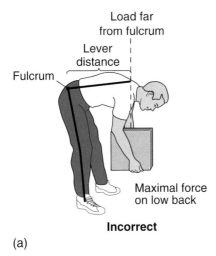

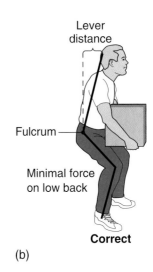

Figure 5-12 How to Lift Objects

(a) Lifting an object from the floor with straight legs and a bent back places significant stress on the lower back, increasing the likelihood of injury. Notice the distance between the box being lifted and the body of the lifter. (b) Lifting an object from the floor with bent legs and a straight back allows the lifter to keep the box close to the body, which places the majority of stress on the legs rather than on the lower back.

The spinal column consists of 33 bones (the vertebrae) and represents the only bony connection between the upper and lower halves of the body. Although humans are born with 33 separate vertebrae, by adulthood 5 vertebrae of the sacrum have fused into 1 bone, and the 4 vertebrae of the coccyx have fused into 1 bone, leaving a total of 24 vertebral bones. See Figure 5-13 on page 152, which illustrates the shape and bony structure of the vertebral column.

Located between the bones of the spine are rings of tough, fibrous tissue, the disks, which act as shock absorbers, keeping the vertebrae from rubbing against each other. The spinal column is S-shaped and consists of naturally occurring curves. When these curves are balanced, the body weight is evenly distributed and movement occurs fluidly. Misalignment in these regions applies substantial stress to the concave, or inner, side of the curves. The more pronounced the curves, the greater the stress because of the uneven distribution of weight on the bones and disks.

Approximately 90 percent of all back problems occur in the lumbar region (lower back) of the spine

Just the Facts

Tips for Preventing and Treating Back and Neck Pain

The following behaviors may help alleviate or prevent back and neck pain:

- If you sit, stand, or work in one place for extended periods, periodically walk around for a few minutes and do some simple stretching exercises.

- If your job requires long periods of standing, you can reduce the stress on your lower back by placing one foot and then the other on a small stool for a few minutes at a time. This rounds the spine and reduces lower-back stress. You can also shift your weight from one foot to the other.

- If you drive for long periods, sit comfortably and make sure you can easily reach the dash, pedals, and steering wheel. You can also try placing a small pillow behind your lower back. Also, stop the vehicle every two to three hours to take a short stretch break.

- Exercise regularly to develop the abdominal muscles and to stretch the back muscles.

- Stretch the back muscles and hamstrings at least three times per week.

- Maintain a healthy body weight.

- Bend at the knees while lifting objects, so that your legs do most of the work.

- Do not smoke cigarettes, because they contribute to the degeneration of the spine.

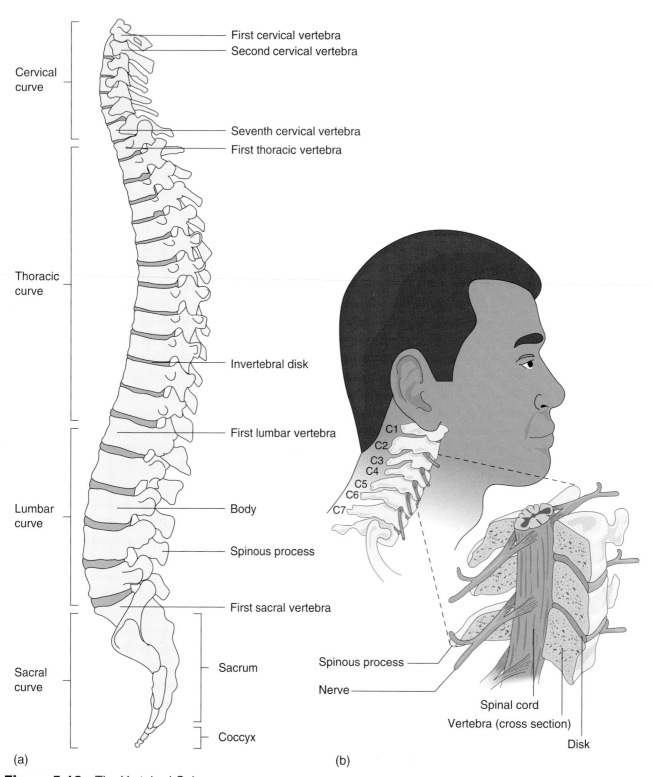

Figure 5-13 The Vertebral Column

(a) The complete column viewed from the left side. Note that the vertebrae of the sacrum are fused into one bone, and those of the coccyx have also fused into one bone. (b) The vertebrae of the cervical curve from the right side.

because that region carries the weight of the torso (the trunk of the human body). The lower back is most vulnerable to strains, as well as other problems, because it is subjected to the greatest amount of physical stress.[22]

Fatigue causes the pelvis to tilt forward when a person is standing, increasing stress on the spinal column and its supporting structures. Wearing high-heeled shoes does the same thing.

Summary

- *Flexibility* refers to the range of motion at a joint or series of joints and is specific to each joint.
- Factors that influence flexibility of a joint are the bony structure, the amount of tissue at the joint, the skin, and the elasticity of the muscles, tendons, and ligaments at the joint.
- Flexibility is influenced by age, gender, and physical activity.
- The maintenance of flexibility of the hamstrings and lower-back muscles is important in the prevention of lower-back pain.
- Normal body weight and good posture are also necessary for a healthy back.
- Ballistic stretching is counterproductive to improving joint elasticity and may contribute to injury.
- Static stretching is the recommended type of exercise. Stretches should be held for 15 to 30 seconds and repeated at least three times.

- Stretching should not be painful, only mildly uncomfortable.
- Stretching exercises can be performed daily.
- Proprioceptive neuromuscular facilitation is the most effective but most difficult form of stretching.
- Proprioceptive neuromuscular facilitation combines passive movement with isometric contractions.
- The goniometer is the most widely used device to measure flexibility.
- Lower-back pain is one of the most common reasons for visiting a physician.
- Factors associated with lower-back and neck pain include excess weight; poor posture; inactivity; fatigue; weak abdominal muscles; the wearing of high heels; stress; cigarette smoking; weak, inflexible back and hamstring muscles; incorrect lifting; work or sports injuries; and disease.

Review Questions

1. Explain why flexibility is such an important component of health-related fitness.
2. Discuss the steps to take when developing a flexibility program.
3. What concepts are necessary to understand about stretching?
4. Distinguish among static, ballistic, and PNF stretching.
5. Discuss the guidelines that should be followed for safe and effective stretching.
6. What factors are associated with lower-back and neck problems?
7. Describe the proper lifting technique for preventing back injury.
8. Discuss the role of repetitive movements in the development of upper-back and neck pain.
9. What can an employer and an employee do to reduce the potential for repetitive motion injuries?

References

1. Alter, M. J. 1996. *Science of flexibility.* Champaign, IL: Human Kinetics.
2. Nieman, D. C. 2003. *Exercise testing and prescription.* New York: McGraw-Hill.
3. Knudson, D. V., P. Magnusson, and M. McHugh. 2000. Current issues in flexibility fitness. *PCPFS Research Digest* 3 (June): 1–8.
4. American College of Sports Medicine. 1998. Position stand on exercise and physical activity for older adults. *Medicine and Science in Sports and Exercise* 30(6):992–1008.
5. American College of Sports Medicine. 1998. Position stand on the recommended quantity and quality of exercise for developing and maintaining cardiorespiratory and muscular fitness and flexibility in adults. *Medicine and Science in Sports and Exercise* 30(6):975–91.
6. American College of Sports Medicine. 2000. *ACSM's guidelines for exercise testing and prescription.* 6th ed. Philadelphia: Lippincott Williams and Wilkins.
7. Brehm, B. A. 2003. Stretching and flexibility: Changing ideas regarding benefits. *Fitness Management* 19 (February): 19.
8. McGill, S. M. 2001. Low back exercises: Prescription for healthy back and recovery from injury. In *ACSM resources manual.* 4th ed. Edited by J. L. Roitman. Philadelphia: Lippincott Williams and Wilkins.
9. Bryant, C. X., and J. A. Peterson. 1998. Treating and preventing low back pain. *Fitness Management* 14(4): 52–54.
10. Johns Hopkins University. 1998. Can religion be good medicine? *Johns Hopkins Medical Letter* 10(9):3.
11. University of California at Berkeley. 1998. Tai chi: Smooth, balanced, low-impact. *University of California at Berkeley Wellness Letter* 15(2):6.

12. Tai chi chuan. September 2004. *Wikipedia* (http://en.wikipedia.org/wik/tai_chi).

13. Harvard University. 1998. The ultimate mind-body workout. *Harvard Health Letter* 24(2):4–5.

14. Weil, A. 2004. Yoga stretches its reach. *Dr. Andrew Weil's Self Healing,* July, 1.

15. Fredette, D. M. 2001. Exercise recommendations for flexibility and range of motion. In *ACSM resources manual.* 4th ed. Edited by J. L. Roitman. Philadelphia: Lippincott Williams and Wilkins.

16. Malkin, M. 2004. Warming up, cooling down and stretching. *Fitness Management* 20 (January): 30–32.

17. Corbin, C. B., and R. P. Pangrazi. 1998. *Physical activity for children: A statement of guidelines.* Reston, VA: NASPE.

18. Hale, B. S., and B. D. Franks. 2001. *Get fit: A handbook for youth ages 6–17.* Washington, DC: The President's Council on Physical Fitness and Sports.

19. Johns Hopkins University. 2001. Stretching out the benefits of exercise. *Johns Hopkins Medical Letter Health After 50* 13(2):6–7.

20. Prentice, W. E. 1999. *Fitness and wellness for life.* New York: WCB/McGraw-Hill.

21. Editors. 2004. Save your neck. *Body and Soul,* September, 26–27.

22. Kostuik, J. P., and S. Margolis. 2004. *Back pain and osteoporosis—the Johns Hopkins White Papers.* Baltimore, MD: Johns Hopkins Medicine.

23. Ylinen, J., et al. 2003. Active neck muscle training in the treatment of chronic neck pain in women: A randomized controlled trial. *Journal of the American Medical Association* 289: 2509–16.

24. U.S. Department of Health and Human Services. 2000. *Healthy people 2010.* 2d ed. Washington, DC: U.S. Government Printing Office.

25. American Academy of Orthopedic Surgeons. September 2004. Low back Pain (http://orthoinfo.aaos.org/brochure/thr_report.cfm?).

Suggested Readings

Huggins, C. E. September 2004. Regular stretching may improve sports performance. *Reuters Health* (http://story.news.yahoo.com/news?).

This article discusses the role of stretching exercises in preventing injuries and improving physical performance. Most studies that were reviewed indicated that stretching before physical performance does not prevent injuries, nor does it improve performance, and, in fact, it hinders performance in activities that require strength and power.

Malkin, M. 2004. Warming up, cooling down and stretching. *Fitness Management* 20 (January): 30–32.

This article defines *warm-up, cooldown,* and *stretching.* It discusses the difference between warm-up and stretching and discusses the most common stretching types and when stretching exercises produce the best results.

Robbins, G., D. Powers, and S. Burgess. 1999. *A wellness way of life.* Boston: McGraw-Hill.

A portion of Chapter 3 in this text is devoted to the enhancement of flexibility. The chapter covers benefits, cautions, principles, guidelines, types of flexibility and basic flexibility exercises.

Stretching and flexibility—How to stretch. September 2004. (www.bath.ac.uk/masrib/stretch/streching_5html).

This article discusses the risks and benefits of stretching, as well as risky stretches. It discusses when to stretch, exercise order, stretching with a partner, stretching to increase flexibility, pain and discomfort, overstretching, and the elements of a good stretch.

Stretching flexibility exercises 1: What science has to say about the performance benefits of flexibility training. September 2004. *Google Search Library* (www.pponline.co.uk/encyc/0203.htm).

This article discusses the latest research findings regarding how and why stretching should be a part of everyone's physical fitness program. It discusses static and dynamic flexibility training and the transfer of each to sports performance. It also identifies categories of sports that do not benefit from flexibility training.

6

Forming a Plan for Good Nutrition

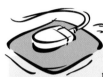

Online Learning Center

Log on to our Online Learning Center (OLC) for access to these additional resources:

- Chapter key term flashcards
- Learning objectives
- Additional goals for behavior change
- Concentration game
- Self-scoring chapter quizzes

- Additional lab activities

The OLC also offers Web links for study and exploration of wellness topics. Access these links through **www.mhhe. com/anspaugh6e**, click on Student Center, click on Chapter 6, and then click on Web Activities.

Goals for Behavior Change

- Decrease or increase your intake of the energy nutrients to meet dietary recommendations.
- Craft a nutrition profile that identifies your intake of essential nutrients and highlights your dietary strengths and shortcomings.
- Formulate a plan for implementing the Dietary Guidelines for Americans that addresses your dietary shortcomings.
- Identify and practice specific strategies for improving your diet.

Key Terms

amino acids
antioxidants
botanicals (phytomedicinals)
calorie
carbohydrate loading (glycogen loading)
complex carbohydrates
Daily Values (DVs)
Dietary Reference Intakes (DRIs)
enhanced food
essential nutrients
folate
foodborne illness
free radicals
functional foods

Glycemic Index (GI)
Glycemic Load (GL)
hydrogenation
legumes
low-carb
macronutrients
micronutrients
minerals
monounsaturated fat
net carb
nutrient density
Olestra
phytochemicals
polyunsaturated fat
Recommended Dietary Allowances (RDAs)
saturated fat

trans fatty acids
vitamins

vitamin supplements
water toxicity

Objectives

After completing this chapter, you will be able to do the following:

- Describe the functions and purposes of the essential nutrients.
- Discuss ways to apply the dietary guidelines for Americans.
- Explain the role of nutrients that are not classified as essential, such as fiber, phytochemicals, and botanicals, but that are thought to have unique health benefits.
- Determine your RDA for protein, carbohydrates, fat, and saturated fat.

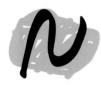utrition has captured the interest of Americans perhaps more than any other topic related to fitness and wellness. Whether concerning antioxidants or phytochemicals, homocysteine or cholesterol, omega-3 fatty acids or trans fatty acids, HDLs or LDLs, low-fat or low-carb, nutrition issues make headlines in both scientific journals and popular magazines, and everybody seems to be an expert. So much is written by so many people that it is difficult to know what and whom to believe.

This chapter presents basic concepts of the science of *nutrition*, the study of nutrients and the way the body processes them, to guide you through the maze of nutrition information. The concepts presented here are within the framework of *Dietary Guidelines for Americans* and should provide you with a basis for sound nutritional planning.

Nutrition and Health

The relationship between nutrition and health has changed dramatically during the last 50 years. The deficiency diseases of the past, such as scurvy and rickets, have been replaced by diseases of dietary excess and imbalance. Chief among such excess is the disproportionate consumption of foods high in fat, often at the expense of foods high in complex carbohydrates, fiber, and other substances conducive to good health. Americans' dietary practices contribute substantially to the burden of preventable illness and premature death and are associated with 4 of the 10 leading causes of death.[1] Coronary heart disease, stroke, and noninsulin-dependent diabetes mellitus have long been connected to nutrition. A growing body of research has also linked cancer to nutrition.[2]

Another important change in nutrition is the new set of standards for expressing dietary intake of nutrients. Previously, **Recommended Dietary Allowances (RDAs)**, which were established in the early 1940s, served as the major standard. In the 1990s, however, experts concluded that the original intent of the RDAs, to prevent nutrient deficiencies, did not adequately address today's major health problems. Consequently, **Dietary Reference Intakes (DRIs)** emerged as the framework for nutrition recommendations and now replaces RDAs as the major umbrella term (see Just the Facts: Why Change RDAs?). DRIs include several sets of standards, including RDAs, Adequate Intakes (AIs), Tolerable Upper Limits (ULs), Estimated Energy Requirements (EERs), and **Daily Values (DVs)** (see Just the Facts: The ABCs of Nutrition Acronyms).

Also changing is the definition of *essential* (required) nutrients. *Phytochemicals* (plant chemicals, also called phytonutrients), *phytomedicinals* (plants with medicinal benefits), and *antioxidants* (compounds that generally prevent the oxidation of substances in food or the body)

are the essential nutrients of the twenty-first century. A countless number of studies exploring the benefits of these nutrients may have dramatic effects on future dietary guidelines.

While the hallmark of the American diet is excess, the low intake of some foods and nutrients also causes concern. Here are a few examples:

- U.S. adults over age 60 consume about 735 mg a day of calcium, about one-half of the recommended amount.[5]
- Seven percent of U.S. toddlers and 10 percent of girls and women ages 12 to 49 are deficient in iron.[6] Iron deficiency is the most prevalent nutritional deficiency worldwide.[7]
- U.S. adults consume 14 to 15 grams of fiber per day, 10 grams short of dietary recommendations.[8]
- Only 3 percent of Americans consume at least three daily servings of vegetables, with at least one serving being dark green or orange vegetables.[1]
- Only 28 percent of Americans consume at least two servings of fruits a day.[1]

Just the Facts

The ABCs of Nutrition Acronyms

- *Dietary Reference Intakes (DRIs):* DRIs is the umbrella term under which all nutrition standards and acronyms fall. It replaces RDAs as the universal acronym for presenting nutrient recommendations and standards. Nutrition standards within the context of DRIs follow.

- *Recommended Dietary Allowance (RDA):* The RDA represents the nutrient intake that is sufficient to meet the needs of nearly all healthy people in an age and gender group. If an RDA is set for a particular nutrient, aim for this intake.

- *Adequate Intake (AI):* An RDA for a nutrient can be set only if there is sufficient information on the need for that nutrient. Presently, there is not enough information on some nutrients, such as calcium, vitamin D, copper, fluoride, biotin, fiber, and essential fatty acids, to set such a precise standard. For these and other nutrients, the DRIs include a category called Adequate Intake (AI). If an RDA is not set for a nutrient, aim for this intake.

- *Tolerable Upper Limits (ULs):* ULs represent the safe upper limit of a nutrient from total intake of food, including dietary intake, fortified food, and supplements, to avoid the possibility of adverse health effects.

- *Estimated Energy Requirements (EERs):* RDAs and AIs address nutrient needs. EERs provide an estimate of the dietary energy intake that is predicted to maintain energy balance in a healthy adult of a defined age, gender, and weight.

- *Daily Values (DVs):* DVs are nutrient standards used on food labels. Since RDAs and AIs are gender- and age-specific, there are too many categories to be used on a food label. DVs serve as a condensed system for allowing consumers to compare their intake of vitamins, minerals, protein, and other dietary components, such as cholesterol, fiber, and carbohydrates, to recommended intakes. DVs are set at or close to the highest RDA or the AI standard presented in the various age and gender categories for a specific nutrient.

SOURCES: Wardlaw, G., J. Hampl, and R. DiSilvestro. 2004. *Perspectives in nutrition.* 6th ed. New York: McGraw-Hill.

Institute of Medicine. 2002. *Dietary Reference Intakes for energy, carbohydrate, fiber, fat, fatty acids, cholesterol, protein, and amino acids.* Washington, DC: The National Academies Press.

Fortunately, improving your diet is not difficult. You don't have to give up your favorite foods to achieve a healthy diet. For many people, cutting back on less healthful foods and making small dietary changes may profoundly affect health and wellness. It is never too late to benefit from dietary improvements. The easy availability of many healthy options makes dietary improvement a realistic goal for most Americans.

Essential Nutrients

Food is made up of six classes of nutrients, including carbohydrates, fat, protein, vitamins, minerals, and water. The energy-yielding nutrients (carbohydrates, fat, and protein) are called **macronutrients** because they are required by the body in larger amounts than that of vitamins and minerals, referred to as **micronutrients.** These nutrients are called **essential nutrients** because they cannot be made by the body and, therefore, must be supplied through the diet. Some experts list fiber as a seventh nutrient, although technically some fibers are carbohydrates and are usually listed with the carbohydrates. Carbohydrates, fat, and protein are called *energy nutrients* because they provide energy (calories) to the body to regulate chemical processes. (See Table 6-1 on page 166.)

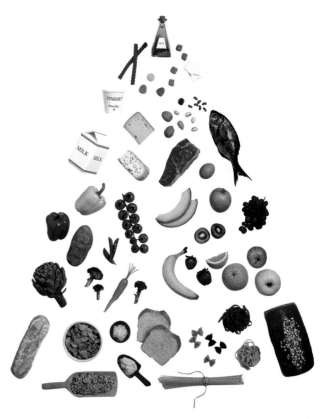

Eating a variety of foods is the best way to ensure that your diet is nutritionally balanced. Have you tried an unfamiliar food lately?

Table 6-1 Thirty-three Essential Nutrients: Daily Values for People over 4 Years of Age and Safe Upper Limits for Selected Nutrients

Nutrient	Unit of Measurement	Daily Value	Upper Limit*
Fat[†]	Gram	31	
Saturated fatty acids[†]	Gram	< 13	
Protein[†]	Gram	71	
Cholesterol[‡]	Milligram	< 300	
Carbohydrate[†]	Gram	210	
Fiber	Gram	38	
Biotin	Milligram	0.35	
Calcium	Milligram	1,300	2,500
Chloride	Milligram	2,300	3,600
Chromium	Microgram	45	
Copper	Microgram	1,300	10,000
Folate	Microgram	600	1,000
Iodine	Microgram	290	1,100
Iron	Milligram	27	45
Magnesium	Milligram	420	350[§]
Manganese	Milligram	6	11
Molybdenum	Microgram	50	2,000
Niacin	Milligram	18	35
Pantothenic acid	Milligram	7	
Phosphorus	Milligram	1,250	4,000
Potassium	Milligram	4,700	
Riboflavin	Milligram	1.6	
Selenium	Microgram	70	400
Sodium	Milligram	1,500	2,300
Thiamin	Milligram	1.4	
Vitamin A	Retinol Equivalents	1,300	3,000
Vitamin B_{12}	Microgram	2.8	
Vitamin B_6	Milligram	2	100
Vitamin C	Milligram	120	2,000
Vitamin D	Microgram	15	50
Vitamin E	Milligram	19	1,000[‖]
Vitamin K	Microgram	120	
Zinc	Milligram	13	40

Daily Values (DVs) were established as a condensed system for presenting generic standards on food labels. These standards are applicable to ages 4 years old through adulthood. DVs are set at or close to the highest RDA, DRI, and/or AI standard seen in the various age and gender categories for a specific nutrient. While DVs are not to be confused with RDAs, they allow consumers to compare their intake to desirable or maximum intakes. The DVs on food package labels have yet to be updated to reflect the current state of knowledge. For example, the DRI for vitamin C was recently increased to 90 mg for adults and 120 mg for women during lactation but remains at 60 mg on food labels.

* Safe upper limits have not been established for many nutrients because of insufficient research information.

[†] No RDA has been set for these nutrients except protein. Cholesterol is not classified as an essential nutrient because the body makes it on its own. The values listed are based on a 2,000-calorie diet, with a caloric distribution of 30% from fat (one-third of this total from saturated fat), 60% from carbohydrate, and 10% from protein.

[‡] Based on recommendations of federal agencies.

[§] Refers to upper limit only from nonfood sources (i.e., supplements).

[‖] 1,100 is upper limit of synthetic vitamin E; 1,500, natural vitamin E.

SOURCES: Wardlaw, G., J. Hampl, and R. DiSilvestro. 2004. *Perspectives in nutrition.* 6th ed. New York: McGraw-Hill.

Institute of Medicine. 2002. *Dietary Reference Intakes for energy, carbohydrate, fiber, fat, fatty acids, cholesterol, protein, and amino acids.* Washington, DC: The National Academies Press.

∿∿∿∿∿ Just the Facts ∿∿∿∿∿

Estimating Calorie Source

Carbohydrates, fats, and protein yield 4, 9, and 4 calories per gram, respectively. These values can be used to estimate the percent of calories by energy source of a food. For example, a turkey sandwich on white bread yields 24 grams of protein, 14 grams of fat, and 29 grams of carbohydrate. Column 2 times column 3 produces the number of calories for each energy source. Total calories in a turkey sandwich equal 338. Percent protein is determined by dividing protein calories by total calories. Repeat the procedure for carbohydrates and fat. Conclusion: 28 percent of the calories in a turkey sandwich come from protein, 34 percent from carbohydrates, and 38 percent from fat.

(1) Energy Source	(2) Calories/gram	(3) Turkey Sandwich	(4) Calories	(5) %
Protein	4	24 grams	96	28
Fat	9	14 grams	126	38
Carbohydrate	4	29 grams	116	34
Total			**338**	**100**

Water and fiber are nonnutrients and are part of a healthy diet.

Calories

Food energy is expressed in kilocalories. A kilocalorie equals 1,000 calories of heat energy. A **calorie** is the amount of heat required to raise the temperature of a gram of water by 1° C. Common reference to kilocalories usually excludes the prefix *kilo*, mainly for convenience. A gram of carbohydrates provides 4 calories (kilocalories) of energy, a gram of protein also provides 4 calories, a gram of fat provides 9 calories, and a gram of alcohol (not an essential nutrient) provides 7 calories. These values can be used to estimate the source of calories of a food (see Just the Facts: Estimating Calorie Source).

The recommended diet for Americans emphasizes complex carbohydrates as the main source of energy. Between 45 and 65 percent of calories should come from carbohydrates, with no more than 10 to 25 percent from simple sugar. No more than 20 to 35 percent of calories should come from fat; 10 to 35 percent of calories should come from protein.[3] The typical American diet, however, excluding alcohol, consists of 52 percent carbohydrates, 33 percent fat, and 15 percent protein[9] (Figure 6-1, page 168). While significant improvements have been made, Americans' diets are still high in fat calories and low in carbohydrate calories. You can tell how your calorie sources compare with dietary recommendations by completing Assessment Activities 6-3 and 6-4.

Carbohydrates

There are three types of carbohydrates: sugars, starches, and fiber. Sugar and starches provide 4 calories per gram. Fiber refers to the substances in food that resist digestion. Fiber has no calorie value because it's not absorbed. Most of the carbohydrates are plant-based. Grains, vegetables, fruits, and legumes are examples. The simplest form of carbohydrates is sugar, also called *monosaccharide*. Monosaccharides include glucose and fructose (fruit sugar). Fructose is the sweetest of simple sugars. Disaccharides are double sugars, meaning that they are pairs of chemically linked monosaccharides. In this group of sugars are sucrose, or table sugar; lactose, or milk sugar; and maltose, or malt sugar.

Starches, also called *polysaccharides*, are **complex carbohydrates.** Whole-grain, high-fiber starches are the preferred source of carbohydrates. A diet high in starch is likely to be lower in fat, especially saturated fat and cholesterol; lower in calories; and higher in fiber. An added benefit of starch consumption over simple sugar consumption is that it helps the body maintain a normal blood sugar level through a slower, more even rate of digestion and glucose absorption. It takes one to four hours for the body to digest starch. This is one reason athletes involved in endurance activities, such as marathons, load up on complex carbohydrates before competition.

All carbohydrates are broken down in the intestine and converted in the liver into glucose. Glucose is blood sugar carried to cells, where it is used for energy. Glucose

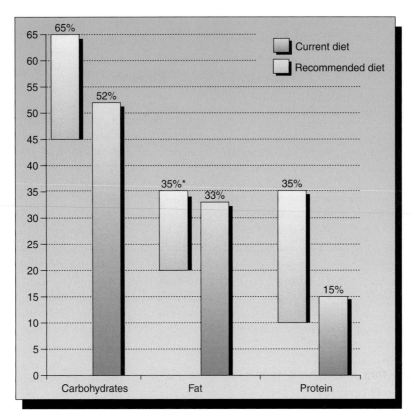

Figure 6-1 Comparison of Recommended and Actual Diets

Both diets are for Americans 20 years and older and exclude alcohol. Recommendations for carbohydrates and protein are minimums; the recommendation for fat is a maximum. Carbohydrates include sugars. Experts recommend a maximum of 35 percent fat calories if most of it is polyunsaturated and/or monounsaturated fat.

in excess of the body's need for energy is stored in limited amounts as glycogen in the muscles and the liver for future use; when glycogen stores are satisfied, glucose is converted to fat.

Many weight-conscious people mistakenly avoid starches, thinking that they are high in calories. Starch foods are often made fattening when they are prepared. For example, a baked potato without additives yields a modest 90 calories. Adding fat in the form of butter, sour cream, margarine, or cheese adds substantially to the calories of a potato.

Recommended carbohydrate intake

Between 45 and 65 percent of the calories in your diet should come from carbohydrates. For 1,500 calories, that translates into 169 to 244 grams of carbohydrates a day (see Just the Facts: Converting Carbohydrate Calories to Carbohydrate Grams). On the surface, it may appear that 169 to 244 grams of carbohydrates are excessive when considering that people on low-carbohydrate diets often consume less than 100 grams. This is a misconception. Carbohydrates have been much maligned because popular diets, such as the Atkins Diet,

ᴖᴖᴖJustᴖtheᴖFactsᴖᴖ

Converting Carbohydrate Calories to Carbohydrate Grams

If you are on a 1,500-calorie diet, approximately how many carbohydrate calories and carbohydrate grams are recommended?

Solution

1. Multiply total calories times the recommended 45% to 65%.

   a. $1,500 \times .45 = 675$ carbohydrate calories
   b. $1,500 \times .65 = 975$ carbohydrate calories

2. Divide carbohydrate calories by 4 (carbohydrates produce 4 calories/gram).

   a. $675 \div 4 = 169$ grams of carbohydrates
   b. $975 \div 4 = 244$ grams of carbohydrates

Conclusion: Between 169 and 244 grams of carbohydrates are recommended for a healthy person on a 1,500-calorie diet.

South Beach Diet, and Zone Diet, claim a carbohydrate-restricted diet is the key to successful weight loss. Adding fuel to the claim are the findings of studies reported in medical journals that indicate that people who are on low-carbohydrate diets lose weight and at the same time achieve positive changes in cholesterol and triglyceride levels. In many respects, "low-carb" has replaced "low-fat" as the nation's nutrition mantra. Low-carbohydrate diets do produce weight loss, but so do low-fat diets or any other diet that lowers caloric intake. Chapter 8 discusses the claims of low-carbohydrate diets in more detail, but it is sufficient to state that, in terms of losing weight, the real issue is how many calories are consumed, not whether the calories come from carbohydrates or fats. *Low-carb* is not necessarily synonymous with *low-calorie*. Neither does *low-carb* have the same meaning as net carb, a term often used to promote a food as low in carbohydrate (see Just the Facts: Low Carbs vs. Net Carbs). It is also important to remember that the usual context for low-carbohydrate diets is weight loss, not nutrition. From the perspective of good nutrition, carbohydrates should be the primary source of energy because they are a major source of vitamins, minerals, fiber, and other nutrients good for health.

Vegetables, fruits, and grain products are high in carbohydrates. They are low in fat, depending on how they are prepared and what is added to them at the table. Meat and animal products are low in carbohydrates, with the exception of lactose (milk sugar) in dairy products. Most Americans of all ages eat fewer than the recommended servings of fruits, vegetables, and whole-grain foods. An estimate of your carbohydrate intake can be determined by completing Assessment Activity 6-1.

There are important differences among carbohydrates. Foods that contain simple or refined carbohydrates, such as white bread, white rice, potatoes, sweetened soft drinks, candies, and sweets, are usually low in nutrients and high in simple sugar, and because they are quickly and easily digested they cause a surge in blood sugar levels and then rebound with a dramatic drop in blood sugar a few hours later. These are the carbohydrates that should be consumed in limited amounts. On the other hand, complex carbohydrate foods are loaded with nutrients and fiber, are digested slowly, and are associated with consistent blood sugar levels. These are the carbohydrates that should be emphasized in the diet.

Easy ways to add whole-grain, high-fiber carbohydrates include switching from white rice to brown rice, opting for whole-grain breads, snacking on dried fruit, and using legumes as a base for soups. Complex carbohydrates, such as whole-grain bread, cereal, rice, and oats, along with fruits and vegetables, form the foundation of a nutritious diet.

Just the Facts

Low Carbs vs. Net Carbs

Low Carbs

The term *low-carb* is splashed on food package labels and restaurant menus to imply that a product is lower in carbohydrates than normally expected. This may be true but it may also be misleading. **Low-carb** implies that a food is low in carbohydrate. In reality, *low-carb* is an ambiguous term because it may differ from one product to another and from one manufacturer to another. Currently, the Food and Drug Administration has not developed a definition for low-carb foods. A low-carb food may be lower in carbohydrates than its regular-packaged counterpart but still higher in carbohydrate than a competing brand. Also, low-carb does not necessarily mean low-calorie. The only way to know for sure is to read the label and comparison shop.

Net Carbs

The term *net carbs* refers to the total grams of carbohydrate per serving after subtracting grams of fiber and sugar alcohols. The reason manufacturers list net carbs on a package label is to promote a food as low-carb, although it may be high in carbohydrates. Take a blueberry muffin* that supposedly contains 35 grams of carbohydrates. It might be advertised as low-carb because it contains only 10 *net grams* of carbohydrates. Through the advancements of food technology, 25 grams of sugar are replaced with sugar alcohols and refined grains with isolated fibers and resistant starches. Chemically, these ingredients are carbohydrates, but they move through the small intestine without being absorbed.[10] As a result, they are subtracted from the total carb count. On the positive side, because sugar alcohols pass through the small intestine and are digested in the large intestine, they do not elevate blood sugar and insulin levels as much as regular sugar. On the negative side, like sugar, they still contain calories. From a weight-loss perspective, a calorie is a calorie; total calories have to be monitored regardless of their source.

* Actual nutrient content (including carbohydrates) may vary from this example.

Protein

Protein is different from carbohydrates and fats in that it contains nitrogen as well as carbon, hydrogen, and oxygen. Because of their unique chemical structures, proteins contain the basic materials that help the body form muscles, bones, cartilage, skin, antibodies, some hormones, and all enzymes. Protein is also an energy

Table 6-2   Comparison of Selected Legumes

Serving/1 Cup	Calories	Protein (grams)	Fat (grams)	Iron (milligrams)*	Fiber (grams)
Soybeans, dry	274	68	37	29	17
Lentils, dry	649	54	2	17	59
Kidney beans	208	14	0	3	8
Black beans	200	14	0	4	14
Chickpeas	448	28	2	2	22
Peanuts, raw	832	38	72	6	14

* Rounded to nearest whole number.

nutrient, yielding 4 calories per gram. As a source of energy, however, protein is inefficient because it must first be processed by the liver and kidneys. Proteins generally directly supply little of the energy the body uses, except during prolonged exercise.[3]

The building blocks of protein are chemical structures called **amino acids.** There are approximately 20 amino acids: 11 can be produced in the body, and 9 must be supplied by the diet.[3] The latter are called *essential amino acids.* A *complete protein* is one that contains all the essential amino acids. A *high-quality protein* is a complete protein that contains the essential amino acids in amounts proportional to the body's need for them. Meat, fish, poultry, eggs, milk, and cheese are examples of high-quality, complete protein sources. Water-packed canned tuna is the most protein-dense food, with 80 percent of its calories as protein.[3]

An *incomplete protein* does not contain all the essential amino acids in the proportions needed by the body. Generally, plant protein sources are incomplete. This has important implications for *vegans,* people who limit their diets to plant sources, because protein synthesis operates on the all-or-none principle. That is, the body cannot make partial proteins, only complete ones. If an amino acid is supplied by one source in a smaller amount than is needed, the total amount of protein made from the other amino acids will be limited. It is necessary to combine protein sources from cereal and grains with legumes to obtain all essential amino acids from plant sources. The practice of combining amino acids from various plant sources is called *protein complementing.*

One plant protein source unique among sources of amino acids is **legumes.** Legumes come from plants with seed pods that split on two sides when ripe, such as black-eyed peas; chickpeas (garbanzo beans); lentils; soybeans; and black, red, white, navy, and kidney beans. Some nuts, such as peanuts, are also legumes. Legumes are high in fiber and minerals and a nutritionally dense food (see Table 6-2).

A legume that is singled out in the health literature because it contains all of the essential amino acids is soybean. Once used primarily in the United States to feed livestock, soy protein is now recognized as a healthy food for humans. Soybeans are good sources of protein, folate, omega-3 fatty acids, minerals (such as iron), and fiber. Health benefits associated with the consumption of soybean products include lower cholesterol,[3] lower diastolic blood pressure, and improved cognitive function.[11] A possible reason for soy's benefits is that, by eating more soy, people consume fewer animal products. Another reason is that soy protein contains *phytoestrogens,* estrogen-like plant substances. Phytoestrogens unique to soybeans are called *isoflavones.* Isoflavones may supply extra estrogen for estrogen-deficient women and provide some relief for women experiencing menopausal symptoms. However, women with breast cancer or a family history of breast cancer are warned not to increase soy consumption without first talking to their physicians because isoflavones can also stimulate the growth of breast cancer cells, especially after menopause.[3]

Soy is available in a variety of foods. Tofu, soy milk, soy nuts, and soy powder, which can be mixed into smoothies, scrambled into omelets, and baked into bread, are several examples.

Nuts are another good plant source of protein. Some experts claim that nuts are the best-kept secret in nutrition. Ounce for ounce, nuts have as much protein as beef.[12] Nuts also contain vitamin E, magnesium, potassium, folate, vitamin B_6, niacin, copper, zinc, fiber, phytochemicals, and isoflavones. They are high in fat but almost all of that fat is unsaturated. Because they are high in calories, they must be consumed with an eye for serving size. An ounce of nuts (an amount that fits in the palm of the hand) provides about 160 to 180 calories.[3] Consumed in moderation, and in the place of other foods rather than in addition to other foods, nuts can contribute to a healthy diet.

Recommended protein intake

For most people, the Recommended Dietary Allowance of protein is 0.36 grams per pound of body weight, or

54 grams for a 150-pound person and 72 grams for a 200-pound person. Growing children, pregnant or lactating women, and people recovering from illness require additional protein. You can estimate your protein intake by completing Assessment Activity 6-1.

Exercise and other physical activities can change the body's need for protein (nutrition needs associated with physical activity are discussed separately in this chapter), but enough protein is usually already consumed. When more protein is consumed than is needed by the body, it is converted into energy or stored as fat. High protein intake may cause the body to excrete calcium and put excessive strain on the kidneys to excrete into the urine the excess nitrogen supplied by the protein.[3] Although the kidneys of most healthy people can handle nitrogen excess easily, diseased kidneys have more difficulty. This is why people with kidney failure are placed on low-protein diets and why people who go on high-protein diets to lose weight (see Chapter 8) are encouraged to drink large quantities of water to flush the kidneys.

Fat

Fats are oils, sterols (such as cholesterol), waxes, and other substances that are not water-soluble. Fat is an essential component of all cells. Fats help synthesize and repair vital cell transport and absorb fat-soluble vitamins. Fat stored as adipose tissue provides insulation and a ready source of energy. As an energy source, fat yields 9 calories per gram.

Basic fat facts

Fat, also called *lipid*, is a compound made by chemically bonding fatty acids to glycerol to form glycerides. When three fatty acids are hooked to glycerol, the fat compound is a triglyceride. Almost 95 percent of fat stored in the body is a triglyceride, with the remaining 5 percent consisting of other glycerides and cholesterol. Scientific literature usually refers to triglycerides when it discusses fat. As an energy nutrient, fat yields 9 calories per gram regardless of its chemical makeup.

Chemically, fats are chains of carbon atoms strung together with hydrogen atoms. If a fat is a **saturated fat,** the carbon chain carries all the hydrogen atoms it can. If it is an unsaturated fat, there is room in the carbon chain for more hydrogen. If the fat is a **monounsaturated fat,** there is room for two hydrogen atoms. If the fat is a **polyunsaturated fat,** there is room for four hydrogen atoms. If it is highly polyunsaturated, there is room for many more hydrogen atoms.

Many people mistakenly assume that the word *polyunsaturated* on a food label means that the fat in the food is not saturated, but because of food-processing techniques, this assumption may be incorrect. If the words *hydrogenated* or *partially hydrogenated* are on the food label, the food contains varying amounts of saturated fat. Because fats are less stable, they are prone to spoilage. Consequently, for many foods, manufacturers use a chemical process called **hydrogenation,** in which hydrogen atoms are added to the unsaturated or polyunsaturated fats to make them more saturated and more resistant to spoilage. This process of hydrogenating food yields a new type of fat not found in nature called **trans fatty acids** (see Just the Facts: How Much Trans Fatty Acid Is in Food? on page 172). Trans fatty acids are saturated fats commonly found in margarine, fried fast foods, cookies, cakes, and many other foods made with shortening. Some scientists believe that trans fatty acids, even those originating from a polyunsaturated food source, are as detrimental to health as saturated animal fat. High levels of these fats raise LDL cholesterol, lower HDL cholesterol, and adversely affect the body's response to insulin.[13]

Saturated and unsaturated fats can be differentiated by their appearance. Saturated fat is typically solid at room temperature. Lard, fat marbled in meat, and hardened grease from a skillet are good examples. Polyunsaturated fats are usually liquid at room temperature. Examples are safflower and corn oils. Solid vegetable shortenings are partially hydrogenated and have a soft consistency. Coconut oil, palm kernel oil, and palm oil are exceptions. They are vegetable oils and are liquid at room temperature, but they are among the most saturated of fats.

Fish oils are among the most unsaturated fats available. They are roughly twice as unsaturated as vegetable oils. They do not harden, even at low temperatures. Their unsaturation has created special interest in relation to heart disease. Fatty acids in cold-water seafood, such as salmon, mackerel, sardines, herring, anchovies, whitefish, bluefish, swordfish, rainbow trout, striped bass, Pacific oysters, and squid, consist of omega-3 fatty acids, thought to be effective in lowering cholesterol and triglyceride levels and reducing clot-forming rates, thereby reducing the risk for heart disease. Health experts believe omega-3s offer such protection against heart disease that two servings a week are recommended regardless of risk factors.[2]

Olestra

Olestra is a synthetic fat that has the flavor and taste of real fat but contains no calories. It cannot be digested or absorbed and, therefore, passes through the digestive system unaltered.

While consumption of Olestra in small amounts is unlikely to cause problems in healthy adults, several side effects have been reported. Olestra can cause abdominal cramps and loose stools. It also inhibits the absorption

Just the Facts

How Much Trans Fatty Acid Is in Food?

In 2006, manufacturers will be required to include the number of grams of trans fatty acids present when listing the number of grams of saturated fat on package labels.[14] If a serving of a food has 10 grams of saturated fat and 4 grams of trans fatty acids, the number 14 will appear in the listing for saturated fat. A footnote saying how many of the grams are trans fat will appear at the bottom of the label.

To determine how much trans fat is in food, it is necessary to have a complete breakdown of the food's fat content. For example, a popular low-saturated-fat margarine contains 10 grams of total fat, including 2 grams of saturated fat, 1.5 grams of polyunsaturated fat, and 2 grams of monounsaturated fat. Adding the amounts of these three fats and subtracting them from the total leaves about 4.5 grams unaccounted for. These grams probably represent trans fatty acids.

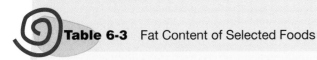

Table 6-3 Fat Content of Selected Foods

Food	Fat/(g)	Total**	Saturated	Monounsaturated	Polyunsaturated
			Percentage of Total Calories from Fat*		
Egg, whole, raw	5.01	64	19	25	8
Butter (pat)	11.4	100	67	31	4
Margarine, regular, hard (stick)	91.0	100	20	45	32
Cheese, cream (1 ounce)	9.9	90	57	25	3
Cheese, cheddar (1 cup)	37.5	74	47	20	2
Cheese, cottage (1 cup)	10.1	39	25	11	1
Milk, whole (1 cup)	8.2	49	30	14	2
Milk, skim (1 cup)	1.0	6	4	1	Trace***
Frankfurter (2 ounces)	16.6	82	33	40	3
Bologna, pork (slice)	4.6	72	26	36	8
Flounder, baked (0.8 ounce)	1.9	9	Trace	Trace	Trace
Fish sticks (1 ounce)	3.4	39	10	18	10
Tuna, canned, oil-packed (3 ounces)	6.9	38	8	10	17
Tuna, canned, water-packed (3 ounces)	2.1	7	Trace	Trace	Trace
Ground beef (3 ounces)	19.2	65	25	28	3
Steak, broiled, sirloin (2 ounces)	4.89	56	24	26	2
Pork chop, broiled (3 ounces)	22.3	62	23	29	7
Chicken breast, fried, flour-coated (7 ounces)	17.4	36	10	14	8
Beans, navy (1 cup)	2.1	4	Trace	Trace	3
Potato (baked)	0.06	1	Trace	Trace	4
Potato chips (1.5 ounces)	13.0	61	16	11	31
Ice cream, vanilla, regular (1 cup)	22.5	48	28	14	2
Apple (raw, unpeeled)	0.5	6	1	Trace	2
Danish pastry	13.6	50	14	29	4

* Rounded off to the nearest whole number.

** Includes undifferentiated fats.

*** *Trace*, less than 0.9% of fat.

Table 6-4 Maximum Fat, Saturated Fat, and Trans Fatty Acid Grams for Selected Caloric Intakes*

Daily Caloric Intake	Total Fat Grams per Day		Total Saturated Fat and Trans Fatty Acid Grams per Day	
	35% Level	20% Level	10% Level	7% Level
1,000	39	22	11	8
1,500	58	33	17	12
2,000	78	44	22	16
2,500	97	56	28	19
3,000	117	67	33	23

* If a person on a 1,500-calorie diet wants to restrict fat intake to no more than 20% of calories, the limit is 33 grams (1,500 × 0.20 = 300 total fat calories; 300 ÷ 9 = 33). Saturated fat intake at the 7% level is restricted to 12 grams (1,500 ÷ 0.07 = 105 saturated fat calories; 105 ÷ 9 = 12).

of the fat-soluble vitamins A, D, E, and K and the absorption of carotenoids, substances thought to aid the immune system in warding off some cancers, heart disease, and eye problems. To counter the effects of Olestra on the absorption of important nutrients, some snack foods are fortified with fat-soluble vitamins.

Relying on fat substitutes, such as Olestra, can help reduce fat in your diet. However, because a product has less fat does not mean it is also low in calories. Experts speculate that the reduction in calories associated with low-fat foods made with Olestra is unlikely to reduce obesity significantly because Olestra is not yet used in foods that contribute the most fat to our diets—high-fat meats.[9]

Cholesterol

Cholesterol, a waxy substance that is technically a steroid alcohol found only in animal foods, is probably the most researched blood lipid. High levels of cholesterol are usually included among the major risk factors for cardiovascular disease. (For information on cholesterol, see Chapter 2.)

Recommended fat intake

To many people, *fat* has negative connotations and is viewed almost as a toxin, but as stated earlier, fat is an essential nutrient. Experts recommend a diet that includes a total fat intake of 20 to 35 percent of total calories. No more than 10 percent of fat calories should come from saturated and/or trans fatty acids.[2]

The advice to consume no more than 20 to 35 percent of calories as fat does not apply to infants and toddlers below the age of 2 years. During the early stages of development, fat is critical to the development of the brain, spine, and central nervous system, so children's intake of fat should not be greatly restricted.[3]

Saturated fat is consistently associated with heart disease. It is the major dietary contributor to total blood cholesterol levels, even more than cholesterol intake. Many associations have also been made between dietary fat and certain types of cancer, notably breast, prostate, and colon cancer. Another health problem related to high fat intake is obesity. Little energy is used to transfer fat from foods to fat storage; the body requires only 3 calories to store 100 calories of dietary fat as fat tissue, compared with 23 to 27 calories to digest 100 calories of carbohydrates. Fat also yields more than twice as many calories as do protein and carbohydrates.

Most Americans have an excessive fat intake and are challenged to make changes in both the amount and type of fat eaten. In trying to lower fat intake, people should not reduce fat calories to less than 20 percent of total calories without the supervision of a physician.[2] When fat makes up less than 20 percent of calories, carbohydrate intake increases and the result is an increase in blood triglyceride levels, which is not a healthful change.[3] Table 6-4 presents a quick reference of maximum fat intake for selected caloric intakes. Figure 6-2 on page 174 compares the saturated, monounsaturated, and polyunsaturated content of dietary fats. You can estimate your personal maximum fat intake by completing Assessment Activity 6-2. You can also learn how fatty your eating habits are by completing Assessment Activity 6-5.

Saturated Fat. Experts agree that saturated fats need to be reduced in the American diet. Diets rich in saturated fats unquestionably increase the risk for heart disease and some cancers. Assessment Activity 6-2 will help you estimate your maximum saturated fat intake. It is recommended that no more than 10 percent of total calories come from saturated fat and/or trans fatty acids.[15] This amounts to less than 12 grams per 1,000 calories.

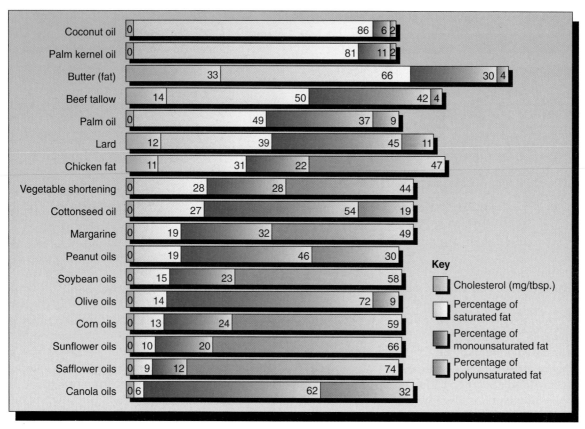

Figure 6-2 Comparison of Dietary Fats

Monounsaturated Fat. Monounsaturated fats are liquid at room temperature and include olive oil, canola oil, and peanut oil. When monounsaturated fats are substituted for saturated fats, a person's blood fat profile usually improves and the risk factors associated with heart disease and some forms of cancer are reduced. Monounsaturated fats should comprise half of total fat intake.[2]

Although the diet of people in Mediterranean countries is higher in fat than that of Americans, the incidence of heart disease and stroke in those countries is much lower. The main difference is that the Mediterranean diet is high in monounsaturated fat, usually from the consumption of olive oil. This has prompted some scientists to suggest that Americans adopt this pattern of eating.

Polyunsaturated Fat. There are two main types of polyunsaturated (poly) fats: omega-6 and omega-3. The omega-6s make up 90 percent of poly fats in the American diet and come primarily from plant oils, such as soybean, corn, sunflower, and safflower oils, as well as from nuts and seeds. Omega-6 provides linoleic acid, an essential fatty acid. The omega-3s come primarily from seafood and provide linolenic acid, another essential fatty acid. The consumption of omega-6s and omega-3s is associated with cardiovascular benefits, including the reduction of blood clotting, prevention of abnormal heart rhythms, and lowering of levels of total cholesterol and LDLs. Recommended daily intakes of linoleic acid are 17 grams for men and 12 grams for women. The respective daily recommendations of linolenic acid are 1.6 and 1.1 grams. Fish should be consumed at least twice a week.[3]

Trans Fatty Acids. Trans fatty acids start out as unsaturated fats but become like saturated fats because of the hydrogenation process. In high amounts, these fatty acids are associated with risk factors similar to those linked to saturated fats. The consumption of trans fatty acids represents a significant health issue. Consumption of trans fatty acids should be held to a minimum. No more than 10 percent of calories should come from a combination of saturated fats and trans fatty acids.

Vitamins

Vitamins are organic compounds (they contain carbon) that are necessary in small amounts for good health. The body can break vitamins down, but it cannot

Table 6-5 Vitamins: Food Sources and Wellness Benefits

Vitamins	Food Sources	Wellness Benefits
Fat-Soluble Vitamins		
1. Vitamin A	Liver, carrots, eggs, tomatoes, dark green and yellow-orange vegetables and some fruits	Healthy skin and mucous membranes, improved night vision, defense against infections, antioxidant benefits (from carotenoids)
2. Vitamin D	Fish oils and fortified milk, exposure to sunlight	Maintenance of blood levels of calcium and phosphorus, promotion of strong bones and teeth, possible reduction of risk for osteoporosis
3. Vitamin E	Plant oils (corn, soybean, safflower, etc.), nuts, seeds	Formation of red blood cells, use of vitamin K, antioxidant benefits
4. Vitamin K	Green vegetables, liver	Promotion of blood clotting, contribution to bone metabolism
Water-Soluble Vitamins		
5. Vitamin C (ascorbic acid)	Citrus fruits, green vegetables	Promotion of healthy gums and teeth, iron absorption; maintenance of normal connective tissues, help in wound healing, antioxidant benefits
Vitamin B Complex		
6. Thiamine (B_1)	Whole grains, legumes, liver, nuts	Carbohydrate metabolism, nerve function
7. Riboflavin (B_2)	Dairy products, liver, enriched grains, spinach	Energy metabolism, production of red blood cells, improved health of skin and eyes
8. Niacin	Nuts, grains, meat, fish, mushrooms	Energy metabolism, fat synthesis, fat breakdown, lowering of cholesterol (when prescribed in large doses)
9. Pyridoxine (B_6)	Whole grains, meat, beans, nuts, fish, liver	Protein metabolism, possible immunity boost in the elderly, homocysteine metabolism
10. Pantothenic acid	Whole grains, dried beans, eggs, milk, liver	Energy metabolism, fat synthesis, production of essential body chemicals
11. Vitamin B_{12}	Animal foods, dairy products, seafood	Folate metabolism, nerve function, formation of red blood cells, homocysteine metabolism
12. Biotin	Cheese, egg yolks, mushrooms, grains	Glucose production, fat synthesis
13. Folate B_9 (folic acid)	Green, leafy vegetables; liver; beans; grains; citrus fruits	DNA synthesis and protein metabolism, reduction of risk for certain birth defects, homocysteine metabolism

produce them, so vitamins have to be supplied in the diet. Unlike carbohydrates, fats, and proteins, vitamins yield no energy. Instead, some serve as catalysts that enable energy nutrients to be digested, absorbed, and metabolized. Some vitamins also interact with minerals. For example, vitamin C facilitates iron absorption, vitamin D improves calcium absorption, and thiamin requires the mineral magnesium to function efficiently.

Vitamins are either water-soluble or fat-soluble (see Table 6-5). Water-soluble vitamins include vitamin C and vitamin B complex. They are present in the watery components of food, distributed in the fluid components of the body, excreted in the urine, needed in frequent small doses, and unlikely to be toxic except when taken in megadoses (very large quantities).

Fat-soluble vitamins include vitamins A, D, E, and K and are found in the fat and oily parts of food. Because they cannot be dissolved and absorbed in the bloodstream, these vitamins must be absorbed into the lymph with fat and transported in lipoproteins. When consumed in excess of the body's need, fat-soluble vitamins are stored in the liver and fat cells. Their storage makes it possible for a person to survive for months or years without consuming them. At least three of the fat-soluble vitamins (A, D, and K) may even accumulate to toxic levels. Megadoses of these vitamins should be avoided.

Antioxidant vitamins

Three vitamins (vitamins C and E and plant pigments known as carotenoids) are classified as **antioxidants**—protective substances that help neutralize the activity of free radicals. **Free radicals** are naturally produced chemicals that arise from normal cell activity. Whenever the body uses oxygen or is exposed to a toxin, such as cigarette smoke, it forms free radicals. These unstable chemicals can damage cells throughout the body. They may damage a cell's DNA in ways that lead to cancer, interact with cholesterol in the bloodstream and form oxidized LDL (see Chapter 2), cause cataracts and rheumatoid arthritis, and be a factor in the physiological changes associated with the aging process. Excess free radical production is thought to contribute to many diseases.[2] Anything that interferes with the destructive effects of free radicals offers a health advantage.

Foods can supply nutrients with antioxidant properties. Vitamins C and E, the mineral selenium, and the carotenoids (including beta-carotene) are well-known antioxidants. A common cooking practice illustrates this antioxidant effect. Some foods, such as bananas, peaches, apples, and potatoes, quickly turn brown when exposed to air. However, when such foods are dipped in lemon or orange juice, the vitamin C in the juice acts as an antioxidant and prevents browning.

Each antioxidant serves a different purpose, but all of them work closely together. For example, vitamin C helps regenerate vitamin E once it has become oxidized.[2] This illustrates the importance of a diet that supplies sufficient amounts of all of the antioxidants rather than focusing exclusively on one.

Should Americans take supplements of antioxidant vitamins? Information from the research community is inconclusive. Until recently, the evidence in support of vitamin supplements was so compelling that many scientists were beginning to believe that antioxidant vitamin supplements could be a highly effective, relatively inexpensive, and risk-free form of preventive medicine.

But now after hundreds of studies on antioxidants and disease risk, the value of taking large doses of antioxidant supplements is still unclear.[16] It may be several years before large-scale studies provide more definitive conclusions. Even then, it is unlikely that studies will ever establish a cause-and-effect relationship between antioxidants and chronic diseases. There are too many factors to consider. For example, people who eat plenty of fruits and vegetables may also lead healthy lifestyles overall. Fruits and vegetables also contain thousands of plant chemicals, many beginning to show promise against disease. Consequently, some scientists advocate patience until scientific consensus is reached, and they do not recommend taking supplements at this time. Other scientists believe that thousands of Americans may die prematurely of heart disease and cancer before a consensus develops and that the ground swell of evidence, despite some inconsistencies, supports taking antioxidants now.

Presently there is only one strategy to combat disease that no scientist would dispute: Eat more produce. Fruits and vegetables are high in fiber and low in fat and contain hundreds of substances that have the potential to improve health—not just the few compounds that have been isolated and packaged as supplements. In all the research that has been done on diet, antioxidants, and disease, the strongest and most consistent pattern has been that eating a variety of fruits and vegetables produces benefits. The daily consumption of five to nine servings of fruits and vegetables is a good goal for most people. Emphasize dark green vegetables and orange, red, and yellow fruits and vegetables. Dark-pigmented fruits and vegetables are excellent sources of antioxidant vitamins and many other nutrients. Consume them together. It is possible that the beneficial effects of antioxidants occur when they are eaten in combination with each other. Don't take supplements of the antioxidant selenium. The difference between an adequate and a toxic dose of selenium is very small.[2]

In preparing food for consumption, remember that vitamin content is easily compromised. Improper storage; excessive cooking; and exposure to heat, light, and air may reduce the vitamin content in food.

Vitamin C

Vitamin C, also called *ascorbic acid*, is essential to the formation of collagen, a protein used to form all the connective tissues of your body. It is required in the breakdown and absorption of some amino acids and other minerals (such as iron) and in the formation of some hormones. It may also help the immune system prevent infections. As an antioxidant, it may play a role in prevention of heart disease. It is unclear whether the heart-protective benefit of vitamin C is associated with the intake of vitamin C supplements or if the benefits are restricted to the interaction of nutrients in vitamin C–rich foods.

Contrary to popular opinion, vitamin C does not prevent the common cold. Scientifically controlled studies reveal no difference in the incidence of colds among vitamin C users and nonusers. On a positive note, however, some studies suggest that large doses (about 2,000 mg a day) can reduce the severity and duration of a cold's symptoms slightly.[17]

The RDA of vitamin C is 90 mg for men and 75 mg for women. Smokers need an additional 35 mg. The Tolerable Upper Limit is 2,000 mg. That much, however, might also cause diarrhea and kidney stones in susceptible people.[18] Advocates of increased vitamin C often recommend intakes of 200 mg or more.[19] Still, an intake of 200 mg/day can be achieved by food intake. Good food sources of vitamin C include broccoli, cantaloupe, citrus, peppers, potatoes, strawberries, apricots, kiwifruit, cauliflower, Brussels sprouts, and tomatoes.

Megadoses (over 2,000 mg) of vitamin C offer little benefit to the body and may be harmful. As a water-soluble vitamin, vitamin C doses in excess of the body's requirement are excreted through the kidneys. In other words, the body can absorb only so much. For those who absorb excess iron, supplements of vitamin C could be dangerous. Large intakes may also produce errors in the results of some diagnostic tests (such as the hemoccult test, which tests for blood in the intestines).

Carotenoids

More than 600 carotenoids are found in nature. They give fruits and vegetables their yellow, orange, and red colors. They're also abundant in dark green vegetables. Three of the major carotenoids (alpha-carotene, beta-carotene, and beta-cryptoxanthin) can be converted by the body into vitamin A and are referred to as *provitamin A*. Until recently, beta-carotene was thought to offer the most health-protecting antioxidant effect. However, after studies showed that the incidence of lung cancer increased in smokers who took beta-carotene supplements, researchers concluded that beta-carotene is not the main protector.

One carotenoid currently being studied for its antioxidant potency is lycopene, the predominant carotenoid in the blood and in the prostate gland in males. It cannot be converted to vitamin A, but it has twice the antioxidant potency of beta-carotene. Benefits attributed to lycopene are a reduced risk for some cancers, especially those of the digestive tract and the prostate. The best source of lycopene is tomatoes.

Currently, carotenoid supplements, including beta-carotene and lycopene, are not recommended. Carotenoids interact with one another, and supplemental doses of one carotenoid may impair the absorption of others. Instead, eat a variety of vegetables and fruits to get a mix of carotenoids. Five servings a day of fruits and vegetables that are mostly yellow-orange, red, or dark green are recommended. It is likely that carotenoids are more beneficial to health when they are consumed together from food than when packaged separately, as in a supplement.

Vitamin E

Vitamin E is a fat-soluble vitamin; it plays a role in the formation of red blood cells and maintenance of nervous tissues, and it aids in the absorption of vitamin A. Claims that vitamin E improves the skin, heals scars, prevents stretch marks, slows the aging process, and increases fertility are more folklore than fact.

Vitamin E is an antioxidant that may boost immunity. Animal studies show that vitamin E is associated with an increase in antibodies that produce protective responses to diseases such as hepatitis B, tetanus, flu, the common cold, and upper respiratory infections.[20] Studies are underway to determine if the same benefits transfer to humans. The strongest evidence for cancer protection is among male smokers. Several studies have found that vitamin E lowers the risk for prostate cancer.[21] Vitamin E is also being studied for its role in improving cognitive function, with an eye toward protecting against or delaying the onset of Alzheimer's disease. In a study of more than 4,700 men and women, aged 65 and older, those who took vitamin E and vitamin C supplements together suffered less Alzheimer's disease. In the same study, however, those who took either vitamin alone showed no protective effect. Researchers speculated that the synergy between E and C produced the positive results.[22] Previous studies that reported cardiovascular health benefits are now under question.

The RDA of vitamin E is 15 mg (22 International Units, or IU). The Tolerable Upper Limit is 1,000 mg. Food sources include nuts, vegetable oils, and fortified cereals. Studies and clinical trials typically administer vitamin E in supplemental amounts of at least 45 mg (100 IU). The effect of consuming vitamin E from food versus obtaining comparable levels through supplements is difficult to determine because dietary vitamin E intake rarely reaches the supplemental level. For example, 1 ounce of almonds, a good source of this nutrient, contains only about 2 mg of vitamin E. Low-fat diets are especially scarce in vitamin E.

Experts are divided in their opinion about taking supplements of vitamin E. If you choose to take a supplement, select the natural form, rather than the synthetic, because it is absorbed more easily into the body. The label for natural vitamin E should read "d-alpha tocopherol." Synthetic vitamin E is labeled "di-alpha tocopherol."

Folate, vitamin B$_6$, vitamin B$_{12}$

Folate is a part of the vitamin B complex and combines with vitamins B$_6$ and B$_{12}$ to form parts of DNA and RNA and to make heme, the iron-containing protein in red blood cells. These three also assist in the metabolism of amino acids. The term **folate** refers to the natural form of the vitamin found in foods. *Folic acid* refers to the synthetic form of the vitamin found in supplements and fortified food.[3] Folic acid is about twice as potent as folate. Vitamins B$_6$ and B$_{12}$ are plentiful in foods, and few people, with the possible exception of strict vegetarians,

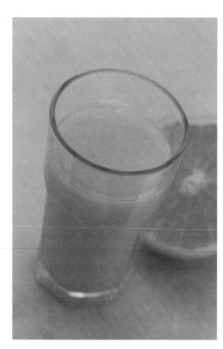

Antioxidant vitamins from foods such as citrus fruits may help protect young and old alike from heart disease and cancer.

need to worry about deficiencies. With advancing age, some people have trouble producing stomach acids in sufficient quantities to separate vitamin B_{12} from foods. They have no trouble absorbing B_{12} from supplements because it is not attached to food, so older people may also need to supplement their diets with B_{12}. Good sources of these vitamins are meat products, dairy products, eggs, spinach, whole-wheat bread, and breakfast cereals.

Folate, as its name implies, is found in foliage—leafy vegetables, such as lettuce and spinach. It is also found in citrus fruits, whole-grain bread, fortified cereals, and liver. Of the three B vitamins mentioned here, folate is the one in which Americans are most likely to fall short.

Because folate has been associated with a reduction in the chances of neurological birth defects, such as spina bifida, a woman planning a pregnancy may be advised by her physician to eat foods rich in folate and possibly to take a supplement. In an effort to reduce the incidence of these birth defects, food fortification guidelines were established in 1998 that require food manufacturers to fortify certain grain products, such as flour, bread, and cereal, with folic acid.

Current interest in folate was sparked by studies that demonstrated that people whose blood levels were low in folic acid had high homocysteine levels. Homocysteine is an amino acid that plays a role in the formation of two other amino acids, cysteine and methionine. To work properly, these amino acids require three B

vitamins—folate, B_6, and B_{12}. If these vitamins are in short supply, homocysteine levels might rise.[23] High homocysteine levels are thought to increase the risk for heart disease (see Chapter 2). The compound has also been implicated in several other diseases, including osteoporosis, cancer, diabetes mellitus, dementia, Alzheimer's disease, and neurological disorders.[24,25]

The best way to lower homocysteine concentrations is to consume enough B vitamins with an emphasis on folate. The RDA of folate is 400 micrograms (mcg) and is easily achievable in the diet. Multivitamin supplements usually have 400 mcg of folic acid. Megadoses of folate should be avoided to prevent the possibility of a false negative for anemia (too few blood cells) caused by a vitamin B_{12} deficiency. If you take folate supplements, tell your physician, so that the appropriate tests can be ordered.

Vitamin supplements

Advertisements proclaim that vitamins provide energy, promote wellness, and prevent disease and that taking more results in more energy and better health. Consequently, many Americans take one or more **vitamin supplements** in multiple and single doses, in both natural and synthetic forms. Vitamins do facilitate energy release from carbohydrates, fats, and proteins, but they do not provide energy. It is not possible to survive on water and vitamins.

Should you take a vitamin supplement? The scientific community is divided in its answer to this question. One position is that healthy adults who eat a variety of foods do not need them. Another position acknowledges the reality that Americans don't usually get their RDAs of vitamins and minerals[26] in their diet and a multivitamin supplement provides a form of insurance. Most multivitamin supplements contain some of the essential minerals plus the RDA of all the essential vitamins, except biotin and vitamin K, which are easy to obtain from foods. Taking a multivitamin supplement can help fill nutritional gaps in the typical American diet, although the practice is no substitute for eating a balanced diet.[2] If you take a supplement, consume it with food. Food facilitates the absorption and interaction of nutrients in a multivitamin supplement.

Although healthy people don't need vitamin supplements if they are eating a balanced diet, there are several situations[27] in which a vitamin or mineral supplement may be called for:

If you are age 65 or older, you may need supplements of vitamins B_6, B_{12}, and D because of the difficulty in absorbing these vitamins with advancing age. Women, especially those not taking estrogen, may require more calcium and vitamin D to protect against osteoporosis.

If you are dieting, consuming fewer than 1,000 calories a day, you may benefit from a vitamin and mineral supplement.

If you have a chronic illness, such as cancer or AIDS, or a disease of the digestive tract, it may interfere with normal digestion and absorption of nutrients and justify your use of vitamin and mineral supplements.

If you smoke, you may need vitamin C supplements.

If you drink excessive alcohol, you may suffer from poor nutrition and the alcohol may interfere with the absorption and metabolism of vitamins.

If you are pregnant and lactating (breast-feeding), supplements of folic acid, iron, and calcium may be recommended for you.

If you are a vegetarian, you may need additional vitamin B$_{12}$. Calcium and vitamin D supplements may also be warranted if your milk intake and sun exposure are limited.

Vitamin supplements are sometimes needed by people with irregular diets or unusual lifestyles or by people following certain weight-reduction regimens or strict vegetarian diets. In addition, infants and pregnant and lactating women may need supplements. When taken as supplements, vitamins should be viewed as medicine and, therefore, should be recommended by a physician.

When shopping for supplements, it is easy to be misled by advertising hype and inaccurate labels. Americans spend billions annually for vitamin, mineral, and herbal supplements. Much of this expenditure goes toward products with no scientifically proven health value. Consequently, it is important for consumers to be discriminating in their purchase of supplements. To that end,

- Shop for supplements that carry the letters *USP* on the label. These conform to the standards set by the U.S. Pharmacopoeia, a nonprofit, nongovernmental agency that establishes drug standards.
- If you take antioxidants for their health benefits, shop by price.
- Look for an expiration date that shows how long the supplement will retain its potency.
- Avoid supplements that claim to have a "sustained release." The delayed release may prevent the nutrients from being absorbed.
- Don't be influenced by most health store advertisements. Remember, if you need a supplement, it's most likely to be a multivitamin.

Minerals

Minerals are simple but important nutrients. As inorganic compounds, they lack the complexity of vitamins, but they fulfill a variety of functions. For example, sodium and potassium affect shifts in body fluids,

calcium and phosphorus contribute to the body's structure, iron is the core of hemoglobin (an oxygen-carrying compound in the blood), and iodine facilitates production of thyroxine (a hormone that influences metabolic rate).

There are 20 to 30 important nutritional minerals. Minerals should be consumed in smaller amounts than amounts of energy nutrients and water. Minerals present in the body and required in large amounts (more than 100 mg, or 0.02 teaspoon, per day) are called *major minerals* or *macrominerals.* They include, in descending order of prominence, calcium, phosphorus, potassium, sulfur, sodium, chloride, and magnesium. Major minerals contribute 60 to 80 percent of inorganic material in the human body.

Minerals required in small amounts (less than 100 mg per day) are called *trace minerals* or *microminerals.* There are more than a dozen trace minerals, the best known being iron, zinc, and iodine (see Just the Facts: Minerals on page 180).

Some minerals are similar to water-soluble vitamins in that they are readily excreted by the kidneys, do not accumulate in the body, and rarely become toxic. Others are like fat-soluble vitamins in that they are stored and are toxic if taken in excess.

Minerals are different from vitamins; they are indestructible and require no special handling during food preparation. The only precautions that need to be taken are to avoid soaking minerals out of food and throwing them away in cooking water.

Major minerals are abundant in the diet; therefore, deficiencies are highly unlikely, especially if a variety of foods are included. If a deficiency in major minerals does occur, it is most likely to be a calcium deficiency, especially among women. Average daily calcium intake for women of all ages is 765 mg, far short of the recommended adequate intake of 1,000 to 1,300 mg. For men the daily intake of calcium averages 966 mg.[28] The following are some tips for increasing your calcium intake:

- Try to consume as much calcium as possible from food. Skim milk and low-fat dairy products are excellent sources of calcium and are fortified with vitamin D. Most people who eschew dairy products don't get enough calcium.[29] Nondairy sources include sardines, shellfish, dark greens, almonds, dried beans, and fortified orange juice.
- Use calcium supplements to compensate for a calcium shortfall. Getting enough calcium from food requires consuming the equivalent of a quart of milk per day. As a result, many people benefit from an over-the-counter calcium supplement.
- Calcium is best absorbed in doses of 500 mg or less, taken with meals.[2] The best type of calcium supplement is calcium carbonate, available in common antacids.[29]

ᨊᨊ Just the Facts ᨊᨊ

Minerals

The following are some basic facts about minerals.

Major (Macro) Minerals

Types: calcium, phosphorus, potassium, sulfur, sodium chloride, and magnesium

Trace (Micro) Minerals

Types: iron, iodine, zinc, selenium, manganese, copper, molybdenum, cobalt, chromium, fluorine, silicon, vanadium, nickel, tin, cadmium

Minerals of Special Concern*

Calcium

Wellness benefits: contributes to bone and tooth formation, general body growth, maintenance of good muscle tone, nerve function, cell membrane function, and regulation of normal heartbeat

Food sources: dairy products, dark green vegetables, dried beans, shellfish

Deficiency signs and symptoms: bone pain and fractures, muscle cramps, osteoporosis

Iron

Wellness benefits: facilitates oxygen and carbon dioxide transport, formation of red blood cells, production of antibodies, synthesis of collagen, use of energy

Food sources: red meat (lean); seafood; eggs; dried beans; nuts; grains; green, leafy vegetables

Deficiency signs and symptoms: fatigue, weakness

Sodium**

Wellness benefits: maintains proper acid-base balance and body fluid regulation, aids in formation of digestive secretions, assists in nerve transmission

Food sources: processed foods, meats, table salt

Deficiency signs and symptoms: restlessness, fatigue, diminished strength. Deficiency is rare in the United States.

* Calcium and iron are of special concern because deficiencies are likely to exist, especially among women and children.

** Sodium is of concern because of the potential for overconsumption.

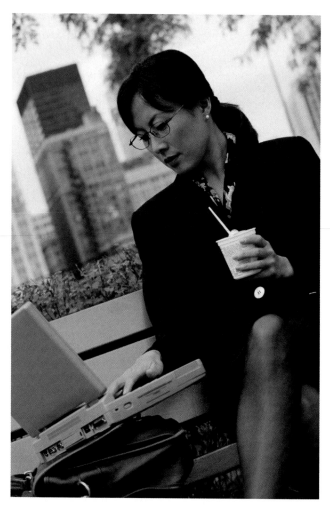

Starting your day with low-fat dairy products, such as milk and yogurt, is a good way to add calcium to your diet.

- Take calcium supplements with meals. Calcium is best dissolved and absorbed in stomach acids secreted during mealtime.
- Look for calcium-fortified foods. A cup of calcium-fortified orange juice, for example, contains about the same amount of calcium as a cup of milk and is absorbed more easily.
- Get the recommended intake of vitamin D. Vitamin D is necessary for the body to absorb calcium. (See Just the Facts: Vitamin D: the Hidden Epidemic.)
- If you're taking other supplements or medicines, check with your physician or pharmacist. Calcium can interfere with the absorption of iron, zinc, and certain medicines.

Of the various trace minerals, iron is of concern to nutritionists because certain groups are at risk of having low iron levels. These include young children and early teens; menstruating women; and people with conditions that cause internal bleeding, such as ulcers or intestinal diseases.[3]

Iron deficiency in the diet is responsible for the most prevalent form of anemia in the United States. Iron deficiency hampers the body's ability to produce hemoglobin, a substance needed to carry oxygen in the blood. A lack of hemoglobin can cause fatigue and weakness and

﹏ Just the Facts ﹏

Vitamin D: The Hidden Epidemic

Vitamin D is an essential nutrient required to maintain the body's calcium stores. In the absence of vitamin D, calcium cannot be absorbed.

Vitamin D is called the sunshine vitamin because it is made in the skin on exposure to 15 minutes of sunlight. Surprisingly, vitamin D deficiencies are common, although they may go unnoticed. Consequently, vitamin D deficiencies are often referred to as the "hidden epidemic," especially among housebound adults. Reasons for vitamin D deficiencies include, in part, the growing concern about skin cancer, a sedentary indoor lifestyle, and a poor diet. Milk is fortified with vitamin D and is a good source of the nutrient. Other food sources include fatty fish, fortified soy, and fortified cereals. A daily multivitamin supplement can help meet vitamin D requirements when diet and sun exposure are inadequate.[2] If you are supplementing your diet with extra calcium, don't overlook the body's need for vitamin D.

can even affect behavior and intellectual function. Proper infant feeding through the use of iron-fortified milk or breast-feeding is the best safeguard against iron deficiency in infants. Among adolescents and adults, iron intake can be improved by increasing consumption of iron-rich foods, such as lean red meats, fish, certain kinds of beans, dried fruits, iron-enriched cereals and whole-grain products, and foods cooked in a cast-iron skillet. For some people, especially premenopausal women with inconsistent diets, iron supplements may be justified. In addition, consuming foods that contain vitamin C enhances the body's ability to absorb iron.

Iron deficiency is rare among healthy men and postmenopausal women. Even strict vegetarians can get iron in sufficient amounts by consuming legumes, dark green leafy vegetables, and fortified breads and cereals. However, it is possible to get too much iron. Some studies report that high iron levels may be linked to heart disease, but the jury is still out on this issue. Also, some people have a rare genetic disorder called *hemochromatosis*, which permits an unhealthy buildup of iron. Iron overload may cause liver cancer, heart disease, diabetes, sterility, or other complications.

Zinc is a trace mineral that has received widespread publicity because of its link to the common cold. Early studies reported that zinc lozenges cured the cold within hours. The results of follow-up studies, however, are mixed and suggest that earlier claims of the cold-prevention benefits of zinc may have been prema-

ture. While zinc is essential for proper functioning of the immune system, too much can interfere with the body's use and absorption of other essential minerals, such as iron and copper. Also, excess zinc can lower HDL cholesterol.[3]

Selenium is another trace mineral that may offer unique health benefits. It is an antioxidant associated with a reduced risk for various cancers. An increase in the intake of selenium is thought to lower the chances of developing lung, colon, and other cancers. Because the results of studies of selenium as an anticancer nutrient are mixed, experts do not recommend selenium supplements at this time. Human studies are underway to determine if the health benefits of extra selenium intake can be confirmed. Fish, meats, eggs, and shellfish are good animal sources of selenium. Grains and seeds grown in soils containing selenium are good plant sources. Most adults get enough selenium in their diet. Excess selenium can be toxic. Daily intakes as low as 1 to 3 mg can cause toxicity symptoms if taken for many months.[3]

Water

Next to air, water is the substance most necessary for survival. Most everything in the body occurs in a water medium. Although people can live without vitamins and minerals for extended periods, death results within a few days without water.

Water makes up about 60 percent of the body's weight. Every cell in the body is bathed in water of the exact composition that is best for it. Even tissues that are not thought of as "watery" contain large amounts of water. For example, water makes up about 75 percent of brain and muscle tissues; bone tissue and fat tissue are about 20 percent water. As a rule, the bodies of men contain more water than do the bodies of women because men have more muscle tissue and muscle tissue holds more water than fat tissue, which is more prominent in the bodies of women.

Water performs many functions. It is vital to digestion and metabolism because it acts as a medium for chemical reactions in the body. It carries oxygen and nutrients to the cells through blood, regulates body temperature through perspiration, and lubricates the joints. It removes waste through sweat and urine, protects a fetus, and assists in respiration by moistening the lungs to facilitate intake of oxygen and excretion of carbon dioxide. It also assists with constipation relief and provides satiety, thus serving as a deterrent to the overconsumption of food.

Although most water intake comes from beverages, solid foods also make a significant contribution (see Just the Facts: Bottled Water Comes with Many Names, page 182). Most fruits and vegetables are more than 80 percent water, meats are 50 percent water, bread is 36 percent water, and butter is approximately 20 percent water.[3]

Just the Facts

Bottled Water Comes with Many Names

If you don't like your water from the tap, you can buy purified water, spring water, mineral water, distilled water, and drinking water by the bottle, six pack, or case. Are there differences among the various types of bottled water? There are, but you almost need a dictionary to sort the differences. The following is a brief description of the common types of bottled water.[30]

- *Distilled water* comes from the stream of public water that has been boiled.

- *Drinking water* is public or municipal water, such as tap water, and comprises 25 percent of bottled water. If the water comes directly from the tap without any treatment, the label has to identify the public source it comes from. If the water has been treated, no disclosure is required.

- *Mineral water* is spring water that naturally contains at least 250 milligrams of dissolved minerals (such as magnesium and calcium) per liter.

- *Purified water* has been treated with distillation, ion-exchange, reverse osmosis, or a similar process.

- *Sparkling water* is spring water that contains carbon dioxide gas (as in cola beverages).

- *Spring water* comes from underground formations beneath the earth's surface. It makes up about 75 percent of the bottled water sold in the United States. Theoretically, spring water is protected from pollution.

How much water should you drink? Until recently, the answer was to drink at least 8 to 12 cups of fluids a day. The Institute of Medicine recently changed its recommendation on water consumption. While water needs vary according to climate and physical activity levels, the current recommendation is to respond to your thirst reflex (see Chapter 3). Fluid intake, driven by thirst, allows maintenance of hydration status and total body water at normal levels (see Real-World Wellness: How Can You Tell If You're Getting Enough Water?).[31] Beverages, colas, alcoholic beverages (in moderation), and food all contribute to the body's need for water. One way to monitor water intake is to check the color and odor of urine. Dark yellow instead of pale urine is a sign of insufficient water intake, as is urine with a very strong odor,[3] understanding, at the same time, that medicines and vitamin supplements can cause dark urine.

Under normal circumstances, too much water cannot be consumed because the body is efficient at getting rid of what it does not need. *Water intoxication,* the

Real-World Wellness

How Can You Tell If You're Getting Enough Water?

Experts say that thirst is a good indicator of when and how much water to drink. But what if I'm a heavy sweater and lose an inordinate amount of water? How can I be sure that I'm properly hydrated?

The thirst mechanism is not always reliable during strenuous physical activities. The following guidelines will help you determine whether to increase your fluid intake.[3]

- Weigh yourself before and after a workout. This will provide a gauge for determining how much water was lost during exercise and how much to replace.

- Replace at least 75 percent of the weight loss, especially as weight loss approaches 2 to 3 percent. Three cups of water are recommended per pound. For example, someone who weighs 200 pounds and loses 4 pounds (2 percent) during a workout should consume 9 cups of water to be sufficiently hydrated (4 pounds × 3 cups/pound = 12 cups × .75 = 9 cups).

- Check the color of your urine. If it is dark and has a strong odor, you probably need more water.

consumption of more water than the kidneys can excrete, is possible, though rare. It can lead to serious side effects, such as headache, blurred vision, cramps, convulsions, and possibly death. An excessive amount would have to approach many quarts each day. Very few people are at risk of drinking too much water.[3]

Other Nutrients with Unique Health Benefits

In addition to the six classes of essential nutrients, many other substances in food contribute to health. Interest in these substances has sparked interest in enriched food, fortified food, functional food, nutraceuticals, botanicals, herbs, and fiber (see Just the Facts: Enhanced Foods). Many of these substances promote health and prevent illness; many more fall far short of their claims. New discoveries and recent developments in these areas have outpaced the scientific community's ability to monitor, test, and confirm various claims. Until these claims can be validated, the public should assume an attitude of skepticism. While many of the chemical compounds in food promise to promote health, taken indiscriminately they may do more harm than good. The exception is fiber, for which most claims are backed by years of solid evidence.

ᔋᔋ Just the Facts ᔋᔋ

Enhanced Foods

The term *enhanced foods* refers to foods that have been modified and or supplemented for the purpose of achieving or facilitating a health benefit. As an umbrella term, *enhanced foods* includes enriched food, fortified food, functional food, nutraceuticals, and genetically modified food.[2,3]

Enriched food. Food that has been supplemented with naturally occurring nutrients often lost or compromised during processing. The addition of the vitamins thiamin, niacin, riboflavin, and folate and the mineral iron to bread is an example.

Fortified food. Food that has been supplemented with nutrients in excess of what was originally in the food or were not present. Three examples include milk fortified with vitamin D, orange juice fortified with calcium, and breakfast cereals fortified with 100 percent of the RDA for certain vitamins and minerals.

Functional food. Food that contains nutrients good for health beyond traditional benefits. For example, tomatoes are good sources of many vitamins and minerals. They also contain another substance beyond vitamins and minerals, called lycopene, that may help prevent some forms of cancer. Therefore, tomatoes can be called a functional food.

Nutraceuticals. Functional foods that have been modified to produce druglike effects. Fruit juice with added herbs, such as ginkgo biloba or echinacea, is an example. When foods are consumed primarily for their medicinal value, they are viewed as nutraceuticals.

Genetically modified food. Food that has been altered at the genetic level to improve health benefits or to make it hardier.

Phytochemicals, Phytonutrients

Phytochemicals, also called phytonutrients, are plant chemicals that exist naturally in all plant foods. Chemically, they are not vitamins, minerals, fiber, or any of the energy nutrients. Rather, they are the hundreds of thousands of active compounds found in small amounts in vegetables and fruits. Although phytochemicals have not been traditionally classified as essential nutrients, scientists believe that they might play an important role in preventing various diseases. For example, populations that consume higher amounts of fruits and vegetables have a lower risk for cancer.[32] Some phytochemicals have a structure similar to the body's natural forms of estrogen. These compounds are called *phytoestrogens* (or *plant estrogens*), and when ingested by way of the diet, they may reduce the potentially harmful effect of the more potent, naturally occurring estrogens often associated with breast and prostate cancer.[2] Although phytochemicals have largely been studied for their role in cancer prevention, researchers are exploring the relationship of phytochemicals to many other diseases, including cardiovascular disease, osteoporosis, diabetes, and hypertension.

There is a great deal of excitement in nutrition and food sciences about the potential of phytochemicals in health promotion. The reported health benefits of several phytochemicals are highlighted in Table 6-6 (page 184). As scientists continue to isolate, identify, and study specific plant chemicals, it is likely that the place of such chemicals in disease prevention will become more important.

Botanicals (Phytomedicinals) (Herbs)

Plants used medically are technically called **botanicals** or **phytomedicinals**. The popular literature usually refers to them as *herbs*. Herbs number in the thousands; however, few are backed by well-conducted research studies similar to those used to test over-the-counter drugs in the United States. Herbs, however, are not regulated as drugs; instead, they are classified as dietary supplements. There is considerable debate about their effectiveness and safety. Consequently, some experts refer to the dietary supplement industry as the "Wild West." The names, food sources, and health claims of several popular herbs are presented in Just the Facts: Some Common Herbs Sold as Nutritional Supplements on page 185. Herbs are not to be confused with hormone supplements, such as melatonin, DHEA (dehydroepiandrosterone), and DMSO (dimethylsulfoxide). Unlike herbs, extracted from plants, these are synthetic compounds. The purported health benefits of these hormones have not yet been proved.

If you decide to take an herb, here are some tips:

- Check with your physician before taking herbs, especially for serious conditions. Inform your physician of herbs you are taking, as you would for prescribed medicines. There are many potential interactions with other supplements and medicines.
- Avoid using herbs if you are pregnant or nursing.
- Check the label for the abbreviation *USP*. This means that the manufacturer has met the stringent guidelines of the U.S. Pharmacopoeia, ensuring the quality, strength, purity, and consistency of the product. The letters *NF*, which stands for *National Formulary*, also ensure that the product meets minimum standards. Presently, only a handful of

Table 6-6 Health Benefits of Selected Phytochemicals, Phytonutrients

Phytochemical/ Phytonutrient	Food Source	Possible Benefit
Allyl sulfide	Garlic, onions, leeks, chives	Decreases reproduction of tumor cells; facilitates excretion of carcinogens; blocks nitrite formation in stomach
Caffeic acid	Fruits	Facilitates excretions of carcinogens
Capsaicin	Hot peppers	Acts as an antioxidant; inhibits carcinogenesis
Coumarin	Citrus fruit, tomatoes	Prevents blood clotting; stimulates anticancer enzymes
Dithiolthione	Cruciferous vegetables	Stimulates anticancer enzymes
Phytoestrogen (isoflavones)	Soybeans, dried beans	Helps prevent breast cancer by stopping the estrogen produced by the body from entering cells
Flavonoids	Fruits, vegetables, red wine, grape juice, green tea	Act as an antioxidant
Phenolic acids (ellagic acid, ferulic acid)	Fruits, grains, nuts	Prevent DNA damage in cells; bind to iron, which may inhibit the mineral from creating free radicals; bind to nitrites in the stomach, preventing them from being converted into nitrosamines
Indoles, isothiocynates, sulforaphane	Cruciferous vegetables	Stimulate anticancer enzymes
Limonene	Citrus fruits	Stimulates anticancer enzymes
Phytic acid	Grains	Binds to iron, which may inhibit the mineral from creating cancer-causing free radicals
Terpenes (lycopene, lutein, carotenoids)	Tomatoes, watermelon, sweet potatoes, carrots, spinach, cantaloupe	Neutralize free radicals and help repair DNA

herbs have been subjected to review using USP standards.

- Do your homework. Read about the herb; ask your pharmacist for information. There are several Web sites that provide helpful information:

    U.S. Pharmacopoeia: **www.usp.org**
    American Botanical Council: **www.herbalgram.org**
    The Herb Research Foundation: **www.herbs.org**

- Monitor your body's response. Start with a lower than recommended dose. Stop taking an herb if you have an adverse reaction.
- Don't expect miracles. Herbs take longer to work than prescribed and over-the-counter medicines.
- Take specific herbs for specific needs. Avoid taking herbs continuously.

Fiber

One advantage of a complex carbohydrate diet is that it will likely be high in fiber unless the foods are refined or highly processed.

Fiber (formerly called *roughage*) is a general term that refers to the substances in food that resist digestion. The amount of fiber in a food is determined by its plant source and the amount of processing it undergoes.

In general, the more a food is processed, the more the fiber is broken down or removed and the lower its fiber content.

There are two kinds of fiber: *soluble fiber* dissolves or swells in hot water, and *insoluble fiber* does not dissolve in water. From a practical, dietary perspective, it is unnecessary to distinguish between the two types of fiber. Every plant food usually contains a mixture of fiber types, and there is significant overlap in the health benefits of soluble and insoluble fiber-rich foods.[34] Good sources of soluble fiber are fruits, vegetables, and grains (see Table 6-7 on page 186). Good sources of insoluble fiber are wheat bran, whole grains, dried beans, and most fruits and vegetables, especially those eaten with the skin (see Just the Facts: Sample Ingredient List for a Whole-Grain Food on page 186).

Health benefits of fiber

Dietary fiber is an important part of a healthy diet. To quote a leading nutrition expert, "It's hard to eat a high-fiber diet that isn't healthy."[20] Health benefits include a reduced risk for heart disease, improvement in blood sugar control, prevention and relief of constipation, and reduced risks of developing precancerous polyps in the

~~~~~~~~~~ Just the Facts ~~~~~~~~~~

Some Common Herbs Sold as Nutritional Supplements

The following are possible benefits and problems[3,33] of various herbs:

- Black cohosh

  Possible benefits: reduce, relieve symptoms of menopause

  Potential problem: mild gastrointestinal distress, nausea, fall in blood pressure

- Cranberry

  Possible benefits: prevention or treatment of urinary tract infections

  Potential problem: concentrated cranberry tablets may increase the risk for kidney stones

- Echinacea

  Possible benefits: immune booster for colds, flus, and respiratory infections

  Potential problem: some allergic reactions reported in people with autoimmune disorders, such as lupus or multiple sclerosis

- Feverfew

  Possible benefits: prevention and treatment of migraines and associated nausea

  Potential problem: a potential allergen for people sensitive to ragweed

- Garlic

  Possible benefits: may promote antibacterial, antifungal, and antiviral activity, including those associated with the common cold; may have cardiovascular benefits

  Potential problem: in excess, possible interactions with other herbs and/or medicines

- Ginger

  Possible benefits: treatment of motion sickness, nausea, indigestion

  Potential problem: may aggravate gallstones, heartburn; acts as a blood thinner

- Ginkgo biloba

  Possible benefits: may improve memory and mental functioning; acts as an antioxidant; aids blood flow to the brain and to the legs

  Potential problem: acts as a blood thinner; may cause gastrointestinal upset, headaches, allergic skin reactions

- Ginseng

  Possible benefits: may enhance immunity

  Potential problem: may increase blood pressure; may cause headaches and skin problems

- Glucosamine and chondroitin

  Possible benefits: may stimulate cartilage growth and relieve pain associated with arthritis and stiff joints

  Potential problem: reduced insulin secretions

- Saw palmetto

  Possible benefits: may improve urinary flow in men with enlarged prostate

  Potential problem: may cause inaccurate readings on PSA tests

- Soy isoflavones

  Possible benefits: reduce postmenopausal symptoms, prevent breast or prostate cancer, promote cartilage formation, decrease joint inflammation, prevent bone loss, and act as a mild antidepressant

  Possible problem: mild headaches

- St. John's wort

  Possible benefits: may alleviate mild to moderate depression

  Potential problem: not useful for severe depression; may cause complications with prescription antidepressants

- Valerian

  Possible benefits: treatment for insomnia, mild anxiety, restlessness

  Potential problem: may cause complications with sedatives or antidepressants

---

intestines. High-fiber diets may also be a key strategy for weight management because fiber delays stomach emptying, which, in turn, promotes a feeling of *satiety*, or fullness, and diminishes the appetite.

If you are not accustomed to eating fiber-rich foods, gradually add them to your diet over time, following these suggestions:[2,36,37]

- Eat whole-wheat bread rather than white bread. Look for bread that provides at least 3 grams of fiber per slice.
- Look for whole grains, such as whole wheat, on food labels. Foods "made with whole-wheat flour" are mostly refined. Wheat flour and unbleached wheat flour are not whole-grain. Color is not an

Table 6-7 Fiber Content of Selected Foods

Food	Fiber (g)
Fruits	
Apple, with peel	4.2
Banana	3.3
Blackberries (1 cup)	9.7
Dates, chopped (1 cup)	15.5
Grapes	1.0
Orange	2.9
Peach, peeled	2.0
Pear, with skin	4.9
Prunes, dried, pitted (10)	13.5
Raisins, seedless (1 cup)	9.6
Breads	
Oatmeal (1 cup)	0.86
Pumpernickel (1 slice)	1.33
Rye (1 slice)	1.65
Wheat (1 slice)	1.40
White (1 slice)	0.68
Whole-wheat (1 slice)	3.17
Cereals	
All-Bran (1/3 cup)	10.1
Bran Chex (2/3 cup)	5
Bran flakes (2/3 cup)	5
Cheerios (1 1/4 cup)	3
Corn flakes (1 cup)	1
Grape-nuts (1 1/4 cup)	2
Life (2/3 cup)	3
Raisin Bran (1/2 cup)	4
Rice Krispies (1 cup)	Trace
Shredded Wheat (1 biscuit)	3
Vegetables	
Baked potato, with skin	4.4
Carrot	2.0
Cauliflower (1/2 cup)	1.3
Corn, canned (1/2 cup)	6.3
Garbanzo beans (1 cup)	8.6
Green beans (1 cup)	3.1
Greens (1 cup)	2.9
Lima beans (1 cup)	9.2
Navy beans (1 cup)	16.5
Split peas (1 cup)	16.4
Tomato	2.2

Just the Facts

Sample Ingredient List for a Whole-Grain Food[35]

- Ingredients: whole-wheat flour, water, high fructose corn syrup, wheat gluten, soybean and/or canola oil, yeast, salt, honey
- Note: "Wheat flour," "enriched flour," and "degerminated corn meal" are not whole grains.

- Use raspberries as a topping for ice cream and yogurt.
- Snack on an unpeeled fruit.
- Top your salads and casseroles with a whole-grain cereal, such as Shredded Wheat.
- Eat the skin on your potato.
- Include beans in soups and vegetable salads.
- Eat more legumes.

How much fiber?

Most Americans consume 14 to 15 grams of fiber per day.[3] The daily recommendation is 25 to 35 grams of fiber if under age 50 and 20 to 30 grams of fiber if over age 50.[2] This is based on 14 grams of fiber per 1,000 calories. Most Americans have trouble meeting this recommendation because of their heavy intake of meat products. Meat provides little or no fiber; consequently, only vegetarians are likely to get enough fiber. Eating naturally high-fiber foods, such as whole grains, fruits, vegetables, and beans, is a good way to increase fiber intake. Starting or ending the day with a high-fiber cereal is another convenient way to increase your consumption not only of fiber but also of many vitamins and minerals. Check food labels, which identify the amount of fiber per serving.

As with most other nutrients, fiber can be consumed in excess. Indiscriminate consumption of fiber may interfere with the body's ability to absorb other essential nutrients. A person who eats bulky foods but has only a small capacity may not be able to take in enough food energy or nutrients. A high intake of dietary fiber, such as 60 grams per day, also requires a high intake of water.[3]

Putting Nutrition to Work

Nutrition is a complex science and involves the study of thousands of nutrients and a countless number of possible interactions, all of which take place at the cellular level. Many of the results of nutritional practices, good or bad, take years or even decades to become apparent. Fortunately, it isn't necessary to be a biochemist to

indication of whole grain. Bread can be brown because of molasses or other ingredients.
- Substitute brown rice, millet, and bulgur wheat for white rice and potatoes.
- Snack on popcorn instead of potato chips (popcorn is a whole grain).
- Eat whole fruit instead of drinking juice.

understand and follow nutritional practices that promote health and prevent the early onset of many health problems. The benchmark for developing a plan for good nutrition is the 2000 *Dietary Guidelines for Americans*.[35] (See This Just In, page 210.) These guidelines recommend that, to stay healthy, persons aged 2 years and older should follow the ABCs for good health: *A*im for fitness, *B*uild a healthy base, and *C*hoose sensibly. The ABCs provide the framework for 10 specific dietary guidelines:

- *To aim for fitness,*
  - Aim for a healthy weight.
  - Be physically active each day.
- *To build a healthy base,*
  - Let the pyramid guide food choices.
  - Choose a variety of grains daily, especially whole grains.
  - Choose a variety of fruits and vegetables daily.
  - Keep food safe to eat.
- *To choose sensibly,*
  - Choose a diet low in saturated fat and cholesterol and moderate in total fat.
  - Choose beverages and foods to moderate intake of sugars.
  - Choose and prepare foods with less salt.
  - If consuming alcoholic beverages, do so in moderation.

Aim for a Healthy Weight

A healthy weight is key to a long, healthy life. To be at their best, adults need to avoid gaining weight, and many need to lose weight. Being obese increases the risk for many chronic diseases. The achievement and maintenance of a desirable body weight and composition are complex issues and are treated separately in this text. For a complete discussion of the principles of balancing food intake with physical activity for evaluating and maintaining desirable body composition, refer to Chapters 7 and 8.

Be Physically Active Each Day

Aim to accumulate at least 60 minutes of moderate physical activity most days of the week, preferably daily.[4] If you already get 60 minutes of physical activity daily, you can gain even more health benefits by increasing the amount of time you are physically active or by taking part in more vigorous activities. No matter what activity you choose, you can do it all at once or spread it out over two or three times during the day.

A moderate physical activity is any activity that requires about as much energy as walking 4 to 5 miles in an hour. Choose activities that you enjoy and that you can do regularly. Some people prefer activities that fit into their daily routine, such as gardening or taking extra trips up and down stairs. Others prefer a regular

Wellness on the Web
Behavior Change Activities

Put "Pyramid Power" to Work for You

When you want to plan a nutritionally balanced diet, your best bet is to eat a variety of foods according to the federal government's Food Guide Pyramid. You can use the pyramid to determine how many servings from each food group to include in your diet; it's also a great way to ensure that you consume the Recommended Dietary Allowances (RDAs) of essential nutrients each day. To use an interactive Food Guide Pyramid, go to **www.mhhe.com/anspaugh6e**. Go to Student Center, Chapter 6, Wellness on the Web, then Activity 1. Place your mouse on any portion of the pyramid and click to obtain a list of foods and the appropriate portions for each food group.

Diet Facts—or Fiction?

Can you lose weight on a grapefruit diet? Should you eat after 6 p.m.? Does gelatin make your nails hard? Are some vegetables and fruits negative-calorie foods? Nutrition has captured the interest of Americans more than perhaps any other aspect of fitness and wellness. Whether it's HDLs or LDLs, fat or fiber, phytochemicals or vitamins, nutritional issues make headlines in both scientific journals and popular magazines, and everyone seems to be an expert. Go to **www.mhhe.com/anspaugh6e** to discover the "Top Ten Diet Myths." Go to Student Center, Chapter 6, click on Wellness on the Web, then on Activity 2.

exercise program, such as a physical activity program at their worksite. Some do both. All contribute to an active lifestyle. The important thing is to be physically active every day. The more exercise you get, the better. If you don't get any exercise at all, any amount of physical activity will yield health benefits. Incorporate physical activity into your lifestyle, so that it is fun and sustainable. If you are already physically active, the goal is one of maintenance and consistency. From a health perspective, achieving a level of fitness that permits you to engage in exercise that is equivalent to a daily 3-mile brisk walk promotes health, prevents the premature onset of many chronic conditions, and provides an extra bonus for people trying to manage their weight by burning about 2,000 calories a week.[38]

The benefits of exercise are discussed throughout this text; specific principles and applications of exercise and physical activity are discussed in depth in Chapters 3, 4, and 5.

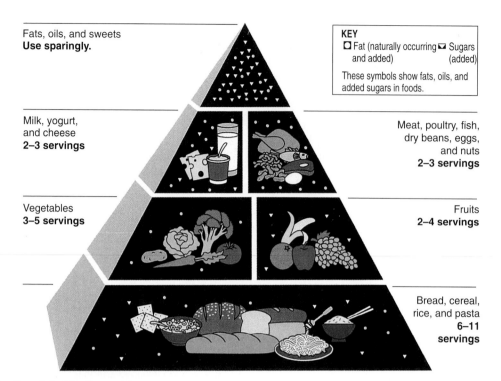

Figure 6-3 Food Guide Pyramid

Children, teenagers, and adults under 25 years of age should choose three servings from the milk, yogurt, and cheese group. Specific serving amounts for each group can be found in the USDA Food Guide on pages 211 and 212.

Let the Food Guide Pyramid guide food choices

Variety and moderation are the essence of a healthy diet. The best way to ensure a varied and moderate diet is to use the Food Guide Pyramid as the foundation for food selection.

Variety. The Food Guide Pyramid (FGP) (Figure 6-3) portrays dietary guidelines in picture form and provides a structure for dietary planning by recommending the number of servings for each food group. (See This Just In, page 210.) Variety is the cornerstone of the FGP (see Just the Facts: Variety: The Cornerstone of a Healthy Diet). The largest area of the pyramid is the base, which calls for 6 to 11 servings of grain products. Foods from this group make up about 40 percent of the daily diet. The next largest areas of the FGP are the fruit and vegetable groups. Together, grain products, fruits, and vegetables make up nearly three-fourths of the recommended diet. The top of the pyramid allows for a smaller number of servings from meat or meat substitutes and dairy products. About 25 percent of the servings in your daily diet should come from foods in these groups. No recommendations are given for the number of servings of fats, oils, and sweets. The advice is to consume these sparingly.

As helpful as the FGP is for meal planning, it has received some criticism (see Just the Facts: The Food

〰 Just the Facts 〰

Variety: The Cornerstone of a Healthy Diet

A plethora of studies link a specific nutrient to good health. But the study of an isolated nutrient, when removed from its original food source, often yields misleading results and sometimes does more harm than good. For example, beta-carotene has long been reputed as a nutrient that prevents lung cancer. In a famous 1994 study, however, male smokers who took a 20-mg supplement of beta-carotene surprisingly ended up with a higher incidence of lung cancer than the placebo group. As a result, the study was stopped midstream. Researchers concluded that, if beta-carotene prevents and/or delays lung cancer, it does so in combination with other foods.

The only sure way to realize the benefits of various nutrients is to eat a variety of foods. No single nutrient or food can supply all of the essential nutrients in the right proportion needed by the body. Variety is the essence of a healthy diet and may be the only practical way of making sure you're getting the full healthful effects of various nutrients.

Just the Facts

The Food Guide Pyramid Is Not Perfect

The Food Guide Pyramid (FGP) was introduced in 1992 and is widely recognized as the standard for planning a sound diet. Still, it is not without criticism. The U.S. Department of Health and Human Services and the U.S. Department of Agriculture have commissioned the Dietary Guidelines Advisory Committee to review the FGP, solicit feedback from experts, and submit new recommendations, as needed (see the new USDA Food Guide on pages 211 and 212). Suggestions, criticisms, and problem areas under review include the following.[40]

The FGP should:

1. Place more emphasis on whole grains.
2. Differentiate between foods in the meat and beans group.
3. Differentiate between unsaturated fats and oils and saturated fats.
4. Set a ceiling for the consumption of trans fatty acids.
5. Emphasize nutrient-dense choices of fruits and vegetables and other groups that are typically under consumed.
6. Provide dietary recommendations that meet the standards for vitamin E and vitamin D.
7. Express food recommendations in household measures, such as cups and ounces, rather than in servings.
8. Include food recommendations for vegetarians.
9. Include physical activity in the food guidance.
10. Include water and other fluid intake in recommendations.
11. Encourage greater consumption of legumes.
12. Include fortified soy products in the milk group. Increase the amounts recommended in the milk group.
13. Include fortified foods or supplements in the food recommendations.

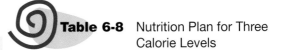

Table 6-8 Nutrition Plan for Three Calorie Levels

	Calorie Level*		
	1,600	2,200	2,800
Grain group servings	6	9	11
Vegetable group servings	3	4	5
Fruit group servings	2	3	4
Milk group servings†	2–3	2–3	2–3
Meat group servings‡	5	6	7
Total fat (g)	53	73	93
Percent fat calories	30	30	30
Total added sugars (tsp.)§	6	12	18

* 1,600 calories is appropriate for many sedentary women and some older adults; 2,200 calories is appropriate for most children, teenage girls, active women, and sedentary men (women who are pregnant or breast-feeding may need more). For teenage boys, many active men, and some very active women, 2,800 calories is appropriate.

† Women who are pregnant or breast-feeding, teenagers, and young adults to age 24 need 3 servings.

‡ Meat group amounts are in total ounces.

§ From candy, desserts, soft drinks, and other sweets.

SOURCE: Wardlaw, G., J. Hampl, and R. DiSilvestro. 2004. *Perspectives in nutrition.* 6th ed. New York: McGraw-Hill.

Guide Pyramid Is Not Perfect). One important omission is any reference to fluid intake. Another criticism is of its lack of guidance for people who don't eat a typical American diet. For that reason, other food pyramids have been developed that meet the needs of alternative diets, such as those of ovolactovegetarians. One such version is presented later in this chapter.

The FGP identifies a range of servings for the food groups. The number of servings that fits your needs depends on your required number of calories. Your calorie requirements depend on many factors, including age, gender, height, weight, activity level, health status, and pregnancy (see Wellness for a Lifetime: The Nutrient Gap on page 190). Three calorie levels, along with the corresponding recommended number of servings, are presented in Table 6-8.

Serving size

What counts as a serving depends on the food and how it is prepared. Sorting through serving sizes can be confusing. One ounce of a ready-to-eat cereal, for example, counts as a serving. This is equivalent to 1/2 cup of cooked cereal. One slice of bread is equivalent to one-half of a bagel. The fruit group is more confusing. One whole piece of fruit is the same as 1/2 cup of chopped fruit or 3/4 cup of fruit juice. The only sure way to determine serving size is to check food package labels.

Moderation. Moderation is another important characteristic of the healthy diet. There is a place in the diet for almost any food if it is consumed prudently—the FGP doesn't label food "good" or "bad." Some foods do have a higher **nutrient density** than others, meaning they yield a higher ratio of nutrients to calories, but all foods contribute to nutrition (see Just the Facts: Nutrient Density on page 191). Moderation means exercising good judgment regarding quantity and frequency. It doesn't mean avoidance. The idea that a particular food is good or bad can be destructive to anyone trying to eat more

Wellness for a Lifetime

The Nutrient Gap

It has been estimated that as many as 25 percent of Americans 60 and older are malnourished. They do not suffer from nutritional diseases, such as scurvy or pellagra; rather, they consume insufficient amounts of key nutrients that have a direct effect on health and body function. Older adults usually expend less energy to meet the demands of their lifestyle than do their younger peers and therefore require fewer calories. This presents a dilemma because, as their need for energy decreases, their need for nutrients increases or stays the same. Unfortunately, a decrease in caloric intake is usually associated with a decrease in key nutrients. There is a gap between what older adults need and what they get from food, as shown in the following table.[39]

Nutrient	What They Need (Age 50+)	How They're Doing	Why Adults Age 50+ Need It
Calcium	1,200 mg	The average intake is 400–600 mg.	The capacity to absorb calcium declines with age.
Folate	400 µg	Only one-fourth of older adults get 400 µg.	Reducing homocysteine levels becomes more important as heart disease risks increase.
Riboflavin	1.1 mg, women 1.3 mg, men	Only one-third get enough.	The body's need is the same throughout adulthood.
Vitamin B_6	1.5 mg, women 1.7 mg, men	50–90% don't get enough.	The body's metabolism changes with age.
Vitamin B_{12}	2.4 µg	20% of adults over 60 and 40% over 80 are deficient.	Increased difficulty in absorbing vitamin B_{12} comes with age.
Vitamin D	400 IU, ages 51–69 600 IU, 70+	The average intake is 100–125 IU.	Decreased ability of skin to synthesize vitamin D from sunlight comes with age.

healthfully. For example, a person with rigid attitudes who thinks that cheesecake is "bad" and then indulges in eating it might think, I am bad, I have no willpower, and I am a weak person. The behavioral result might be a cheesecake binge, because the forbidden nature of the food makes it harder to resist. A more positive approach is to understand that cheesecake is not "bad" and that eating a slice does not make the eater a bad person.

Another reason for moderation is that even nutritionally dense foods can be consumed in excess. The interaction of the various substances in food can cause one nutrient to overpower or nullify the effects and benefits of another. The body's processes may be compromised or the nutrients in foods may interfere with the desired effects of medicines. Following are several examples of the negative effects of excessive consumption of various nutrients:

- Too much protein from animal sources may cause the body to lose extra calcium.[3]

- Botanicals such as garlic, ginger, and ginseng, when combined with vitamin E, fish oils, or blood-thinning medicines (e.g., aspirin, Coumadin), may inhibit the blood-clotting mechanism of the body and cause internal bleeding.[33]
- Megadoses of vitamin A can cause birth defects.
- Megadoses of vitamin C can cause diarrhea, nausea, abdominal cramps, and headache.[3]
- Excessive intake of vitamin D causes too much calcium to move from the bones to the blood and then to the urine, through which it is excreted from the body.[3]
- High intake of folate may mask the symptoms of pernicious anemia, a condition associated with a vitamin B_{12} deficiency.
- Excess niacin may aggravate glucose intolerance associated with noninsulin-dependent diabetes.
- Foods high in vitamin K, such as broccoli, spinach, and turnip greens, may neutralize the effectiveness of blood-thinning medicines.

Just the Facts

Nutrient Density

A key strategy for eating well is to select foods that offer significant amounts of nutrients but small numbers of calories. If a particular food has a high ratio of nutrients to calories, it is a nutritionally dense food. You can determine the nutrient density of food by adding the percentages of the RDA for the essential nutrients and dividing by the number of calories per serving (see the following example). The higher the score, the higher the nutrient density. The concept of nutrient density can help the health-conscious and weight-conscious person make informed choices.

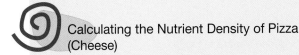
Calculating the Nutrient Density of Pizza (Cheese)

Calories	RDA %	354
Protein	28	
Vitamin A	19	
Vitamin C	20	
Thiamin	25	
Riboflavin	29	
Niacin	19	
Calcium	33	
Iron	15	
Total		**188**

Nutrient density = 53% (188 ÷ 354 × 100)

These examples are not meant to discourage your consumption of a particular food. Each food offers a unique contribution to health. Vitamin D, for instance, is required for calcium metabolism; however, too much of it may result in a depletion of calcium. Moderation is an important concept that applies to essential nutrients, just as it applies to nutrients with bad reputations. Choosing foods from the FGP, with an emphasis on variety and moderation, not only satisfies the body's need for essential nutrients but also helps prevent problems associated with dietary excess. A longitudinal study at Harvard University that followed more than 100,000 people for 8 to 12 years concluded that people who eat a good diet have a 10 to 20 percent lower risk for major disease (and a 30 to 40 percent lower risk for heart disease) than people who eat a poor diet.[41] A good diet was described as daily consumption of five servings of vegetables, four servings of fruit, and fiber from cereals and breads; consumption of more fish and poultry than beef, pork, and lamb; one serving of nuts; no more than two or 3 grams of trans fat; and a multivitamin.

Choose a Variety of Grains Daily, Especially Whole Grains

Grain products (bread, cereal, rice, and oats) help form the foundation of a nutritious diet. They are rich in vitamins, minerals, complex carbohydrates, dietary fiber, and other substances essential for good health. The FGP recommends at least six servings per day, more for older children, teenagers, adult men, and active women.[35] Unrefined, whole-grain foods should be emphasized over refined grain products—white bread, white rice, white flour, and pasta. Refined grains are not good sources of fiber. Remember, it's hard to eat a high-fiber diet that isn't healthy.

Meeting this dietary guideline is a formidable challenge to most Americans. For example, in planning meals, Americans often think first of the entrée, which is typically a meat dish. This is usually true whether we're eating at home or dining out. The FGP challenges us to reverse this approach by thinking of plant products first.

The vegetarian alternative

The importance of a plant-based approach to eating is evidenced by the fact that a properly planned vegetarian diet is now viewed as a healthful and acceptable way of meeting all nutritional needs. Some vegetarians avoid all animal products, including dairy products, poultry, eggs, and fish. Others include eggs and milk products but exclude fish, poultry, and red meat. There are many variations of vegetarian diet. The more common types are presented in Table 6-9 (page 192).

With the exception of vegans, most types of vegetarians have little trouble getting all of the essential nutrients, including protein. Milk products, eggs, fish, and poultry are sources of complete, high-quality protein. *Vegans*, who eat all-plant diets, need to be discriminating in their food selections because most plants are sources of incomplete protein. One notable exception, as mentioned earlier, is soy protein. Vegans who don't consume soy products need to combine complementary foods, such as grains and legumes, to obtain all of the essential amino acids.

The nutritional problem most likely to occur in a strict vegetarian diet is a deficiency in vitamin B_{12}, which occurs naturally only in animal products. Vegans can get vitamin B_{12} by taking a supplement or consuming food fortified with B_{12}. Vitamin D is another potential problem to the vegan if he or she has limited exposure to the sun. Milk products, fortified with vitamin D, are about the only dietary source of vitamin D. However, the body can produce adequate amounts of this vitamin if the skin receives sufficient exposure to sunlight.

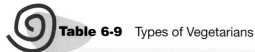

Table 6-9 Types of Vegetarians

Type	What Is Excluded from Diet	What Is Included in Diet
Vegans	All animal products	Fruits, vegetables, grains, legumes, nuts, and seeds
Lactovegetarians	Eggs, fish, poultry, and meat	Milk products and fruits, vegetables, grains, legumes, nuts, and seeds
Ovolactovegetarians	Fish, poultry, and meat	Eggs (*ova*), milk products (*lacto*), fruits, vegetables, grains, legumes, nuts, and seeds
Pescovegetarians	Poultry and meat	Fish (*pesco*), eggs, milk products, fruits, vegetables, grains, legumes, nuts, and seeds
Pollovegetarians	Red meat	Poultry (*pollo*), fish, eggs, milk products, fruits, vegetables, grains, legumes, nuts, and seeds
Semi- or demi-vegetarians	Same as vegan, except meat may be eaten occasionally	Same as vegan

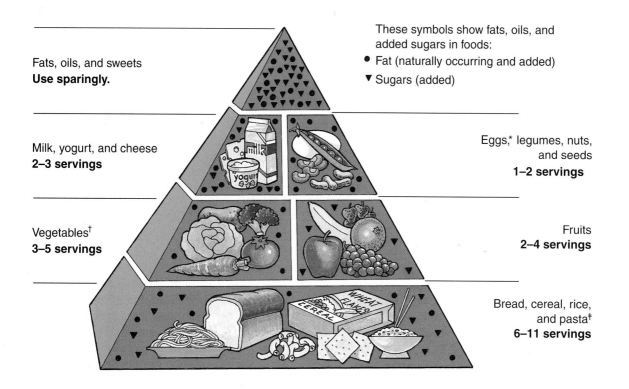

*Lactovegetarians can omit eggs from this pyramid.
†Include one dark green or leafy variety daily.
‡One serving of a vitamin- and mineral-enriched cereal is recommended.

Figure 6-4 Food Pyramid for Ovolactovegetarians
Base serving sizes on those listed for the Food Guide Pyramid (contains about 75 g of protein and 1,650 calories).

During periods of limited sunlight exposure, vegans may need to take vitamin D supplements. Other essential nutrients richly supplied by animal products and thus of concern to vegans, such as riboflavin, iron, zinc, and calcium, can be easily derived from a variety of plant sources.

Figure 6-4, a food pyramid for ovolactovegetarians, presents a helpful plan for people trying to avoid meats. The recommended number of servings of grains, fruits, vegetables, and milk products is identical to the recommended amounts in the Food Guide Pyramid. The major difference is the exclusion of meat in favor of legumes, nuts, seeds, and eggs. Lactovegetarians can omit eggs from this pyramid.

Following are some practical tips for adding fruits, vegetables, and grains to the diet that should be helpful for people opting for a meatless meal, choosing to eat vegetarian for a day, or favoring vegetarianism as a lifestyle:

- Start off the day with fruit juice.
- Add fruit to a salad.
- Serve fruit for dessert.
- Have a smoothie (blend fruit juice, ice, and a banana).
- Add fruit to cereal.
- Eat cereal as a snack.
- Eat vegetable snacks.
- Aim for a colorful plate, with dark green, yellow, and red vegetables.
- Increase the number of vegetables in a salad by adding tomatoes, carrots, cucumbers, peppers, spinach, or broccoli.
- Eat a vegetable pizza.
- Make a soup with leftover vegetables.
- Eat an all-vegetable meal.
- Mix legumes with a salad.
- Try a new fruit or vegetable.
- Top fat-free frozen yogurt with low-fat granola and berries.
- Top salad with whole-wheat cereal.

A properly selected vegetarian diet has many health benefits (see Just the Facts: Health Benefits of a Vegetarian Diet). People who have health conditions associated with diets high in fat and saturated fat and low in folate, carotenoids, phytochemicals, and antioxidants stand to benefit from a plant-based diet.

ᨳᨰ Just the Facts ᨳᨰ

Health Benefits of a Vegetarian Diet

As a group, vegetarians have lower morbidity and mortality rates from several chronic degenerative diseases than do nonvegetarians.[42] Typically, vegetarian diets are lower in fat and saturated fat and have higher concentrations of nutrients (vitamins, minerals, and phytochemicals) associated with health benefits. Following are some of the benefits of a vegetarian diet over a nonvegetarian diet:

- Lower cholesterol level
- Reduced risk for heart disease
- Lower incidence of hypertension
- Fewer complications and lower mortality from Type 2 diabetes mellitus
- Reduced incidence of cancer

Choose a Variety of Fruits and Vegetables Daily

Fruits and vegetables are key parts of a nutritious diet. To promote health, at least two servings of fruits and three servings of vegetables should be consumed daily. Fruits and vegetables provide essential vitamins and minerals, fiber, phytochemicals, antioxidants, and other substances good for health. They are naturally low in fat and calories and are filling. Some are high in fiber, and many are quick to prepare and easy to eat.

In choosing fruits and vegetables, aim for variety. Try many colors and kinds. Choose any form: fresh, frozen, canned, dried, juices. All forms provide vitamins and minerals, and all provide fiber except for most juices.

One way to cultivate a taste for a variety of vegetables and fruits (and grain products) is to acquire a taste for ethnic food. The typical diets of many other countries favor grains, fruits, and vegetables and place less emphasis on animal fats. However, watch out for the Americanization of ethnic foods. For example, the traditional Italian pasta dish comes with a tomato-based sauce containing small amounts of meat or meatballs on the side, served with crusty Italian bread or pizza with an extra-thick crust and a mere sprinkle of tomato sauce, herbs, and cheese. Americanized, the same pasta dish comes with less pasta, more creamy sauces, and more meat and is served with buttery garlic toast or pizza with a thin crust, pepperoni, sausage, olives, and extra cheese. For additional comparisons, see Just the Facts: Do You Eat Real Ethnic Food? on page 194.

Keep Food Safe to Eat

Americans face a paradox: We are urged to eat more fruits, vegetables, fish, and poultry, but we are warned about contamination and foodborne illness. **Foodborne illness** is a condition caused by eating food that contains harmful bacteria, toxins, parasites, viruses, or chemical contamination (see Just the Facts: Foodborne Illness: Food Sources and Symptoms on page 195). More than 76 million cases of foodborne illness occur in the United States each year, causing about 5,000 deaths.[3] These illnesses are difficult to prevent because they involve different kinds of organisms infecting foods of all types grown in many parts of the world.

With the exception of hepatitis A, the organisms that cause foodborne illness are bacterial. For most of them, treatment consists of hydration and the administration of antibiotics. Other types of organisms are involved in foodborne illnesses. Parasites, such as *Trichinella spiralis* (found in pork and wild game) and tapeworms (found in beef, pork, and fish), also infect many people. The same is true of fungi, which produce mold spores that yield toxins, such as aflatoxin.

~~~~~~~~~~ Just the Facts ~~~~~~~~~~

Do You Eat Real Ethnic Food?

The typical diets of many other countries tend to contain more high-carbohydrate foods and fewer foods high in animal fats than does the common American diet. However, when ethnic foods are prepared in the United States, especially in restaurants, they are often Americanized by the inclusion of larger portions of meat and cheese and the addition of sauces. What follows are descriptions of some traditional, high-carbohydrate ethnic foods and their higher-fat, Americanized versions. Which versions of these ethnic foods do you tend to eat?

Chinese

- Traditional: large bowl of steamed rice with small amounts of stir-fried vegetables, meats, and sauces as condiments
- Americanized: several stir-fried or batter-fried entrées in sauces, with a small bowl of fried rice on the side

German

- Traditional: large portions of potatoes, rye and whole-grain breads, stew with dumplings, and sauerkraut
- Americanized: fewer potatoes, less bread, more sausage and cheese

Japanese

- Traditional: large bowl of steamed rice with broth-based soups containing rice noodles, vegetables, and small amounts of meat

- Americanized: tempura (batter-fried vegetables and shrimp), teriyaki chicken, oriental chicken salad with oil-based dressing

Italian

- Traditional: large mound of pasta with tomato-based sauce containing small amounts of meat or meatballs on the side, served with crusty Italian bread or pizza with an extra-thick crust and mere sprinkle of tomato sauce, herbs, and cheese
- Americanized: less pasta, more creamy sauces, and more meat, served with buttery garlic toast or pizza with a thin crust, pepperoni, sausage, olives, and extra cheese

Mexican

- Traditional: mostly rice, beans, and warmed tortillas and lots of hot salsa and chiles
- Americanized: crispy fried tortillas, extra ground beef, added cheese, sour cream, and guacamole (avocado dip)

Middle Eastern

- Traditional: pita bread (round bread), pilaf (rice dish), hummus (chickpea dip), shaved slices of seasoned meat, diced vegetables, and yogurt-based sauces, all seasoned with garlic
- Americanized: meat kebabs, salads drenched in olive oil, less bread and pilaf

---

Most foodborne illnesses can be prevented by observing some basic rules for storing, handling, and preparing food:

- Avoid cross-contamination: Do not prepare foods in an unclean sink and do not allow utensils that have come into contact with an unclean surface to touch food.
- Wash hands when first starting to handle food and after handling garbage or dirty dishes.
- Use separate cloths, sponges, and towels for washing dishes, wiping counters and tabletops, wiping hands, and drying clean dishes.
- Measure the temperature of cooked or held foods to make sure they're hot enough to destroy bacteria (see Figure 6-5 on page 196).
- Do not consume foods whose "use-by" dates have expired.
- Transfer leftovers from deep pots and casseroles to shallow pans before refrigeration to speed cooling (and thereby slow bacterial growth).

- Quickly freeze or refrigerate all ground meat and other perishable foods after shopping.
- Wash hands, utensils, and work areas with hot, soapy water after contact with raw meat to keep bacteria from spreading. Also wash your hands after using the bathroom; diapering a child; using the telephone; handling garbage; or touching your face, your hair, or other people.
- Keep the refrigerator temperature below 40° F (37° F is optimal). Keep the freezer at or below 0° F.
- Wash whole produce. This includes melons and citrus fruits before cutting them open, to prevent the transfer of bacteria from the fruit's skin to the edible part.
- Wash or sanitize cutting boards between each use.
- Store meat products in containers separate from fruits and vegetables.
- Flip steaks with tongs or a spatula rather than with a fork during cooking. Unlike ground beef, in which bacteria are mixed throughout the meat during the

∿∿∿∿∿Just the Facts∿∿∿∿∿

Foodborne Illness: Food Sources and Symptoms

Following is a short list of organisms that are common culprits of foodborne illness, along with their food sources and symptoms.

Staphylococcus toxins are usually present in meats, poultry, egg products, tuna, potato and macaroni salads, and cream-filled pastries. Symptoms occur 2 to 6 hours after exposure and include diarrhea, vomiting, nausea, and abdominal cramps. Recovery normally takes place in 24 to 36 hours.

Salmonella infections are associated with eggs, poultry, meat, dairy products, seafood, and fresh produce. Symptoms usually occur within 6 to 48 hours and include nausea, vomiting, abdominal cramps, diarrhea, fever, headache, and sometimes a rash. *Salmonella* infections may be serious, even fatal, in infants, the elderly, and the sick.

Clostridium botulinum, usually referred to as *botulism*, occurs in an anaerobic environment, such as in canned goods, and affects low-acid foods, such as green beans, mushrooms, spinach, olives, and beef. Symptoms occur 12 to 36 hours after exposure and affect the central nervous system. Paralysis and death may follow. Infected food usually has an odor. Avoid canned goods that show any signs of damage.

Campylobacter jejuni contamination is linked to raw and undercooked poultry, unpasteurized milk, and untreated water. Symptoms usually occur in 2 to 5 days and include diarrhea, fever, abdominal pain, nausea, headache, and muscle pain. Infections may last 7 to 10 days.

E. coli O157:H7 is typically present in undercooked and raw ground beef, raw milk, lettuce, untreated water, and unpasteurized fruit juices. Symptoms include severe abdominal pain and cramping and diarrhea (first watery, then bloody).

Listeria monocytogenes is associated with soft cheeses, poultry, fish, and raw meats and vegetables. The illness causes flulike symptoms, including fever, and may progress to fatal infections of the blood and central nervous system.

Hepatitis A virus comes from contaminated fecal material from people who harvest, process, or handle food, including workers on farms, in food-processing plants, and in restaurants. Symptoms, which may not occur for several weeks, include fever, nausea, abdominal discomfort, and sometimes jaundice. The infection is usually mild, though symptoms can be severe.

---

grinding process, steak harbors bacteria only on the surface. Sticking a fork into meat before it is cooked injects the interior with bacteria from the outside.

- Cook fish until it flakes with a fork.
- Put your sponge or scouring pad in the dishwasher every time you run it. Or microwave your sponge on high for 30 to 60 seconds.
- Don't store raw foods on the refrigerator shelf above ready-to-eat foods.
- Don't thaw frozen food on the kitchen counter or at room temperature. Thaw frozen food in the refrigerator or microwave.
- Don't eat hamburgers or any other form of ground beef until the juices run yellow, with no trace of pink left. A single hamburger may contain meat from hundreds of animals, creating an increased risk for contamination.[43] (The color of the meat isn't a reliable indicator of doneness. Check the juice.)
- Don't let juice from raw meat, poultry, or fish drip on your hands or any fresh foods in your grocery cart.
- Don't consume unpasteurized milk and juice or foods made with raw eggs.
- Don't use tasting utensils that have touched food under preparation.

- Don't grill, barbecue, broil, or pan-fry meats, poultry, or fish at extremely high temperatures. (Grills can reach temperatures in excess of 640° F. Ovens roast at a temperature of 350° F.) Cooking meats at high temperatures promotes the formation of heterocyclic amines,[44] HCAs. HCAs are thought to be carcinogenic. Boiling, steaming, poaching, stewing, and microwaving do not produce HCAs.
- Don't serve or transport cooked food on the plate used for raw meat.
- Don't store raw fish in your refrigerator for more than 24 hours. Raw poultry or ground beef will keep for 1 to 2 days and raw red meat for 3 to 5.
- Reheat leftovers thoroughly to at least 165° F.[35]

Choose a Diet That Is Low in Saturated Fat and Cholesterol and Moderate in Total Fat

Some dietary fat is needed for good health. Fats supply energy and essential fatty acids and promote absorption of the fat-soluble vitamins. Whether from plant or animal sources, fat contains more than twice the number of calories as its carbohydrate and protein

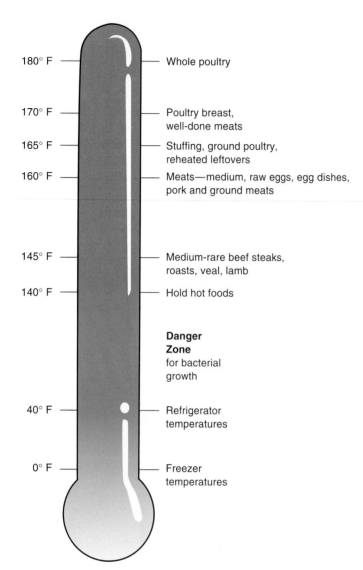

180° F	Whole poultry
170° F	Poultry breast, well-done meats
165° F	Stuffing, ground poultry, reheated leftovers
160° F	Meats—medium, raw eggs, egg dishes, pork and ground meats
145° F	Medium-rare beef steaks, roasts, veal, lamb
140° F	Hold hot foods
	Danger Zone for bacterial growth
40° F	Refrigerator temperatures
0° F	Freezer temperatures

Figure 6-5 How Hot Is Hot Enough?

These recommended safe cooking and storage temperatures are not intended for processing, institutional, or food service preparation.

SOURCE: U.S. Department of Health and Human Services. 2000. *Nutrition and health: Dietary guidelines for Americans.* Washington, DC: U.S. Government Printing Office.

equivalents. Fats are represented in the apex of the FGP; *Dietary Guidelines for Americans* calls for no servings of fat because the body's need for essential fatty acids is easily satisfied by foods in the other food groups. Perhaps one of the greatest shortcomings of the American diet is the abundance of fat. Compounding this problem is that fat is usually consumed at the expense of fruits, vegetables, and grains. For many people, reducing both the amount and the type of dietary fat eaten is a formidable challenge. Table 6-4 presented a quick reference of maximum fat intake for selected caloric intakes. You can estimate your personal

maximum fat intake by completing Assessment Activity 6-2. You can learn how fatty your eating habits are by completing Assessment Activity 6-5.

Tips for reducing dietary fat

The following are some suggestions for reducing total dietary fat consumption, lowering saturated fat intake, and replacing saturated fats with unsaturated fats:

- Assess your fat intake. Complete the assessments at the end of this chapter, along with those in the nutrition software that accompanies this text, to determine your fat intake. Compare your fat intake with the recommendations in Table 6-4.
- Read labels and become familiar with the fat content of food. Try to identify foods that should be consumed in limited amounts; also identify foods that are low in fat (see Table 6-3).
- Become familiar with sources of saturated, monounsaturated, and polyunsaturated fats (see Figure 6-2).
- Check for the presence of trans fatty acids by reading the fine print on food labels. Look for the word *hydrogenated* or *partially hydrogenated* to identify foods that should be consumed in limited amounts.
- Limit meat, seafood, and poultry to no more than 5 to 7 ounces per day.
- Eat chicken or turkey (without the skin) or fish instead of red meat in most meals.
- Substitute one or two meals of fish per week for red meats. Choose fish high in omega-3 fatty acids and low in saturated fat, such as Atlantic cod, haddock, salmon, shrimp, scallops, sardines, tuna, red snapper, and trout.
- Choose lean cuts of meat, trim all the visible fat, and throw away the fat that cooks out of the meat.
- Substitute meatless or low-meat main dishes for regular entrées.
- Substitute legumes for meat one or two times per week.
- Eat a vegetarian diet at least one day a week.
- Use no more than 5 to 8 teaspoons of fats and oils per day for cooking, baking, and preparing salads.
- Choose foods that contain fewer than 3 grams of fat per 100-calorie serving.
- Choose foods that contain less than 1 gram of saturated fat per 100-calorie serving.
- Use low-fat dairy products (whole milk has more than eight times the fat calories of skim milk).
- Substitute pureed fruit, such as applesauce, when cooking from a recipe that calls for cooking oil (equal substitution).
- Use soft margarine in place of hard margarine.
- Use liquid or spray margarine when possible.
- Serve dressings and condiments (for salads, potatoes, etc.) on the side. Try to cut these servings in half.

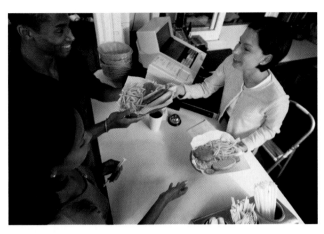

Even if your weight is healthy, too many high-fat take-out dinners may mean too few fruits and vegetables.

- Avoid fried foods. Substitute another cooking method (baking, grilling, broiling, or roasting) for frying.
- Eat more vegetables and fruits.
- Eat low-fat foods that have a high satiety value, such as whole grains and high-fiber foods.
- Substitute olive oil or canola oil for margarine, butter, or lard.
- Try to add diversity to your diet. Cultivate a taste for low-fat ethnic foods.
- Avoid a "forbidden fruit" approach to food selection. Any food can be enjoyed in moderation. If you consume an unusually high-fat food or meal, try to compensate with more prudent choices during the week.

Choose Beverages and Foods to Moderate Your Intake of Sugars

Sugars are carbohydrates and a source of energy (calories). Dietary carbohydrates also include the complex carbohydrates (starch) and dietary fiber. During digestion, all carbohydrates except fiber break down into sugars.[35] Americans eat sugars in many forms, and most people enjoy the taste of sugars. Some sugars are used as natural preservatives, thickeners, and baking aids in foods. Most of the simple sugar eaten by Americans has been added to foods and beverages during processing and manufacturing. A food is likely to be high in sugars if one of the following is listed first or second in the ingredients list on a food label: brown sugar, corn sweetener, corn syrup, fructose, fruit juice concentrate, glucose (dextrose), high-fructose corn syrup, honey, invert sugar, lactose, maltose, molasses, raw sugar, sucrose (table sugar), or syrup. Many foods contain a combination of sugars.

Dietary guidelines recommend that sugar consumption be limited to 10 to 25 percent of total calories. On average, Americans get 20 percent of their calories from added sugar.[45] Recent studies indicate a 22 percent increase in sugar consumption among Americans since 1962; 80 percent of this increase comes from sugared beverages.[46]

The major health problem associated with a high sugar intake is dental caries (cavities). The main offenders are sweet and gummy foods. They stick to the teeth and supply bacteria with a steady source of carbohydrate from which to make acids that can dissolve tooth enamel. Foods that promote caries are termed *cariogenic*.

Contrary to popular belief, there is little or no evidence that high sugar intake causes hyperactivity in children, heart disease, diabetes, or obesity. If that were the case, most Americans would have all of these conditions. The major nutritional problem of a high-sugar diet occurs when sugar is substituted for more nutritionally dense foods. When this happens, the result may be insufficient vitamin and mineral intake.

Sugar intake, Glycemic Index, Glycemic Load

Some health experts are exploring the relationship between blood sugar and chronic diseases from a different angle. It has been observed that sugar and starch cause a surge of glucose into the bloodstream. The glucose, in turn, stimulates the pancreas to make insulin, the hormone that converts glucose to energy. The **Glycemic Index (GI)** is a scale that assesses blood sugar surges associated with a particular food. More precisely, the Glycemic Index calculates how high blood sugar rises in the two hours after eating a high-carbohydrate food (specifically, enough to provide 50 grams of carbohydrates), compared with what happens after eating a 50-gram serving of white bread or 50 grams of glucose, each of which earns 100 on the GI scale.[47] Foods with a high GI theoretically result in quicker blood sugar surges in comparisons with foods with lower GI. **Glycemic Load (GL)** is based on the same concept but takes into account how much food is usually consumed and, for that reason, is regarded as a better indicator of a food's effect on blood sugar surges. GL is calculated by multiplying the carbohydrate grams in a serving of food times its Glycemic Index. By combining the Glycemic Index with the amount of food eaten, the Glycemic Load produces a value that is less likely to be misleading. For example, one slice of whole-wheat bread has a Glycemic Index score of 69, one point short of the "high" classification, but a Glycemic Load score of 9, a "low" score.[48] In this example, the high Glycemic Index score might incorrectly influence you to avoid whole-wheat bread, when, in actuality, its Glycemic Load score is low and accurately indicates that it is a good choice. Studies indicate that people who consistently eat foods with a high Glycemic Load are at greater risk of developing Type 2 diabetes, cardiovascular disease, and certain cancers.[48] GI and GL values are not included on food labels because there are many complicating factors involved in carbohydrate metabolism. But the Glycemic Load does give a more complete picture of a food's effect on blood sugar levels and eventually may turn out to be a more useful concept than is the chemical classification of carbohydrate as simple or complex, or as sugars or starches.

Choose and Prepare Foods with Less Salt

Salt contains about 40 percent sodium by weight and is widely used in the preservation, processing, and preparation of foods. Sodium is an essential mineral, but it is one that Americans consume in excess. Average daily consumption of sodium is 3,735 milligrams,[9] almost eight times the minimum requirement of 500 milligrams (one-tenth of a teaspoon) and almost double the 2,400 milligrams considered adequate.[3] The main health problems associated with consumption of too much sodium are hypertension, osteoporosis, and stomach cancer. Of the three, hypertension, discussed in Chapter 2, is the most common problem. Sodium contributes to the development of osteoporosis because it pulls calcium from bones and causes the kidneys to excrete calcium. Sodium contributes to stomach cancer because it irritates the stomach lining, causing cells to replicate themselves, increasing the odds of cancer-cell initiation.

The majority of sodium consumed is in the form of hidden salt added during the processing of food. Just how much sodium is in a processed food can be determined by reading the package label.

Taste buds cannot always judge salt content. Some foods that taste salty may be lower in salt content than foods that do not. For example, peanuts taste salty because the salt is on the surface where the taste buds immediately detect it. However, cheese contains more salt than peanuts or potato chips, and chocolate pudding contains even more salt. To cut down on salt consumption, you should do the following:

- Avoid adding salt before tasting food.
- Add little or no salt to food at the table.
- Season food with sodium-free spices, such as pepper, allspice, onion powder, garlic, mustard powder, sage, thyme, and paprika.
- Avoid smoked meats and fish.
- Cut down on canned and instant soups.
- Read labels for sodium content, especially on frozen dinners or pizza, processed meat, processed cheese, canned or dried soup, and salad dressing. When

shopping for canned and processed foods, select foods with no more than 200 mg of sodium per 100 calories.
- Eat plenty of fruits and vegetables high in potassium, calcium, and magnesium. These minerals may help keep blood pressure down.

If You Drink Alcoholic Beverages, Do So in Moderation

Dietary Guidelines for Americans defines *alcohol moderation* as no more than one drink per day for women and no more than two drinks per day for men.[35] This limit is based on differences between men and women in both weight and metabolism. (A drink is defined as 12 ounces of beer, 5 ounces of wine, or 1.5 ounces of 80-proof spirits.) The allowance for women is smaller because women, on average, are smaller than men; they have less muscle and, therefore, less water than men (so alcohol does not get diluted as well in their bodies); and they have less of an enzyme that breaks down alcohol before it reaches the bloodstream. A maximal level of alcohol consumption has not been set for women during pregnancy, so pregnant women and women who have a high chance of becoming pregnant should not use alcohol.

From a health perspective, alcohol has both advantages and serious risks. On the one hand, it is associated with drunken-driving injuries and deaths, cirrhosis of the liver, and a host of social ills caused by alcoholism. On the other hand, when consumed in moderate amounts as recommended by *Dietary Guidelines*, it offers protection from heart disease and stroke in some people, even more so than does abstinence. Population studies show a 30 percent reduction in coronary risk among moderate drinkers, compared with abstainers. The data are similar in men and women.[2]

Another benefit of alcohol is enhanced brain function. Light to moderate alcohol consumption (one to three drinks daily) cuts the risk of developing dementia in people over age 55 by over 40 percent.[49] Like many issues related to nutrition, moderation is the key. Too much of a good thing may do more harm than good. For example, in the case of dementia, while moderate consumption of alcohol offers some protective effect, too much alcohol increases the risk for dementia.[50] Several theories have been advanced to explain alcohol's benefit: It may improve blood levels of high-density lipoproteins, and it may serve as a blood thinner by inhibiting the blood-clotting mechanism often associated with atherosclerosis. Contrary to popular belief, wine does not appear to offer any advantage over other forms of alcohol.

The health benefits of alcohol consumption are short term. That is, excessive consumption on one occasion followed by long periods of abstinence does not provide protection from heart disease, strokes, and/or dementia. Instead, the benefits occur on a daily basis. Occasional users and previous consumers of alcohol no longer experience the benefits of alcohol when consumption ceases.[51]

Regardless of alcohol's potential health benefits, experts don't recommend alcohol consumption for everyone. Some people have medical, religious, and personal reasons for abstaining. People with uncontrolled hypertension, liver disease, pancreatitis, or strong family histories of addiction should avoid alcohol. The same is true for women during pregnancy. Also, some medicines may have a potentiating effect when taken with alcohol. For women there is also some concern about the link between moderate consumption of alcohol and breast cancer.[2] Remember that the health benefits associated with alcohol come from a moderate level of consumption. Alcohol consumption in excess of that recommended in *Dietary Guidelines* can cause a variety of health problems that outweigh the potential benefits. As is the case with many health issues, moderation serves as the guiding principle for alcohol consumption.

Other Nutrition Issues of Concern

Nutrition and Pregnancy

Good nutrition is crucial to a successful pregnancy, and a healthy pregnancy starts before conception. Alcohol consumption, smoking, an inadequate diet, dietary excesses of some nutrients, drug abuse, and the interactions of a host of medicines are some of the factors that may threaten a pregnancy even before conception is known or confirmed. Poor health habits throughout pregnancy, especially during the first three months, can harm the mother and developing baby. Although genetic and environmental influences introduce some risk factors beyond the mother's control, there is a considerable amount of medical advice about weight gain and the nutritional needs unique to pregnant women.

Weight gain

Adequate weight gain for a mother is one of the best predictors of pregnancy outcome. A weight gain of 25 to 35 pounds is recommended for most women and yields optimal health for both mother and fetus if pregnancy lasts at least 35 weeks. To accommodate the extra demands for energy, the expectant mother needs to increase her caloric intake by about 300 calories daily, particularly after the third month of pregnancy.[3] Inadequate weight gain can lead to many problems. It is important to monitor weight throughout the pregnancy. Large

fluctuations in the recommended weight-gain pattern should be brought to the attention of the health care provider.

Nutrient needs

The RDAs for many nutrients increase during pregnancy:[3]

- The protein RDA increases by 25 grams daily.
- Because of its role in DNA synthesis, folate is a crucial nutrient during pregnancy. The RDA for folate during pregnancy increases to 600 µg per day. Folate deficiencies have been linked to some neural tube birth defects, such as spina bifida. The increased need for folate can be achieved through the diet or a prenatal vitamin and mineral supplement.
- Iron intake should double during the final six months of pregnancy to achieve the RDA of 27 milligrams per day. The extra iron is needed to synthesize the additional hemoglobin required during pregnancy and to provide iron for the developing fetus. Women often need an iron supplement if their typical iron intake is marginal. Iron deficiencies during pregnancy may threaten the health of both the baby and the mother.
- Calcium is needed during pregnancy for skeletal and tooth development of the fetus, especially during the last three months, when growth of these tissues is most prolific. The DRI for calcium is 1,000 to 1,300 mg. A prenatal supplement usually contains 200 mg of calcium.
- The zinc RDA increases 35 percent (to 15 milligrams) during pregnancy to satisfy the requirements for growth and development of the fetus. Foods rich in protein also supply zinc. Zinc deficiencies increase the chance of a low-birth-weight baby.
- Prenatal supplements may contribute to a successful pregnancy for some women and, with the possible exception of vitamin A, provide benefits that outweigh potential risks. Because of its role in cell differentiation, megadoses of vitamin A from both supplements and dietary sources are associated with birth defects, particularly when the vitamin A is consumed during the first three months of pregnancy. It is recommended that women set their limit of vitamin A according to the RDAs.

Slight modifications of the recommended servings in the Food Guide Pyramid should satisfy women's unique nutritional needs during pregnancy. The major differences involve adding a serving of food from two food groups: the milk group and the meat group. Women who practice either ovolactovegetarianism or lactovegetarianism generally do not have difficulty meeting their nutritional needs during pregnancy. Vegans, on the

Table 6-10 Two High-Carbohydrate Preactivity Meals

	Calories	Protein (grams)	Fat (grams)	Carbohydrate (grams)
Menu 1				
White bread, 2 slices	123	4	2	22
Peanut butter, 1 tbsp.	95	4	8	3
Grape jelly, 1 tbsp.	56	0	0	14
2% milk, 1 cup	125	8	5	12
Orange, 1 medium	60	1	0	15
Meal total	459	17	15	66
Menu 2				
Vegetable lo mein (soft noodles with stir-fried vegetables), 2 cups	352	11	15	47
Fresh papaya, 1 cup	54	1	0	14
Herbal iced tea, sweetened with honey, 12 oz.	56	0	0	13
Meal total	462	12	15	74

The timing of the preactivity meal depends on the amount of calories consumed. Allow four hours for a big meal (about 1,200 calories), three hours for a moderate meal (about 800 to 900 calories), and an hour or less for a snack (about 300 calories).[3]

other hand, must plan their diets carefully to ensure adequate amounts of protein, vitamin D, vitamin B_6, iron, calcium, zinc, and vitamin B_{12}. Vegans need to increase their intake of grains, beans, nuts, and seeds to supply the required amounts of nutrients. In addition, supplements of vitamin B_{12}, iron, and calcium along with a multipurpose prenatal supplement will probably also be necessary.[3]

Nutrition and Physical Activity

The relationship between physical activity and nutrition is obvious. The ability to engage in physical activity, whether it is low-intensity and recreational or high-intensity and competitive, is influenced by dietary intake. Conversely, nutritional needs change, depending on the type, intensity, and duration of activity. Nutrition and athletic performance are complex subjects involving not only the science of nutrition but also the sciences of biochemistry and physiology. While a presentation of the intricacies of sports nutrition is beyond the scope of this text, the following information should help you plan to meet your nutrient needs when you participate in regular physical activities.

Type of activity and energy source

The body's use of carbohydrates, fats, and protein for energy depends on the type of activity and the level of physical fitness. For high-intensity, anaerobic activities lasting for only a minute or less, such as a 100-yard

sprint, carbohydrates are the major fuel source. For aerobic activities lasting from several minutes to four or five hours, a combination of carbohydrates, fats, and protein provides fuel for work. If the activity is intense, such as that of a runner trying to achieve a personal best in a 1-mile run, carbohydrates will be in greater demand. If the activity is moderately intense, such as jogging or brisk walking, fats and carbohydrates are used evenly. If the activity lasts more than a few minutes and is less intense, such as easy walking, fat becomes a major source of energy.[3] Energy from protein is minimal during most activities because protein functions as a fuel source primarily after carbohydrate fuel is depleted, such as might occur in activities of long duration (such as long-distance running), and then its contribution accounts for only about 3 to 10 percent of the energy. In general, carbohydrates are the main fuel source for both anaerobic and high-intensity aerobic activities; fat is the main fuel source for prolonged, low-intensity exercise; and protein is a minor fuel source, primarily for endurance activities.[52]

Recommended sources of energy

The diet of a physically active person should favor carbohydrates. The body is capable of converting carbohydrates to a usable form of energy more quickly and more efficiently than it can fats or protein. As a general rule, dietary intake of carbohydrates should account for 55 to 70 percent of the energy.[52] Tables 6-10 and 6-11 present

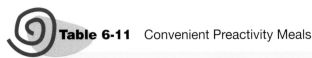

Table 6-11 Convenient Preactivity Meals

	Energy Content
Breakfast (McDonald's)	
Hot cakes with syrup and margarine	900 cal
Orange juice, 2 servings	67% from carbohydrates
English muffin (whole) with 2 tsp. margarine and 2 tsp. jam	(150 g)
• • •	
Cheerios, 3/4 cup	450 cal
Low-fat milk, 1 cup	82% from carbohydrates
Blueberry muffin	(92 g)
Orange juice, 1 serving	
Lunch or Dinner (Wendy's)	
Chili, 8-oz. portion	900 cal
Baked potato with sour cream and chives	65% from carbohydrates
Chocolate Frosty, 10 oz.	(150 g)
• • •	
Grilled chicken sandwich	425 cal
Cola, 12 oz.	65% from carbohydrates
	(70 g)

some high-carbohydrate meal options that are appropriate as preactivity meals. An increase in carbohydrate intake should be accompanied by a decrease in fat intake.

Carbohydrate loading provides some advantages for athletes participating in intense aerobic events lasting more than 60 minutes or in shorter events repeated over a 24-hour period. **Carbohydrate loading** (also called **glycogen loading**) is the practice of increasing carbohydrate intake for 6 days before an event while decreasing exercise duration.[3] The purpose of carbohydrate loading is to increase the availability of glycogen stores in the muscles. A typical regimen[3] consists of a carbohydrate intake of 45 to 50 percent of calories during the first 3 days, followed by a carbohydrate intake of 70 to 80 percent of calories during the next 3 days. At the same time, the duration of workouts is gradually decreased. For example, a 60-minute workout on the sixth day before an athletic event is decreased to 40, 40, 20, and 20 minutes, respectively, on the following days. The sixth day is a day of rest. Carbohydrate loading is unnecessary if the physical activity event lasts less than 60 minutes.[52]

Carbohydrate loading is not a substitute for training. Preparation for a "personal best" requires substantial commitment, time, energy, sacrifice, training, and probably sweat. Carbohydrate loading may improve

performance for some people for some events. However, some athletes report negative affects. The only way to know for sure is trial and error during training.

Protein supplement

Many physically active people, especially athletes, have the mistaken notion that intense physical activities impose a greater than usual demand for protein. This idea stems partly from the perception that, if a modest amount of a nutrient is good for you, large amounts must be even better and partly because protein is needed for the synthesis of new tissue. Both of these ideas can lead to mistaken conclusions. What athletes and others engaged in intense activities need is not extra protein but extra carbohydrates. The body's need for protein is biologically driven and any excess in this amount is inefficiently converted to energy or stored as fat.

Two exceptions to this protein guideline occur for athletes engaged in endurance sports and athletes starting weight training programs. The recommendations for protein range from 1.2 to 1.4 grams of protein per kilogram of body weight for the athlete. For athletes beginning a weight training program, 1.6 to 1.8 grams of protein per kilogram of body weight is recommended.[3] This represents a substantial increase of the RDA for protein. Experts disagree about the importance of excessive protein intake for weight training.

Vitamins and minerals

Vitamin and mineral needs of the physically active person are about the same as those of the sedentary person. People who exercise usually eat more than sedentary people do and therefore get more vitamins and minerals. Contrary to popular belief, especially among athletes, there is no need to take vitamin and mineral supplements if adequate servings of food from the FGP are consumed. Two exceptions are athletes on low-calorie diets (fewer than 1,200 calories/day) and vegetarian athletes. In these cases, taking vitamin and mineral supplements and consuming fortified food, such as breakfast cereals, are recommended.[53]

If a mineral deficiency occurs, it is most likely to involve iron and calcium, especially for women athletes. A deficiency of either of these minerals not only impairs athletic performance but also may lead to serious medical conditions. Dietary intake of these two minerals should be monitored regularly.

Fatty acids and activity

Most of the body's energy reserve is in its fat stores. When fat stores are broken down, fatty acids move through the bloodstream and enter muscle cells, where they are converted to energy. Well-trained muscles have a greater capacity to execute this conversion process and the ability to burn more fat. Thus, improved physical fitness causes more fat to be used for energy.[3,52] Also, the body's use of fat stores is affected by the duration of the activity. Prolonged activities (lasting more than 20 minutes) cause fat storage to be tapped for energy, particularly when the activity remains at a low intensity level. Unlike carbohydrate stores, which are limited, an unlimited amount of fatty acids is available to sustain the energy needs of low-intensity activities. Weight-conscious people interested in physical activity as a strategy for using fat, therefore, are better served by low-intensity to moderate-intensity activities that can be endured for a long period.

Fluid intake and activity

Consuming the right amount of fluids before, during, and after physical activity, which is addressed in Chapter 3, is crucial for the regulation of body temperature and the dissipation of heat.

Food Labels

The FDA oversees the labeling of food products other than meat and poultry. Virtually all processed and packaged foods are required to have uniform labels. These foods include processed meat and poultry, regulated by the USDA. Guidelines for voluntary labeling of raw vegetables and fruits and fish are also available and will likely be displayed in most supermarkets.

Food labels must indicate the manufacturer and the packer or distributor; declare the quantity of contents, either by net weight or by volume; and list the common name of each ingredient in descending order of prominence. Information about those nutrients most closely associated with chronic disease risk factors—the amount of total fat, saturated fat, cholesterol, sodium, sugar, dietary fiber, total carbohydrate, and protein—must also be included.

Labels are divided into two parts (Figure 6-6) and present information according to generic standards called Daily Values (DVs). Daily Values are benchmarks for evaluating the nutrient content of foods. They express this content as a percentage of a 2,000-calorie diet (Recommended Dietary Allowances are not used as the standards because they are age- and gender-specific). Information in the top part of a label will vary according to the contribution one serving of that food makes to the Daily Values listed in the bottom part of the label.

The DV standards located on the bottom panel are the same on all food labels and are based on two calorie levels: 2,000 and 2,500 (Table 6-12). This means that total fat intake should be fewer than 65 grams for a 2,000-calorie diet and fewer than 80 grams for a 2,500-calorie

diet. Dividing the nutrient content listed in the top panel by the DVs listed in the bottom panel yields the percent Daily Value for one serving. For example, a serving of mac 'n' cheese contains 15 grams of fat, or 23 percent of the Daily Value of 65 g for a person on a 2,000-calorie diet. With the application of simple arithmetic, you can calculate the Daily Value percents for any food with a breakdown of nutrient content.

Standard food labels are useful if daily caloric intake is approximately 2,000 or 2,500 calories and if the goal is to conform to minimum dietary recommendations. If your diet calls for significantly more or less of a nutrient, your DVs will differ. If that is the case, keep track of the total amount of a nutrient. For example, if you are on a 1,500-calorie diet and are trying to limit fat intake to 20 percent, keep a running total of fat grams to determine when 33 g have been reached.

In the past, manufacturers often used labeling ploys to deceive consumers. Currently, the FDA has approved health claims that link the following foods and diseases.[3]

- Calcium-rich foods and reduced risk for osteoporosis
- Low-sodium and high-potassium foods and reduced risk for high blood pressure and stroke
- Low-fat diet and reduced risk for cancer
- Diet low in saturated fat and cholesterol and reduced risk for heart disease
- High-fiber foods and reduced risk for some cancers
- Soluble fiber in fruits, vegetables, and grains and reduced risk for heart disease
- Soluble fiber in oats and psyllium seed husk and reduced risk for heart disease
- Fruit- and vegetable-rich diet and reduced risk for cancer
- Folate-rich foods and reduced risk for neural tube defects
- Less sugar and reduced risk for dental caries
- Low saturated fat and low cholesterol diet that includes 25 grams of soy protein and reduced risk for cardiovascular disease
- Omega-3 fatty acids from oils present in fish and a reduced risk for cardiovascular disease
- Margarines containing plant stanols and sterols and a reduced risk for cardiovascular disease

The FDA has defined commonly used words describing calories, sodium, sugar, fiber, fat, and cholesterol in food. For example, when the word *free* is highlighted on a package in reference to calories, it means that the product yields fewer than 5 calories per serving; in reference to sodium, it means the product contains fewer than 5 milligrams; and in reference to fat, it means the product contains less than 0.5 grams. When *light* or *lite* is used on a package label, it means that the product has one-third fewer calories or 50 percent less fat than a

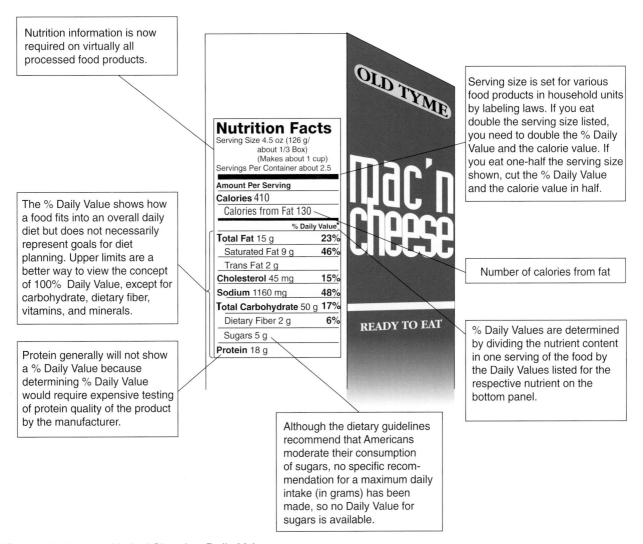

Nutrition information is now required on virtually all processed food products.

The % Daily Value shows how a food fits into an overall daily diet but does not necessarily represent goals for diet planning. Upper limits are a better way to view the concept of 100% Daily Value, except for carbohydrate, dietary fiber, vitamins, and minerals.

Protein generally will not show a % Daily Value because determining % Daily Value would require expensive testing of protein quality of the product by the manufacturer.

Serving size is set for various food products in household units by labeling laws. If you eat double the serving size listed, you need to double the % Daily Value and the calorie value. If you eat one-half the serving size shown, cut the % Daily Value and the calorie value in half.

Number of calories from fat

% Daily Values are determined by dividing the nutrient content in one serving of the food by the Daily Values listed for the respective nutrient on the bottom panel.

Although the dietary guidelines recommend that Americans moderate their consumption of sugars, no specific recommendation for a maximum daily intake (in grams) has been made, so no Daily Value for sugars is available.

Nutrition Facts
Serving Size 4.5 oz (126 g/about 1/3 Box)
(Makes about 1 cup)
Servings Per Container about 2.5

Amount Per Serving
Calories 410
Calories from Fat 130

% Daily Value*

Total Fat 15 g	23%
Saturated Fat 9 g	46%
Trans Fat 2 g	
Cholesterol 45 mg	15%
Sodium 1160 mg	48%
Total Carbohydrate 50 g	17%
Dietary Fiber 2 g	6%
Sugars 5 g	
Protein 18 g	

Figure 6-6 Food Label Showing Daily Values

Food labels provide information about those nutrients most associated with chronic disease risk factors.

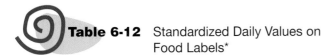

Table 6-12 Standardized Daily Values on Food Labels*

	Calorie Levels	
	2,000	**2,500**
Total fat	< 65 g	< 80 g
Saturated fat	< 20 g	< 25 g
Cholesterol	< 300 mg	< 300 mg
Sodium	< 2,400 mg	< 2,400 mg
Total carbohydrates	300 g	375 g
Fiber	25 g	30 g

* The Daily Values on food package labels have not yet been updated to reflect the current state of knowledge (see Table 6-1).

similar product. *Low-calorie* foods can have no more than 40 calories per serving; *low-fat* foods can have no more than 3 grams of fat per serving. *Healthy* means that a food meets the criteria for low fat and low saturated fat, does not exceed maximum levels for sodium and cholesterol, and contains at least 10 percent Daily Value for at least one of the following: vitamins A and C, calcium, iron, protein, or fiber. The word *organic* can be used only on raw products grown without added hormones, pesticides, or synthetic fertilizers and on processed foods that contain 95 percent organic ingredients. The food label may display the USDA organic seal.

Freshness dates have also been defined. Phrases such as *Best Before, Better If Used Before*, and *Best If Used By* tell how long food will retain its best flavor or quality. The food is still safe to eat after the printed date, but it might become stale or change somewhat in taste or texture. The *Expiration, Use By,* or *Use Before* date, which appears on refrigerated foods, provides the deadline for consumption. A product past its expiration date is no longer of sufficient quality and should not be eaten. The *Sell By* date is usually found on highly perishable foods with a particularly short shelf life, such as meat, milk, and bread. It indicates the last day the product should appear on a supermarket shelf.

In 2006, food labels will also include information about trans fat. Trans fat will be listed directly under the line for saturated fat. This new requirement acknowledges the evidence that trans fat, saturated fat, and dietary cholesterol raise low-density lipoprotein cholesterols and increase the risk for coronary heart disease.

Consumer interest in low-carb foods has motivated the food industry to feature the words *low-carb* and *net carbs* on many package labels. Unlike the terms *low-fat* and *low-sodium,* which are defined by the FDA, there are no guidelines or definitions for *low* or *net* carbohydrates. The use of these terms should be regarded with caution.

Even with the improvements in label laws, the unwitting consumer can still be misled. A brand of margarine changed its name from *Brand . . . Light* to *Brand . . . Light Taste*—manufacturers can still use *light* to describe taste, texture, or color. The makers of a brand of brownie mix claim that it is low-fat. But the fine print says that the low-fat designation pertains only to each serving of the mix alone. Once an edible brownie is created by adding vegetable oil, its fat-gram content more than triples. Some foods promise fruit or other ingredients but deliver only flavor. One brand of strawberry frozen yogurt has no real strawberries, despite pictures on the label of real strawberries; a brand of blueberry pancakes has no berries. Clearly, although labels have improved dramatically during the past several years, they still fall short in several areas. Deception in old labels was more obvious; today's labels challenge consumers to apply a higher level of discrimination to sort between fact and fantasy.

Changes in American Eating Patterns

Changes in the American family are mirrored in the trend toward convenience-food eating. For many families, time is a precious commodity that has a dramatic influence on how, where, when, and what people eat. Family meals at home are being replaced by a quick-stop, eat-on-the-go trend. Dining out has become a part of the quintessential American lifestyle, with about 45 percent of all food dollars spent on meals away from home each day.[3] In terms of good health, this is a questionable trend when considering that the more people eat out the more calories, fat, and sodium they consume.

Not only do many people eat away from home, but they also skip meals. This is a questionable practice. The idea that skipping meals, for example, facilitates weight loss is dabatable. Often, it has the opposite effect by encouraging binge eating, increased snacking, or overcompensatory eating. Skipping breakfast is troublesome in that the body is denied a source of energy to replace carbohydrate stores used during the night's sleep. It should be of little surprise, therefore, that midmorning sluggishness is a common experience of students and workers.

Snacking

Snacking refers to consuming food between the three main meals of the day. Most Americans have at least one snack per day, and snack foods represent one of the fastest-growing markets in the food industry. From a nutrition point of view, snacking is neither good nor bad. The three meals a day standard is based more on social custom than on physiology. The issue is not the time or frequency of eating but what is eaten. Nutritionally dense foods eaten as snacks are as good for health as they are when consumed as meals. The converse is also true; foods low in nutrient density eaten at mealtime are as worthless as when they are eaten as snacks. With the exception of foods restricted for medical reasons, all foods can contribute to a healthful diet. Problems occur when a person's diet is dominated by foods low in nutrient density. Rather than rule out snacking, consume snack foods that enhance wellness. The most direct way to improve snacking behavior is the most obvious one: Purchase and make nutritionally dense foods available (see Real-World Wellness: Snack Ideas).

From a nutritional viewpoint, the criticisms of fast-food eating are the same as those of the rest of the American diet: too much fat, too many calories, too much sodium, and not enough complex carbohydrates and fiber. The average meal of a cheeseburger, milkshake, and fries supplies about 1,500 calories, 43 percent of which come from fat. Chicken and fish are as fatty as other protein sources offered by fast-food restaurants because they are breaded and fried. Frying has the same effect on potatoes. Milkshakes get most of their calories from sugars. The Food Composition Table located in the appendix of this text provides detailed information that can be used to compare many fast-food menu items.

Eating at fast-food restaurants does not have to be a nutritionally worthless activity. Many restaurants are aware that Americans are more knowledgeable about the nutrient content of food and are demanding wholesome, safe, and nutritious foods. Consequently, there has been a trend toward more nutritious menus, including salad, pasta, and potato bars. Guided by good judgment

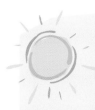

Real-World Wellness

Snack Ideas

After completing a thorough three-day dietary analysis, I was surprised to learn that the key to improving my overall nutritional profile is to make changes in my snack food choices. My meals are fairly well balanced, but my snacks are typically high in fat, high in sodium, high in sugar, and low in nutrient density. What are some examples of nutritionally dense snacks?

The following snacks are surprisingly flavorful and satisfying and will help you improve your overall nutrition:

- Fresh raw vegetables served with a cottage cheese dip
- Fresh fruit, prewashed and cut into bite-size pieces
- Fruit dipped in yogurt
- Bagels topped with reduced-fat cream cheese
- Breadsticks
- Air-popped popcorn seasoned with herbs
- Frozen fruit-juice bars
- Low-fat frozen yogurt
- Pita chips with salsa
- Pretzels
- Rye crisps or rice cakes spread with a little peanut butter or low-fat cheese
- Broth-based soup
- Cereal (low-sugar, low-fat)
- Shelled sunflower seeds
- Gelatin with added fruit
- English muffins
- Flour tortillas with canned chili and grated low-fat cheese
- Pita bread topped with spaghetti sauce and grated low-fat cheese
- Fruit juice with added club soda
- Hot cocoa (low-sugar, low-fat)
- Milkshake made with low-fat milk and frozen fruit

in the choice of foods, an occasional meal at a fast-food chain does not have to compromise a well-balanced diet.

Prepackaged Convenience Dinners

Prepackaged convenience dinners have also become part of the American diet. Consumers spend billions of dollars a year on them, and food manufacturers are constantly turning out new lines. The challenge for health-conscious consumers is to determine which ones fit easily into a nutritious diet.

Prepackaged convenience dinners can be evaluated by applying the following criteria:

- There should be no more than and preferably fewer than 35 percent of calories from fat, and most of the fat calories should come from monounsaturated and polyunsaturated fats.
- There should be no more than 200 milligrams of sodium per 100 calories.
- They should meet at least 40 percent of the RDA for vitamins A and/or C.

Just because a dinner meets these criteria does not necessarily mean that it provides every nutrient. Some meals are likely to be deficient in some nutrients, so foods that will compensate must be added.

Planning a Nutrition Strategy for Wellness

It is not necessary to be a nutritionist to form a nutrition strategy that works for you. A nutrition plan will work only if it is personalized. Several strategies should be helpful in personalizing your nutrition plan.

Assess Your Nutrition

You should take an honest look at your eating choices and analyze your nutrition profile through Assessment Activities 6-3, 6-4, and 6-6 to determine whether you are doing the following:

- Eating a variety of foods every day from the Food Guide Pyramid
- Avoiding high-fat foods (more than the equivalent of 3 grams of fat per 100 calories)
- Including sufficient fiber in the form of whole grains, dried beans, and fresh fruits and vegetables
- Consuming 8 to 12 cups of water (8 ounces each) daily
- Consuming no more than three or four high-sugar desserts or sweets each week
- Restricting your intake of high-salt foods, such as processed meats
- Consuming no more than one or two alcoholic drinks a day and not letting drinking interfere with your appetite

Make Small Adjustments

The principle of changing health behavior is that the smaller the change, the longer it lasts (see Chapter 1). For example, rather than vowing to abstain from eating ice cream, reduce the amount or number of servings at first and substitute a low-fat brand. If your diet is heavy

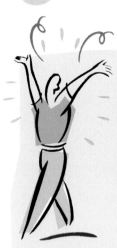

Nurturing Your Spirituality

Enjoy Your Food—the Missing Dietary Guideline

The fast-paced, eat-on-the-run trend among Americans comes with a high price: Fewer and fewer people spend time preparing good, home-cooked meals, and even fewer use mealtime as a time for relaxation and social bonding. Other cultures recognize that mealtime is a key social time of the day and reflect this value in the dietary recommendations health experts offer their citizens:[54]

- In Japan, immediately following the guideline to avoid too much sodium comes the advice "Happy eating makes for a happy family life; sit down and eat together and talk; treasure family taste and home cooking."

- In Great Britain, the first guideline is "Enjoy your food."

- Korea tells its citizens to "Enjoy meals and keep harmony between diet and daily life."

- In Norway, people are told, "Food and joy equal health."

- In Vietnam, the advice is to "Serve a healthy family meal that is delicious and served with affection."

The greatest nutrition challenge for Americans may not be to reduce fat intake or cut back on sodium. It may be to construct a positive view of food and of mealtime. One highly respected nutrition publication reminds us "Healthful eating is about more than eating the right mix of nutrients. It's also about sustaining well-being in a way that can't be measured on a blood test but that is just as important to overall health as vitamins and minerals.[54]

in salt, you can gradually substitute sodium-free seasonings. If you have a sweet tooth, you can try low-sugar snacks. If you eat for fullness, you can prepare less food or leave food on your plate. You should plan an approach that builds on the cumulative effect of many small successes.

Think of balancing your diet over a long period rather than in a day or a meal. Try to meet the dietary guidelines over several days or a week. For example, not every meal needs to contain less than 30 percent fat. Keep portions of favorite high-fat foods small and limit other sources of fat. Check labels to get an idea of what nutrients you are consuming, but don't keep a calculator by your plate. If you eat foods from the Food Guide Pyramid, you will get all the vitamins, minerals, and protein you need.

Choose Foods for Wellness

Choosing foods for wellness means following the Dietary Guidelines for Americans. Your diet should

- Be low in saturated fat (maximum of 8 percent)
- Emphasize complex carbohydrates, such as bread, potatoes, and pasta
- Provide 8 to 12 glasses of water throughout the day
- Provide iron and calcium
- Emphasize fresh fruits and vegetables
- Be low in sugar, salt, alcohol, and caffeine

Finally, make sure when choosing foods for wellness to enjoy what you eat (see Nurturing Your Spirituality: Enjoy Your Food—the Missing Dietary Guideline).

Summary

- The six classes of nutrients are carbohydrates, fat, protein, vitamins, minerals, and water. The nutrients that provide energy in the form of calories are carbohydrates, fat, and protein.
- The recommended diet for Americans in *Dietary Guidelines for Americans* emphasizes complex carbohydrates as the major source of energy. A diet high in complex carbohydrates is likely to be lower in fat, lower in calories, and higher in fiber. A low-carbohydrate diet is not necessarily low in calories.
- The terms *low-carb* and *net carbs* imply that a product is low in carbohydrates. This may be true but it may also be misleading. The FDA has not defined these terms.

- A complete protein is one that provides all of the amino acids in amounts proportional to the body's need for them. Protein sources from animals are complete proteins. Plant sources of complete protein, such as soy protein, come from the legume family.
- One of the greatest shortcomings of the American diet is its excessive intake of fat, especially saturated fat.
- The amount of saturated, monounsaturated, and polyunsaturated fat in foods varies considerably. Most food contains a mixture of these fats.
- The process of hydrogenation increases the saturated fat content of polyunsaturated and monounsaturated fats and yields small amounts of fat not found in nature called trans

fatty acids. No more than 10 percent of calories should come from saturated and/or trans fats.

- Dietary fat intake should favor foods high in monounsaturated fats, such as olive oil, canola oil, and peanut oil.
- The consumption of antioxidant vitamins, especially in fruits and vegetables, is associated with a reduced risk for heart disease and cancer.
- Adequate folate consumption is thought to lower the concentration of homocysteine, an amino acid associated with an increased risk for heart disease.
- Two minerals of special concern are calcium and iron. Most women fall short of the RDA for calcium. People at risk for low iron levels include young children, early teens, menstruating women, and people with health conditions that cause internal bleeding.
- Thirst is a good indicator of when and how much water to drink. One exception is during strenuous physical activity.
- Phytochemicals, or phytonutrients, are plant chemicals found naturally in foods. They play an important role in preventing many diseases.
- Enhanced foods are foods that have been modified and/or supplemented to achieve a health benefit.
- Many botanicals are thought to have health benefits. Because they are considered nutritional supplements and are not regulated with the same rigor as drugs, there is debate about their effectiveness and safety. Twenty to 30 botanicals are backed by well-conducted research.
- Fiber benefits the body by adding bulk to the stool, thus speeding the transit of food through the body, which reduces the chance of developing colon cancer, and lowering blood cholesterol levels.
- A good nutrition plan is one that consists of a variety of foods from the Food Guide Pyramid.
- A food is nutrient dense when it has a high ratio of nutrients to calories.
- Variety and moderation are principles that should most influence eating habits. There is room in the diet for any food as long as it is consumed in moderation in quantity and frequency.
- *Dietary Guidelines for Americans* officially recognizes a vegetarian diet as a healthful and acceptable way of meeting all of our nutritional needs.
- The health benefits of a vegetarian diet include a lower cholesterol level; lower levels of LDLs; reduced incidence of hypertension and lung, colorectal, and breast cancer; and fewer complications from noninsulin-dependent diabetes mellitus.
- Americans consume sugar and sodium in excessive amounts. The major health issue associated with high sugar intake is dental caries; for sodium, it's hypertension.
- Glycemic Index is a scale that indicates the effect of food on blood sugar surges.
- Moderate consumption of alcohol may be beneficial for some people at risk for cardiovascular disease and stroke.
- Pregnancy imposes a greater demand for some nutrients, including protein, vitamin D, folate, iron, calcium, and zinc.
- Carbohydrates are the main source of energy for both anaerobic and high-intensity aerobic activities; fat is the main energy source for prolonged, low-intensity exercise; and protein is a minor fuel source, primarily for endurance activities.
- The risk for foodborne illness can be reduced by preventing cross-contamination of food; by washing hands, fruits, produce, and meats; and by exercising caution in the way food is prepared and stored.
- Food labels provide helpful information about nutrients associated with the common chronic health problems of Americans as well as about essential nutrients.
- The criticisms of snacking and fast-food eating are the same as those of the rest of the American diet: too much fat, sodium, and sugar; too many calories; and not enough complex carbohydrates and fiber.
- Americans are challenged not only to eat more healthfully but also to construct a positive attitude about food and mealtimes.

Review Questions

1. What is meant by "nutritional diseases of the past have been replaced by diseases of dietary excess and imbalance"?
2. What was the rationale for revising the Recommended Dietary Allowances for essential nutrients?
3. Identify three nutrients that most Americans do not consume in sufficient amounts.
4. How many calories are supplied by carbohydrates, fat, and protein? What percent of total calories should come from each of these sources? How does Americans' intake of energy nutrients compare with dietary recommendations?
5. Why are carbohydrates the preferred source of energy?
6. Explain the difference between *low-carb* and *net carb*. Why should the trend toward low-carb foods be regarded with caution?
7. What is the difference between a high-quality, complete protein and a low-quality, incomplete protein?
8. What plant sources of protein are unique in that they are considered complete proteins?
9. What are the differences among saturated, monounsaturated, and polyunsaturated fats? What are some food sources of each? What percent of fat calories should come from each type?
10. What are trans fatty acids? Why should they be avoided?
11. List five dietary practices that will help lower consumption of fat, especially saturated fat.
12. What are the similarities and differences between water-soluble and fat-soluble vitamins?
13. Which vitamins are classified as antioxidants? What is the relationship between antioxidants and health?
14. What role does folate play in preventing disease?

15. Identify three situations or circumstances that would justify the use of a vitamin or mineral supplement.
16. What are phytochemicals? How are they different from botanicals? How do they contribute to health?
17. What two minerals are Americans most likely to be consuming in insufficient amounts? Which segments of the population are most likely to be affected?
18. How much water should be consumed during periods of strenuous physical activity?
19. What are the major health benefits of a high-fiber diet?
20. What is the rationale for the assertion that variety and moderation are the most important principles for a healthy diet?
21. Distinguish among the different types of vegetarianism. Which types are most likely to require some form of vitamin or mineral supplementation? What are the health benefits of a vegetarian diet?

22. Identify four nutrients that pregnant women require in larger amounts than those in the RDAs.
23. How do the intensity and duration of physical activities affect the way the body uses carbohydrates, fat, and protein for energy? What type of physical activity is most conducive to burning fat calories?
24. List six things a person can do to help prevent unnecessary exposure to foodborne illness.
25. Distinguish among the acronyms RDA, DRI, AI, UL, and DV.
26. To what does the Glycemic Index (GI) of food refer? Glycemic Load (GL)? What are the health implications of GI and GL?
27. What are the main criticisms of snacking and fast-food eating?

References

1. U.S. Department of Health and Human Services. 2000. *Healthy people 2010.* 2d ed. With *Understanding and improving health and objectives for improving health.* 2 vols. Washington, DC: U.S. Government Printing Office.
2. Wilder, L. B., L. J. Cheskin, and S. Margolis. 2004. *The Johns Hopkins white papers: Nutrition and weight control for longevity.* New York: Medletter.
3. Wardlaw, G., J. Hampl, and R. DiSilvestro. 2004. *Perspectives in nutrition.* 6th ed. New York: McGraw-Hill.
4. Institute of Medicine. 2002. *Dietary Reference Intakes for energy, carbohydrate, fiber, fat, fatty acids, cholesterol, protein, and amino acids.* Washington, DC: The National Academies Press.
5. Consumers Union. 2004. Stronger bones without the hype. *Consumer Reports on Health* 16(5):1, 4.
6. Tufts Media. 2003. Iron deficiency remains a concern. *Tufts University Health and Nutrition Letter* 21(11):2.
7. International Atomic Energy Agency. 2003. *Improving nutrition through nuclear science.* Austria: International Atomic Energy Agency.
8. Consumers Union. 2003. Are you getting enough fiber? *Consumer Reports on Health* 15(11):7.
9. Wright, J. D., C. Y. Wang, J. Kennedy-Stephenson, and R. B. Ervin. 2003. Dietary intake of ten key nutrients for public health, United States: 1999–2000. *Advance data from vital and health statistics, no. 334.* Hyattsville,

MD: National Center for Health Statistics.
10. Consumers Union. 2004. The truth about low-carb foods. *Consumer Reports* 69(6):12–18.
11. Editors. 2003. More soy findings. *Environmental Nutrition* 26(9):3.
12. Harvard Medical School. 2001. Is it time to stop eating meat? *Harvard Health Letter* 26(11):6.
13. Harvard Medical School. 2003. Nutrition: Conversation with an expert. *Harvard Health Letter* 28(11):6–7.
14. Consumers Union. 2003. New food labels help consumers avoid the worst fats. *Consumer Reports on Health* 15(12):3.
15. *Tufts University Health and Nutrition Letter.* 2003. Trans fatty acid content to be listed on labels. *Tufts University Health and Nutrition Letter* 21(7):2.
16. Editors. 2003. Vitamin E, beta-carotene supplements fail again. *Environmental Nutrition* 26(7):1.
17. Ward, E. 2004. Vitamin C: Still the key for immunity, cancer, heart disease, eye health. *Environmental Health* 27(3):1, 6.
18. *New England Journal of Medicine.* 2003. Vitamin C may help your heart. *HealthNews* 9(10):4.
19. Welland, D. 2003. Vitamins and minerals: Are you getting enough? Too much? Confused? *Environmental Nutrition* 26(3):1, 6.
20. Tufts Media. 2004. Tufts nutrition: Translating the research for use at your table. *Special Supplement to the Tufts University Health and Nutrition Letter* 21(12):1–4.

21. Harvard Medical School. 2004. Vitamins: The quest for just the right amount. *Harvard Health Letter* 29(8):4–5.
22. Aubertin, A. 2004. Research still suggests vitamin E may boost immunity and benefit brain. *Environmental Nutrition* 27(5):1, 4.
23. Consumers Union. 2004. Disease-fighting B vitamins. *Consumer Reports on Health* 16(1):10.
24. Editors. 2004. Elevated homocysteine—Bad to the bones. *Environmental Nutrition* 27(6):1.
25. Golub, C. 2004. B vitamins: Focus on fab three for a healthy heart, mighty memory. *Environmental Nutrition* 27(2):1, 4.
26. Ervin, R. B., J. D. Wright, C. Y. Wang, and J. Kennedy-Stephenson. 2004. Dietary intake of selected vitamins for the United States population: 1999–2000. *Advanced data from vital and health statistics, no. 339.* Hyattsville, MD: National Center for Health Statistics.
27. Consumers Union. 2004. Multivitamins may ward off disease. *Consumer Reports on Health* 16(3):7.
28. Ervin, R. B., C. Y. Wang, J. D. Wright, and J. Kennedy-Stephenson. 2004. Dietary intake of selected minerals for the United States population: 1999–2000. *Advanced data from vital and health statistics, no. 341.* Hyattsville, MD: National Center for Health Statistics.
29. Consumers Union. 2004. Stronger bones without the hype. *Consumer Reports on Health* 16(5):1, 4–5.

30. Schardt, D. 2000. Water, water, everywhere. . . . *Nutrition Action Healthletter* 27(5):1–7.

31. Tufts Media. 2004. New consumption guidelines issued for water, sodium, and potassium. *Tufts University Health and Nutrition Letter* 22(2):1, 4–5.

32. Webb, D. 2003. Phytonutrients: The hidden keys to disease prevention, good health. *Environmental Health* 26(1):1, 6.

33. Center for Science in the Public Interest. 2003. Are your supplements safe? *Nutrition Action Healthletter* 30(9):3–7.

34. Consumers Union. 2003. Are you getting enough fiber? *Consumer Reports on Health* 15(11):7.

35. U.S. Department of Health and Human Services. 2000. *Nutrition and your health: Dietary guidelines for Americans.* Washington, DC: U.S. Government Printing Office.

36. U.S. Department of Agriculture. 2002. Get on the grain train. *Dietary guidelines for Americans no. 267-2.* Washington, DC: U.S. Government Printing Office.

37. Webb, D. 2004. High-fiber, low-carb or sugar-free slices: Which breads are the best? *Environmental Nutrition* 27(5):5.

38. Harvard Medical School. 2004. Exercise your right to health. *Harvard Heart Letter* 14(11):4–5.

39. Tufts Media. 2003. Growing older presents new nutrition challenges. *Tufts University Health and Nutrition Letter* 21(8):1, 8.

40. U.S. Department of Health and Human Services, U.S. Department of Agriculture. 2004. *Dietary guidelines advisory committee meeting, meeting summary, January 28–29, 2004.* Washington, DC: U.S. Government Printing Office.

41. Center for Science in the Public Interest. 2003. The best diet. *Nutrition Action Healthletter* 30(3):9.

42. Forman, A. 2003. So you want to be a vegetarian? EN answers your questions. *Environmental Nutrition* 26(3):2.

43. *New England Journal of Medicine.* 2004. Food irradiation: A recipe for safer food? *Healthnews* 10(6):4–5.

44. Nagao, M., and T. Sugimura. 2000. *Food borne carcinogens: Heterocyclic amines.* Weimar, TX: Culinary and Hospitality Industry Publications Services.

45. Tufts Media. 2004. How much sugar is right? Less. *Tufts University Health and Nutrition Letter* 22(4):3.

46. Popkin, B. M., and S. J. Nielsen. 2003. The sweetening of the world's diet. *Obesity Research* 11(11):1325–32.

47. *Environmental Nutrition.* 2002. Glycemic index: Gateway to good health or grand waste of time. *Environmental Health* 25(11):1, 6.

48. Foster-Powell, K., S. H. A. Holt, and J. C. Brand-Miller. 2002. International table of Glycemic Index and Glycemic Load values: 2002. *American Journal of Clinical Nutrition* 76(1):274–81.

49. Harvard Medical School. 2002. Lift a glass (but not too many) to health. *Harvard Health Letter* 27(6):3.

50. Mayo Clinic. 2003. Alcohol and health. *Mayo Clinic Health Letter* 21(11):4–5.

51. Mukamal, K. J., K. M. Conigrave, M. A. Mittleman, C. A. Camargo, M. J. Stampfer, W. C. Willett, and E. B. Rimm. 2003. Roles of drinking pattern and type of alcohol consumed in coronary heart disease in men. *New England Journal of Medicine* 348(10): 109–19.

52. Nieman, D. 2003. *Exercise testing and prescription: A health-related approach.* 5th ed. McGraw-Hill.

53. Manore, M. M. 2000. Effect of physical activity on thiamine, riboflavin, and vitamin B-6 requirements. *American Journal of Clinical Nutrition* 72(suppl.): 598.

54. *Tufts Media.* 1998. The missing dietary guideline; enjoy your food. *Tufts University Health and Nutrition Letter* 16(5):3.

Suggested Readings

Cooperman, T., W. Obermeyer, and D. Webb, eds. 2003. *Consumerlab.com's guide to buying vitamins & supplements: What's really in the bottle?* White Plains, NY: ConsumerLab.com, LLC.

As an independent testing company, ConsumerLab.com provides objective, concise, and reliable reviews of 20 supplements from B vitamins to valerian. The information includes ingredients, dosages, quality concerns, shopping tips, and warnings. Hundreds of brands are included. This is considered a "must read" by the editors of *Environmental Nutrition* for anyone considering the purchase of a vitamin, a mineral, or an herbal supplement.

Icon Health Publications. 2003. *Antioxidants: A medical dictionary, bibliography, and annotated research guide to Internet references.* San Diego, CA: Icon Health Publications.

This book was created for medical professionals, students, and members of the general public who want to conduct medical research using the most advanced tools available and spending the least amount of time doing so. It gives a complete medical dictionary covering hundreds of terms relating to antioxidants. It provides information on how to obtain reliable information on antioxidants using various Internet resources.

O'Neil, M. S., and D. Webb. 2004. *No-guilt nutrition advice from the "dish divas."* New York: Atria Books.

Registered dietitians M. S. O'Neil and D. Webb present the lowdown on eating out, eating in, entertaining, and getting active. This unique book presents funky food facts, quirky illustrations, and recipes from high-profile chefs. Recipes and advice are based on latest nutrition research without overwhelming the reader with scientific jargon. The highly respected newsletter *Environmental Nutrition* endorses this book.

Wardlaw, G., J. Hampl, and R. DiSilvestro. 2004. *Perspectives in nutrition.* 6th ed. New York: McGraw-Hill.

This book provides in-depth, comprehensive information on all aspects of nutrition. It is an excellent introductory reference in nutrition.

Wilder, L. G., L. J. Cheskin, and S. Margolis. 2004. *Nutrition and weight control for longevity.* Baltimore, MD: Johns Hopkins Medical School.

This 85-page monograph is a concise, no-nonsense presentation on basic nutrition and weight-control facts and guidelines. Written by medical doctors at the highly respected Johns Hopkins Medical School, this book presents guidelines that are backed by recent scientific studies in the medical world. The latest information on fat, carbohydrates, vitamins, minerals, antioxidants, phytochemicals, enhanced foods, organic foods, and food safety is discussed.

Willett, W. C., and P. J. Skerrett. 2002. *Eat, drink, and be healthy: The Harvard Medical School guide to healthy eating.* New York: Free Press.

Walter Willett, Harvard professor and nationally known nutrition researcher, takes issue with the USDA's Food Guide Pyramid. This book maintains that the Food Guide Pyramid puts too much emphasis on red meat and lumps too many different types of carbohydrates together. It also claims that nuts, beans, and healthy oils that have positive effects on health are not emphasized. Dr. Willett offers his own pyramid, which recommends whole grains at most meals; emphasizes plant oils, such as olive, canola, and soy; suggests eating lots of vegetables; and recommends fish, poultry, and eggs over red meat.

☆ This Just In

The much-anticipated revision of the *Dietary Guidelines* is now a reality with the publication of the *Dietary Guidelines for Americans, 2005.* The ten dietary guidelines listed on page 187 have been replaced with 23 "key recommendations" and an additional 18 recommendations for specific population groups. The new guidelines urge Americans to consume fewer calories, incorporate physical activity in their daily routine, and make smarter food choices. Two eating patterns that apply the principles of a healthful diet include the USDA Food Guide (see pages 211 and 212) and the DASH (Dietary Approaches to Stop Hypertension) Eating Plan (see Chapter 2 and the complete plan at www.mhhe.com/anspaugh6e). The Food Guide Pyramid that is presented on page 188 is scheduled for final revision in late 2005 or early 2006; its new name is the USDA Food Guide.

Selected guidelines in *Dietary Guidelines for Americans, 2005* include:

- Consume a variety of nutrient-dense foods and beverages within and among the basic food groups while choosing foods that limit the intake of saturated and trans fats, cholesterol, added sugars, salt, and alcohol.

- Meet recommended intakes within energy needs by adopting a balanced eating pattern, such as the USDA Food Guide or the DASH Eating Plan.

- To prevent gradual weight gain over time, make small decreases in food and beverage calories and increase physical activity.

- Achieve physical fitness by including cardiovascular conditioning, stretching exercises for flexibility, and resistance exercises or calisthenics for muscle strength and endurance.

- Consume a sufficient amount of fruits and vegetables while staying within energy needs. Two cups of fruit and 2½ cups of vegetables per day are recommended for a reference 2,000-calorie intake, with higher or lower amounts depending on the calorie level.

- Choose a variety of fruits and vegetables each day. In particular, select from all five vegetable subgroups (dark green, orange, legumes, starchy vegetables, and other vegetables) several times a week.

- Consume 3 or more ounce-equivalents of whole-grain products per day, with the rest of the recommended grains coming from enriched or whole-grain products. In general, at least half the grains should come from whole grains.

- Consume 3 cups per day of fat-free or low-fat milk or equivalent milk products.

- Consume less than 10 percent of calories from saturated fatty acids and less than 300 mg/day of cholesterol, and keep trans fatty acid consumption as low as possible.

- Choose and prepare foods and beverages with little added sugars or caloric sweeteners, such as amounts suggested by the USDA Food Guide and the DASH Eating Plan.

- Consume less than 2,300 mg (approximately 1 tsp of salt) of sodium per day.

For more information on *Dietary Guidelines for Americans, 2005* go to http://www.healthierus.gov/dietaryguidelines

USDA Food Guide

The suggested amounts of food to consume from the basic food groups, subgroups, and oils to meet recommended nutrient intakes at 12 different calorie levels. Nutrient and energy contributions from each group are calculated according to the nutrient-dense forms of foods in each group (e.g., lean meats and fat-free milk). The table also shows the discretionary calorie allowance that can be accommodated within each calorie level, in addition to the suggested amounts of nutrient-dense forms of foods in each group.

continued

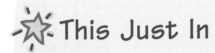

This Just In

continued

Daily Amount of Food from Each Group (vegetable subgroup amounts are per week)

Food Group[1]	Calorie Level											
	1,000	1,200	1,400	1,600	1,800	2,000	2,200	2,400	2,600	2,800	3,000	3,200
	Food group amounts shown in cup (c) or ounce-equivalents (oz-eq), with number of servings (srv) in parentheses when it differs from the other units. See note for quantity equivalents for foods in each group.[2] Oils are shown in grams (g).											
Fruits	1 c (2 srv)	1 c (2 srv)	1.5 c (3 srv)	1.5 c (3 srv)	1.5 c (3 srv)	2 c (4 srv)	2 c (4 srv)	2 c (4 srv)	2 c (4 srv)	2.5 c (5 srv)	2.5 c (5 srv)	2.5 c (5 srv)
Vegetables[3]	1 c (2 srv)	1.5 c (3 srv)	1.5 c (3 srv)	2 c (4 srv)	2.5 c (5 srv)	2.5 c (5 srv)	3 c (6 srv)	3 c (6 srv)	3.5 c (7 srv)	3.5 c (7 srv)	4 c (8 srv)	4 c (8 srv)
Dark green veg.	1 c/wk	1.5 c/wk	1.5 c/wk	2 c/wk	3 c/wk	3 c/wk	3 c/wk	3 c/wk	3 c/wk	3 c/wk	3 c/wk	3 c/wk
Orange veg.	.5 c/wk	1 c/wk	1 c/wk	1.5 c/wk	2 c/wk	2 c/wk	2 c/wk	2 c/wk	2.5 c/wk	2.5 c/wk	2.5 c/wk	2.5 c/wk
Legumes	.5 c/wk	1 c/wk	1 c/wk	2.5 c/wk	3 c/wk	3 c/wk	3 c/wk	3 c/wk	3.5 c/wk	3.5 c/wk	3.5 c/wk	3.5 c/wk
Starchy veg.	1.5 c/wk	2.5 c/wk	2.5 c/wk	2.5 c/wk	3 c/wk	3 c/wk	6 c/wk	6 c/wk	7 c/wk	7 c/wk	9 c/wk	9 c/wk
Other veg.	4 c/wk	4.5 c/wk	4.5 c/wk	5.5 c/wk	6.5 c/wk	6.5 c/wk	7 c/wk	7 c/wk	8.5 c/wk	8.5 c/wk	10 c/wk	10 c/wk
Grains[4]	3 oz-eq	4 oz-eq	5 oz-eq	5 oz-eq	6 oz-eq	6 oz-eq	7 oz-eq	8 oz-eq	9 oz-eq	10 oz-eq	10 oz-eq	10 oz-eq
Whole grains	1.5	2	2.5	3	3	3	3.5	4	4.5	5	5	5
Other grains	1.5	2	2.5	2	3	3	3.5	4	4.5	5	5	5
Lean meat and beans	2 oz-eq	3 oz-eq	4 oz-eq	5 oz-eq	5 oz-eq	5.5 oz-eq	6 oz-eq	6.5 oz-eq	6.5 oz-eq	7 oz-eq	7 oz-eq	7 oz-eq
Milk	2 c	2 c	2 c	3 c	3 c	3 c	3 c	3 c	3 c	3 c	3 c	3 c
Oils[5]	15 g	17 g	17 g	22 g	24 g	27 g	29 g	31 g	34 g	36 g	44 g	51 g
Discretionary calorie allowance[6]	165	171	171	132	195	267	290	362	410	426	512	648

Source: U.S. Department of Health and Human Services and U.S. Department of Agriculture. 2005. *Dietary guidelines for Americans, 2005.* 6th ed. Washington, DC: U.S. Government Printing Office.

Notes for the USDA Food Guide

[1] Food items included in each group and subgroup:

Fruits All fresh, frozen, canned, and dried fruits and fruit juices: for example, oranges and orange juice, apples and apple juice, bananas, grapes, melons, berries, raisins. In developing the food patterns, only fruits and juices with no added sugars or fats were used. *See note 6 on discretionary calories if products with added sugars or fats are consumed.*

Vegetables In developing the food patterns, only vegetables with no added fats or sugars were used. *See note 6 on discretionary calories if products with added fats or sugars are consumed.*

Dark green vegetables All fresh, frozen, and canned dark green vegetables, cooked or raw: for example, broccoli; spinach; romaine; collard, turnip, and mustard greens.

Orange vegetables All fresh, frozen, and canned orange and deep yellow vegetables, cooked or raw: for example, carrots, sweet potatoes, winter squash, and pumpkin.

Legumes (dry beans and peas) All cooked dry beans and peas and soybean products: for example, pinto beans, kidney beans, lentils, chickpeas, tofu. (See comment under meat and beans group about counting legumes in the vegetable or the meat and beans group.)

Starchy vegetables All fresh, frozen, and canned starchy vegetables: for example, white potatoes, corn, green peas.

Other vegetables All fresh, frozen, and canned other vegetables, cooked or raw: for example, tomatoes, tomato juice, lettuce, green beans, onions.

Grains In developing the food patterns, only grains in low-fat and low-sugar forms were used. *See note 6 on discretionary calories if products that are higher in fat and/or added sugars are consumed.*

Whole grains All whole-grain products and whole grains used as ingredients: for example, whole-wheat and rye breads, whole-grain cereals and crackers, oatmeal, and brown rice.

Other grains All refined grain products and refined grains used as ingredients: for example, white breads, enriched grain cereals and crackers, enriched pasta, white rice.

Meat, poultry, fish, dry beans, eggs, and nuts (meat & beans) All meat, poultry, fish, dry beans and peas, eggs, nuts, seeds. Most choices should be lean or low-fat. *See note 6 on*

continued

☆ This Just In

continued

discretionary calories if higher fat products are consumed. Dry beans and peas and soybean products are considered part of this group as well as the vegetable group but should be counted in one group only.

Milk, yogurt, and cheese (milk) All milks, yogurts, frozen yogurts, dairy desserts, cheeses (except cream cheese), including lactose-free and lactose-reduced products. Most choices should be fat-free or low-fat. In developing the food patterns, only fat-free milk was used. *See note 6 on discretionary calories if low-fat, reduced-fat, or whole milk or milk products or milk products that contain added sugars are consumed.* Calcium-fortified soy beverages are an option for those who want a non-dairy calcium source.

[2] Quantity equivalents for each food group:

Grains The following each count as 1 ounce-equivalent (1 serving) of grains: ½ cup cooked rice, pasta, or cooked cereal; 1 ounce dry pasta or rice; 1 slice bread; 1 small muffin (1 oz); 1 cup ready-to-eat cereal flakes.

Fruits and vegetables The following each count as 1 cup (2 servings) of fruits or vegetables: 1 cup cut-up raw or cooked fruit or vegetable, 1 cup fruit or vegetable juice, 2 cups leafy salad greens.

Meat and beans The following each count as 1 ounce-equivalent: 1 ounce lean meat, poultry, or fish; 1 egg; ¼ cup cooked dry beans or tofu; 1 Tbsp peanut butter; ½ ounce nuts or seeds.

Milk The following each count as 1 cup (1 serving) of milk: 1 cup milk or yogurt, 1½ ounces natural cheese such as cheddar cheese or 2 ounces processed cheese. Discretionary calories must be counted for all choices, except fat-free milk.

[3] Explanation of vegetable subgroup amounts: Vegetable subgroup amounts are shown in this table as weekly amounts, because it would be difficult for consumers to select foods from each subgroup daily. A daily amount that is one-seventh of the weekly amount listed is used in calculations of nutrient and energy levels in each pattern.

[4] Explanation of grain subgroup amounts: The whole grain subgroup amounts shown in this table represent at least three 1-ounce servings and one-half of the total amount as whole grains for all calorie levels of 1,600 and above. This is the minimum suggested amount of whole grains to consume as part of the food patterns. More whole grains up to all of the grains recommended may be selected, with offsetting decreases in the amounts of other (enriched) grains. In patterns designed for younger children (1,000, 1,200, and 1,400 calories), one-half of the total amount of grains is shown as whole grains.

[5] Explanation of oils: Oils (including soft margarine with zero *trans* fat) shown in this table represent the amounts that are added to

foods during processing, cooking, or at the table. Oils and soft margarines include vegetable oils and soft vegetable oil table spreads that have no *trans* fats. The amounts of oils listed in this table are not considered to be part of discretionary calories because they are a major source of the vitamin E and polyunsaturated fatty acids, including the essential fatty acids, in the food pattern. In contrast, solid fats are listed separately in the discretionary calorie table (appendix A-3) because, compared with oils, they are higher in saturated fatty acids and lower in vitamin E and polyunsaturated and monounsaturated fatty acids, including essential fatty acids. The amounts of each type of fat in the food intake pattern were based on 60% oils and/or soft margarines with no *trans* fats and 40% solid fat. The amounts in typical American diets are about 42% oils or soft margarines and about 58% solid fats.

[6] Explanation of discretionary calorie allowance: The discretionary calorie allowance is the remaining amount of calories in each food pattern after selecting the specified number of nutrient-dense forms of foods in each food group. The number of discretionary calories assumes that food items in each food group are selected in nutrient-dense forms (that is, forms that are fat-free or low-fat and that contain no added sugars). Solid fat and sugar calories always need to be counted as discretionary calories, as in the following examples:

- The fat in low-fat, reduced fat, or whole milk or milk products or cheese and the sugar and fat in chocolate milk, ice cream, pudding, etc.
- The fat in higher fat meats (e.g., ground beef with more than 5% fat by weight, poultry with skin, higher fat luncheon meats, sausages)
- The sugars added to fruits and fruit juices with added sugars or fruits canned in syrup
- The added fat and/or sugars in vegetables prepared with added fat or sugars
- The added fats and/or sugars in grain products containing higher levels of fats and/or sugars (e.g., sweetened cereals, higher fat crackers, pies and other pastries, cakes, cookies)

Total discretionary calories should be limited to the amounts shown in the table at each calorie level. The number of discretionary calories is lower in the 1,600-calorie pattern than in the 1,000-, 1,200-, and 1,400-calorie patterns. These lower calorie patterns are designed to meet the nutrient needs of children 2 to 8 years old. The nutrient goals for the 1,600-calorie pattern are set to meet the needs of adult women, which are higher and require that more calories be used in selections from the basic food groups. Additional information about discretionary calories, including an example of the division of these calories between solid fats and added sugars, is provided in appendix A-3.

Name _____   Date _____   Section _____

Assessment Activity 6-3

Nutrient Intake Assessment

One way to determine if you are getting sufficient quantities of the proper nutrients is to keep a record of your diet. Ideally, this record will cover a time span of at least one week. However, in this exercise you are asked to assess your dietary selections for only one day. Therefore, choose a day representative of your overall nutritional practices. (Your instructor may ask you to conduct a two- or three-day assessment. In this case, photocopy additional copies of the assessment forms as needed.)

Directions: There are two options for completing this assessment: (1) use the nutrition software that accompanies the textbook or (2) analyze your diet manually by following the instructions and completing the forms in Assessment Activities 6-3 and 6-4. Whichever option you choose, record all of the foods and beverages that you consume during one day, with the exception of vitamin or mineral supplements. Be specific regarding the amount eaten, how it is cooked, and so on. List condiments and seasonings, such as mustard, ketchup, and butter, and dressings and trimmings, such as lettuce, onions, marshmallows, and sugar. The more detailed your record, the more accurate it will be and the more you will learn from it. Remember, the quality of the results is dependent on the quality of the information entered. A carefully and thoroughly prepared dietary recall will yield an accurate nutritional profile.

Instructions for Computer Analysis Using Nutrition Software   Once foods have been listed, you are ready to use the nutrition software that accompanies this text to generate your personal nutrition assessment report. Enter your new User Profile information. When you have completed data entry, print and arrange the results in the following order:

1. User profile with personal information, including height, weight and BMI.
2. Intake of total calories, total fat, saturated and trans fat, mono fat, poly fat, cholesterol, 10 vitamins, and 7 minerals.

3. Nutrient intake, listing foods, and amounts
4. Nutrient spreadsheet
5. Food pyramid breakdown of servings for one day
6. Bar graph showing dietary intake analysis of nutrients and percent RDA
7. Bar graph comparing breakdown of carbohydrates, fat, protein with recommendations
8. Bar graph showing breakdown of fat
9. Nutrition fact box
10. Major source of nutrients for those vitamins and minerals that do not meet the RDAs in #6
11. Summary paragraph describing what you learned about your dietary strengths and deficiencies and what changes are needed to improve your nutrition profile

Instructions for Conducting a Manual Nutrition Assessment   Complete Parts A, B, C, and D. Then proceed to Assessment Activity 6-4.

Part A: Recording Your Nutrient Intake

1. Use the following form to record your dietary selections for one day. Photocopy extra copies of the form as needed.
2. Refer to the Food Composition Table in the appendix and record appropriate values in the spaces provided. For foods not included in the appendix, refer to package labels, if available, to determine nutritive values.
3. Add the values for each nutrient and enter the result in the total column.

Foods for One Day: List in column headings. Photocopy extra copies as needed.

Nutrients							Total
Calories							
Protein (g)							
Carbohydrate (g)							
Fat (g)							
Cholesterol (mg)							
Saturated and trans fat (g)							
Sodium (mg)							
Potassium (mg)							
Iron (mg)							
Vitamin A (RE)							
Vitamin C (mg)							
Thiamin (mg)							
Riboflavin (mg)							
Niacin (mg)							
Calcium (mg)							
Fiber (g)							
Folate (mg)							
Selenium (mg)							

Part B: Are You Meeting the RDA?

1. Transfer the values in the Total column in Part A to the Total column in Part B for the following nutrients.
2. Fill in the DV column with your protein RDA results from Assessment Activity 6-1.

3. Subtract the DV from your totals and indicate your status in the appropriate column. A positive value means that you are meeting the DV for that nutrient; a negative value means that you are deficient in that nutrient.
4. For nutrients with a negative value, identify several specific foods that will eliminate the deficiency. Refer to the Food Composition Table in the appendix.

Nutrient	Total	DV	Status	Food Prescription
Protein		See Assessment 6-1.		
Iron		18 mg		
Vitamin A		1,000 RE		
Vitamin C		60 mg		
Thiamin		1.5 mg		
Riboflavin		1.7 mg		
Niacin		20 mg		
Calcium		1 g		
Folate		400 mg		
Selenium		70 mg		

Part C: Are You Meeting the DVs?

1. Transfer the values in the total column from part A to the total column in Part C for the following nutrients. (Refer to Assessment Activities 6-1 and 6-2 for your personal DV for fat, saturated fat, and carbohydrate.)

2. Compare the DV listed with your totals. Indicate your status by subtracting the DV value from your value. Note that some values are maximum and should not be exceeded; others are goals that serve as minimums.

Nutrient	Total	DV*	Status
Fat		See Assessment 6-2.[†]	
Saturated fat/trans fat		See Assessment 6-2.[†]	
Cholesterol		300 mg[†]	
Sodium		2,400 mg[†]	
Carbohydrate		See Assessment 6-1.[‡]	
Fiber		25 g	
Potassium		3,500 mg (goal)	

* DV based on 2,000-calorie diet.

[†] Maximum.

[‡] Goal.

Part D: What Did You Learn?

Write a summary paragraph describing what you learned about your dietary strengths and deficiencies and what changes are needed to improve your nutrition profile.

_____

_____

_____

_____

_____

_____

_____

_____

_____

_____

_____

_____

_____

Name _____ Date _____ Section _____

Assessment Activity 6-4

How Does Your Diet Compare with the Recommended Diet?

Directions: The recommended guidelines suggest that carbohydrate calories should make up at least 55 percent of the diet (including complex carbohydrates and sugar), fat calories should be less than 30 percent, and protein calories should be 15 percent. The purpose of this assessment is to compare your diet with these recommendations. First convert your caloric intake to percentages as follows.

Percent Carbohydrate Calories Your carbohydrate intake (refer to total carbohydrate intake from Part A, Assessment Activity 6-3) multiplied by 4 equals your carbohydrate calories:

_____ g × 4 = _____ carbohydrate calories

Your carbohydrate calories divided by total calories (refer to Part A, Assessment Activity 6-3) multiplied by 100 equals percent carbohydrate calories:

_____ carbohydrate calories ÷ _____ total calories × 100 = _____ %

Draw a bar on the graph to indicate percentage of carbohydrate calories.

EXAMPLE: For a person on a 2,000-calorie diet who consumed 175 grams of carbohydrate,

175 × 4 = 700 carbohydrate calories
700 ÷ 2,000 = 0.35
0.35 × 100 = 35%

Percent Protein Calories Your protein intake (refer to total protein intake from Part A, Assessment Activity 6-3) multiplied by 4 equals protein calories:

_____ g × 4 = _____ protein calories

Your protein calories divided by total calories (refer to Part A, Assessment Activity 6-3) multiplied by 100 equals percent protein calories:

_____ protein calories ÷ _____ total calories × 100 = _____ %

Draw a bar on the graph to indicate percentage of protein calories.

EXAMPLE: For a person on a 2,000-calorie diet who consumed 100 grams of protein,

100 × 4 = 400 protein calories
400 ÷ 2,000 = 0.20
0.20 × 100 = 20%

Percent Fat Calories Your fat intake (refer to total fat intake from Part A, Assessment Activity 6-3) multiplied by 9 equals your fat calories:

_____ g × 9 = _____ fat calories

Your fat calories divided by total calories (refer to Part A, Assessment Activity 6-3) multiplied by 100 equals percent fat calories:

_____ fat calories ÷ _____ total calories × 100 = _____ %

Draw a bar on the graph to indicate percentage of fat calories.

EXAMPLE: For a person on a 2000-calorie diet who consumed 100 grams of fat:

100 × 9   = 900 fat calories
900 ÷ 2,000 = 0.45
0.45 × 100 = 45%

Example Profile The following graph shows the percentages for the example as the yellow bar below the recommended amount, shown as a red bar.

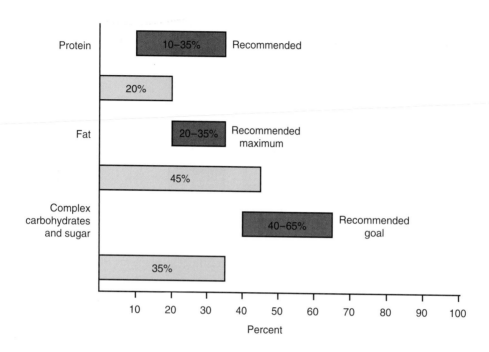

Your Profile Complete the bars with amounts calculated for your diet:

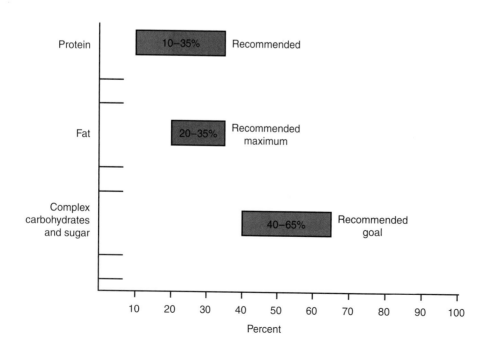

Name _____ Date _____ Section _____

Assessment Activity 6-6

Eating Behaviors to Consider

Directions: Answer the following questions to reveal information about your eating habits, how you developed certain tastes, and your attitude about various foods.

1. When was the last time you tried a new food? What was the food? What were the circumstances? _____

2. What new foods have you learned to eat during the past year? _____

3. Name the foods that have been on your "will not try" list (that is, foods that you will not eat under any circumstances). _____

4. What special events do you celebrate in some way with food? _____

5. Where is your favorite place to eat? _____

6. If you were to go on an eating binge, what foods would you be most likely to eat? _____

7. Describe in detail your favorite meal. _____

8. Do you consider yourself a slow eater, moderately fast eater, or gulper? What do you think is responsible for your eating pattern? _____

9. To what extent, if any, are your eating habits related to stress? Emotions? _____

10. What do you consider to be your good eating habits? Poor eating habits? _____

7

Understanding Body Composition

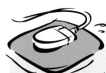

Online Learning Center

Log on to our Online Learning Center (OLC) for access to these additional resources:

- Chapter key term flashcards
- Learning objectives
- Additional goals for behavior change
- Concentration game
- Self-scoring chapter quizzes

- Additional lab activities

The OLC also offers Web links for study and exploration of wellness topics. Access these links through **www.mhhe.com/anspaugh6e**, click on Student Center, click on Chapter 7, and then click on Web Activities.

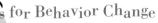

Goals for Behavior Change

- Use Table 7-5 to calculate your body mass index and interpret your results.
- Make a commitment to either maintain your existing weight or select a healthier weight.
- Formulate a long-range plan to achieve or maintain an ideal body weight and improve your body composition.

Key Terms

amenorrheic
body composition
body mass index (BMI)

obesity
overfat
overweight

Objectives

After completing this chapter, you will be able to do the following:

- Define *body composition.*
- Define *essential fat* and *storage fat.*
- Define and differentiate between *obesity* and *overweight.*
- Discuss the health implications of regionally distributed fat.

- Discuss the limitations of height/weight tables for weight management.
- Calculate body mass index and interpret the results.
- Describe hydrostatic weighing, bioelectrical impedance, and skinfold measurements as methods for determining body composition.

he body is composed of fat mass and fat-free mass. **Body composition** is the ratio between the two. Fat-free weight includes all tissues—muscle, bone, blood, organs, fluids—exclusive of fat. Fat is found in the organs (such as the brain, heart, liver, and lungs) and adipose cells.[1] Adipose cells are fat cells located subcutaneously (beneath the skin) and surrounding various body organs. They are an insulator against heat loss and a protection for the internal organs against trauma. The majority of body fat is found in adipose cells, where it acts as a vast storage depot for energy.

A certain amount of fat is required for normal biological functions. This is referred to as *essential fat.* Essential fat is located in the bone marrow, organs, muscles, and intestines; it is a component of cell-membrane structure as well as of brain and heart tissue. The amount of essential fat in the male and female bodies differs. Essential fat constitutes 3 to 5 percent of the total weight of men and 8 to 12 percent of the total weight of women.[2] Total body fat includes adipose fat plus essential fat.

The higher female requirement for essential fat is directly related to fertility and childbearing. Women whose body fat drops below essential requirements, such as gymnasts, ballerinas, long-distance runners, and anorexics, often become **amenorrheic;** that is, they stop having a menstrual cycle. The period of infertility continues until they gain weight and their essential fat is restored. In both genders, essential fat represents a minimal threshold, or lower limit, for the maintenance of health.

Obesity

Obesity, or overfatness, is gender-specific. For men, **obesity** is defined as body fat equal to or greater than 25 percent of total body weight, and for women, it is equal to or greater than 32 percent of total body weight.[3] These values are arbitrary because the point at which fat storage increases health risks has not been determined. Contributing further to the confusion is the fact that methods of assessing the amount of body fat are indirect, and each contains a degree of measurement error. Another complicating factor is that all obesity is not the same. The distribution of body fat in the abdominal area is highly correlated with illness and premature death.[4] A discussion of this topic occurs later in the chapter.

Acceptable body fat percentages have been derived from young adult subjects, and these standards have been applied to all age groups—age-specific standards have yet to be determined, and it is possible that such standards will vary somewhat with age. The results of studies of young adults demonstrate that fat typically ranges from 20 to 30 percent for young females and 10 to 20 percent for young males.[1] These data have led many authorities to suggest that body fat values of 25 percent for females and 15 percent for males are acceptable.

However, more recent body fat health standards based on age and gender allow for an increase in percent body fat with age. This allowance amounts to a trade-off in risks for chronic diseases, especially for women. Low body fat among middle-aged women is associated with losses of bone mineral content, which can lead to osteoporosis and bone fractures. However, leanness, or low body fat, helps protect these women against heart disease. It is best for women to be lean enough to prevent heart disease yet not so lean as to risk the development of osteoporosis. This is particularly problematic for small-framed women, whose bone mineral content is already low. See Tables 7-1 and 7-2 for recommended body fat percentages for women and men of different ages. These are only recommendations designed to recognize differences between males and females, and increasing age is taken into account. Whether these recommendations are accepted or rejected by the scientific community will become evident in the near future. See also Nurturing Your Spirituality: Setting Realistic Fitness and Weight-Loss Goals.

 Table 7-1 Recommended Body Fat Percentages for Women

Age	Essential Fat %	Minimal Fat %	Recommended Fat %	Obese Fat %
Over 56	8–12	10–12	25–38	> 38
35–55	8–12	10–12	23–38	> 38
34 or younger	8–12	10–12	20–35	> 35

> greater than

Adapted from Lohman, T. G., L. B. Houtkooper, and S. B. Going. 1997. Body composition assessment: Body fat standards and methods in the field of exercise and sports medicine. *ACSM Health Fitness Journal* 1:30.

Table 7-2 Recommended Body Fat Percentages for Men

Age	Essential Fat %	Minimal Fat %	Recommended Fat %	Obese Fat %
Over 56	3–5	5	10–25	> 28
35–55	3–5	5	10–25	> 28
34 or younger	3–5	5	8–22	> 25

> greater than

Adapted from Lohman, T. G., L. B. Houtkooper, and S. B. Going. 1997. Body composition assessment: Body fat standards and methods in the field of exercise and sports medicine. *ACSM Health Fitness Journal* 1:30.

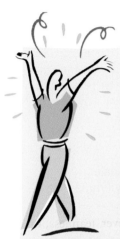

Nurturing Your Spirituality

Setting Realistic Fitness and Weight-Loss Goals

Success in any endeavor requires the establishment of long-term goals. Goals that are challenging and worthwhile but not impossible to accomplish are the keys to success. For instance, it would be unrealistic to expect to run a marathon after a few months of sporadic training or to lose 30 pounds in one month and keep it off.

A more feasible approach is to set realistic short-term goals that can be accomplished relatively easily and quickly. The accomplishment of these will provide the feedback you need to stay on track and the reinforcement to continue the program.

Attainable, realistic goals for exercise should be consistent with the American College of Sports Medicine guidelines for exercise, and realistic weight loss should not exceed 1.5 to 2 pounds per week. People often throw themselves into exercise with a vengeance, as if to wipe out years of inactivity with a frenzied few weeks of activity. The same degree of impatience surfaces with weight-loss attempts.

The following guidelines increase the likelihood of succeeding with exercise and weight loss:

1. Genetics is responsible for 40 to 50 percent of the factors that determine how aerobically fit we may become.[4,5] We can achieve our aerobic potential with regular exercise, but world-class endurance performances are beyond the reach of most of us. Exercise and enjoy it, be as good as you can, and be satisfied with a significant accomplishment. You should be encouraged to know that you are in the select 15 percent of the adult population who exercise regularly and vigorously.

2. Genetics is responsible for 25 percent of the factors that lead to overweight and obesity.[6] Although this represents a substantial influence, authorities are convinced that overweight individuals inherit only the *tendency* to become overweight or obese.[7] Our physical activity patterns and eating habits determine whether genetic history becomes destiny.

3. For weight loss or physical fitness, participate in moderate physical activity (preferably low impact if you are a beginner) that builds exercise into your daily life, such as mowing the lawn, washing the car by hand, and climbing stairs instead of taking elevators; plus participate in a structured exercise program (walking, walking/jogging, cycling, swimming, aerobics, etc.). Thirty minutes or more of exercise per day, preferably five days per week, plus eating nutritious meals based on the Food Guide Pyramid, will improve physical fitness and produce sensible weight loss that can be maintained for life.

4. Avoid the inflexible pursuit of artificial aesthetic ideals and aim for reasonable goals. Don't pressure yourself to achieve your goals too rapidly. Remember, healthy eating and sensible, regular exercise are for a lifetime, not just a few weeks or months. Let the body changes that result from this lifestyle occur slowly, and you will be able to enjoy them for a lifetime.

Taking care of your body does not result in instant health. To make real changes in your lifestyle, you must change the way you think. You must do more than nurture your body; you must nurture your mind as well.

Overweight

Overweight refers to excessive weight for height without consideration of body composition. Because the term *overweight* makes no allowances for body composition, it is a poor criterion for determining the desirability of weight loss. For example, a well-muscled person may be overweight but lean in regard to body fat. By American social standards, such body mass is healthy, aesthetically pleasing, and desirable. It is also possible for a person to be well within the norms for total body weight but **overfat**; that is, such a person

Real-World Wellness

Practical Ways to Estimate Overweight and Obesity

What are some practical techniques I can use to determine whether I'm overweight or obese that don't require much time, a technician, or sophisticated measuring equipment?

Practical sources for measuring overweight and overfatness rely on subjective observations and other sensory information. These estimates do not quantify, in a real sense, the extent of the problem, should one exist.

Our mirrors supply us with visual feedback. Stand naked in front of a full-length mirror and, as objectively as possible, observe the shape of your body, determine where fat has accumulated, and estimate the amount of muscle you have. Use a tape measure to measure the circumference of your waist and hips. Your hips should be larger than your waist. While you have the tape measure in your hands, measure the circumference of your ankle according to the directions in Table 7-3. This will estimate your skeletal size, or frame size. People with large frame sizes can carry more weight than can people of the same height with small frame sizes. Knowing your frame size may help you more accurately interpret the results from the bathroom scale in conjunction with height/weight charts.

A few years ago the slogan "pinch an inch" became popular. If you can pinch an inch at various sites on the body, you are probably somewhat overweight.

The fit of your clothes will provide other clues. If your pants or dress size is increasing steadily, you are gaining weight. Conversely, if the sizes are getting smaller, you are successfully losing weight, changing your body composition, or both. If you are not consciously trying to lose

weight and don't need to lose but are doing so, anyway, this could be a sign of emerging disease and should be evaluated by a physician.

There is always the feedback you receive from other people. They may tell you that you appear to have either gained or lost some weight. Their perceptions may or may not be correct, but your size has led them to their conclusions.

After all is said and done, remember this: About 40 percent of men are dissatisfied with their appearance and two-thirds of young women between 13 and 19 years think they weigh too much. Millions of normal-weight Americans, particularly young women, are also attempting to lose weight.

We are preoccupied with thinness in the United States. Beauty is in the eye of the beholder, but the vision has been distorted by Madison Avenue's preoccupation with excessive leanness. We need to be realistic and understand that excessive leanness is not within the grasp of most people, nor should it be. Thinness does not always go hand in hand with robust health.

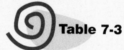

Table 7-3 Measurement of Ankles to Determine Body Frame Size

Measure the ankle at the smallest point above the two bones that protrude on each side of the ankle. The tape measure should be pulled very tightly. Read the tape measure in inches and see the table for an interpretation.

Gender	Small Frame	Medium Frame	Large Frame
Male	< 8 inches	8–9¼ inches	> 9¼ inches
Female	< 7½ inches	7½–8¾ inches	> 8¾ inches

carries a large proportion of body weight in the form of fat rather than lean tissue. Overfat is unhealthy and, according to American social standards, unattractive.

See Real-World Wellness: Practical Ways to Estimate Overweight and Obesity.

Regional Fat Distribution

Deposition of fat varies among people. The amount of fat and the storage sites are influenced by heredity and gender (Figure 7-1). After puberty, women generally deposit fat in the buttocks, hips, breasts, and thighs. These preferential sites are largely dictated by the female hormone estrogen.[7] This tendency is known as the *gynoid*, or feminine, pattern of fat deposition. Gynoid fat is not confined exclusively to women; a few men deposit fat in this configuration as well.

Because they produce little estrogen, men usually deposit minimal amounts of fat in the female pattern. Instead, they store fat primarily in the abdomen, lower back, chest, and nape of the neck. Some women store fat this way as well. After menopause, estrogen production decreases and the prevalence of *android* fat deposition increases.

Although the general claim is that *android*, or masculine, pattern of fat deposition (sometimes called *central fat*) is harmful, newer evidence indicates that not all android fat is equal.[8,9] Intra-abdominal fat, stored deep within the abdominal cavity, carries a much higher risk than does subcutaneous abdominal fat, stored directly beneath the skin. Physical activity tends to reduce intra-abdominal fat as well as subcutaneous fat. Moderately intense physical activities, such as gardening and casual walking, may not improve one's

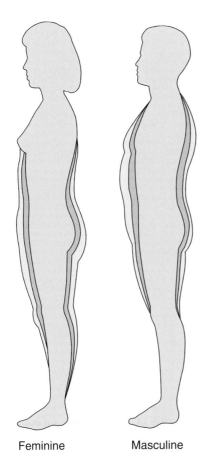

Feminine   Masculine

Figure 7-1 Feminine Versus Masculine Deposition of Fat

cardiorespiratory endurance, but when coupled with modest caloric restriction, they can decrease abdominal fat.

The waist-to-hip ratio (WHR) is a simple method for determining the distribution of body fat. It requires an accurate measurement of the circumference of the waist at the narrowest point between the rib cage and the navel and of the hips at the largest circumference of the hip/buttocks region. The waist measurement is then divided by the hip measurement. The resulting value may be interpreted by comparing the WHR with the following standard:[10]

- Males: A WHR greater than 0.9 indicates an excessive amount of upper-body fat. Acceptable levels are less than 0.9.
- Females: A WHR greater than 0.8 indicates an excessive amount of upper-body fat. Acceptable levels are less than 0.8.

The WHR has been criticized for failing to recognize factors other than abdominal fat, such as skeletal size and muscle mass in the buttocks. An ex̶ ̶ ̶ ̶ ̶ ̶ vened by the National Heart ̶ ̶ ̶ ̶ ̶ ̶ ̶ ̶ ̶ ̶ ̶ ̶ ̶ ̶ ̶ ̶ ̶ in 1998 concluded that a ci̶ ̶ ̶ ̶ ̶ ̶ ̶ ̶ ̶ ̶ ̶ ̶ ̶ ̶ ̶ure of only the waist is more highly prea̶ ̶ ̶ ̶ disease risk than is the WHR.[11] For males, a high waist circumference is

greater than 40 inches, and for females it is greater than 35 inches. The power of waist circumference to predict heart disease is unaffected by height, and its predictive power is increased if combined with a body mass index greater than 25kg/m^2. **Body mass index (BMI)** is the ratio of body weight to height calculated in kilograms per meter squared (kg/m^2) (BMI = wt[kg]/ht[m^2]). See Wellness on the Web on page 232.

The android pattern of fat deposition is related to an increase in the risk for heart disease, stroke, Type 2 diabetes, and some forms of cancer.[7] There are several reasons for this increased risk. First, enzymes in abdominal adipose cells are active, so fat moves in and out easily. In sedentary people, abdominal fat enters the bloodstream and is routed directly to the liver, where it becomes the raw material for the manufacture of very low-density lipoprotein (VLDL) triglycerides. Later these are converted to low-density lipoprotein cholesterol (LDL-C), and this increases the risk for cardiovascular disease. Conversely, active people direct abdominal fat to the muscles, where it is used as fuel for physical work.

Second, abdominal fat cells are larger than other fat cells. Large fat cells are associated with blood glucose (sugar) intolerance and excessive amounts of insulin in the blood. Such an environment is conducive to the development of Type 2 diabetes because the cells' receptor sites become resistant to insulin. Higher than normal amounts of insulin must be secreted to transport sugar from the blood to the cells, but excessive insulin remains in the blood. The body's cells continue to resist insulin, so blood sugar also remains high. This sequence of events is characteristic of glucose intolerance, or poor regulation of sugar. Over the years these factors can lead to Type 2 diabetes. A person does not have to be excessively overweight to be at risk for Type 2 diabetes; it is enough that fat be concentrated in the abdominal region. This pattern of fat deposition increases the risk of developing Type 2 diabetes 10 to 15 times.[12] Extra fat that accumulates in the hips (gynoid pattern) also increases the risk, but only 3 to 4 times.

Third, excessive insulin in the blood interferes with the removal of sodium by the kidneys, possibly leading to hypertension. Concurrently, the high circulating level of insulin stimulates the overproduction of epinephrine and norepinephrine, both of which raise the blood pressure. This cluster of disorders—high blood pressure, high blood sugar (glucose intolerance), high blood lipids (cholesterol and triglycerides), and abdominal obesity—has deadly consequences. Researchers refer to this combination as *syndrome X* or *metabolic syndrome*.[13]

̶ ̶ ̶ good news about android fat is that it is more easily removed from the body than is fat stored in the gynoid pattern. Fat stored in the feminine pattern is highly resistant to removal from its storage depots. Losing gynoid fat usually requires calorie restriction and exercise. Even the best effort may not result in the removal

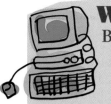

Wellness on the Web
Behavior Change Activities

What's Your BMI?

Body mass index (BMI) is not everyone's favorite number. Why? Because it provides an acceptable estimate of the proportion of our body weight that's composed of fat. Although knowing your BMI is more fun if you're fit, don't be discouraged if you're not there yet—use this useful measure to help you achieve your desired level of fitness. BMI is the ratio of body weight in kilograms to height in meters squared. There are several body mass index protocols, all of which represent attempts to adjust body weight to derive a height-free measure of body fat. Although BMI doesn't provide an estimate of percent body fat, it's far more useful than height/weight tables. Calculate your BMI easily and quickly by going to www.mhhe.com/anspaugh6e. Click on Student Center, Chapter 7, Wellness on the Web, then Activity 1. Type in the information requested; then click on "calculate" to view your BMI.

Is There Really an "Ideal Weight"?

Your "ideal weight," if there is such a thing, depends on a host of factors: your gender, age, height, and frame size, to name the most prominent. Instead of agonizing over outdated height and weight tables published years ago by insurance companies, turn to the experts on the Internet. You can calculate your ideal weight painlessly by going to the Web site mentioned previously and clicking on Activity 2. Type in the information requested, then click on "calculate," and view your ideal weight.

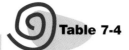

Table 7-4 Disease Risk Based on Body Mass Index (BMI) and Waist Circumference

Class	BMI (kg/m²)	Disease Risk Based on Waist Circumference*	
		Men ≤ 40 in.** Women ≤ 35 in.	Men > 40 in.** Women > 35 in.
Underweight	< 18.5**		
Normal	18.5–24.9		
Overweight	25.0–29.9	Increased	High
Stages of Obesity			
I	30.0–34.9	High	Very high
II	35.0–39.9	Very high	Very high
III	> 40	Extremely high	Extremely high

* Disease risk is for cardiovascular disease, hypertension, and Type 2 diabetes.

** Increased waist circumference may be a marker for an elevated risk even for people of normal weight.

Adapted from National Heart, Lung, and Blood Institute. 1998. *Obesity education initiative expert panel clinical guidelines on the identification, evaluation, and treatment of overweight and obesity in adults.* Washington, DC: National Heart, Lung, and Blood Institute.

of enough fat from the lower half of the body to satisfy the dieter. Lower-extremity fat is stubborn and much more difficult to lose than is upper-body fat.

Methods for Measuring Body-Weight Status

Height/Weight Tables

Optimal body weight is not necessarily reflective of optimal body composition. This was illustrated by a comparison of young and middle-aged men within 5 percent of their ideal weight as determined by height, weight, and frame-size charts. Although both groups were within the ideal range, the middle-aged subjects had twice the amount of fat as the young subjects.[10]

Height/weight tables do not measure body composition. They act as a standard for total body weight based on height and gender without regard to the composition of weight. Some of the height/weight tables also require

users to know their body frame sizes. One method for determining body frame size was presented in Real World Wellness: Practical Ways to Estimate Overweight and Obesity earlier in the chapter. These tables are poor criteria for the establishment of weight-loss recommendations.

Body Mass Index

Another method for measuring body-weight status is to calculate body mass index. As previously mentioned, body mass index is the ratio of body weight in kilograms to height in meters squared. There are several body mass index protocols, all of which originate from height/weight measurements. These protocols represent an attempt to adjust body weight to derive a height-free measure of obesity. Although BMI does not provide an estimate of percent body fat and although BMI uses height/weight data, it is more useful than the height/weight tables[14] and it can be used to compare population groups. It also correlates fairly well ($r = 0.70$) with percent fat derived from underwater weighing.[7] "r" is a coefficient of correlation between two variables; in this particular case, it is between BMI and underwater weighing.

In June 1998, the American Heart Association added *obesity* to its list of major controllable risk factors for heart disease.[15] Obesity is now viewed as a chronic disease that represents a "dangerous epidemic" in this country. Later the same month, The National Heart, Lung, and Blood Institute (NHLBI) issued its initial clinical recommendations on obesity (see Table 7-4). A panel of 24 experts commissioned by the NHLBI conducted an extensive review of the research literature on obesity and concluded that people with BMIs of 25.0 to 29.9 kg/m² should be classified as overweight.[16] The panel recommended that people whose BMIs fall in this category should attempt to lose weight if they have two or more weight-related risk factors for illness. These include high blood pressure, diabetes, impaired glucose tolerance, and a waist circumference of greater than 40 inches for men and greater than 35 inches for women.

People whose BMIs are 30 kg/m² and higher are considered to be obese, and the panel advises these people to make serious attempts to lose weight.[16] According to the new BMI guidelines, approximately 65 percent of Americans are currently overweight.[17] This figure was recently reported by the Centers for Disease Control and Prevention. This value reflects the increasing number of Americans who have become overweight, up 10 percent, compared with the recent past.

There are two major limitations to using BMI measurements: (1) The technique is misleading for people with greater than average muscle mass because it measures overweight rather than overfat and (2) the results are difficult for the general public to interpret, and the average person does not know how to apply BMI values to weight loss. The first limitation is easily surmounted. People with large amounts of muscle tissue should be directed to use a technique such as skinfold measurements or underwater weighing to measure their body composition.

The second limitation is more challenging. Follow these guidelines to establish and interpret BMI measurement. Calculate BMI taking care to accurately measure weight and height. Weigh yourself in the morning after voiding and prior to breakfast. Wear light clothing and no shoes. For the height measurement, take off your shoes and stand with your back against a flat wall with your heels, buttocks, shoulders, and head against it. Have another person establish your height by using an object that has a right angle, such as a carpenter's square, a textbook, a clipboard on edge, or any other rigid item that is rectangular and has a 90° angle. The person doing the measuring should place the right angle against the wall and slide it down to the top of your head, mark the wall at the bottom of the right angle, and use a tape measure to measure from the mark to the floor.

The simplest way to calculate BMI is to bypass the formula and to use Table 7-5. Find your height in the left

Table 7-5 Calculating Body Mass Index (BMI)

Each entry gives the body weight in pounds for a person of a given height and BMI. Pounds have been rounded off. To use the table, find the appropriate height in the far-left column. Move across the row to a given weight. The number at the top of the column is the BMI for that height and weight.

Height (Inches)	19	20	21	22	23	24	25	26	27	28	29	30	35	40
58	91	96	100	105	110	115	119	124	129	134	138	143	167	191
59	94	99	104	109	114	119	124	128	133	138	143	148	173	198
60	97	102	107	112	118	123	128	133	138	143	148	153	185	211
61	100	106	111	116	122	127	132	137	143	148	153	158	191	218
62	104	109	115	120	126	131	136	142	147	153	158	164	191	218
63	107	113	118	124	130	135	141	146	152	158	163	169	197	225
64	110	116	122	128	134	140	145	151	157	163	169	174	204	232
65	114	120	126	132	138	144	150	156	162	168	174	180	210	240
66	118	124	130	136	142	148	155	161	167	173	179	186	216	247
67	121	127	134	140	146	153	159	166	172	178	185	191	223	255
68	125	131	138	144	151	158	164	171	177	184	190	197	230	262
69	128	135	142	149	155	162	169	176	182	189	196	203	236	270
70	132	139	146	153	160	167	174	181	188	195	202	207	243	278
71	136	143	150	157	165	172	179	186	193	200	208	215	230	286
72	140	147	154	162	169	177	184	191	199	206	213	221	258	294
73	144	151	159	166	174	182	189	197	204	212	219	227	265	302
74	148	155	163	171	179	186	194	202	210	218	225	233	272	311
75	152	160	168	176	184	192	200	208	216	224	232	240	279	319
76	156	164	172	180	189	197	205	213	221	230	238	246	287	328

BMI (kg/m²) — Body Weight (Pounds)

Wellness for a Lifetime

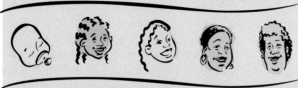

Body Composition of Children and Adolescents

The body composition of children changes during the growth process. It has been well established that obese children and adolescents have a higher probability of becoming obese adults than do normal-weight children and that dramatic changes in body fat and body composition can occur during the peripubertal years (the time before, during, and after puberty). The proportion of body fat in young children ranges from 10 to 15 percent, with boys toward the lower end and girls toward the upper.[18]

Body fat generally increases in adolescent boys and girls and continues to do so into young adulthood, so that the percentage of fat in males increases to 15 to 20 percent, whereas that of females increases to 20 to 25 percent. As we age, the percentage of fat continues to increase while muscle mass decreases. By middle age, fat accumulation exceeds 25 percent of the total weight of many men and 30 percent of the total weight of many women. The reason is a growing disparity between energy intake (food consumption) and energy expenditure (level of physical activity). We become less active with age.

Television, computers, automobiles, elevators, escalators, remote controls, golf carts, riding mowers, and a lack of quality physical education programs in the public schools have diminished the energy expended by American children and adults.

Skinfold measurements made on children and adolescents in the 1960s and 1970s have been compared with those made on similar subjects in the 1980s. A trend surfaced in this comparison, indicating that a systematic increase in body fat percentage had occurred during the interim.[2] There is not a generally accepted definition of *obesity* that distinguishes it from overweight among children and adolescents.[19] Therefore, the term *overweight* is used to determine cutoff points at which health can be negatively affected. In 2000, the incidence of overweight among children (aged 6 to 11) was 15.3 percent and among adolescents (aged 12 to 19) was 15.5 percent. An additional 15 percent of children and 14.9 percent of adolescents were just below the cutoff point for being overweight.

One study examined the relationship between body fatness and health status among children and adolescents.[1] The risks for high blood pressure, high total and LDL cholesterol (the harmful form), and low HDL cholesterol (the protective form) were associated with body fat above 25 percent for men and 30 percent for women. These levels have subsequently been proposed as useful health standards for those between 6 and 18 years of age.

---

column and move across to your weight in the same row. The number at the top of this column is your BMI. For example, a man who is 71 inches tall and weighs 200 pounds has a BMI of 28 kg/m². This man is in the "overweight" category. How much weight would he need to lose if he wanted to achieve a BMI of 24 kg/m²? He can easily calculate this from the table. Find the column with the desired BMI of 24 kg/m² and drop down in the table to the row with his height (71 inches). He should weigh 172 pounds to achieve a BMI of 24 kg/m². Then subtract his desired weight (172 pounds) from his current weight (200 pounds). He needs to lose 28 pounds to reach his goal. Turn to Assessment Activity 7-1 to calculate your BMI and your desired body weight.

Measurement of Body Fat

The only direct means to measure the fat content of the human body is to perform chemical analysis on cadavers. The information obtained from cadaver studies has been used to develop indirect methods for estimating fat content. Because these estimates are indirect, they contain some degree of measurement error and should be interpreted accordingly. These indirect methods are commonly used in exercise physiology laboratories and fitness and wellness centers. See Wellness for a Lifetime: Body Composition of Children and Adolescents.

Selected Methods for Measuring Body Composition

Underwater Weighing

Underwater weighing, one of the most accurate of the measurement techniques, involves weighing subjects both on land and while completely submerged in water (Figure 7-2).

Whole-body density is calculated from body volume according to Archimedes' principle of displacement.

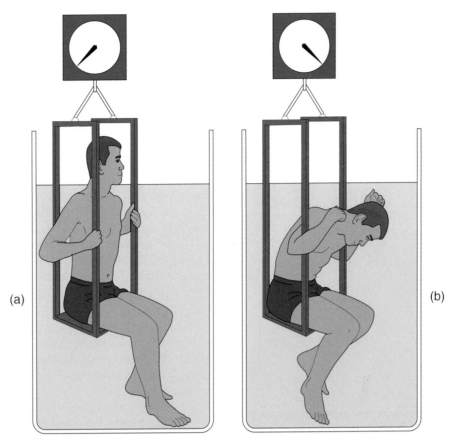

Figure 7-2 Underwater Weighing Apparatus

(a) The subject is in the ready position for underwater weighing. (b) The subject is being weighed.

Several thousand years ago, Archimedes discovered that a body immersed in water loses an amount of weight equal to the weight of the displaced water. The loss of weight in water is directly proportional to the volume of the water displaced or the volume of the body that displaces that water. The density of bone and muscle is higher than that of water and tends to sink. The density of fat is lighter than water and tends to float. Therefore, people with more muscle mass weigh more in water than do those who have less. Formulas have been developed that use weight on land and weight in water to determine the percent of the total weight that consists of fat.

Underwater weighing has an inherent error of measurement that can be minimized when the residual volume of air (the air left in the lungs after a maximal expiration) is accurately measured. If residual air is measured, the error is approximately 2.7 percent.[10] Accuracy also depends on the subject's ability to exhale maximally on each trial and to sit still while completely submerged for 6 to 10 seconds.

The equipment required for underwater weighing includes an autopsy scale with a capacity of approxi-

mately 9 kg (about 20 lbs.). The scale is suspended over a tank of water at least 4 feet deep. The subject sits suspended chin-deep, exhales completely, and bends forward from the waist until entirely submerged. This position is maintained for 6 to 10 seconds to allow the scale to stabilize. Five to 10 trials are required, and the underwater weight is attained by averaging the 3 heaviest readings. The subject's net underwater weight is calculated by subtracting the weight of the seat, its supporting structure, and a weight belt (if needed) from the gross underwater weight. Percent body fat can be calculated from body density by using appropriate formulas.

Bioelectrical Impedance Analysis

Bioelectrical impedance analysis (BIA) is a relatively new and simple method of determining body composition. The equipment is portable and computerized but fairly expensive. It is safe, noninvasive, quick, and convenient to use (Figure 7-3, page 236). Additionally, it does not require a high degree of technical skill, it

Recent advances in BIA instrumentation have improved the technique.[2] The newer instruments use multiple frequency bioelectrical impedence analysis (MFBIA), which seems to be less susceptible to the hydration status of subjects. As a result, a better estimate of lean body mass can be achieved.

Bioelectrical impedance analysis is as accurate as skinfold measurements, provided potential error sources are controlled.[2,10] The main sources of error are the hydration state of the subject and the prediction equation used. Hydration is affected by eating, drinking fluids, urination, and exercise, and it significantly influences the results. Technician error is relatively minor, provided standard procedures for electrode placement and body position of the subject are followed. To reduce error, the temperature of the testing room should be comfortable, and the following guidelines should be given to subjects the day before they are scheduled for testing:

- No eating or drinking within 4 hours of the test
- No exercise within 12 hours of the test
- No urination within 30 minutes of the test
- No alcohol consumption within 48 hours of the test
- No diuretic medicines within 7 days of the test

Skinfold Measurements

Skinfold measurements are one of the least expensive and most economical methods of measuring body composition. The cost of skinfold calipers can be as low as $10. Computerized models, however, can run as high as $600. The most accurate calipers maintain a constant jaw pressure of 10 g/mm^2 of jaw surface area.

The thumb and index finger are used to pinch and lift the skin and the fat beneath it. The caliper is placed beneath the pinch (Figures 7-4 through 7-8). Tables 7-6 and 7-7 (pages 239 and 240) show how to convert the sum of millimeters of skinfold thickness to percentage of body fat. When performed by skilled technicians, skinfold measurements correlate well (.70–.90) with body density calculated from underwater weighing.[20]

As suggested by the American College of Sports Medicine, these guidelines should be followed when taking skinfold measurements:[20]

1. All measurements should be made on the right side of the body.
2. The caliper heads should be placed about 1/4 to 1/2 inch below the thumb and index finger, perpendicular to the fold, and halfway into the length of the fold.
3. The pinch should be held continuously while reading the caliper.

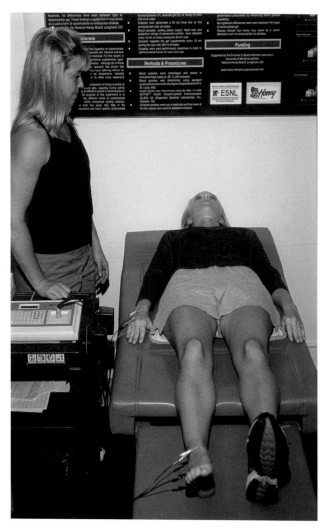

Figure 7-3 Bioelectrical Impedance Analysis

intrudes less on the subject's privacy than other methods, and it is generally more comfortable.

The most common application of BIA employs a harmless, low-level, single-frequency electric current. This current is passed through the body of the person being measured via electrodes attached to specific sites on the right hand and foot, as shown in Figure 7-3. Impedance represents resistance to the transmission of an electrical current. Impedance is least in lean body tissues because of their high water content (approximately 73 percent water). Water is an excellent conductor of electricity. Conversely, fat contains only 14 to 22 percent water and is resistant to electrical flow.[2]

A major limitation of BIA is that it does not accurately estimate fat-free mass in very lean or very fat subjects. Body fatness is generally overestimated for lean subjects and underestimated in obese subjects.

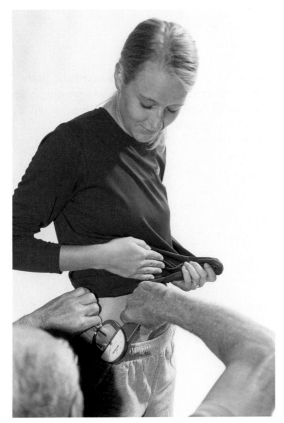

Figure 7-4 Suprailium Skinfold Measurement

Take a diagonal fold above the crest of the ilium, or upper portion of the hip bone, directly below the midaxilla (armpit).

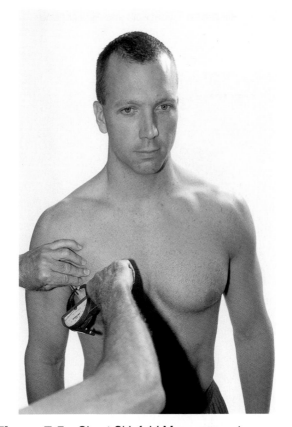

Figure 7-5 Chest Skinfold Measurement

Take a diagonal fold half the distance between the anterior axillary line and the nipple.

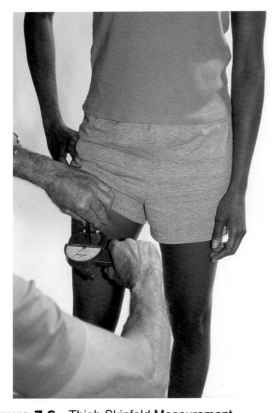

Figure 7-6 Thigh Skinfold Measurement

Take a vertical fold on the front of the thigh midway between the hip and the knee joint. The midpoint should be marked while the subject is seated.

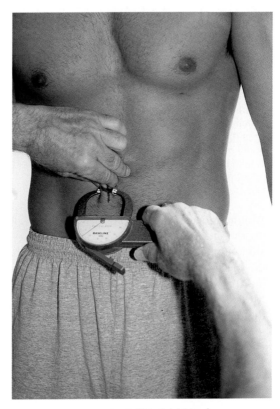

Figure 7-7 Abdominal Skinfold Measurement

Take a vertical fold about 1 inch from the navel.

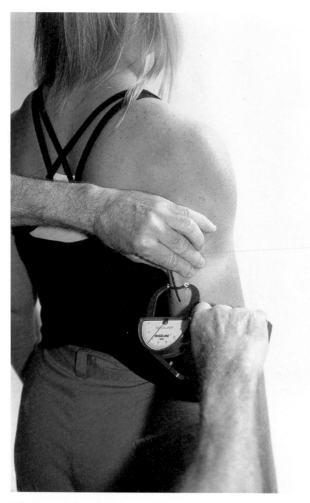

Figure 7-8 Triceps Skinfold Measurement

Take a vertical fold on the midline of the upper arm over the triceps, halfway between the acromion and olecranon processes (tip of the shoulder to the tip of the elbow). The arm should be extended and relaxed when the measurement is taken. All skinfold measurements should be taken on the right side.

4. Wait no more than one to two seconds before reading the caliper.
5. Take duplicate measures at each site, and retest if the measures are farther than 1 to 2 millimeters (mm) apart.
6. Measure each of the sites one time, and then repeat the measurements again. This will allow time for the skinfold to return to normal before the next measurement.

Determining Desired Body Weight from Body Fat

Calculating desirable body weight is a simple procedure when the percentage of body fat is known. The following

example is for a 148-pound woman whose body fat is equal to 30 percent of her total body weight, based on her skinfold measurements. She wishes to reduce her body fat to 23 percent.

Find fat weight (FW) in pounds:

$$
\begin{aligned}
\text{FW (lbs.)} &= \frac{\text{Body weight (BW) (lbs.)} \times \% \text{fat}}{100} \\
&= \frac{148 \text{ lbs.} \times 30}{100} \\
&= \frac{4{,}440 \text{ lbs.}}{100} \\
&= 44.4 \text{ lbs.}
\end{aligned}
$$

Find lean weight (LW) in pounds:

$$
\begin{aligned}
\text{LW (lbs.)} &= \text{BW} - \text{FW} \\
&= 148 \text{ lbs.} - 44.4 \text{ lbs.} \\
&= 103.6 \text{ lbs.}
\end{aligned}
$$

Find desirable body weight (DBW) in pounds:

$$
\begin{aligned}
\text{DBW (lbs.)} &= \frac{\text{LW (lbs.)}}{1.0 - \% \text{ fat desired}} \\
&= \frac{103.6 \text{ lbs.}}{1.0 - 0.23} \\
&= \frac{103.6 \text{ lbs.}}{0.77} \\
&= 134.5 \text{ lbs.}
\end{aligned}
$$

The method for calculating desirable body weight based on percent body fat is relatively effective if the subject does the following:

- Exercises to maintain muscle tissue
- Loses no more than 1.5 pounds per week
- Is evaluated for body fatness two or three times during the weight-loss period
- Understands that indirect measurements of body fatness contain some error

Complete Assessment Activity 7-2 to determine your desirable body weight.

Air-Displacement Plethysmography

Air-displacement plethysmography is one of the more recent methods developed to measure body composition through densiometry techniques. In lieu of being submerged in water, subjects sit inside a precisely calibrated chamber, marketed commercially as the BodPod (Figure 7-9, page 241), where they displace air instead of water.[21,22] Preliminary investigations have shown that this method of assessing body composition is highly

Table 7-6 Percentage of Fat Estimated for Men (Sum of Chest, Abdomen, and Thigh Skinfolds)

Sum of Skinfolds (mm)	Age to Last Year								
	Under 23	23–27	28–32	33–37	38–42	43–47	48–52	53–57	Over 57
8–10	1.3	1.8	2.3	2.9	3.4	3.9	4.5	5.0	5.5
11–13	2.2	2.8	3.3	3.9	4.4	4.9	5.5	6.0	6.5
14–16	3.2	3.8	4.3	4.8	5.4	5.9	6.4	7.0	7.5
17–19	4.2	4.7	5.3	5.8	6.3	6.9	7.4	8.0	8.5
20–22	5.1	5.7	6.2	6.8	7.3	7.9	8.4	8.9	9.5
23–25	6.1	6.6	7.2	7.7	8.3	8.8	9.4	9.9	10.5
26–28	7.0	7.6	8.1	8.7	9.2	9.8	10.3	10.9	11.4
29–31	8.0	8.5	9.1	9.6	10.2	10.7	11.3	11.8	12.4
32–34	8.9	9.4	10.0	10.5	11.1	11.6	12.2	12.8	13.3
35–37	9.8	10.4	10.9	11.5	12.0	12.6	13.1	13.7	14.3
38–40	10.7	11.3	11.8	12.4	12.9	13.5	14.1	14.6	15.2
41–43	11.6	12.2	12.7	13.3	13.8	14.4	15.0	15.5	16.1
44–46	12.5	13.1	13.6	14.2	14.7	15.3	15.9	16.4	17.0
47–49	13.4	13.9	14.5	15.1	15.6	16.2	16.8	17.3	17.9
50–52	14.3	14.8	15.4	15.9	16.5	17.1	17.6	18.2	18.8
53–55	15.1	15.7	16.2	16.8	17.4	17.9	18.5	19.1	19.7
56–58	16.0	16.5	17.1	17.7	18.2	18.8	19.4	20.0	20.5
59–61	16.9	17.4	17.9	18.5	19.1	19.7	20.2	20.8	21.4
62–64	17.6	18.2	18.8	19.4	19.9	20.5	21.1	21.7	22.2
65–67	18.5	19.0	19.6	20.2	20.8	21.3	21.9	22.5	23.1
68–70	19.3	19.9	20.4	21.0	21.6	22.2	22.7	23.3	23.9
71–73	20.1	20.7	21.2	21.8	22.4	23.0	23.6	24.1	24.7
74–76	20.9	21.5	22.0	22.6	23.2	23.8	24.4	25.0	25.5
77–79	21.7	22.2	22.8	23.4	24.0	24.6	25.2	25.8	26.3
80–82	22.4	23.0	23.6	24.2	24.8	25.4	25.9	26.5	27.1
83–85	23.2	23.8	24.4	25.0	25.5	26.1	26.7	27.3	27.9
86–88	24.0	24.5	25.1	25.7	26.3	26.9	27.5	28.1	28.7
89–91	24.7	25.3	25.9	26.5	27.1	27.6	28.2	28.8	29.4
92–94	25.4	26.0	26.6	27.2	27.8	28.4	29.0	29.6	30.2
95–97	26.1	26.7	27.3	27.9	28.5	29.1	29.7	30.3	30.9
98–100	26.9	27.4	28.0	28.6	29.2	29.8	30.4	31.0	31.6
101–103	27.5	28.1	28.7	29.3	29.9	30.5	31.1	31.7	32.3
104–106	28.2	28.8	29.4	30.0	30.6	31.2	31.8	32.4	33.0
107–109	28.9	29.5	30.1	30.7	31.3	31.9	32.5	33.1	33.7
110–112	29.6	30.2	30.8	31.4	32.0	32.6	33.2	33.8	34.4
113–115	30.2	30.8	31.4	32.0	32.6	33.2	33.8	34.5	35.1
116–118	30.9	31.5	32.1	32.7	33.3	33.9	34.5	35.1	35.7
119–121	31.5	32.1	32.7	33.3	33.9	34.5	35.1	35.7	36.4
122–124	32.1	32.7	33.3	33.9	34.5	35.1	35.8	36.4	37.0
125–127	32.7	33.3	33.9	34.5	35.1	35.8	36.4	37.0	37.6

compatible with underwater displacement. The difference in body fat measured between the two methods was a scant 0.3 percent.

The BodPod has several advantages over underwater weighing: (1) The measurement takes only about five minutes, (2) the system is easy to operate, (3) the device is mobile, (4) minimal technical training is required due to the menu-driven software, and (5) it may more effectively accommodate special populations, including, but not limited to, the disabled, the obese, children, the elderly, and nonswimmers afraid to submerge completely in a water tank. This technique seems to have a great

Table 7-7 Percentage of Fat Estimated for Women (Sum of Triceps, Suprailium, and Thigh Skinfolds)

Sum of Skinfolds (mm)	Age to Last Year								
	Under 23	23–27	28–32	33–37	38–42	43–47	48–52	53–57	Over 57
23–25	9.7	9.9	10.2	10.4	10.7	10.9	11.2	11.4	11.7
26–28	11.0	11.2	11.5	11.7	12.0	12.3	12.5	12.7	13.0
29–31	12.3	12.5	12.8	13.0	13.3	13.5	13.8	14.0	14.3
32–34	13.6	13.8	14.0	14.3	14.5	14.8	15.0	15.3	15.5
35–37	14.8	15.0	15.3	15.5	15.8	16.0	16.3	16.5	16.8
38–40	16.0	16.3	16.5	16.7	17.0	17.2	17.5	17.7	18.0
41–43	17.2	17.4	17.7	17.9	18.2	18.4	18.7	18.9	19.2
44–46	18.3	18.6	18.8	19.1	19.3	19.6	19.8	20.1	20.3
47–49	19.5	19.7	20.0	20.2	20.5	20.7	21.0	21.2	21.5
50–52	20.6	20.8	21.1	21.3	21.6	21.8	22.1	22.3	22.6
53–55	21.7	21.9	22.1	22.4	22.6	22.9	23.1	23.4	23.6
56–58	22.7	23.0	23.2	23.4	23.7	23.9	24.2	24.4	24.7
59–61	23.7	24.0	24.2	24.5	24.7	25.0	25.2	25.5	25.7
62–64	24.7	25.0	25.2	25.5	25.7	26.0	26.7	26.4	26.7
65–67	25.7	25.9	26.2	26.4	26.7	26.9	27.2	27.4	27.7
68–70	26.6	26.9	27.1	27.4	27.6	27.9	28.1	28.4	28.6
71–73	27.5	27.8	28.0	28.3	28.5	28.8	29.0	29.3	29.5
74–76	28.4	28.7	28.9	29.2	29.4	29.7	29.9	30.2	30.4
77–79	29.3	29.5	29.8	30.0	30.3	30.5	30.8	31.0	31.3
80–82	30.1	30.4	30.6	30.9	31.1	31.4	31.6	31.9	32.1
83–85	30.9	31.2	31.4	31.7	31.9	32.2	32.4	32.7	32.9
86–88	31.7	32.0	32.2	32.5	32.7	32.9	33.2	33.4	33.7
89–91	32.5	32.7	33.0	33.2	33.5	33.7	33.9	34.2	34.4
92–94	33.2	33.4	33.7	33.9	34.2	34.4	34.7	34.9	35.2
95–97	33.9	34.1	34.4	34.6	34.9	35.1	35.4	35.6	35.9
98–100	34.6	34.8	35.1	35.3	35.5	35.8	36.0	36.3	36.5
101–103	35.3	35.4	35.7	35.9	36.2	36.4	36.7	36.9	37.2
104–106	35.8	36.1	36.3	36.6	36.8	37.1	37.3	37.5	37.8
107–109	36.4	36.7	36.9	37.1	37.4	37.6	37.9	38.1	38.4
110–112	37.0	37.2	37.5	37.7	38.0	38.2	38.5	38.7	38.9
113–115	37.5	37.8	38.0	38.2	38.5	38.7	39.0	39.2	39.5
116–118	38.0	38.3	38.5	38.8	39.0	39.3	39.5	39.7	40.0
119–121	38.5	38.7	39.0	39.2	39.5	39.7	40.0	40.2	40.5
122–124	39.0	39.2	39.4	39.7	39.9	40.2	40.4	40.7	40.9
125–127	39.4	39.6	39.9	40.1	40.4	40.6	40.9	41.1	41.4
128–130	39.8	40.0	40.3	40.5	40.8	41.0	41.3	41.5	41.8

deal of promise. The major disadvantage is its cost—approximately $34,000.

Dual-Energy X-Ray Absorptiometry (DEXA)

Dual-energy X-ray absorptiometry was originally developed to measure bone mineral density, but advances in technology have allowed for the quantifica-tion of fat and lean tissue as well. DEXA uses an X-ray generator and two energy levels as the source radia-tion. The subject lies on a table while a series of trans-verse scans are made 1 centimeter (cm) apart from head to toe. This system allows for the simultaneous measurement of bone mineral, fat, and nonbone lean tissue. The radiation exposure is very low and techni-cians can stay in the room while the procedure is in progress (see Figure 7-10).

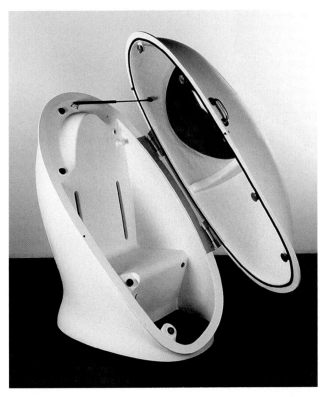 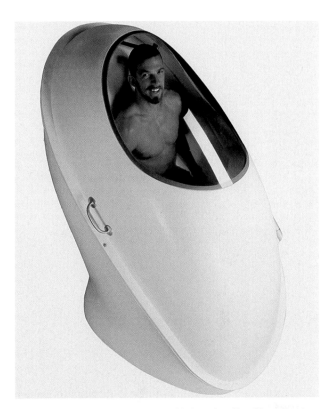

Figure 7-9 A Subject Prepared for Air-Displacement Plethysmography Measurement Using the BodPod Body Composition System

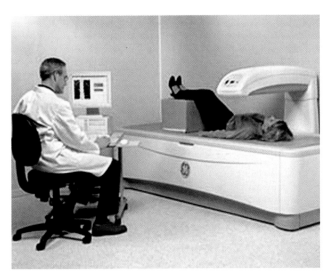

Figure 7-10 The Dual-Energy X-Ray Absorptiometry (DEXA) System

The advantages of DEXA are the following:

1. The subject's participation role is to simply lie on a table while the scan is in progress.
2. The procedure takes 10 to 20 minutes.
3. The elderly, the young, and the disabled can be measured with this technique.
4. It estimates bone mineral, fat, and nonbone lean tissue at the same time.

Research indicates that DEXA provides accurate and reliable estimates of body composition.[23,24] But its use is possibly limited by its price, which runs $75,000 to $150,000. Also, some authorities suggest that the equations used to assess body composition need some refinement.

Summary

- Essential fat is necessary for normal biological function.
- Men carry 3 to 5 percent of their weight in the form of essential fat; women carry 11 to 14 percent of their weight as essential fat.
- *Obesity* is defined as overfatness.
- Men are obese when fat constitutes 25 percent or more of the body's weight, and women are obese when fat constitutes 32 percent or more of the body's weight.
- The majority of women store fat in the hips, buttocks, thighs, and breasts (gynoid fat).
- The majority of men store fat in the abdomen, lower back, chest, and nape of the neck (android fat).
- Height/weight tables are limited and poor instruments for weight-loss recommendations.
- Body mass index correlates fairly well with percent fat derived from hydrostatic weighing.
- A high body mass index correlates with hypertension, high total cholesterol, low HDL cholesterol, high serum triglycerides, and poor glucose tolerance.
- Bioelectrical impedance is a safe, quick, and relatively accurate method for assessing percent body fat.
- Skinfold measurements are one of the most economical methods of measuring body composition in terms of the cost of equipment and the time required to determine percent body fat.
- Underwater weighing is still considered the "gold standard" for measuring body composition.
- Air-displacement plethysmography is one of the newest techniques for measuring body composition, and it correlates highly with underwater weighing.
- DEXA is an accurate method for measuring body composition.

Review Questions

1. What is essential fat, and how is it distributed in men and women?
2. How would you define *obesity* and *overweight*?
3. At what level of fat deposition does obesity become a health hazard for men and women?
4. What are *gynoid obesity* and *android obesity*? Which is a greater health risk and why?
5. What are the limitations of height/weight tables for recommending weight loss?
6. What is body mass index, and how is it classified for men and women?
7. How are underwater weighing, bioelectrical impedance, and skinfold measurements used to determine percent body fat?
8. How is healthy body weight determined when the percent body fat is known?

References

1. Going, S., and R. Davis. 2001. Body composition. In *ACSM's resource manual*. 4th ed. Edited by J. L. Roitman. Philadelphia: Lippincott Williams and Wilkins.
2. Robergs, R. A., and S. O. Roberts. 2000. *Fundamental principles of exercise physiology*. New York: McGraw-Hill.
3. American College of Sports Medicine. 1995. *ACSM's guidelines for exercise testing and prescription*. 5th ed. Baltimore, MD: Williams and Wilkins.
4. Powers, S. K., and E. T. Howley. 2004. *Exercise physiology*. New York: McGraw-Hill.
5. Wilmore, J. H., and D. L. Costill. 2004. *Physiology of sport and exercise*. Champaign, IL: Human Kinetics.
6. Bouchard, C. 1991. Heredity and the path to overweight and obesity. *Medicine and Science in Sports and Exercise* 23:285–91.
7. Grillo, C. M., and K. D. Brownell. 2001. Interventions for weight management. In *ACSM's resource manual*. 4th ed. Edited by J. L. Roitman. Philadelphia: Lippincott Williams and Wilkins.
8. Shirai, K. April 2004. Obesity as the core of the metabolic syndrome and the management of coronary heart disease. *Medscape* (www.medscape.com/viewarticle/472666_print).
9. Wong, S. L., et al. 2004. Cardiorespiratory fitness is associated with lower abdominal fat independent of body mass index. *Medicine and Science in Sports and Exercise* 36 (March): 286–91.
10. Nieman, D. C. 2003. *Exercise testing and prescription*. New York: McGraw-Hill.
11. National Heart, Lung, and Blood Institute. 1998. *Obesity education initiative expert panel clinical guidelines on the identification, evaluation, and treatment of overweight and obesity in adults*. Washington, DC: National Heart, Lung, and Blood Institute.
12. Bryant, C. X., and J. A. Peterson. 1998. Determining ideal body weight. *Fitness Management* 14(7):24.
13. American Diabetes Association. April 2004. The metabolic syndrome (www.diabetes.org/utils/printthispage.jsp?PageID=).
14. Blair, S. N., et al. 1995. Changes in physical fitness and all-cause mortality. *Journal of the American Medical Association* 273(14):1093.
15. Editors. 1998. Guidelines call more Americans overweight. *Harvard Health Letter* 23(10):7.
16. Editors. 1998. Should fewer calories be in your future? *Tufts University Health and Nutrition Letter* 16(6):8.
17. Flegal, K., et al. 2002. Prevalence and trends in obesity among U.S. adults 1999–2000. *Journal of the American Medical Association* 288:1723–27.
18. Williams, M. A. 2001. Human development and aging. In *ACSM's resource manual*. 4th ed. Edited by J. L. Roitman. Philadelphia: Lippincott Williams and Wilkins.
19. U.S. Department of Health and Human Services. 2003. *Statistics related to*

overweight and obesity. Washington, DC: NIH Publication No. 03-4158.

20. American College of Sports Medicine. 2000. *ACSM's guidelines for exercise testing and prescription.* 6th ed. Philadelphia: Lippincott Williams and Wilkins.

21. McCrory, M. A., et al. 1995. Evaluation of a new air displacement plethys- mography for measuring human body composition. *Medicine and Science in Sports and Exercise* 27:1686–91.

22. Wagner, D. R., V. H. Heyward, and A. L. Gibson. 2000. Validation of air displacement plethysmography for as- sessing body composition. *Medicine and Science in Sports and Exercise* 32:1339–44.

23. Kohrt, W. M. 1998. Preliminary evi- dence that DEXA provides an accurate assessment of body composition. *Journal of Applied Physiology* 84: 372–77.

24. Salamone, L. M., et al. 2000. Measure- ment of fat mass using DEXA: A vali- dation study in elderly adults. *Journal of Applied Physiology* 89:345–52.

Suggested Readings

Cheline, A. J. 2003. The business of body composition. *Fitness Management* 19 (September): 24–26.

This article defines body composition, identifies and discusses several of the more popular methods for assessing body composition, and discusses the ben- efits associated with its measurement.

Nieman, D. C. 2003. *Exercise testing and prescription.* 5th ed. New York: McGraw-Hill.

Chapter 5 in this text is entirely devoted to body composition. The author pre- sents a very thorough review, which in- cludes the use of elementary height/ weight techniques to very sophisticated techniques such as magnetic resonance imaging (MRI), computed tomography (CT), and total body electrical conduc- tivity (TOBEC).

Petroni, M. L., et al. 2003. Feasibility of air plethysmography (BOD POD) in morbid obesity: A pilot study. *Acta Diabetolog- ica* 40 (suppl. 1): S59–S62.

This pilot study was conducted to deter- mine whether air plethysmography would be a successful technique for cal- culating percent body fat in morbidly obese subjects. Extremely overfat people such as these are difficult to measure. The researchers concluded that air plethysmography is a suitable method to use for this population.

Powers, S. K., and E. T. Howley. 2004. *Ex- ercise physiology.* 5th ed. New York: McGraw-Hill.

A portion of Chapter 18 is devoted to body composition. These respected scien- tists define *body composition* and identify and describe more than a dozen methods for measuring body composition.

Wilmore, J. H., and D. L. Costill. 2004. *Physiology of sport and exercise.* 3d ed. Champaign, IL: Human Kinetics.

A portion of Chapter 14 is devoted to body composition and body type. The need for body composition is explained and a number of assessment techniques are presented.

8

Achieving a Healthy Weight

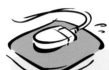

Online Learning Center

Log on to our Online Learning Center (OLC) for access to these additional resources:

- Chapter key term flashcards
- Learning objectives
- Additional goals for behavior change
- Concentration game
- Self-scoring chapter quizzes

- Additional lab activities

The OLC also offers Web links for study and exploration of wellness topics. Access these links through **www.mhhe. com/anspaugh6e**, click on Student Center, click on Chapter 8, and then click on Web Activities.

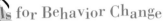

Goals for Behavior Change

- Compare physical characteristics of your ideal body image with your actual body image.
- Estimate caloric expenditure for your basal metabolism and physical activity level.
- Adjust your caloric intake and physical activity as necessary to achieve a healthy weight.
- Formulate a plan for achieving a healthy weight.

Key Terms

anorexia nervosa
bariatric surgery
basal metabolic rate (BMR)
binge-eating disorder
body dysmorphic disorder (BDD)
bulimia nervosa
caloric deficit
caloric expenditure
caloric intake
diet resistance
fasting
female athlete triad

gastroplasty
hyperplasia
hypertrophy
liposuction
novelty diets
overcompensatory eating
set point
thermic effect of food (TEF)
very low-calorie diets (VLCDs)
weight cycling
weight maintenance

Objectives

After completing this chapter, you will be able to do the following:

- Define *obesity* and *overweight*.
- Differentiate between hypertrophic and hyperplastic development of adipose cells.
- Identify and discuss the health aspects of obesity.
- Discuss biological and behavioral causes of obesity.
- Discuss the relationship of genetics, setpoint, overeating, and physical activity to body shape, fat distribution, and obesity.
- Define, identify, and distinguish among various forms of eating disorders and disordered eating.
- Calculate the caloric cost of physical activities.
- Compare and contrast dieting and physical activity as strategies for weight management.
- Identify principles of weight management.

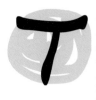

heoretically, achieving a healthy weight is a simple issue: A person balances **caloric intake**, calories supplied by food, with **caloric expenditure**, calories expended by physical activity and metabolism. In practice, however, people vary considerably in their responses to caloric intake and caloric expenditure. No two people have identical experiences with dieting or physical activity regimens. Some people who chronically face weight problems eat no more and sometimes less than their normal-weight peers. Conversely, some normal-weight people have voracious appetites and do not expend any more calories than their overweight peers.

How can this be explained? Are the differences due to heredity, metabolism, or errors in reporting food intake and physical activity expenditures? Although on the surface body weight appears to be a function of the basic laws of nature (caloric intake vs. caloric expenditure), in truth it is a complex issue still not fully understood by medical experts. For many people, self-improvement goals involving weight management are achievable and

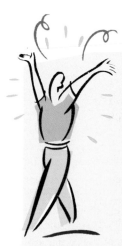

Nurturing Your Spirituality

Body Image Is About More Than Losing Weight[1,2,3]

Body image involves our perception of and about our bodies. For most Americans, this perception is not positive. The majority of Americans are unhappy with their physical appearance and even more are dissatisfied with their body weight. This is particularly true for young women who are willing to subject themselves to elective surgery to improve some aspect of their appearance. Cosmetic surgery is one of the fastest-growing medical specialties, as unprecedented numbers of women and even young girls submit to "the knife" to remove wrinkles, get rid of fat, enlarge breasts, or change any number of facial features.

Why are so many people unhappy with their appearance or weight? Why do people tend to focus on their physical imperfections? Why does such a large discrepancy exist between the ways people see their bodies and the ways others see them? Body-image studies identify the following factors as being responsible for negative body images:

- The media's preoccupation with thinness as the trademark for beauty
- The plethora of messages in the media about the prevalence of obesity
- Disapproving messages from others
- Physical changes, such as pregnancy
- Chronic illness
- Childhood teasing
- Weight gain
- Sexual abuse
- Cultural pressures

What are the costs of an exaggerated negative body image? People who are deeply troubled about their appearance or preoccupied with selected physical "flaws" often limit their social activities; may not be assertive at work, at school, or in personal relationships; may experience difficulty in forming a positive sexuality; may engage in high-risk behaviors; and often become victims of unrealistic fad diets. Studies of adolescents indicate that body dissatisfaction is the single strongest predictor of eating disorders and excessive dieting. Extreme cases may involve a psychological disorder called **body dysmorphic disorder (BDD)**. People with this condition are so preoccupied with what they see as a disfiguring flaw that they avoid social activities, including school and work.

Although self-improvement is a worthy goal for many people, when it comes to body image it is important to separate nature from nurture, heredity from environment. The challenge for many people with negative body images is to set realistic goals about what can be changed and to accept what can't be changed. Every one of us has a natural, unique size and shape. While it is true that more and more Americans are challenged to lose weight, it is important to remember that our self-esteem depends on accepting the physical features unique to each of us. Losing weight is not likely to change physical features that set us apart from others. Changing what and how we think about our bodies can be healthier than constantly working to change our body weight and shape by diet and exercise. Having a positive body image is not just about losing weight.

SOURCES: Veale, D. 2004. Body dysmorphic disorder. *Postgraduate Medical Journal* 80(940):67–71.

Tiggemann, M., and D. Hargreaves. 2003. The effect of "thin ideal" television commercials on body dissatisfaction and schema activation during early adolescence. *Journal of Youth and Adolescence* 32(5):367–74.

Mayo Foundation for Medical Education and Research. 1998. Body image: What do you see in the mirror? [**www.mayohealth.org/ mayo/9704/htm/body_ima.htm**].

worthwhile. For others, formulating weight-management goals means first constructing a realistic view of body image (see Nurturing Your Spirituality: Body Image Is About More Than Losing Weight). This chapter addresses some of the complexities of body weight issues and presents basic principles for achieving a healthy weight.

Americans' Obsession with Body Weight

Americans are preoccupied with their body weight. Books that offer creative but questionable advice for losing weight invariably become best sellers and add fuel to the next diet craze. The diet industry hawks far-out gadgets and gimmicks ranging from lipo-slim briefs, which supposedly massage away cellulite, to aroma pens, inhalants that come in banana, green apple, and peppermint, claimed to squelch hunger pangs. At any given time, a large percentage of women and men are on a diet, often several a year. Even children are getting the message that dieting is fashionable—a large number of elementary-aged girls are on a diet, although only 16 percent are obese.[4]

The evidence for this obsession can be found in advertisements and the news. Numerous television celebrities have engaged in special diet or weight-loss programs. Both the print and video media show countless numbers of advertisements that associate supersvelte body images with almost every imaginable product. Consumers demand low-calorie versions of every consumable food, and much of this demand is motivated more by the desire to achieve an unobtainable physique than by health reasons. Consumers have been observed counting the number of calories even in a dose of laxatives. The term *calorie anxiety* applies to many Americans. Even health magazines and professional journals reinforce this preoccupation by featuring headlines of diet articles or diet studies on their covers. If some new diet finding is released by the scientific community, it will surely be headlined on national and local news shows and will quickly be followed by numerous feature stories, many of which produce misleading claims. A recent example is Americans' fascination with low-carb diets and the subsequent explosion of printed and video materials related to this dieting strategy.

For some people, the obsession with weight is so intense that it causes serious body-image problems; distorts their self-esteem; and eventually leads to eating disorders, conditions almost unheard of 30–40 years ago. Extreme cases may involve body dysmorphic disorder (BDD).[1] If a slight flaw in appearance is present, the person's concern is markedly excessive. This preoccupation leads to compulsive checking and questioning; inappropriate surgeries; and occasionally, self-inflected injury.

These symptoms, in turn, may lead to social isolation. This preoccupation is not to be confused with the "normal" dislikes many people associate with one of their physical features. People often complain about the shape of their noses, the size of their ears, or skin blemishes. However, these dislikes do not seriously limit anyone's life. BDD goes far beyond mere dislike into the realm of distress and serious perceptual distortion.

The effects of weight obsession may be more subtle. Some people develop aversive attitudes toward food, eating, and mealtime. Rather than serving as a source of pleasure and enjoyment, the eating experience becomes a constant test of willpower, which rarely yields positive results. For too many people, attitudes about appearance, body weight, and food combined with the ubiquitous messages and body images promulgated by the media form a vicious cycle of guilt, denial, and unhappiness. For example, the body mass index of Miss America winners has steadily decreased over time; during the past three decades, most winners had a body mass index in the "underweight" category (less than 18.5).[5] In contrast, the average body mass index of an American woman ranges from 24 to 27 ("high normal weight" to "overweight" category). A very small percentage of the population genetically fits the typical model's body mass index zone. The rest of the population is left with unobtainable and unrealistic body images. The challenge for many people is to construct a realistic view of their bodies while maintaining positive attitudes toward food and formulating reasonable strategies to address the weight problem (see Assessment Activity 8-1).

Defining the Problem

For many Americans, weight loss is a healthy goal. Losing weight often means reducing the risk of developing common chronic health problems. However, many people who are not overweight and have good body composition try to lose weight. For them, losing weight offers no health benefits and may even be harmful.

The number of people who stand to benefit from weight loss is at an all-time high. New standards established by the National Institutes of Health (NIH) and the World Health Organization define a healthy weight as a BMI equal to or more than 18.5 and no more than 24.9 (see Chapter 7). Being overweight, or preobese, is defined as having a BMI of 25 or higher; *obesity* is defined as having a BMI of 30 or higher. Extreme obesity occurs when BMI is 40 or higher.[6] (See Just the Facts: When Is Overweight the Same as Obesity? on page 252.) By these definitions, 34 percent of adults are overweight but not obese; 30.5 percent of adults are obese.[7] Nearly two-thirds of American adults are overweight or obese. These figures are significantly higher than comparison

∼∽ Just the Facts ∽∼

When Is Overweight the Same as Obesity?

A body mass index (BMI) of 25 or higher defines *overweight*. A BMI of 30 or higher defines *obesity*. It seems, therefore, that the difference between these two classifications is objective and clear-cut. In reality, these two terms are sometimes misunderstood or misinterpreted.

BMIs of 25 and 30 fall at the 85th and 95th percentile, respectively. Some researchers refer to the 95th percentile as overweight and others refer to it as obesity. The Centers for Disease Control and Prevention (CDC) avoids using the word *obesity* and identifies every child and adolescent above the 85th percentile as overweight. The American Obesity Association, on the other hand, uses the 95th percentile as a criterion for obesity because it corresponds to a BMI of 30 and it serves as a marker for when children and adolescents should have an in-depth medical assessment.[7]

When is overweight the same as obesity? Look for information about BMI or percentile rank. If BMI is 30 or higher or is at the 95th percentile, technically and medically, it is obesity, even though it may be called overweight.

figures for each of the previous decades since data have been collected. During the past 25 years, the prevalence of overweight adults has increased nearly 50 percent; the prevalence of obesity has more than doubled. Adults are not the only ones overweight or obese. About 15.5 percent of adolescents (ages 12 to 19) and 15.3 percent of children (ages 6 to 11) are obese.[8] Obesity prevalence among children has more than doubled and among adolescents more than tripled since 1976. These dramatic increases suggest that obesity is epidemic in the United States, regardless of age.

Americans are getting heavier for two reasons: too little energy going out (as exercise) and too much energy going in (as food). The majority of Americans are sedentary; at the same time, they are consuming extra calories. Overall, 59 percent of adults 18 years of age and over don't participate in any leisure-time periods of vigorous physical activity lasting 10 minutes or more per week.[9] What do children and adults do in their leisure? For many, watching television is a favorite pastime. This has significant implications for adults and children alike because large-scale health studies indicate that the risk for obesity increases 23 percent for

each 2-hour increment in daily television watching.[10] The impact on children is obvious when considering that they spend more time watching television than doing any other activity except sleeping. In addition to promoting a sedentary lifestyle, television viewing is also associated with poor food selections.[11] Food products that dominate commercial messages are predominantly low in nutritional value, particularly in children's programming.

Although BMI provides a basis for classifying levels of overweight and obesity, it is not without its limitations (see Chapter 7). It is also important to remember that BMIs of 25 and 30 (for overweight and obesity, respectively) are not precise points on a scale that, when exceeded, magically increase a person's risk for health problems. For example, although a BMI of 29.9 does not technically fall into the category of obesity, it is a small step away from the "magic number" of 30, the cutoff point for obesity. For all practical purposes, a BMI of 29.9 carries the same risk for obesity as a BMI of 30.

Health Aspects of Obesity

In declaring obesity a disease, the NIH signaled a new approach toward obesity. Medical experts no longer regard being obese as a failure of willpower. Instead, obesity is considered a chronic disease. This is a radical departure from traditional thinking. Like any other chronic disease, obesity is a complex issue with multiple causes and diverse treatments. No single cause and effect relationship has been established that accounts for the wide variance in eating and activity patterns among the obese. What we know today about obesity is the tip of the iceberg and represents a small portion of this evolving and growing medical field.

One aspect of obesity that has not changed is its medical consequences. Morbidity occurs more frequently and with greater severity and mortality occurs at an earlier age among obese people than among those of normal weight.[12] Experts believe that obesity will soon overtake tobacco as the leading preventable cause of premature death in the United States.[13] (See This Just In on page 21.) Obesity has a profound effect on life span, especially in middle-aged adults. A 2003 analysis of the Framingham Heart Study suggests that middle-aged adults who are overweight or obese have shorter life expectancies than normal-weight adults. Forty-year-old men and women who are obese but do not smoke are likely to die 6 to 7 years earlier on average than their normal-weight peers. Obese smokers are likely to die 13½ years sooner than normal-weight smokers.[14] Another 2003 study by researchers at Johns Hopkins found that obesity in young adults is associated with the greatest reduction in life expectancy.[14] The magnitude of the risk for morbidity and premature death is dependent on the degree of obesity and the distribution and location of excess fat cells. Fortunately, losing as little as 10 percent of body weight can yield significant improvement in health and self-esteem.[14] This is often referred to as a *healthier weight*. Although a person might not achieve a BMI below 25, he or she might still be healthier after a small, permanent degree of weight loss.

Obesity is highly correlated with coronary heart disease and stroke. LDL cholesterol, which contributes to the development of atherosclerosis, is associated with obesity. Hypertension is also related to obesity. Many lifestyle factors are related to hypertension but, overall, obesity is considered the one with the most influence.[5] Many hypertensive people experience a decline in systolic and diastolic blood pressures during the early stages of a weight-loss program.

Obesity is also a major risk factor for some forms of cancer. The American Cancer Society estimates that extra body weight accounts for 14 percent of all cancer deaths in men and 20 percent in women.[15] Topping the list are colorectal, uterine, breast, esophageal, and kidney cancer.[5,14,15]

About 80 percent of people with Type 2 diabetes are overweight. For many people with Type 2 diabetes, oversized fat cells interfere with or resist the body's use of insulin.[5] In the absence of insulin, the cells cannot make full use of circulating blood sugar (glucose), so the affected person develops *hyperglycemia,* or high blood sugar, as a result of glucose remaining in the bloodstream. Sustained levels of blood glucose lead to full-blown Type 2 diabetes. Type 2 diabetes linked to obesity often disappears as weight is lost. Even if diabetes persists after weight loss, the body's need for insulin often drops dramatically.

Other conditions associated with obesity include osteoarthritis, gallbladder disease, excessive acid reflux, and sleep apnea. *Sleep apnea* is a condition characterized by loud snoring and brief halts in breathing. It is thought to be caused by the accumulation of fat in the upper airway, which interferes with breathing.

Obesity, combined with high blood sugar, hypertension, and abnormal blood fat levels, is highly related to a condition referred to as *metabolic syndrome* (see Chapter 2). Nearly one-fourth of American adults have metabolic syndrome, which increases the risk for diabetes, heart disease, and stroke.[14]

For some people, the first symptom of strain placed on the body by excess fat is shortness of breath. As fat accumulates, it crowds the space occupied by organs. Some people cannot sit comfortably because of fat accumulation in their abdomens. In a sitting position, a person's lungs have limited space in which to expand.

Postsurgical complications occur more often in overweight people than in those who are not overweight.

Wounds don't heal as well or as fast. Infections are more common.

In addition to suffering from medical hazards, some obese people suffer psychological stress, depression, social discrimination, and reduced income. They pay higher premiums for health insurance or are denied coverage. Obese children are often ridiculed by their normal-weight peers. Armed forces personnel are forced out of the military if they gain weight beyond an acceptable level.

The link between obesity and chronic disease is well established, but evidence has emerged indicating that the *distribution* of fat is equally important to the development of disease. Studies have confirmed that abdominal fat is associated with a higher rate of heart attack and stroke than is fat distributed around the hips and thighs (see Chapter 7). Guidelines for doctors now suggest that, in addition to calculating BMI, they should assess waist circumference. A waist measurement of 40 inches or higher in men and 35 inches or higher in women is considered a predictor of health risks.[14] (See Just the Facts: Waist Size Matters at www.mhhe.com/anspaugh6e Student Center, Chapter 8, Just the Facts.)

In summary, the medical community clearly concurs that the health risks and complications of obesity are associated with premature death. Overweight is also associated with premature death but not to the same degree as obesity. The extent to which a person is overweight, coupled with other lifestyle factors, has an important influence on the risk of contracting obesity-related diseases or conditions. Overweight people who participate in vigorous physical activities, for example, may have lower risk for premature death than their normal-weight peers. Many experts suggest that, while participation in physical activity may not make the overweight skinny, it does make them healthier (see Just the Facts: Can You Be Fat and Fit? on page 254). While there is some debate among medical experts about the health effects of being overweight, there is a consensus opinion that maintaining a physically active lifestyle is associated with good health, regardless of body weight status.

Weight Loss: A New Attitude Emerges

The term *weight loss* lacks specificity, and it is often used in such a way to imply that indiscriminate weight loss—of body fluids, protein, and fat—is desirable. A more appropriate weight-related goal is to measure success by the amount of fat lost, not by weight loss. The term *weight loss* should be replaced by the more specific term *fat-weight loss*.

Until recently, advice to overfat people was imprecise. For example, the suggestion to "cut back on calories"

~~~Just the Facts~~~

Can You Be Fat and Fit?

Overweight men as a group are less physically fit and have a higher death rate than their normal-weight peers. But what about overweight men who are fit? Researchers at the Cooper Institute of Aerobics Research in Dallas, Texas, revealed some surprising results when they examined the weight and fitness levels of almost 22,000 men, ranging in age from 30 to 83. They found that being unfit, regardless of one's weight status, increased the risk for death 2.24 times beyond those in the "fit and of normal weight" reference group.[16] What surprised them the most was that fit but overweight men suffered fewer deaths by all causes than unfit but normal-weight men. In other words, it is better to be physically fit and overweight than to be unfit and normal weight. In this study, *fitness* was defined as the equivalent of 30 minutes a day of moderate-intensity activity—briskly walking a couple miles a day at a 15-minute-per-mile pace.

reinforces the misconception that diet alone can lead to fat-weight loss. Successful weight management is rarely the result of following a diet or counting calories for a specific period. Successful weight management usually requires a lifelong lifestyle change. The loss or gain of body weight, the development of fat cells, and the causes of obesity are complex issues related to the interaction of three factors—heredity, diet, and exercise.

Development of Obesity

The body consists of 30 to 40 billion adipose cells (fat cells) that provide storage space for extra energy. Adipose cells can be viewed as collapsible, thin-walled containers with unlimited storage capacities (Figure 8-1). In prehistoric humans, large fat stores developed when food was available in spring and summer, and this proved biologically advantageous when winters were long and harsh and food was scarce. Energy stored in fat cells could be tapped for use later. This is not the case today. Food is available year-round for most Americans and surplus fat storage is not advantageous.

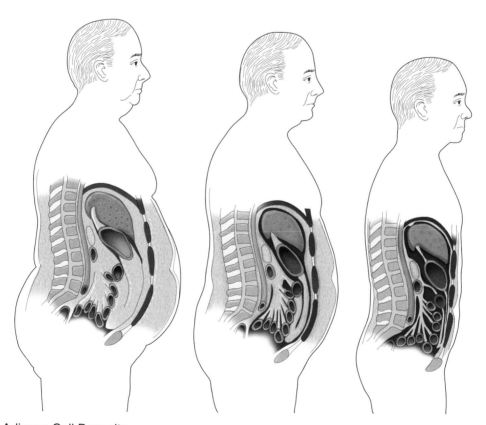

Figure 8-1 Adipose Cell Deposits

Adipose (fat) tissue can be deposited in many areas of the body. Losing fat and building lean muscle tissue boost metabolism, reduce strain on the hips and knees, and may prevent lower-back pain.

Just the Facts

Classification of Obesity

There are several types of obesity, each resulting from different causes:

- Juvenile-onset obesity: Caused by an increase in both the number (hyperplastic) and size (hypertrophic) of fat cells

- Adult-onset obesity: Caused primarily by an increase in size of fat cells (hypertrophic)

- Other types of obesity: Caused by endocrine and/or genetic disorders, such as hypothyroidism, brain tumors, and Turner's syndrome

Obesity occurs when adipose cells increase excessively in size (**hypertrophy**), in number (**hyperplasia**), or both. Obesity that results from an increase in the size of fat cells is hypertrophic, obesity that results from an increase in the number of fat cells is hyperplastic, and obesity that results from an increase in both is hypertrophic/hyperplastic.

Adipose cells follow a normal pattern of growth and development. When obesity develops in infancy or childhood (juvenile-onset obesity), more adipose cells develop, and each cell grows greatly, resulting in hypertrophic/hyperplastic obesity. When obesity develops in adulthood (adult-onset obesity), a normal number of adipose cells usually develops, but each cell contains a large amount of fat (see Just the Facts: Classification of Obesity). As obesity progresses, adult-onset obesity can be both hyperplastic and hypertrophic.[5] Once developed, fat cells do not disappear in the adult state.

Adipose cells have a long life span. If adult obesity is both hypertrophic and hyperplastic, is it more difficult to lose weight than if adult obesity is due to hypertrophy alone? Some evidence indicates that an increased number of fat cells increases the body's reluctance to reduce fat stores. The needs of adipose cells may require that they store at least nominal amounts of fat. More fat cells would then result in more fat storage, complicating efforts to lose weight. The longer a person remains obese, the more difficult it is to correct the problem.

Gender differences in depositing fat become noticeable during and after puberty. Men distribute fat primarily in the upper half of the body, and women tend to deposit it in the lower half. The percentage of fat in the body reaches peak values during early adolescence for boys and then declines during the remainder of adolescent growth. Girls experience a continuous increase in the percentage of fat from the onset of puberty to age 18–20.

From approximately 2 years of age, obese children develop a greater number of fat cells than do children of normal weight. Although it is widely believed that obese children become obese adults, most obese adults were not obese as children.[17] The large majority of obesity is thought to be adult-onset obesity. Still, childhood obesity should not be ignored, since about 33⅓ percent of obese preschool children, 50 percent of school-age children, and about 80 percent of obese adolescents become obese adults.[17] Significant weight gain generally begins either between ages 5 and 7 or during the teenage years.[5]

Causes of Obesity

The laws of thermodynamics state that energy cannot be destroyed; it is used for work or converted into another form. Accordingly, the progressive accumulation of stored fat in the body is the result of consumption of more calories (energy) than are expended. Food energy in excess of the body's need results in storage of fat in adipose cells (Figure 8-2, page 256). This relationship is demonstrated in almost all people. Excessive caloric intake and deficient energy expenditure are responsible for most obesity. What is more difficult to explain, however, is the difference among people's responses to the laws of energy conservation and expenditure. Two people may be overfed the same number of calories and yet differ in the amount of weight gained, even if their activity levels are held constant. What accounts for these differences? The answer suggests that obesity is a complex issue, involving both biological and behavioral theories.

Biological Theories

Age, metabolism, gender, disease, heredity, and set point, the body's internal signal for the level of fatness it tries to defend, are biological factors that influence body weight and obesity. As people age, their amount of muscle tends to drop, and fat accounts for a greater percentage of their body weight. Metabolism also slows naturally with age. Together these changes reduce calorie needs, often adding an extra pound a year after age 35.[3] Women usually have higher fat-to-muscle ratios than men because of the influence of hormones unique to fertility and the female reproductive system. Also, men typically have higher muscle-to-fat ratios than women, which increases metabolism and caloric expenditure. Diseases that affect the thyroid gland may have a dramatic impact on body weight. An overactive thyroid gland (hyperthyroidism) increases the resting metabolic rate (RMR) and may cause weight loss. Conversely, an underactive thyroid gland (hypothyroidism) lowers RMR and may lead to overweight or obesity.

Infections may also be a factor in obesity. This is not altogether unexpected because a number of chronic

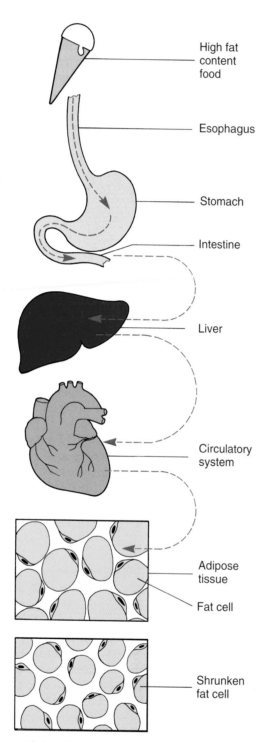

High fat
content
food

Esophagus

Stomach

Intestine

Liver

Circulatory
system

Adipose
tissue

Fat cell

Shrunken
fat cell

Figure 8-2 Fat Storage

Fat can be manufactured in the body from any food and
stored when caloric intake exceeds expenditure. Fat
droplets travel to the liver from the stomach and intestines
and then enter the circulatory system, where they are delivered to the cells and organs. Excess fats are stored in adipose tissue. When more energy is needed, fats are
released from adipose cells. If the energy needs continue,
the cells shrink.

conditions have been connected to viral and/or bacterial
infections. Atherosclerosis and ulcers are two examples.
Viral infections have been shown to cause obesity in animals. It will take years of research to determine if there
is a link between viruses and weight gain in humans.

The two major biological explanations of obesity are
heredity and set point. Although they are interrelated,
they are discussed separately here.

Heredity

The study of obesity lends itself to the classic question of
nature versus nurture, heredity versus environment. Does
obesity run in families? If so, is it caused by eating habits
learned from family influence or by genetic influence?

Studies of adoptees and identical twins help reveal
the influence of the genetic component of obesity. In
classic longitudinal studies when researchers follow
adoptees over time, they find that their body weight
classification resembles that of their biological parents,
rather than that of their adoptive parents, even though
they learned and practiced the lifestyles of their adoptive
parents.

Identical twins are excellent subjects for these studies
because they have identical genetic makeups. Any physical differences that occur can be attributed to environmental and/or lifestyle factors. Classic longitudinal studies
of identical twins consistently reveal a strong genetic influence.[5] When comparing height, weight, and BMI,
identical twins follow similar patterns. Each member of
the pair can be expected to gain the same amount of
weight at approximately the same time in life. The simi-
larity in identical twins is twice that observed in fraternal twins (twins who emanate from separate eggs that
do not have identical genes).

The connection between heredity and obesity is also
confirmed in studies that correlate the prevalence of
childhood obesity with the prevalence of obesity in parents. Eighty percent of children born to two obese parents will themselves become obese, compared with 40
percent of children born to one obese parent and 14 percent of children born to nonobese parents.[14] Studies
support the idea that obesity and fat deposition are significantly influenced by heredity.

In addition to influencing body weight, heredity influences body shape. Body shape generally falls into
one of three categories: ectomorph, endomorph, and
mesomorph (see Just the Facts: Body Shapes). Most
people are a combination of all three, with a tendency
to be more like one or two of them. If a person's body
shape strongly favors a particular classification, the
person cannot realistically hope to attain another
body type. It would be more appropriate for such a
person to seek changes in body composition that reduce fat weight regardless of body-shape tendencies.

Just the Facts

Body Shapes

According to somatotype (body-type) experts, there are three classic body shapes. Most people are a combination of all three. The body shapes/body types are as follows:

Ectomorphic	*Ectomorphs* have long, thin body frames; are slender; and have a low capacity for fat storage.
Endomorphic	*Endomorphs* have rounded physical features and large frames. Of the three classic body shapes, they have the greatest capacity for fat storage.
Mesomorphic	*Mesomorphs* have muscular, athletic body frames with an ability to store fat that falls in between ectomorphs and endomorphs.

Shape acceptance is essential in constructing a realistic view of body weight.

Another factor that helps explain the connection between heredity and obesity surfaced with the discovery of *leptin*, a hormone made in fat cells by a gene called *ob* (for its connection with obesity), often referred to as the *fat gene*. Leptin senses when fat cells are satisfied and signals the hypothalamus to suppress appetite. The hypothalamus is a part of the brain that regulates such functions as heart rate, blood pressure, body temperature, and food and water intake. Scientists hypothesize that obesity occurs for one of three reasons: (1) The gene fails to produce enough leptin, (2) the body's cells do not recognize leptin, or (3) the body develops a resistance to leptin. The prevailing theory is the hypothalamus is resistant to leptin, thus denying the brain of the usual signals to suppress appetite. In the absence of this signal, appetite continues regardless of intake.[14] It is too early to know if the leptin connection is a true medical breakthrough or another false alarm, and experts warn against the idea that leptin is the magic key for weight loss. Even if human studies confirm the connection, leptin will still be a pharmaceutical adjunct to diet and exercise, not a replacement for them.

Set point theory

The set point theory of weight control also reflects the role of genetics. Proponents of this theory suggest that the body works to maintain a certain weight. More specifically, each person has an internal **set point** for fatness, sometimes called the *adipostat*, which seems to regulate the body by adjusting hunger, appetite, food intake, and energy expenditure. Researchers have demonstrated that human and animal subjects put on low-calorie or high-calorie diets lose and gain only to a certain level. When the diet ends, food consumption increases and they return to their approximate original weight.

How the body determines its set point is not known. One hypothesis is that the body is able to adjust its energy expenditure by adjusting its metabolism. Gordon Wardlaw, well-known nutrition author, provides an analogy and explanation.[18] The analogy is to view set point as a coiled spring: The farther you stray from your usual weight, the harder the force acts to pull you back to that weight. When dieters lose weight, their metabolism slows down. When they gain weight, metabolism increases.

There is physiological evidence to support the set point explanation. If energy intake is reduced, the blood concentration of thyroid hormone falls, and the metabolic rate slows. In addition, lower body weight decreases the energy cost of activity and the total energy used by muscle tissue falls because some of these tissues are also lost. In addition, the enzyme used by fat cells and muscle cells to take up fat from the bloodstream often increases its activity. Through these changes, the body resists further weight loss.[5]

If a person overeats, in the short run the metabolic rate tends to increase because total body mass increases. This causes some resistance to further weight gain. People often recognize the body's resistance to weight loss when dieting but do not think much about the resistance to weight gain after eating a big holiday meal. However, in the long run, resistance to weight gain is much less than resistance to weight loss.[5] When a person gains weight and stays at that weight for a while, the body tends to defend the new weight.

Can a person change his or her set point? Proponents of the set point theory think that the set point does shift over time in response to behavioral factors: Eating a high-fat diet tends to raise the set point for fatness, and regular physical activity tends to lower it. This shift may be so slight and gradual as to go unnoticed for years.

Some proponents of the set point theory suggest that, because some people are genetically programmed to have unwanted pounds, efforts to eliminate fat with diet, exercise, or both are doomed. The body can shut down its calorie-losing mechanism by lowering metabolism and can stimulate appetite to the point that a person must have food (see Nurturing Your Spirituality: Nature Versus Nurture—Make Peace with Obesity or Take Action on page 258).

Other proponents of the set point theory argue that vigorous regular exercise brings about physiological changes in muscle that speed up metabolism and lower the set point, thereby lowering the level of fat the body

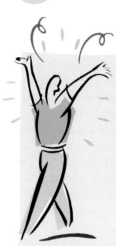

Nurturing Your Spirituality

Nature Versus Nurture—Make Peace with Obesity or Take Action

Very few health issues fuel the debate about nature vs. nurture better than obesity. Genetic factors account for anywhere between 30 and 70 percent of weight differences between people, depending on which medical expert you ask. In addition, each one of us appears to have a built-in set point for fatness, which the body tries to maintain, and when we stray too far from this set point certain biological changes occur to return us to our natural weight. The genetic and set point explanations of obesity give validity to the argument that obesity is beyond individual control. Therefore, since we can't do anything about it, why fight it? Would it not be better to make peace with our body-weight status and go about the process of enjoying life, rather than constantly doing battle with obesity, inevitably losing the battle, and feeling demoralized because of it?

Arguments against genetics and the set point theory maintain that people become obese because of lifestyle choices. For some people, obesity is caused by physical inactivity or poor dietary habits; for others, obesity is explained by social, emotional, or physical environmental factors; for still others, all of these factors apply. Proponents of nurture as the cause of obesity maintain that, while nature may provide a predisposition, or set point, for fatness, it is behavior, or what we choose to do, that determines our level of fatness.

What are we to conclude about the debate between nature and nurture, genetics and behavior, as causes of obesity, especially when all of the explanations seem plausible? It's helpful to remember several things: First, obesity is a complex disease; second, obesity is influenced by so many variables that it will likely be years before genetic and environmental factors are clearly understood; third, any attempt to oversimplify obesity is probably born out of misinformation or naiveté; and fourth, causes of obesity are theories, not proven facts.

If you are obese, or you appear to be predisposed to obesity, what's the bottom line? In the final analysis, we must assume responsibility for weight maintenance ourselves. There is little to be gained by blaming genetics or pointing a finger at biological factors for which we have little control. Rather than getting stuck in denial, blame, or rationalization and never taking action to manage our weight, we are better served by a can-do and will-do attitude, realizing that we can take steps to improve health and promote weight maintenance, even if we are obese or can't lose weight.

will accept and defend. Exercise induces the body to stabilize at a lower body weight, precisely what dieters try to do. Proponents of the set point theory argue that, while exercise cannot negate heredity, it can modify it. Obesity need not be destiny (see This Just In on page 286).

Behavioral Theories

Behavioral explanations of obesity include excessive caloric intake (overeating) and lack of physical activity (hypokinesis).

Overeating

The basic laws of nature require that calories be consumed before energy can be stored as excess weight. The body cannot make energy on its own. For the obese and overweight, therefore, caloric intake is an important issue, especially considering that Americans are consuming more calories today than in the past. Caloric consumption averages 400 calories per day more than it did 20 years ago and 500 calories more than it did 25 years ago.[19] This is equivalent to 3 to 4 pounds per month and 41 to 51 pounds per year of extra calories.

Does the increased caloric consumption of Americans apply to all people or just to people with obesity? This has been a controversial question, and researchers fall into two camps regarding this issue. One camp suggests that obese people eat no more and sometimes less than normal-weight people. They maintain that blaming obesity on a lack of willpower is unfair and oversimplifies the facts. The body of the obese person is more efficient at converting calories to adipose cells for reasons beyond his or her control, such as genetic predisposition or higher set point for fatness. Stated another way, obese people may not eat more than normal-weight people; they just consume more calories than are required by their bodies.

The other camp claims that obese people do eat more than normal-weight people; the problem, they argue, is a discrepancy in reporting food intake. In one study, 86 percent of women underestimated their intake by 621 calories; 60 percent of men underestimated their intake by 581 calories. The farther people were from what they considered to be their ideal weight, the more likely they were to underreport. For every pound a person was above ideal weight, the underreporting error increased

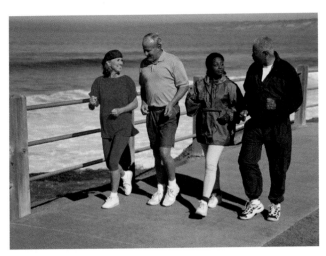

Exercising with a friend is a fun way to stay active and keep your weight in check.

by 7 calories.[20] This helps explain the difficulty some people have losing weight despite repeated attempts. They may be consuming more calories than they realize. According to these researchers, the phenomenon referred to as **diet resistance,** the inability to lose weight by dieting, has little to do with innate biological factors.

High fat intake

Although researchers are divided on the issue of overeating, they tend to agree that the abundance of food high in fat and calories is a major factor in the prevalence of obesity in the United States. In his review of the literature on obesity—a review that included more than 300 citations from the scientific literature—David C. Nieman, exercise scientist at Appalachian State University, wrote, "Of all the current theories attempting to explain the epidemic of obesity in most Western societies, the high dietary fat intake hypothesis is most widely accepted by experts."[17] Overweight people tend to eat a higher-fat diet than do people of normal weight. Ounce for ounce, fat yields more than double the number of calories than protein or carbohydrates do (9 calories versus 4). Calories from fat also appear to be more readily converted to body fat than are calories from carbohydrates and protein.

Excess carbohydrates are converted to glycogen in the liver and muscle. The body can store only a limited amount of glycogen. This is not true for fat. Fat cells are distributed throughout the body. Whereas carbohydrate storage is carefully regulated, fat storage is not, allowing a high degree of expansion. Given the sedentary lifestyles of most Americans, glycogen stores are rarely exhausted. The reality for too many people is that they burn carbohydrates and store fat.

The **thermic effect of food** (TEF) represents the amount of energy required by the body to digest,

absorb, metabolize, and store nutrients. Dietary fat has less of a thermic effect than does carbohydrate or protein and can thus be easily stored as adipose tissue. The body expends 0 to 5 calories of energy to process 100 calories from fat, compared with 20 to 30 calories to process 100 calories from protein and 5 to 10 calories from carbohydrates. Between 5 and 10 percent of total body energy goes to support the TEF.[5] For example, after a meal containing 1,000 calories, the body uses 50 to 100 calories to process the meal. The TEF helps explain why studies consistently show that, when adults and children overeat and consume high amounts of dietary fat, they tend to gain weight. Conversely, when the intake of dietary fat is low and the intake of protein, carbohydrate, and fiber is high from nutrient-dense foods, desirable body weight is more readily achieved.[17]

Portion sizes and volume eating

Americans' obsession with fat grams and low-carbohydrate diets is misplaced because the real issue is less about the type of food eaten and more about the quantity of food eaten. Food producers and eating establishments are cashing in on our quest to get a better value for the dollar. *Supersized, all-you-can-eat, buffet-style eating,* and a *meal in a sandwich* are some of the catch phrases used to increase business. When it comes to calories, the phrases are not all hype (see Just the Facts: Restaurant Dining and Supersized Calories on page 260). Bloated portions are the norm and have given rise to descriptive magazine headlines, such as "Portion Distortion,"[21] "Runaway Portion Sizes,"[22] and "Serving-Size Sprawl."[23] Restaurant portions have more than doubled over the past 20 years.[24] The problem with large serving sizes is that we tend to eat what is served. This is as true for beverages as it is for solid food (see Just the Facts: Solids Calories vs. Liquid Calories at **www.mhhe.com/anspaugh6e** Student Center, Chapter 8, Just the Facts). When people are served larger portions of food, they eat more because most people eat whatever portion size they're served.[15] People get accustomed to large amounts and feel cheated when served a normal portion. The challenge for many people is to overcome the "I'm going to eat what I pay for" attitude. Usually, this means now, rather than later.

Signs in supermarkets can also encourage people to buy more food. A consumer planning to purchase one carton of ice cream is likely to return home with two cartons if the product is priced at two for $10 instead of at $5 each. When grocers suggest the purchase of a specific number of items, shoppers are more likely to buy more than the one or two they intended to buy.

Eating out also contributes to volume eating. While restaurants are serving food in larger portions than in the past, Americans are eating at restaurants more than

∿Just the Facts∿

Restaurant Dining and Supersized Calories

Americans are overwhelmed with supersized servings of food, especially when eating out. A medium-size baked potato served at a fast-food restaurant weights 7 ounces, compared with the typical potato, which weighs 4 ounces; a medium bagel weighs 4 ounces, double the size listed in food composition tables; a medium muffin is 6 ounces, triple the size of regular muffins; a double hamburger at one popular fast-food restaurant has almost three times the number of calories as its single hamburger counterpart; a serving of BBQ ribs and fries at another national chain restaurant consists of 15 ounces of meat and 70 french fries (the FDA says a serving of fries numbers 10); a pasta serving at one popular restaurant consists of 8 cups of pasta and 6 ounces of sausage (this is equivalent to 16 servings, or two days' worth, of carbohydrates and 2 to 3 servings of meat); and one casual dining restaurant offers a no-frills entrée that weighs as much as the Manhattan *Yellow Pages*.

Exacerbating the problem of supersized portions served at restaurants is that Americans are eating out more than before. For most Americans, the more they eat out, the more calories they consume. People who eat out at least 13 times a month consume on average 32 percent more calories than those who eat out fewer than 5 times a month.[19]

These two trends, eating food in supersized portions and eating out, are recipes for creeping weight gain. The challenge for most people when eating out is to ask for small portions; another option is to eat modest amounts of food and take the rest home.

half a tub of popcorn, whether it was medium or jumbo, which held twice as much as the medium tub. The researchers concluded that people often eat about 50 percent more of pleasure foods, such as candy, chips, and popcorn, when they come in bigger packages. With other foods, the increase is usually about 25 percent.[24]

Hypokinesis

Obesity is in large part caused by the sedentary lifestyle of most Americans. Scientific improvements have led to modern conveniences and labor-saving devices that decrease the need for physical activity. Advancements in technology make it possible to bank, shop, and even complete college courses without leaving the desktop computer. Devices such as mechanized golf carts have made leisure activities less strenuous. Each new invention fosters a receptive attitude toward a life of ease. The mechanized way is generally the most expedient way in the time-oriented American society. Exercise for fitness is now separate from other parts of life. Even when people do exercise during their leisure time, their total daily energy expenditure still falls far short of what was typical several decades ago. The average sedentary person usually expends only 300 to 800 calories a day in physical activity, most of this through informal, unplanned types of movement.[17] Some experts believe that lack of physical activity is the factor that distinguishes the obese from people of normal weight.

The general decline in physical activity and fitness is correlated with the rise in obesity. When physical activity levels of overweight people are compared with those of normal-weight people, normal-weight people are about twice as active as their overweight peers. Obese men informally walk an average of 3.7 miles per day, whereas normal-weight men walk 6 miles; obese women walk 2 miles per day, and normal-weight women walk 4.9 miles.[17]

To state that obese people are less physically active than normal-weight people is one thing; to claim that lack of physical activity causes obesity is different. Researchers are not clear which comes first: Does obesity lead to physical inactivity or does physical inactivity lead to obesity? The cause and effect nature of the relationship between these two factors has yet to be determined and is complicated by the fact that energy expenditure from exercise differs very little between the obese and the normal weight. Because of their extra weight, the obese expend more energy when they participate in physical activity. In other words, even though they exercise less, they expend more energy in the course of activity. For this reason, overeating is considered by most experts to be more important than inactivity as a determinant of obesity.[17] Still, there is general agreement that exercise is vital to the success of

ever before. In a long-term study conducted at the University of Minnesota, people who ate more frequently at fast-food restaurants consumed more calories and gained more weight than those who ate less frequently at such restaurants.[21] In another study, which included 3,700 young adults over the course of 15 years, Harvard researchers found that eating fast food more than twice a week increased the risk for obesity.[21]

Do people eat more when food is packaged in larger quantities? In trying to answer this question, researchers gave either a 1- or a 2-pound bag of M&Ms plus either a "medium" or a "jumbo" movie theater–sized tub of popcorn to participants. On average, participants ate 112 M&Ms from the 1-pound bag and 156 from the 2-pound bag. Likewise, the average person ate roughly weight maintenance. In its guidelines on the treatment of obesity, the National Heart, Lung, and Blood Institute (NHLBI) notes that, according to randomized, controlled trials, physical activity among overweight and obese people reduces abdominal fat "only modestly or not at all." But don't dismiss exercise. It is the number one way to prevent weight gain.[25]

Dieting and Exercise: Strategies for Weight Maintenance or Weight Loss

To maintain weight, caloric intake must be balanced by caloric expenditure. To lose weight, a person has to achieve a **caloric deficit,** in which the number of calories burned exceeds the number of calories consumed. This is the basic principle of weight management. It is simple and straightforward, and it includes three obvious strategies: (1) the restriction of caloric intake by dieting, (2) the increase of caloric expenditure through physical activity, and (3) a combination of dieting and physical activity. What is not so easy to explain is how two people can respond so differently to dieting and exercise weight-loss strategies. Complex forces, many of which are still not clearly understood, influence the success of weight-management/weight-loss efforts.

The loss of 1 pound of body fat requires a caloric deficit of 3,500 calories. (The loss of 1 pound of adipose tissue yields more than 1 pound of body weight because fat storage includes some lean support tissue—muscle, connective tissues, blood supply, and other body components.) A caloric deficit of 3,300 calories results in a loss of 1 pound of body weight.[5] A loss of 1 pound of body fat per week is a good goal and requires an average daily caloric deficit of 500 calories. A caloric deficit of more than 500 calories per day, unless medically supervised, borders on the extreme and is difficult to sustain over long periods. A loss of 2 pounds of body fat per week is considered a maximum goal.

Body fat loss in excess of 2 pounds per week is not practical for most people. For example, diets that promise a fat-weight loss of 10 pounds per week require a caloric deficit of 35,000 calories per week; that is an average of 7,000 calories per day. For that kind of caloric deficit, a person would have to go to the extremes of fasting while running two marathons in one day. Weight loss in excess of a couple of pounds per week usually involves lean tissue weight, which should be retained, and fluid weight, which needs to be replaced to prevent health consequences ranging from dehydration to electrolyte imbalance.

A desirable long-term goal for a person needing to lose weight is 1 to 2 pounds per week until about 10 percent of excess weight is lost. The emphasis should be on a slow, steady weight loss rather than on a rapid weight loss. Once this goal is reached, the dieter should go into maintenance for about six months before attempting more weight loss.[5] For example, a 250-pound person should go into a six-month maintenance program after losing 25 pounds. This conservative approach to weight loss is likely to yield health improvements while promoting a more stable, consistent body weight.

Dieting

Statistics show that dieting is the method of choice for most Americans trying to lose weight. Although dieting usually works only temporarily, most people who fail to maintain weight loss are willing to try again. Many people seek the miraculous diet that will transform them from fat to thin, preferably with minimal effort and in the shortest time possible.

The success rate of diet-only strategies is dismal. Only 5 percent of people who lose weight keep it off for at least a year, a standard definition of weight-loss success.[26] Some recent findings, however, suggest that this estimate may be too low. A study of 32,213 dieters revealed that 25 percent of them successfully lost 10 percent of their weight and kept it off for at least a year.[27] While 25 percent may not seem very impressive, if it holds true in future studies, it is much more encouraging than the bleak 5 percent. Still, the consensus opinion among experts favors the more conservative 5 percent success rate. Typically, one-third of the weight lost during dieting is regained within the first year, and almost all weight lost is regained within three to five years.[5] Maintaining postdiet weight is one of the major failures of weight loss through dieting because dieters do not learn the habits and behaviors needed to remain at the new weight. As a result, they lose and regain weight many times in their lives. This pattern of repeated weight loss and gain, known as **weight cycling,** *yo-yo dieting,* and *seesaw approaches* to weight loss, is potentially harmful and counterproductive (see Just the Facts: Yo-Yo Dieting and Toxicity: Another Reason to Lose Weight Slowly and Keep It Off on page 262).

The consequences of weight cycling are numerous. The most immediate negative effect is rebound weight gain. Typically, weight gained after dieting includes not only the weight that was lost but additional weight as well. After years of yo-yo dieting, many dieters experience a weight-gain pattern that takes on a stair-step effect, increasing in small but noticeable increments with each successive effort. In addition, the weight regained is in the form of adipose tissue, whereas the weight that was lost consisted of a mixture of adipose and muscle tissue. The result of weight cycling is not only extra weight but also extra fat weight. Weight cycling is also

ᐱᐱᐱJust the Factsᐱᐱ

Yo-Yo Dieting and Toxicity: Another Reason to Lose Weight Slowly and Keep It Off

Repeated weight loss and gain, known as yo-yo dieting, has long been associated with numerous physical consequences. Recently scientists discovered another problem. When weight is lost, the body apparently triggers the release of toxins stored in its fat cells.[29] These toxins enter the bloodstream and exert adverse effects on the nervous system and some are known carcinogens. Blood samples taken during periods of dramatic weight loss reveal that blood levels of toxins increase as much as fivefold. This can become significant with the repeated weight loss of yo-yo dieting. Toxins gradually clear from the bloodstream as weight stabilizes. The implication is that people who are constantly on and off a diet subject themselves to another risk. To avoid this risk, the key is to lose weight gradually and keep it off.

ᐱᐱᐱJust the Factsᐱᐱ

Should Weight Maintenance Be Your Goal?

The average weight gain of Americans over 10 years is approximately 8 pounds, a little less than 1 pound per year.[5] Few of us would become overly concerned with a 1-pound weight gain over the course of a year. Most of us probably wouldn't even notice a gain of just 1 pound and, if we did, would prefer to view it as a temporary occurrence that would even out over time. However, we would probably notice a 16-pound weight gain 20 years later or a 24-pound weight gain 30 years later. But by that time eating habits and activity patterns are deeply entrenched in our being and more difficult to change. For many adults, weight maintenance, or weight stability, is a preferred goal. If, after an 8-pound weight gain over 10 years, a 30-year-old adult focuses on weight maintenance, creeping obesity can be prevented with very slight changes in lifestyle. For example, a daily drop of 100 calories in food intake is not much and can be as little as one serving of a sweetened beverage. The result is a 700-calorie deficit over the course of a week; 3,500 calories, or 1 pound, in five weeks; and a little more than 10 pounds in a year. A modest plan of this nature won't sell books or make headlines and it doesn't promise huge weight loss. But it is doable and will be an effective strategy for curbing the weight gain cycle of the previous decade.

associated with negative psychological effects. Dieting failures diminish self-confidence; low self-confidence dampens enthusiasm and makes it harder to keep off extra weight.

The high recidivism rate of diet-only programs coupled with the negative effects of weight cycling seems to negate dieting as a strategy for losing weight. The reality, however, is that weight loss requires a caloric deficit, and limiting food intake is the most direct and immediate way to get results. The mistake people tend to make with most diet-only strategies is to set unrealistic goals. They want to lose too much weight and they want to lose it immediately. An ideal approach is to lose weight at the same rate as weight is gained. For most people, this involves a plan of modest dietary restrictions implemented over a period of months or years, rather than days or weeks. Weight-loss goals structured according to the guidelines mentioned are more likely to be successful.

A better goal for many people is weight maintenance, or weight stability. **Weight maintenance** is consistently maintaining weight within certain limits between any two points in time. There is no universally accepted definition of *weight limits*, though some researchers use a ±5-pound standard.[5] The concept of weight maintenance is not popular, doesn't make headlines, and doesn't require weight loss. For people with creeping weight gain, however, it will curb the tendency to gain weight over time (see Just the Facts: Should Weight Maintenance Be Your Goal?).

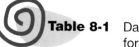

Table 8-1   Daily Calorie Goals for Weight Loss[28]

Weight of Dieter (Pounds)	Daily Calorie Goal	
	Men	Women
250 or less	1,400	1,200
251–300	1,600	1,400
301 or more	1,800	1,600

SOURCE: Mayo Foundation for Medical Education and Research. 2001. Healthy weight: A process of changing your lifestyle habits. *Mayo Clinic Health Letter* 19(1):1–2.

In diet-only strategies, the caloric intake should not drop below 1,200 per day in women or 1,400 per day in men (see Table 8-1). Gender differences in caloric intake are due to differences in physical activity patterns, metabolism (from more or less muscle tissue), and size. Because fat is more than twice as energy dense as carbohydrates, many experts recommend concentrating on limiting fat

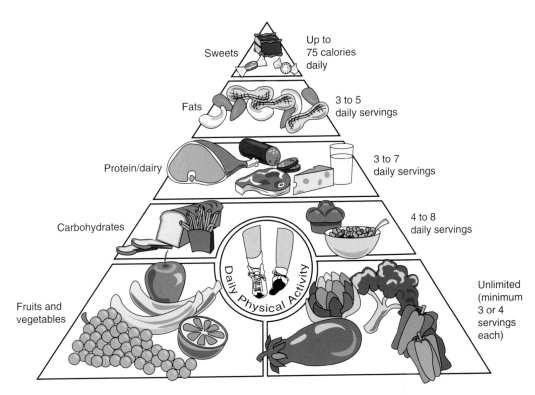

Sweets — Up to 75 calories daily

Fats — 3 to 5 daily servings

Protein/dairy — 3 to 7 daily servings

Carbohydrates — 4 to 8 daily servings

Fruits and vegetables — Unlimited (minimum 3 or 4 servings each)

Daily Physical Activity

Figure 8-3 Mayo Clinic Healthy Weight Pyramid

The Mayo Clinic Healthy Weight Pyramid shows you where to focus when selecting foods that help promote healthy weight. What's more, you'll never be hungry with this dining approach.

intake rather than on counting calories. If an eating plan calls for a caloric intake below 1,200 calories for women and 1,400 calories for men per day, discuss it with your health care provider. You may need to take vitamin and/or mineral supplements. One last caveat for people frustrated because they can't lose weight on a 1,200- or 1,400-calorie diet: If you can't lose weight at this caloric level, you probably don't need to lose weight. You might be better served by reexamining your reasons for losing weight.

In structuring a diet, some modification in the Food Guide Pyramid (FGP) is recommended (see Chapter 6). Figure 8-3 presents the Mayo Clinic Healthy Weight Pyramid and recommends food selections that start first with fruits and vegetables.[28] At least four servings of vegetables and at least three servings of fruit are recommended each day, but you are allowed to eat an unlimited number of servings of both. Next in ascending order is the carbohydrate group (grains, pasta, etc.) with four to eight servings recommended. This represents a 33 percent reduction in the number of servings of carbohydrates in comparison with the FGP. Whole-grain, high-fiber foods are the preferred source of carbohydrates. Protein and dairy foods are combined as one food category, with a recommendation of three to seven servings.

The Mayo Clinic Healthy Weight Pyramid emphasizes foods that promote both healthy weight and good nutrition. Hunger should not be an issue with this approach. Also, in the center of the pyramid is the recommendation to engage in physical activity on a daily basis.

Very low-calorie diets

Very low-calorie diets (VLCDs) are diets containing fewer than 800 calories a day. They are considered extreme diets (food is usually replaced with a powdered supplement) and should be viewed as a medical intervention. Typically, VLCDs are undertaken under medical supervision and administered in hospital/clinic settings for a period of three to four months and include counseling, behavior management, nutrition and dieting classes, and support groups. Often, they include an exercise program. Once the diet is completed, dieters on a VLCD gradually return to food intake.

VLCDs are usually recommended for people with a BMI of 35 or higher or whose obesity is threatening to their health and who are unable to lose weight through dieting and exercise.[14] People who have insulin-dependent diabetes mellitus, liver disease, kidney disease, or a history of heart disease are warned against this method of losing weight.

For people who can stay on them, VLCDs produce dramatic reductions in weight. Still, they are not a panacea. About 25 percent of people who start a VLCD drop out of the program.[14] Like most extreme dieting programs, VLCDs have a high failure rate. As a result, VLCD programs are worthless without careful attention paid to long-term maintenance that incorporates newly learned eating patterns.[14]

Low-fat diets

Low-fat diets are potentially effective techniques for losing weight. With its high caloric yield and almost unlimited capacity for storage, fat is a major threat to weight maintenance. Consequently, Americans are fixated on fat-free or low-fat foods. The assumption is that, if a food is low in fat, it is also low in calories. As a result, although Americans are consuming fewer fat calories percentagewise, they are consuming more total calories from all sources and are getting heavier. (Actual fat intake remains the same as it was during the past 10 years.) Percentagewise, it dropped because of an increase in total calories consumed.

Low-fat foods and overcompensatory eating

Although diet experts advocate restricting fat calories, low-fat diets have not been effective for many dieters because of **overcompensatory eating.** This occurs when the consumption of low-fat foods is accompanied by an increase in total calories. Researchers at Pennsylvania State University demonstrated this point when, on separate occasions, they gave a group of women two kinds of yogurt: One was labeled *high-fat,* and one was labeled *low-fat.* The ingredients were manipulated, so that both kinds of yogurt had the same number of calories. A comparison group of women was given the same, but unlabeled, yogurt. Thirty minutes after consuming the yogurt, the women ate lunch. After eating the yogurt labeled *low-fat,* subjects compensated by taking in more calories during lunch than they did when they consumed the yogurt labeled *high-fat.* This pattern of overcompensatory eating was not observed for the comparison group who ate the unlabeled yogurt. The researchers concluded that, when the women ate yogurt labeled *low-fat,* they rationalized that they could indulge more at lunch. When they didn't know what kind of yogurt they had eaten, they were more tuned in to their bodies' physical cues and naturally adjusted the amount they ate.[30]

The attitude that people can eat what they want, in unlimited quantities, as long as it is fat-free is wrong. Calories do count. Fat-free foods can help people lose weight if they are used properly, if they don't result in overcompensatory consumption of food, and if total calories are kept in line. Some experts recommend that Americans trade in their obsession with low-fat diets for more productive strategies, such as monitoring portion sizes and being more physically active.[31]

The FDA approval of Olestra (Olean) as a fat substitute is partly responsible for the proliferation of low-fat and fat-free foods. Many people unwittingly consume foods in large quantities, thinking that, if it is fat-free, it is also calorie-free. A fat-free product made with Olestra may turn out to have more total calories (from carbohydrates) than a companion product made with typical ingredients, including fat. For that reason, it is important to check labels. The bottom line to look for is total calories. Diets high in Olestra also carry the risk of compromising the body's use of essential nutrients, such as fat-soluble vitamins.

Popular diets

Many diets on the market are nutritionally sound, and many are not. Some are potentially hazardous, and

---

∿ Just the Facts ∿

Outlandish Weight-Loss Promises—What to Do

Quick and unrealistic weight-loss schemes that promise outlandish results are common, and the number of fad diets promoted in print and video media exceeds the FDA's capacity to check claims and promises.[32,33] One newspaper published an advertiser's claim: "Lose 40 pounds by Christmas." The date of the advertisement was November 3, about seven weeks before Christmas. This ad was an example of blatantly misleading advertising. The responsibility for demonstrating "proof" rests with authors and publishers, often motivated more by profits than by credible and reliable information. What can the average consumer do if he or she is exposed to some outrageous claims?

- First and foremost, adopt an attitude of skepticism. If it sounds too good to be true, it probably is. No one diet device or pill can work miracles. Even respectable diet programs require you to eat less and exercise more.

- Call your local chapter of the Better Business Bureau to check claims and reputation before you enlist in a program or buy a product or gadget.

- Register a complaint with the source (newspaper, magazine, television station) of the advertisement.

- If you see a suspect ad, send it to The Director, National Advertising Division, Council of Better Business Bureaus, 70 W. 36th St., 13th Floor, New York, NY 10018.

- And remember, if you don't lose weight with a particular product, don't automatically blame yourself. You may have not failed; the product may have failed you.

many are based on faulty nutritional and physiological concepts. Some require that food be eaten in a certain order and severely restrict foods. Some require medical supervision. Others impose unrealistic caloric restrictions, and still others make promises based more on fantasy than facts. (You can explore a list of popular diets that includes descriptions, the type of weight loss expected, health drawbacks, and pros and cons for each diet on this text's Online Learning Center at **www.mhhe.com/anspaugh6e** Student Center, Chapter 8, Popular Diets.) The Food and Drug Administration (FDA) does not investigate every new fad diet, and many diet plans are published without the FDA's endorsement (see Just the Facts: Outlandish Weight-Loss Promises—What to Do). If a diet is published, it is usually because a publisher sees potential profits from its sales. Publishers know that the advice to "eat fewer calories and increase physical activity" will not sell books, but fad diets with secret ingredients or magic formulas will.

Because fad diets are unlikely to disappear, identifying some of the characteristics and marketing strategies used by diet promoters to appeal to unwitting consumers is helpful.[5] Fad diets

- Promote quick results
- Stress eating one type of food to the exclusion of others
- Emphasize gimmick approaches, such as eating food in a particular order
- Cite anecdotes and testimonials, usually involving well-known people
- Claim to be a panacea for everyone
- Often promote a secret ingredient
- Often recommend expensive supplements
- Rarely emphasize permanent changes in eating habits
- Usually show little concern for accepted principles of good nutrition (see Chapter 6)
- Are usually cynical about the evidence that comes from the scientific community

Dieting is an ineffective weight-management method. The expectation that temporary changes in eating habits will lead to permanent weight loss is unrealistic. Sensible and permanent dietary changes that depend on wise food choices are an excellent way to cut calories and a healthy way to eat. (Table 8-2 demonstrates how to reduce calories that come from fat and cholesterol by making appropriate substitutions.)

 Table 8-2 Food Substitutions That Reduce Fat, Cholesterol, and Calories

Instead of eating . . .	Substitute . . .	To save*
1 croissant	1 plain bagel	35 calories, 10 g fat, 13 mg cholesterol
1 cup cooked egg noodles	1 cup cooked macaroni	50 mg cholesterol
1 whole egg	1 egg white	65 calories, 6 g fat, 220 mg cholesterol
1 oz. cheddar cheese	1 oz. part-skim mozzarella	35 calories, 4 g fat, 15 mg cholesterol
1 oz. cream cheese	1 oz. cottage cheese (1% fat)	74 calories, 9 g fat, 29 mg cholesterol
1 tsp. whipping cream	1 tbsp. evaporated skim milk, whipped	32 calories, 5 g fat
3.5 oz. skinless roast duck	3.5 oz. skinless roast chicken	46 calories, 7 g fat
3.5 oz. beef tenderloin, choice, untrimmed, broiled	3.5 oz. beef tenderloin, select, trimmed, broiled	75 calories, 10 g fat
3.5 oz. lamb chop, untrimmed, broiled	3.5 oz. lean leg of lamb, trimmed, broiled	219 calories, 28 g fat
3.5 oz. pork spare ribs, cooked	3.5 oz. lean pork loin, trimmed, broiled	157 calories, 17 g fat
1 oz. regular bacon, cooked	1 oz. Canadian bacon, cooked	111 calories, 12 g fat
1 oz. hard salami	1 oz. extra-lean roasted ham	75 calories, 8 g fat
1 beef frankfurter	1 chicken frankfurter	67 calories, 8 g fat
3 oz. oil-packed tuna, light	3 oz. water-packed tuna, light	60 calories, 6 g fat
1 regular-size serving french fries	1 medium-size baked potato	125 calories, 11 g fat
1 oz. oil-roasted peanuts	1 oz. roasted chestnuts	96 calories, 13 g fat
1 oz. potato chips	1 oz. thin pretzels	40 calories, 9 g fat
1 oz. corn chips	1 oz. plain air-popped popcorn	125 calories, 9 g fat
1 tbsp. sour-cream dip	1 tbsp. bottled salsa	20 calories, 3 g fat
1 glazed doughnut	1 slice angel-food cake	110 calories, 13 g fat, 21 mg cholesterol
3 chocolate sandwich cookies	3 fig bars	4 g fat
1 oz. unsweetened chocolate	3 tbsp. cocoa powder	73 calories, 13 g fat
1 cup ice cream (premium)	1 cup sorbet	320 calories, 34 g fat, 100 mg cholesterol

* The values listed are the most significant savings; smaller differences are not shown. Weights given for meats are edible portions.

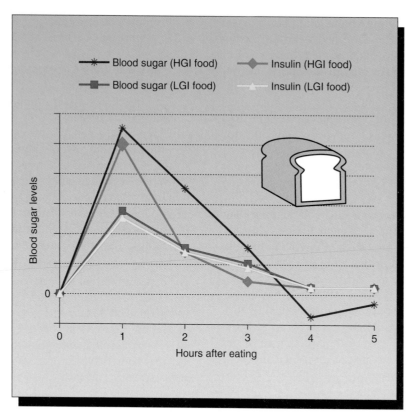

Figure 8-4   Blood Sugar and Insulin Response to High- and Low-Glycemic-Index Foods

Foods with a high Glycemic Index (HGI food)—such as white, refined bread—cause a quick surge of blood sugar and insulin to enter the bloodstream. After three to four hours, blood sugar drops below fasting level ("0"); circulating insulin leads to a hunger reflex and increased appetite. Foods with a low Glycemic Index (LGI food)—such as whole-wheat bread—are digested more slowly and cause less of a surge in blood sugar and insulin; blood sugar keeps pace with circulating insulin, does not drop below the fasting level, and doesn't cause increased appetite.[36]

SOURCE: Consumers Union. 2003. Carbohydrates without fear. *Consumer Reports on Health* 15(10): 1, 4.

Low-carbohydrate diets   The low-carbohydrate diet is the most common form of diet.[5] Without carbohydrates, the liver is forced to produce needed glucose. Once glycogen stores are used, the body calls on protein stores for glucose. Thus, a low-carbohydrate diet results in protein tissue loss. Because protein tissue is mostly water, the dieter loses weight rapidly. When a normal diet is resumed, the protein tissue is replaced along with the weight.

Popular diets that represent some variation of low-carbohydrate diets include Dr. Atkins' New Diet Revolution, Protein Power, Sugar Busters, The Carbohydrate Addict's Diet, Dr. Stillman's Calories Don't Count Diet, the Scarsdale Diet, the Drinking Man's Diet, Four-Day Wonder Diet, and the Air Force Diet.[5,32] Major claims of these diets are that carbohydrates break down into glucose, enter the bloodstream, and trigger the secretion of insulin from the pancreas to convert the glucose into a usable form of energy. Refined carbohydrates with a high Glycemic Index (see Chapter 6), such as white bread, pasta, and white rice, are more easily converted into

glucose than high-fiber carbohydrates with a low Glycemic Index, such as whole grains, vegetables, and legumes. The surge of blood sugar from high-Glycemic-Index foods causes a sudden rush of insulin, which drives blood sugar levels lower than normal. Low blood sugar promotes an appetite for more fast-acting carbohydrates, thus repeating the cycle.[27] (See Figure 8-4.) The net result is that more carbohydrates mean more calories; more calories mean added weight. Low-carbohydrate diets claim to break this cycle by limiting carbohydrate intake. Most of these diets provide a larger allowance for the consumption of protein and fat.

Low-carbohydrate diets have been around since the early 1970s. Until recently, experts debunked them because they were high in promises but low in data. That changed with the recent publication of studies from the medical community. Researchers now suggest that the early criticisms of low-carbohydrate diets may have been partially wrong. Studies conducted at Duke University Medical School and at the University of Cincinnati reported that people on low-carbohydrate diets lost more weight and had better blood fat readings than their peers on low-fat and/or low-calorie diets.[34] These results made headlines and appeared to give the Atkins Diet and other low-carbohydrate diet plans instant credibility. Favorable press from the medical community snowballed with headlines from the print and video media and provided the impetus for the "low-carb" craze. "Low-carb" has replaced "low-fat" as the mantra for dieters. Only time will tell if low-carb diets will live up to their hype (see Just the Facts: Do Low-Carb Diets Live Up to Their Hype?).

What are the pros and cons of low-carbohydrate diets? On the positive side, reducing carbohydrate intake may be an effective strategy for cutting calories, especially since so many nutritionally empty foods, such as many snack foods and sweetened beverages, are loaded with simple sugars. Also, the high fat intake associated with low-carbohydrate diets may facilitate weight loss because it makes food more satisfying and filling, which

helps keep the carbohydrates out of the diet and therefore the calories down.[34] On the negative side, many low-carbohydrate diets don't discriminate among types of fat. This is a mistake because the consumption of saturated fats and trans fatty acids are associated with numerous health detriments. Fat consumption, regardless of diet regimen, should favor monounsaturated and polyunsaturated fats (see Chapter 6). Another negative is that low-carbohydrate diets restrict the intake of many foods (fruits, vegetables, whole grains) that are good for health.

The American Heart Association does not recommend low-carbohydrate diets because they are associated with health risks, including cardiac, renal, bone, and liver abnormalities.[35] They may also lead to *ketosis,* an abnormal state that occurs in uncontrolled diabetes and starvation. Ketosis occurs when there is a high concentration of *ketone bodies.* Ketone bodies come from the incomplete breakdown of fat. In the absence of glucose

Just the Facts

Do Low-Carb Diets Live Up to Their Hype?

With the publication of favorable results from the medical community, the popularity of low-carb diets has exploded. The findings of recent studies indicate that many people on low-carb diets lose weight and, at the same time, experience improvements in their blood fat profile. LDL cholesterol improves, triglyceride levels drop, and HDL cholesterol increases—all favorable responses. In other words, people can consume foods that are high in calories (fat and meat products) and lose weight if they seriously restrict their consumption of carbohydrates. To meat lovers, this seems too good to be true.

More recent studies muddy the water regarding the claims of low-carb diets:

- An analysis of 107 studies published on low-carbohydrate diets in the past 35 years found one consistent theme: low caloric intake. The average intake was 1,100 calories per day for a period of four to five months. Researchers concluded that calories and duration, not carbs, were the key factors.[37] Contrary to popular opinion, low-carb diets don't allow people to eat all they want and lose weight.

- People on low-carbohydrate diets lose weight faster than those on low-fat diets, but they end up in a statistical tie after a year. Low-carb dieters experience most of their weight loss during the first six months and then level off or, in some cases, regain some of the lost weight; low-fat dieters catch up with them by steadily and continuously losing weight.[38,39]

- Improvements in the blood profile of low-carb dieters may be due to weight loss rather than a low intake of carbohydrates. (Weight loss is known to reduce blood cholesterol regardless of diet strategy.[40]) In other words, further studies may reveal nothing unique about the relationship between low-carb diets and blood cholesterol levels. Only time will tell.

- Researchers are uncertain if HDL cholesterol improvements associated with low-carb diets are, in fact, beneficial. There is some evidence that the increased HDL seen with high-saturated-fat diets are actually more like LDL cholesterol.[40] This causes concern about the long-term safety of this diet strategy.

- The effectiveness of low-carb diets dwindles with time. Most people who go on low-carb diets don't stick with them very long.[41] About 40 percent of people enrolled in low-carb studies drop out.[42]

- Foods packaged as *low-carb* may have as many calories as their regularly packaged versions. *Low-carb* is not an approved term of the Food and Drug Administration and therefore has no legal definition.[43]

- Low-carb, high-protein diets can threaten the health of the kidneys, particularly in people with moderate to severe kidney disease.[44]

(because of low carbohydrate intake), the body is without its most basic form of energy. Fatty acids flood into the bloodstream and eventually form ketone bodies. The heart, muscles, brain, and other vital organs begin to use ketone bodies for energy. This is an adaptive response of the body that spares some of the body's protein breakdown.[5] However, if the concentration of ketone bodies is too high, the blood becomes highly acidic, a condition called *acidosis*. Acidosis indicates a disturbance of the body's acid-base balance and is associated with potentially serious health consequences.[35]

Novelty diets

Novelty diets are the classic fad diets typically based on gimmicks. Often the gimmicks are explained with scientific terminology. A novelty diet promotes certain nutrients, foods, or combinations of foods as having unique, magical, or previously undiscovered qualities. The rationale behind some of these diets is that the dieter eats only a certain food for so long; eventually gets bored; and, theoretically, ends up by consuming fewer calories. Some low-carbohydrate diets are also novelty diets.

Novelty diets, like most other extreme diets, don't work if success is judged by weight maintenance. Once dieters reach their goal, they usually regain the weight on resuming previous eating patterns. Some novelty diets espouse views that are misleading, even absurd. A well-known nutrition expert explains: "The most bizarre of the novelty diets proposes that 'food gets stuck in your body.' Fit for Life, the Beverly Hills Diet, and the Eat Great, Lose Weight are examples. The supposition is that food gets stuck in the intestine, putrefies, and creates toxins that invade the blood and cause disease. This is utter nonsense. Nevertheless, the same idea has been promoted in health-food books since the 1800s. Today, Fit for Life suggests that meat eaten with potatoes is not digested and that fresh fruit should be consumed only before noon. These recommendations are absurd. They are gimmicks that appear controversial but are really designed to sell books."[5]

The age-old advice of caveat emptor applies, especially to novelty diets. There is no limit in the creativity of hucksters willing to promote weight-loss products and fad diets, usually at considerable expense to the consumer. It's helpful to be reminded that, if a new diet gimmick sounds too good to be true, it is.

Diet Drugs

If recent history is a good predictor of the future, American dieters can anticipate a new arsenal of drug solutions for losing weight. Drugs that suppress appetite by stimulating the satiety center in the brain have helped many dieters lose weight temporarily. Drugs marketed under the names *fen-phen* (fenfluramine) and *redux*

(dexfenfluramine) during the mid-1990s quickly sold in huge quantities. The popularity of these drugs did not last long, however, because of the plethora of side effects, including death, which eventually led to their withdrawal from the marketplace. Newer appetite-suppressant drugs, such as Meridia (sibutramine), offer another pharmacologic solution for dieters. Although early studies of Meridia are encouraging, the drug is not off the safety hook. Some people on this drug experience dangerous jumps in blood pressure. Because of the potential for adverse side effects, the use of Meridia should be viewed with caution. Additional research is underway to evaluate its safety.[14]

Other classes of drugs include lipase inhibitors (e.g., Xenical), which block the body's absorption of dietary fat; noradrenergics (e.g., Didrex), which inhibit the appetite center in the brain; and antidepressants (e.g., Prozac), which create a feeling of fullness by raising levels of serotonin in the brain.[14]

The so-called new wonder drug for weight loss is Rimonabant. This is a different class of drug that works by inhibiting receptors in the body's endocannabinoid system (EC system). These receptors influence not only cravings that affect food intake but also those associated with cigarette smoking. The EC system plays a critical role in the regulation of food intake and metabolism.[45] Rimonabant is still in the experimental stage of development and won't be available in the United States as either a weight-loss drug or a stop smoking aid until approved by the FDA. Even if it is approved, some experts question the use of taking this drug for a lifetime.

The type of medication prescribed will vary from patient to patient and is dependent on a number of factors, including the physician's preference, the potential side effects, and its contraindications.

Diet drugs are not intended for people who are overweight or marginally obese. Instead, they are intended for the management of severe obesity that does not respond to dieting and exercise regimens and for people whose obesity causes serious health risks that outweigh the possible risks of the medication. Unfortunately, many people are drawn to the quick fix of a drug, and many physicians are willing to provide a prescription.

The reality is that drugs offer only a temporary solution. They do not correct the underlying cause of persistent weight gain. People who take weight-loss medications can anticipate the typical weight cycling effect of other dieting strategies with an added problem: Diet drugs are powerful medicines that tamper with the body's delicate balance of hormones and body chemicals. Except for the severely obese, long-term exposure to diet drugs creates harmful effects that may far outweigh the health benefits of fewer pounds of body weight.

Surgery

The most extreme treatment for obesity is surgery. Surgery to reduce weight is called **bariatric surgery.**[26] Bariatric surgery performed to limit the size of the stomach is called **gastroplasty.**[5] The popular literature often refers to gastroplasty as stomach stapling. Its popularity as an option was given a boost with the development of laparoscopic procedures that require small incisions. There are several variations of gastroplasty; for example, one variation of this surgery decreases the size of the stomach to limit the volume of food that can be processed by the body; another variation involves bypassing the stomach by rerouting the small intestines to a portion of the stomach about the size of a golf ball.[5] The latter method is call *gastric bypass*. There are more than a dozen variations of bariatric surgery, but gastric bypass is the most commonly used procedure (see Figure 8-5).[47] Regardless of the procedure recommended, surgery is a drastic approach to weight loss and is recommended as a last resort for people classified as morbidly obese or for people with significant complications of obesity. Specifically, it is considered a treatment option for people who either have a BMI of 40 or greater or are 100 pounds overweight and have been unable to lose weight through nonsurgical means. It may also be appropriate for people with a BMI between 35 and 40 who have serious obesity-related complications.[14] For many people, the results of bariatric surgery are dramatic, helping people lose 50 to 100 pounds or more.[26] However, there are many disadvantages, including a high morbidity rate

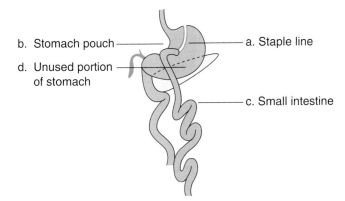

Figure 8-5 Gastric Bypass Surgery

In gastric bypass surgery, the surgeon staples (a) off a large section of the stomach, leaving a tiny pouch (b). Patients simply can't eat as much as they did before surgery, because this small pouch can accommodate only a few ounces of food at a time, and they subsequently lose weight. Additionally, because most of the stomach and some of the small intestine (c) has been bypassed, some nutrients and calories will not be absorbed.

SOURCE: Columbia University Department of Surgery. 2004. Surgical options. (www.columbiasurgery.org/divisions/obesity/surgical_roux.html).

(illness after surgery) and even death. Surgery also requires major, lifelong lifestyle changes.[5]

Liposuction is the surgical removal of fat tissue, but it is not to be confused with gastroplasty. Liposuction is primarily a cosmetic procedure that helps remove stubborn fat deposits. Common sites of liposuction include the abdomen, hips, buttocks, legs, and upper arms. Although the extracted fat cells will not return, weight can still be gained at other sites in the body.[26] Fat removal by liposuction has no proven health benefits. In a study of 15 women who underwent liposuction that removed an average of 36 percent of their abdominal subcutaneous fat tissue, resulting in 20 pounds of weight loss, no improvements in coronary risk factors were observed.[47] Liposuction is typically performed by plastic surgeons.

Diet Supplements and Herbal Remedies

Numerous supplements and herbal versions of prescription drugs used for losing weight are available in health food stores, many drugstores, and online. Some are promoted as "fat burners," while others act as diuretics, stimulants, and/or laxatives.

Conjugated linoleic acid (CLA) is the so-called wonder fat burner because it claims to develop muscle tissue and at the same time reduce fat tissue. CLA is a type of polyunsaturated fat found, in small amounts, in dairy products, beef, and other meats. It is also available as a concentrated dietary supplement. Animal studies reveal promising results. The results of recent human studies are also promising. In a study of 180 healthy overweight volunteers, subjects taking CLA lost an average of 7 percent of total body fat and boosted muscle mass by 1.5 percent.[48] This provided a double-edged benefit: fat loss, muscle gain. In terms of body weight, the CLA group lost only 3 pounds because of the slight increase in muscle mass. Despite these favorable findings, it is still premature to take CLA indiscriminately. For example, in the previously mentioned study, the CLA group experienced an increase in lipoprotein (a) (see Chapter 2). Also, CLA has not been studied in people with obesity-related conditions, such as diabetes, heart disease, and hypertension.[48]

Researchers theorize that CLA works either by helping draw fat out of the body's fat cells or by inhibiting their incorporation of additional fat, thereby redirecting food calories into muscle rather than fat cells.

Some herbs act as diuretics (chemicals that increase urine production), so they can help people lose water weight. Examples are buchu, celery seed, dandelion, juniper, parsley, and uva ursi. Diuretics are not effective for long-term weight loss because they trigger the body's thirst reflex to replace lost fluids. The body eventually

～～ Just the Facts ～～

Ephedra Warnings

The case against the use of ephedra is compelling. Ephedra accounts for 64 percent of all adverse reactions to herbal products reported to the American Association of Poison Control Centers. The distribution of supplements containing ephedra is illegal in Illinois, New York, and California. A federal ban on ephedra is being considered. The National Football League, the National Collegiate Athletic Association, the International Olympics Committee, and Major League Soccer have banned ephedra's use among players.[49]

adjusts to the continued use of diuretic herbs and retains water despite them.

Some herbs are stimulants that reportedly increase metabolism and suppress appetite. Examples are ephedra (in Chinese, *ma huang*) and caffeine. Ephedra (or ephedrine) is viewed as a natural form of fen-phen. To be effective, these herbs have to be taken in such large doses that they often cause unpleasant side effects, such as insomnia, irritability, jitters, elevated blood pressure, rapid heartbeat, seizures, stroke, heart attack, and death.[49] The dangers associated with ephedra are sufficient to have it banned in several states. Despite warnings about the use of ephedra and ephedra-caffeine combinations (see Just the Facts: Ephedra Warnings), they continue to be sold not only as weight loss supplements but also as energy boosters. Ephedra is not recommended for weight loss.

Another group of herbs produces a feeling of fullness and, therefore, inhibits appetite. These are mucilaginous herbs: They absorb fluids, such as might occur in the stomach at mealtime, and expand substantially. The most notable herb in this group is psyllium. Psyllium seed is sold in bulk in herb shops and is available in drugstores as the common bulk-forming laxative Metamucil.

Hot, spicy herbs, such as red pepper and mustard, reportedly increase metabolism, which, in turn, causes more calories to be burned. Hot herbs also stimulate thirst. Researchers who observe weight-loss benefits from these herbs do not know if they are from the herbs' effect on metabolism or if they cause people to fill up on water and, therefore, ingest fewer calories.

The view that herbs are safe because they come from nature is misleading. When packaged in large, concentrated doses and taken as pills or supplements, they should be viewed as drugs with potential side effects. From a medicinal point of view, a major shortcoming of herbs is that they are classified as supplements and,

therefore, are not subjected to the same scientific testing as are FDA-approved drugs. The Federal Trade Commission (FTC) conducted a study on the claims of weight-loss adds, including the use of supplements and herbs, and found that 40 percent of them were definitely false and 55 percent of them were likely to be false.[50] Medical groups usually recommend that herbal weight-loss products be avoided.

Fasting

Fasting, or complete starvation, has been practiced throughout history. Traditionally, people fasted for religious reasons. Although fasting is still used to achieve spiritual enlightenment by some people, a growing number of people fast for dubious physical reasons: to lose weight, to detoxify their bodies of impurities, and to cure everything from allergies to chronic diseases. The physical benefits of fasting have not been demonstrated in carefully planned studies. Most people who are in good health can tolerate a 24-hour fast without a problem as long as they drink plenty of water. However, prolonged fasting can be harmful and even fatal.

Modified fasts that allow for fruit and vegetable juices in addition to water are generally safer. In terms of weight loss, however, fasting is not an effective strategy. Fasting is an extreme action. Like any extreme diet plan, when this one is over, the weight returns. If you are healthy and still choose to fast, don't fast for more than 24 hours and drink plenty of fluids. If you are taking medicines, consult your physician before fasting.[51]

Physical Activity

The optimal approach to weight loss combines mild caloric restriction with regular physical activity. A weight loss of 1 pound per week requires a caloric deficit of 3,500 calories, or 500 calories per day. This can be accomplished by the following:

- Reducing caloric intake by 500 calories per day
- Reducing daily caloric intake by 250 calories and increasing daily energy expenditure 250 calories or any combination that equates to 500 calories per day
- Increasing caloric expenditure via physical activity by 500 calories per day

The last option may be the most difficult for people who are obese or severely overweight. Initially, they may not be able to tolerate the frequency, duration, or intensity of exercise needed to achieve this energy level. A combination of caloric restriction and moderately intense physical activity is most likely to achieve the best result.[52]

Use of calories

One of the obvious benefits of physical activity is that it burns calories. Calories are consumed according to

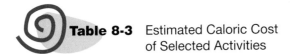

Table 8-3 Estimated Caloric Cost of Selected Activities

Activity	Calories/Min./Lb.*
Aerobic dance (vigorous)	0.062
Basketball (vigorous, full-court)	0.097
Bathing, dressing, undressing	0.021
Bed making (and stripping)	0.031
Bicycling (13 MPH)	0.071
Canoeing (flat water, 4 MPH)	0.045
Chopping wood	0.049
Cleaning windows	0.024
Cross-country skiing (8 MPH)	0.104
Gardening	
Digging	0.062
Raking	0.034
Weeding	0.038
Golf (twosome, carrying clubs)	0.045
Handball (skilled, singles)	0.078
Horseback riding (trot)	0.052
Ironing	0.029
Jogging (5 MPH)	0.060
Laundry (taking out and hanging)	0.027
Mopping floors	0.024
Peeling potatoes	0.019
Piano playing	0.018
Rowing (vigorous)	0.097
Running (8 MPH)	0.104
Sawing wood (crosscut saw)	0.058
Shining shoes	0.017
Shoveling snow	0.052
Snowshoeing (2.5 MPH)	0.060
Soccer (vigorous)	0.097
Swimming (55 yds./min.)	0.088
Table tennis (skilled)	0.045
Tennis (beginner)	0.032
Walking (4.5 MPH)	0.048
Writing while seated	0.013

* Multiply calories/min./lb. by your body weight in pounds and then multiply that product by the number of minutes spent in the activity.

body weight, so heavier people burn more calories per minute than do lighter people for the same activity. Table 8-3 presents the calorie consumption of some physical fitness activities and a few common physical activities. To use it, multiply your body weight by the coefficient in the calories/min./lb. column and then multiply this value by the number of minutes spent participating in the activity. For example, to determine the calories expended by a 170-pound person who walks at 4.5 MPH for 30 minutes, do the following:

1. Multiply body weight by calories/min./lb.:

$$170 \text{ lbs.} \times 0.048 \text{ calories/min./lb.}$$
$$= 8.16 \text{ calories/min.}$$

2. Multiply calories/min. by the exercise time in minutes:

$$8.16 \text{ calories/min.} \times 30 \text{ min.} = 244.8 \text{ calories}$$

If this person performs this exercise daily, 1 pound will be lost in approximately 14 days, or 25 pounds will be lost in 1 year, provided caloric intake is unchanged. The annual weight loss is calculated as follows:

$$3,500 \text{ calories/lb.} \div 245 \text{ calories/day} = 14.29 \text{ days/lb.}$$
$$365 \text{ days/year} \div 14.29 \text{ days/lb.} = 25.5 \text{ lbs./year}$$

Follow the example in Assessment Activity 8-2 and apply the directions to your situation or to a hypothetical situation.

Aerobic exercises, such as walking and cycling, contribute significantly to weight loss. The American College of Sports Medicine (ACSM) emphasizes consistency, adherence, and enjoyment, rather than intensity or mode of exercise when developing a weight-loss plan.[52] A good goal is one that requires an expenditure of 300 calories per day at least three times per week or 200 calories per day at least four times per week. Deconditioned people should start slowly and gradually progress according to the principles of exercise intensity, frequency, and duration discussed in Chapters 3 and 4 in this text. Complete Assessment Activity 8-4 to determine the number of minutes that you should devote to your favorite activities to burn a minimum of 300 calories.

Rather than monitoring calories expended through exercise, the National Academy of Sciences expresses its recommendation in terms of time spent in physical activity. Every person should set a goal of at least 60 minutes of moderate activity each day.[53] (See This Just In on page 286.) This is double the 30-minute recommendation of the surgeon general in 1996 and is motivated primarily by the trend toward excess weight and obesity in the United States. If you have a healthy weight, the original 30-minute recommendation will still be sufficient to provide health benefits. If you need to lose weight or if you have noticed a slow but steady weight gain that needs to be arrested, the 60-minute recommendation should be the goal. Sixty minutes may seem excessive but remember that the effects of exercise are cumulative. While a 60-minute workout may not be realistic for some people, four 15-minute sessions might be. For many people, moderately intense activities, such as a brisk walk, are optimal. The more you walk, the better (21 miles per week versus 9), and distance is more important than speed (walking 3 miles per day versus jogging 2 miles per day).[54,55] (See Just the Facts: Walking for Weight Loss, Weight Maintenance: Think "More Time" on page 272.) A 15-minute walk repeated four times throughout the day will satisfy the 60-minute recommendation and serve as a good strategy for weight loss and/or weight maintenance. For every hour a day devoted to physical activity, such as brisk walking, the risk of developing obesity and diabetes is reduced 24 and 34 percent, respectively.[56] Any physical activity above the amount normally done in a day is a bonus for weight control. Walking upstairs, mowing the lawn, and mopping floors can be combined with a structured exercise program to produce steady, safe weight loss.

If you are sedentary, walking 60 minutes a day may be too much at first. An initial goal of 30 minutes a day (in increments, if preferred) will provide a good foundation for progressively increasing time and distance until a 60-minute-a-day workout can be sustained.

Exercise stimulates metabolism

Basal metabolic rate (BMR) is the energy required to sustain life when the body is in a rested and fasted state. BMR is measured in calories and represents the energy needed to keep the heart, lungs, liver, kidneys, and all other organs functioning. More calories are used to maintain BMR than to perform any other function.

Metabolism is affected by age, gender, nervous system activity, secretions from endocrine glands, nutritional status, sleep, fever, climate, body surface area, and amount of muscle tissue. Because men have more muscle tissue than do women, their BMRs average 5 to 10 percent higher. See Assessment Activity 8-3 to learn how to estimate your BMR.

Muscle tissue stimulates metabolism. Therefore, physical activity is a key strategy for weight management. This is especially true for people as they get older (see Wellness for a Lifetime: Age and Weight Gain Do Not Have to Go Together). The single best way for someone to change his or her metabolic rate is by being more physically active.[57]

The key to weight control

Although scientifically controlled studies have not yet proven that physical activity is instrumental in losing weight, they provide compelling evidence of its importance in weight control and weight-loss maintenance. Most people who lose weight and keep it off exercise daily. Regular physical activity is one of the best predictors for those who are able to maintain weight loss over the long term.[17] Ninety percent of people who lose weight and keep it off do so because they are likely to be exercising enough to burn more than 1,500 calories a week.[58] Thus, although physical activity as a singular strategy has modest effects on weight loss, it is the key strategy for lifelong weight control. Stated more directly, weight maintenance gets easier when people exercise. More importantly, moderate exercise improves health and reduces the risk factors associated with morbidity and mortality for the obese just as it does for normal-weight people.

Exercise intensity and fat loss

In Chapter 6, a distinction is made between the intensity and duration of exercise and the accompanying use by the body of energy nutrients. In general, carbohydrates are the main source of energy for high-intensity exercise, and fat is the main source of energy for low-intensity exercise sustained for a prolonged time. (The body instinctively spares its protein reserve except when needed for activities of exceptional duration.) The fat-burning benefit of low-intensity exercise should be a source of encouragement for people trying to shed extra fat, making exercise a viable option for most people. Walking, gardening, yard work, housework, and golfing (assuming you're walking) burn fat calories.

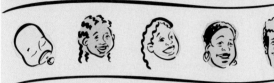

Wellness for a Lifetime

Age and Weight Gain Do Not Have to Go Together

Weight gain is one experience people ages 25 to 65 have in common. From the time people embark on their professional careers until the time they start thinking about retirement, they often experience creeping weight gain, sometimes obesity. Often they blame the aging process. But is creeping obesity a function of biological factors that are part of the aging process, or are other factors involved? Rather than aging, a higher standard of living may be responsible for such weight gain. A higher standard of living usually results in an easier, less active life. Improvements in standard of living go hand-in-hand with labor-saving devices that add convenience and save energy. Many experts believe that weight gain associated with increased age is a function of the subtle changes in metabolism caused by less muscle tissue, which is caused by less physical activity.

Metabolism is an important issue for the weight-conscious person, because 70 percent of our energy is expended to support basic life processes. Muscle tissue burns more energy at rest than does fat tissue, so changes in body composition that favor muscle tissue over fat tissue provide a calorie-burning advantage throughout the day. Conversely, changes in body composition that favor fat over muscle lower the body's metabolism and promote weight gain. Metabolism declines with age, primarily because of the physical inactivity and muscle loss that often accompany aging. The annual decrease in BMR beginning at 25 years of age, though imperceptible, has serious ramifications for weight management and accounts for a significant amount of the weight gained with age. The loss of muscle tissue is equal to 3 to 5 percent every decade after age 25. The subsequent decline in BMR produces changes in body composition. Exercise and physical activities are the keys to weight management because they increase or sustain muscle tissue, thus accelerating metabolism and using calories.

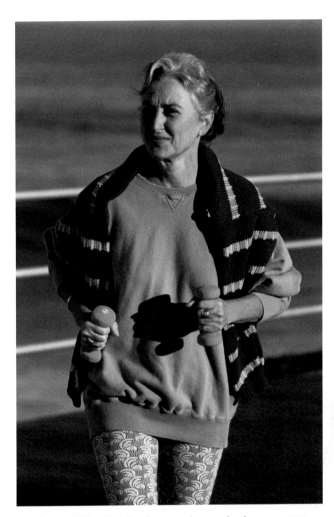

Physical activities that develop muscle can also increase your metabolism.

Does this mean that high-intensity exercises are of little value as a weight-management strategy? The answer is no, because the overall goal is to create a caloric deficit, and calories count regardless of exercise intensity. Physically demanding activities, such as jogging, running, rock climbing, swimming, cycling, and aerobics, burn more total calories than do low-intensity activities if participation time is held constant; they just require a higher proportion of fuel from glycogen stores than from fat. Still, both energy sources are tapped. For example, if you burn 200 calories exercising for a half hour at a low intensity, 41 percent of those calories come from fat, giving you a fat loss of 82 calories. If you exercise for the same amount of time at a high intensity, you burn 375 calories, including 90 fat calories, even though the percentage of energy supplied by fat is only 24 percent. The point of this example is not to discourage participation in low-intensity activities but only to suggest that, if you're in good health and enjoy vigorous exercise, you do not need to limit yourself to low-intensity exercise. Exercising on a consistent basis is the best strategy for managing weight, regardless of intensity level.

Regular Exercise Is the Key to Weight Management: Make It Fun

Whatever kind of exercise you do on a regular basis, it is the best strategy for weight management. If your motivation for exercise is based solely on external factors, such as losing weight or preventing disease, it is unlikely that exercise will become a permanent fixture in your lifestyle. Many experts believe that physical activity is more likely to become a lifestyle pattern if it is motivated by intrinsic factors, such as having fun, feeling pleasure, and feeling good. Losing weight is a good reason to start exercising, but you probably won't sustain exercise unless you learn to enjoy it and to value the way it makes you feel. People who are consistently physically active shift their focus from the outcome (weight loss) to the process of exercise. Regular exercisers want to work out because they like it and it makes them feel better.[59] (For tips on making exercise fun, see Nurturing Your Spirituality: Fun Is the Key to Regular Exercise for Weight Maintenance.) With this approach to exercise, even if weight loss is modest, overall health is improved.

Combining Dietary Modification and Exercise

Because caloric consumption and expenditure are involved in weight management, both should be manipulated to be effective. Combining sensible exercise and sensible changes in eating habits that can be maintained for life is the most effective approach to permanent weight management. Dieting alone can promote significant weight loss, but a substantial component of the weight loss may be lean tissue. Physical activity alone results in modest fat loss and an increase in lean body mass. Combination strategies involving both food restriction and physical activity meet the goals of weight management most effectively: These strategies improve body composition by promoting weight loss, fat loss, and lean-tissue gain.

Behavioral Effects

Some evidence suggests that obese people are more likely than normal-weight people to eat in response to external cues. A clock that says it is suppertime; media messages advertising food and beverages; and the sight, sound, and aroma of food are more apt to elicit eating behavior in the obese. This tendency is the basis of the "externality" hypothesis: If people can learn to eat in response to external cues, they can also learn to recognize cues that stimulate eating behavior, substitute other behaviors for eating, and use techniques that decrease the amount of food eaten. As a result of this training, the response to

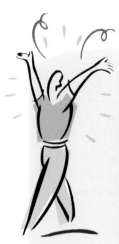

Nurturing Your Spirituality

Fun Is the Key to Regular Exercise for Weight Maintenance

Experts have shifted the paradigm of weight management from counting calories burned in exercise to promoting movement that is social, playful, and pleasurable. If exercise is fun, if it makes you feel good about yourself, and if it provides that mini-vacation each day (a time and place where nothing else interferes), it is more likely to be incorporated permanently into daily living. As noted by one expert, "Inner joy is the key to dutiful exercise. The body fails to persist if the soul is in rebellion."[59]

Do you want to move from an occasional, dreaded workout to one that you look forward to on a regular basis? Following are some tips passed on by others who once were couch potatoes:

- First, examine your likes and dislikes. Think in terms of activities that are fun for you. These may be taking a stroll in a park, working in a flower garden, skating to class, or joining a fitness club.

- Build relationships with people who share your interests and goals. Workout partners often provide incentive and encouragement for working out.

- Tell people if you notice improvements in their energy level and appearance after exercising. Not only will they feel better but so will you, and the compliment will likely be returned at some point.

- Join a fitness club or participate in a structured fitness program that will increase your repertoire of skills and activities.

- Find a comfortable workout environment with a supportive staff.

- Vary your activities. Variety is the antidote for boredom; cross-training is the key for many longtime exercisers.

external cues should be reduced and replaced by attention to internal hunger signals. Many techniques have been developed to assist people in resisting the tendency to eat indiscriminately or to overeat. Generally, these techniques use one or more of the following approaches:

1. *Self-monitoring:* A journal or daily log records food consumption, physical activities, and circumstances related to eating. In a recent study of dieters from two weeks before Thanksgiving until two weeks after New Year's, it was found that participants who were the most consistent in

Real-World Wellness

Behavioral Strategies for Reshaping Your Eating Habits

In Chapter 1, I learned about intervention strategies for changing behavior. In this chapter, I've learned about the importance of gaining control over the tendency to overeat. How can I apply behavioral principles from Chapter 1 to my goal of curbing overeating?

Try the following strategies:

- Eat in a certain place—not in every room of your home.
- Eliminate from your immediate environment all food that can be eaten without careful preparation.
- Always eat at a carefully set place at the table and eat only one helping of planned foods.
- Prepare only enough food for one meal.
- Eat slowly.
- Chew each bite 25 to 50 times.
- Set down your utensils after every mouthful.
- Partway through the meal, stop and relax without eating for two to three minutes.
- Leave some food on your plate at each meal.
- Plan to eat some meals alone. (There is a tendency to overeat in social situations.)
- Eat a carefully balanced diet, so that you are not deprived of a particular food element.

monitoring food intake were also the most successful in losing weight and keeping it off.[60]

2. *Control of precursors to eating:* The events and circumstances that elicit eating and overeating are identified.

3. *Control of eating:* Behavior modification techniques are used to control, change, or modify specific eating behaviors. (See Real-World Wellness: Behavioral Strategies for Reshaping Your Eating Habits.)

4. *Reinforcement through the use of rewards:* Rewards tied to the achievement of behavioral goals are identified and used.

These techniques may be useful especially if they are combined with sensible food choices and exercise.

Eating Disorders and Disordered Eating

Anorexia nervosa (anorexia) and bulimia nervosa (bulimia) are eating disorders familiar to most Americans. More recently, binge-eating disorder and female athlete triad have emerged as health issues that require professional intervention. Full-blown anorexia and bulimia are eating disorders; binge-eating disorder and female athlete triad usually involve disordered eating patterns. The major difference between the two types of conditions is that eating disorders meet certain criteria as outlined by the American Psychiatric Association. Disordered eating, on the other hand, entails mild and short-term changes in eating patterns that occur in relation to a stressful event, an illness, or even a desire to modify the diet for a variety of health and personal appearance reasons.[5] It may involve unnecessary dieting or occasional bingeing and purging.[61] While these conditions share some characteristics, each has some distinctive qualities.

Anorexia Nervosa

The chief characteristic of **anorexia nervosa** is a refusal to maintain a minimally normal weight for age and height. Refusal to eat is the hallmark of the disease, regardless of whether other practices, such as binge-purge cycles, occur. Although specific causes of anorexia have not been identified, a combination of biological, social, and psychological factors contributes to the disorder. Support for an organic influence has centered on the hypothalamus (the portion of the brain reputed to house the appetite center) and the pituitary gland (the master gland of the body). Sociocultural theories focus on the compulsion of adolescent girls to become and remain lean. This exaggerated goal manifests at a time when girls are naturally depositing fat.

Anorexia is characterized by extreme weight loss, amenorrhea (absence of a menstrual period), and a variety of psychological disorders culminating in an obsessive preoccupation with the attainment of thinness. Fortunately, most anorectics recover fully after one experience with the disease. However, the longer a person practices anorexic behaviors, the less the chance for recovery. Just the Facts: Criteria for Diagnosing Anorexia Nervosa (page 276) lists the criteria that have been developed by the American Psychiatric Association for diagnosing anorexia.[62]

When confronted, anorectics typically deny the existence of a problem and the weight-loss behaviors that have resulted in their emaciated physical appearance. They also avoid medical treatment, refuse the well-intended advice of family and friends regarding professional assistance, and submit to treatment only under protest. Anorexia is a subtle disease, and anorectics become secretive in their behaviors. They are evasive, and many hide their disease in deep denial even while undergoing treatment, making the diagnosis especially difficult.

The course of treatment for anorexia is complex, involving a coordinated effort by several health care

∿ Just the Facts ∿

Criteria for Diagnosing Anorexia Nervosa

The American Psychiatric Association[62] has identified the following criteria for a diagnosis of anorexia nervosa:

- Weight change
  - Unwillingness to maintain minimal normal body weight for the person's age and height
  - Weight loss that leads to the maintenance of a body weight that is 15 percent below normal
  - Failure to gain the amount of weight expected during a period of growth, resulting in a body weight that is 15 percent below normal
- Inordinate fear of gaining weight or becoming fat despite being significantly underweight
- Disturbed and unrealistic perceptions of body weight, size, or shape; feeling of being "fat" although emaciated; possible perception of one specific part of the body as "too fat"
- Absence of at least three menstrual cycles for women when they would normally be expected to occur (amenorrheic women have a normal menstrual cycle only during administration of hormone therapy)
- Rigid dieting; maintenance of rigid control in lifestyle; security found in control and order
- Rituals involving food and excessive exercise

Real-World Wellness

Helping a Friend Overcome an Eating Disorder

I suspect a friend of mine is struggling with an eating disorder. How can I help without making matters worse? Are there some Internet resources available?

Try doing the following:

- Talk to the person alone.
- Tell the person why you are concerned.
- Be nonjudgmental; ask clarifying questions; listen carefully.
- Offer to go with the person to talk to someone.
- Encourage him or her to verbalize feelings.
- Show how much you care by asking frequently how the person is doing.
- Show an interest in the person's life outside of eating.
- Enlist the help of a counselor if you think the disorder is severe; however, eating disorders are usually not emergency situations.
- Anticipate and accept that denial and anger are part of the illness.

Avoid doing the following:

- Threaten or challenge the person.
- Give advice about weight loss.
- Get into an argument.
- Try to keep track of the person's food consumption.
- Try to force the person to eat.
- Be patronizing by being overly caring.
- Try to be a hero or rescuer; the person may resent such efforts.

Following are some Internet sites that serve as good resources:

- Eating Disorders Awareness and Prevention, Inc., at **www.edap.org**
- National Eating Disorders Information Centre at **www.nedic.on.ca**
- American Dietetics Association at **www.eatright.org**
- The Center for Eating Disorders at **www.eatingdisorder.org**
- Pale Reflections Weekly Newsletter for Those with Eating Disorders at **www.members.aol.com/paleref/index.html**

specialists. Hospitalization is often required because anorectics may have to be fed intravenously or by some other method if they cannot or will not eat. Medications that stimulate the appetite and medications that calm the patient are usually necessary. Nutritional counseling and psychological counseling—individual, group, and family—are integral components of treatment (see Real-World Wellness: Helping a Friend Overcome an Eating Disorder). Finally, behavior modification techniques are used to help change the perceptions and lifestyle of the anorectic. At this point, no single treatment has proved to be unusually successful in the treatment of anorexic patients.

Bulimia Nervosa

Bulimia nervosa is characterized by alternate cycles of binge eating and restrictive eating. Binge eating is distinguished from ordinary overeating in that it involves the consumption of a large amount of food in a relatively

Criteria for Diagnosing Bulimia

The American Psychiatric Association[62] has identified the following criteria for a diagnosis of bulimia:

- Episodic secretive binge eating characterized by rapid consumption of large quantities of food in a short time; never overeating in front of others

- At least two eating binges per week for at least three months

- Loss of control over eating behavior while eating binges are in progress

- Frequent purging after eating; using techniques such as self-induced vomiting, laxatives, or diuretics; engaging in fasting or strict dieting; or engaging in vigorous exercise

- Constant and continual concern with body shape, size, and weight

- Erosion of teeth; swollen glands

- Purchase of syrup of ipecac

brief time (that is, within a one- to two-hour period) and is accompanied by lack of control. Bingeing is nearly always done in private; in public, the bulimic tends to eat normal or even less than normal amounts. Unlike the occasional splurge almost everyone has, the bulimic becomes compulsive and habitual and often resorts to secretive eating. Binges are usually followed by purging, primarily by self-induced vomiting supplemented with laxatives and diuretics. Some people with this disorder may purge excess energy by *hypergymnasia*, or excessive exercise. The physical ramifications of bulimia include esophageal inflammation, erosion of tooth enamel caused by repeated vomiting, and the possibility of electrolyte imbalances. Psychological ramifications include guilt, shame, self-disgust, anxiety, and depression.

The diagnostic criteria for bulimia are given in Just the Facts: Criteria for Diagnosing Bulimia.[62] These criteria specify that, to be diagnosed a bulimic, a person must vomit at least twice a week for three months. Binge-purge cycles may occur daily, weekly, or in other intervals. Bulimic behaviors range from binge eating frequently or from time to time, binge eating with a feeling of being unable to control food intake, severe restriction of the diet between binge periods, and binge eating followed by purging. Purging in the form of laxatives, vomiting, diuretics, fasting, and excessive exercise follows in the hope that weight gain will be blunted. Because many people with bulimia engage in binge-purge

practices in isolation and because bulimics are often not excessively thin, they cannot be diagnosed easily or by their appearance.

Bulimics are treated similarly to anorectics, except that hospitalization is usually not required. In addition to nutritional and psychological counseling, treatment often includes antidepressive medication because bulimia is associated with clinical depression. Treatment focuses on correcting typical bulimic behaviors, such as "all-or-none" thinking: "If I'm not perfect, I'm a failure, so one slipup—one cookie—justifies a binge." Generally, psychotherapy aims primarily to help a person with self-acceptance and to be less concerned with body weight.[5]

Binge-Eating Disorder

Binge-eating disorder is similar to bulimia in two ways: (1) It involves eating large amounts of food in a short time, and (2) it is accompanied by a sense of lack of control regarding eating. It is different from bulimia in that it is not associated with compensatory behaviors, such as purging, fasting, and excessive exercise. When binge eating occurs on average at least two days a week for six months, it becomes an eating disorder. The American Psychiatric Association has identified additional criteria for this disorder.[62] (See Just the Facts: Criteria for Diagnosing Binge-Eating Disorder.)

Criteria for Diagnosing Binge-Eating Disorder

The American Psychiatric Association[62] has identified the following criteria for a diagnosis of binge-eating disorder:

- Recurrent episodes of eating an amount of food clearly larger than most people would eat in a similar circumstance

- Binge eating that occurs, on average, at least two days a week for six months

- A sense of lack of control over eating

- Binge eating associated with any three of the following:

  - Eating large amounts of food when not feeling hungry

  - Eating alone because of embarrassment over the amount of food eaten

  - Eating much more rapidly than normal

  - Eating far beyond comfort level

  - Feeling guilty or depressed after eating

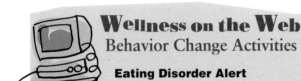

Wellness on the Web
Behavior Change Activities

Eating Disorder Alert

In today's appearance-focused culture, we're all familiar with the terms anorexia nervosa, bulimia nervosa, and binge eating. Although these eating disorders differ markedly from each other in many respects, people who have them share a common trait: an intense fear of becoming overweight. Does this describe you? Whether the answer is yes or no, go to www.mhhe.com/anspaugh6e to complete a self-test that will help you determine whether you have an eating disorder. Click on Student Center, Chapter 8, Wellness on the Web, and then Activity 1. The questions presented involve behaviors and feelings common to persons who have eating disorders. Whatever your results, remember that you and no one else are the final judge of whether you have an eating disorder. If you think you do, you'll find help and support from a wide array of reputable sources.

Boost Your Metabolism—Naturally!

Looking for the magic key to successful weight management? Magic or not, compelling evidence points to the importance of regular exercise in weight control and weight-loss maintenance. People who lose weight and keep it off almost always exercise daily. Studies that attempt to identify predictors of successful weight maintenance point to physical activity as one of the best markers for long-term success. Walking is considered an excellent form of exercise for shedding pounds. To calculate how many calories you burned walking, go to the Web site mentioned previously; then select Activity 2. Enter your weight and the duration of your walk; then select your approximate speed and click on "walk it off" to calculate your calories burned.

Female Athlete Triad

Female athlete triad is a condition marked by three characteristics: disordered eating, *amenorrhea* (lack of menstrual periods), and osteoporosis (low age-adjusted bone density).[5] It most often affects women athletes engaged in appearance-based, weight-based, and endurance sports. The components of the triad are interrelated. Typically the triad begins with disordered eating. Poor nutrition combined with intense training results in an energy deficit. In time, the energy deficit can cause the body to shut down the production of estrogen, which in turn can trigger amenorrhea. The lack of estrogen combined with nutritional deficiencies, particularly in calcium and vitamin D, may seriously compromise bone

density and increase the risk of contracting osteoporosis.[61] Some young women diagnosed with female athlete triad have bones equivalent to those of 50- to 60-year-olds, making them overly susceptible to fractures during both sports and general activities. Much of the bone loss is irreversible.[5] Women with this condition should seek professional help to reduce their preoccupation with food, weight, and body fat; to regain body weight; to establish regular menstrual cycles; and to increase their consumption of food.

Underweight

A small number of people who are not anorexic or bulimic are naturally thin, and some of them are dissatisfied with their appearance. Being underweight presents as much of a cosmetic problem for affected people as obesity does for the obese person. Many underweight people find it more difficult to gain a pound than it is for obese people to lose one.

In their attempts to gain weight, many lean people consume large quantities of food, particularly those rich in calories. Unfortunately, these foods are also high in fat and sugar. This eating pattern is unhealthy for anyone, regardless of body weight. The preferred approach is to combine muscle-building exercises with three well-balanced, nutritious meals supplemented by two nutritious snacks. Increasing caloric intake by 500 calories a day should yield a weight gain of about a pound a week. In doing so, emphasize calorie-rich foods from the Food Guide Pyramid. Whole-grain cereals with nuts and raisins and dried fruits are examples. Also emphasize foods that are good sources of monounsaturated fats. Examples include olive oil and canola oil. Finally, plan an exercise program that includes resistance training. Instead of gaining fat as calories are increased, muscle weight will be added.

The amount and type of weight gain should be closely monitored. Fat stores should not be increased unless the person is extremely thin and on the verge of dipping into stores of essential fat.

Principles of Weight Management: Putting It All Together

The best approach to weight management is the most obvious: maintaining a moderate lifestyle, so that excess weight is not gained. In summary, the basic principles of weight maintenance and weight loss are the following:

1. Avoid the obsession with body weight. Remember that body weight per se is not the most important issue; rather, body composition is. Modest weight gain distributed in the wrong places increases

health risks. Conversely, significant weight gain in the form of muscle tissue enhances health and well-being. You should consider losing weight if it becomes excessive or if you have a family history of disease that may be worsened by excess weight.

2. The most important factor in weight maintenance is physical activity. Americans weigh more now than ever because of sedentary lifestyles. The challenge is either to sacrifice some labor-saving devices and their convenience or to consciously seek opportunities to impose extra physical demands on the body. This may mean choosing the stairs rather than the elevator or walking to class rather than driving. Participating in physical activities on a consistent basis is the best way to prevent excessive weight gain. It is also the best way to maintain weight loss over time. Almost all people who successfully lose weight and keep it off exercise daily. Exercise is the best way to overpower the body's set point for fatness.

   Exercise is just as important to the chronically obese and overweight as it is to those who are trying to lose or maintain weight. Obese people who are fit enjoy the same health benefits as normal-weight people.

   The ACSM recommends a caloric deficit of 500 calories a day to lose 1 pound in a week. This can be achieved by reducing caloric intake by 250 calories and exercising to burn 250 calories. A 250-calorie workout is equivalent to a 2.5-mile walk for most people. Remember, energy expenditure through exercise does not have to occur at one time. The effects of physical activity are cumulative and reinforce the value of activity spread throughout the day. The key issue in exercising is consistency and moderation. Plan an activity program that can be sustained one year and five years from now.

   The National Academy of Sciences recommends a minimum of 60 minutes of physical activity each day (see This Just In on page 286). This can be in the form of a structured exercise program, lifestyle activities (such as housework and/or yard work), and play. It can be done in one setting or in multiple settings. The activity does not have to be intense. Walking at a brisk pace is a good strategy for weight loss and/or weight maintenance.

3. Follow the Mayo Clinic Healthy Weight Pyramid by eating nutrient-dense foods and stress consumption of fruits and vegetables. Calories from fat convert easily to fat, with only 3 percent being lost in the digestive process. By comparison, 25 percent of carbohydrate calories are lost in the process.

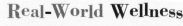

Real-World Wellness

Practical Tips for Coping with Supersized Foods

My friends and I enjoy eating out and prefer fast-food or casual dining restaurants. The local restaurants provide some supersized bargains that fit a college budget. My problem is that I am a volume eater—I eat what is served, usually much more than I need and certainly more than is good for my waistline. But I live on a tight budget and refuse to throw away good food. What are some strategies that will help me manage my tendency for volume eating without being wasteful?

Following are some suggestions for volume purchasing without waste:

- Eat what you need, not necessarily what is served. Take the rest home.

- Share an entrée, an appetizer, or dessert. This saves calories and money. (Some restaurants add a surcharge for sharing meals.)

- Start each day with a plan. Think first of your main meal and work around it. If you're planning a prime rib dinner, for example, favor vegetables and fruits for breakfast and lunch. One serving of prime rib is plenty of meat for one day.

- At a buffet, serve yourself small portions and eat slowly. Give your food time to digest. Emphasize vegetables and fruits in your food selections.

- Ask for a half order of an entrée.

- Order only appetizers.

- When grocery shopping, plan ahead. Make a list of the amount or quantity of each item to buy. Stick to your list.

- If you're watching calories, learn what makes a serving. One small fistful of candy, french fries, or nuts is a serving.

- Picture what you think is a reasonable serving before food is served. If more is served, take it home.

Emphasize fiber in your diet. Because of fiber's high satiety value, people who eat a great deal of it usually consume fewer total calories at mealtime. An added benefit is that fiber may help block the digestion of some of the fat consumed with it. The less fat digested, the less absorbed in the bloodstream.[5]

4. Avoid volume eating. (See Real-World Wellness: Practical Tips for Coping with Supersized Foods.) Calories count, regardless of their source. The

penchant to practice compensatory eating behavior may be especially common among people who choose low-fat and/or low-calorie products. People are eating food in larger quantities. Avoid buffet-style, all-you-can-eat restaurants. People eat more when they are served more.[63] Practice behavioral strategies that make volume eating more difficult. For example, split restaurant entrées with a friend or avoid the practice of cleaning your plate by taking leftovers home. When eating low-fat, low-carb, or low-calorie foods, be aware of the tendency to overcompensate by eating more food. Remember, two servings of a low-fat food that contains 5 grams of fat yields 90 total fat calories and may exceed the number of fat calories in one serving of the regular, high-fat version. The tendency to overcompensate by consuming more calories also applies to beverages. Liquid calories don't have the satiety value of solid food and often result in extra calories. Drink plenty of water and substitute calorie-free beverages or limit calorie-containing beverages.

5. Set realistic goals. Don't be misled by messages and advertisements that promise huge weight loss in a short time. Weight loss per week usually should not exceed 1 to 2 pounds. The ideal approach is to lose pounds at the same rate at which they were gained. In trying to set goals, ask yourself these questions: What is the least I have weighed as an adult, for at least a year? Based on past experiences, what is the most weight I can expect to lose? A weight goal set below your lowest weight or one that was achieved for only a brief period of time following a strenuous diet is not realistic. Adjust your goals upward from your minimum weight. A good goal is to lose 10 percent of your body weight. For a 200-pound person, a good weight loss goal is 20 pounds. Once 10 percent of excess weight is lost, go into maintenance for six months before trying to lose more weight.[5] Losing these first pounds produces the biggest health gains in lower blood pressure, lower blood cholesterol, and lower blood sugar. This is especially true for people with abdominal fat.

6. Make a gradual lifestyle change. Such change represents a calm, deliberate approach, rather than a frenetic "lose it now" attitude. A 200-pound person should exercise, reduce calories, and eat like a 180-pound person to become a 180-pound person. Once the weight is lost, the person must resist reverting to the habits of a 200-pound person. A diet is only successful if the weight does not return.

7. Anticipate a plateau. During the first week of a diet, weight loss comes primarily from loss of protein, glycogen, and water but little fat. As the body adjusts to a diet, fat loss increases. This adjustment takes about a week on a moderate diet and still longer when the diet is severe. Many dieters experience a plateau after about three to four weeks, not because they are suddenly cheating but because they have gained water weight while still losing body fat. If physically active, dieters may gain lean body mass and lose fat while maintaining weight. If weight loss is drastic during the early stages, it induces an adaptive response in the body that slows down metabolism. The body resists drastic change of any sort. Once its internal signals recognize a substantial reduction in caloric intake, it slows down to conserve fuel. After losing 20 to 30 pounds, expect to reach a stable plateau.

8. Avoid diet pills, special formula diets, all-you-can-eat diets, fat-burning concoctions, skin creams, and other fad diets. Some of these fads impose health risks, and others simply don't work; if they do, their results are temporary and lead to weight cycling. The more extreme the diet, the less likely the weight loss will be permanent.

The new generation of diet pills currently being investigated as a potential solution for the chronically obese should be viewed with caution. Even if such pills prove successful, they must be taken for life, and they may have side effects as harmful to health as the extra weight. Many experts are reluctant to endorse a lifelong pharmaceutical solution to obesity.

9. Avoid very low-calorie diets. Such diets decrease RMR up to 20 percent, making weight loss success even harder.[64] The reduction in RMR may partly account for the plateau mentioned in number 7. Diets that cut calories to under 1,200 (if you're a woman) or 1,400 (if you're a man), however, do not allow enough food to be satisfying over the long haul and are unlikely to meet the body's needs for nutrients. Remember, if you can't lose weight at the 1,200- or 1,400-calorie level, you probably don't need to.

10. Develop an eating plan that includes easily obtained foods.

11. Develop a less rigid lifestyle, one that reduces the need to consciously control what is eaten. Maintaining weight loss is the antithesis of counting every calorie. Also, it doesn't matter what time of the day calories are consumed. A calorie is a calorie, regardless of the time (see Just the Facts: A Calorie Is a Calorie).

12. Avoid fasting and restrictive dieting. These practices often lead to a preoccupation with food, weight, and/or dieting. Dieting should allow people to attend parties, eat at restaurants, and participate in normal activities. People erroneously

〰️Just the Facts〰️

A Calorie Is a Calorie

A common misconception is that eating at night facilities weight gain. If this is true, it is because of the amount of calories consumed at night, not the time. When researchers gave overweight women 70 percent of their calories either before noon or closer to dinnertime, it didn't affect their body fat. In a large survey of almost 2,000 people, how much people ate in the evening had no bearing on the extent of their change in weight over 10 years.[68] The body doesn't distinguish between calories consumed in the morning and those consumed at night. A calorie is a calorie.

assume that, if they have eaten just a little bit of a forbidden food, they have crossed the line. Foods are neither good nor bad. Labeling them as such often promotes a denial-guilt-preoccupation cycle, in which one slight deviation from a diet or food choice is interpreted as a failure: A forbidden food is eaten (denial), a sense of relief from restraint leads to a binge, the binge leads to guilt and a feeling of failure, and both denial and guilt exacerbate the preoccupation. The preoccupation leads back to denial and the cycle continues. This cycle exerts considerable pressure on the dieter. To avoid the dissonance that comes with failure, the dieter often abandons attempts to lose weight. Given moderation and discretion, almost any food can be enjoyed. Food is one of life's pleasures, so you need not avoid any one food. If it is high in fat and calories, eat a small portion. If you do not deny yourself, you might not feel compelled to cheat.

13. Avoid meal skipping. One strategy that surprises some dieters with its effectiveness is eating frequent small meals and snacks. The more often a person eats, the less hungry that person feels and the less food that person will eat.[65] Eating five or six times a day—breakfast, a midmorning snack, lunch, an afternoon snack, dinner, and a before-bed snack— might require some retraining. Keep portions small and emphasize fruits and vegetables.

    Resist the temptation to skip breakfast. People who eat a healthy breakfast generally feel less hungry throughout the day and consume fewer calories by the time the day is over.[66,67]

14. Form a buddy system or join a support group. The support and encouragement of a friend or relative are often the difference between success and failure.

15. If you stop smoking, don't be discouraged by subsequent weight gain. If you are a heavy smoker, you can expect on average an increase in weight of 10 pounds. That's not enough to make most smokers obese. From a health perspective, you would have to gain 100 to 150 pounds after quitting to make your health risks as high as when you smoked.[69]

16. Don't indulge yourself in self-blame for past failures. View past dieting attempts objectively as a psychologist would. Focus more on what you learned from past experiences. Most people who are successful at maintaining weight loss are not successful in their first attempt. In studies that track dieters listed in the Weight Control Registry, 90 percent of them are repeaters. In some studies, nearly 60 percent of dieters were found to have made five attempts before achieving success.[60] Rather than blaming yourself, reflect on what you learned about yourself and what worked and didn't work.

17. Weight maintenance may be a more appropriate goal than weight loss. Most people gain weight slowly and progressively over time. The first step (and the only step) for many people creeping into obesity is to stop the pattern of weight gain by stabilizing at the present weight. Weight maintenance, or weight stability, can usually be achieved with slight changes in lifestyle (see Just the Facts: Ten Ways to Cut Back 100 Calories a Day on page 282). Even if weight loss becomes necessary, a history of weight maintenance provides a benchmark for future efforts.

18. Develop your own plan for losing weight. You don't need to enroll in an expensive program. In a study of more than 32,000 dieters, researchers found that those who kept off at least 10 percent of their starting weight for at least a year created their own eating plans. They didn't buy food supplements or follow the advice of a diet guru. They ate lean protein, small quantities of healthful fats, fiber-rich grains and legumes, and plenty of fruits and vegetables, and they exercised regularly.[71]

19. Finally, accept yourself. Before trying to lose weight, determine how great a risk your weight poses to your health. People at risk for chronic conditions, such as hypertension and Type 2 diabetes, for example, often improve dramatically with a modest weight loss. Some people, however, are overweight despite their best efforts to reduce. For such people, striving to attain a certain weight may be futile and even damaging to health. If a person was overweight throughout childhood, chances are that person will never be thin. Be realistic and aim for a healthy weight for you, not for an actor or actress. Not everyone can be skinny. Everyone can try to be healthy.

Just the Facts

Ten Ways to Cut Back 100 Calories a Day

The recommended caloric deficit of 500 calories per day is standard advice for weight-loss programs. What about people trying to achieve weight maintenance or people who are in no hurry to lose weight? A caloric deficit of just 100 calories can result in weight loss, although it takes longer. On the positive side, a deficit of 100 calories is hardly noticeable and is sustainable. The highly respected newsletter *Environmental Nutrition* provides 20 ways to cut 100 calories a day.[70] Following are 10 of them. You can identify many more by comparing the caloric content on food package labels.

1. Substitute 2 tablespoons of jam instead of butter or margarine (100 vs. 200 calories).
2. Order an egg sandwich without the cheese (105 calories per slice).
3. Choose tuna packed in water instead of oil (175 vs. 275 calories per 6 ounces).
4. Substitute fat-free mayo in place of regular mayo (100 vs. 200 calories per 2 tablespoons).
5. Order a 12-ounce (small) beverage in place of a 21-ounce (medium) beverage (110 vs. 210 calories) or choose a sugar-free beverage (0 vs. 210 calories).
6. Choose a medium-sized baked potato over a large one (160 vs. 278 calories).
7. Enjoy two Haagen Dazs chocolate bars in place of 1/2 cup of gourmet ice cream (160 vs. 230 calories).
8. Order a McDonald's regular cheeseburger instead of a Quarter Pounder (330 vs. 430 calories).
9. Snack on a small handful of cashews instead of a large handful (163 calories for 18 nuts vs. 273 for 30 nuts).
10. Make an omelet without the egg yolks (33 vs. 149 calories for two large eggs).

Summary

- Americans' obsession with body weight is evidenced by the large number of women, men, and even children who are unhappy with their physical appearance and willing to subject themselves to elective surgery to improve some aspect of their body.
- A healthy weight is defined as a BMI of 18.5 to 24.9. Overweight occurs with a BMI of 25 or over. Obesity occurs with a BMI of 30 or over. Extreme, or morbid, obesity occurs when BMI is 40 or higher. By these standards, nearly two-thirds of Americans are overweight or obese.
- Obesity is a risk factor for coronary heart disease, stroke, hypertension, LDL cholesterol, some forms of cancer, impaired glucose tolerance, osteoarthritis, gallbladder disease, and sleep apnea.
- Experts believe that obesity will soon overtake tobacco as the leading preventable cause of premature death in the United States.
- Obesity occurs when fat cells increase excessively, either in size (hypertrophy) or in number (hyperplasia). Most obesity is adult-onset and caused by hypertrophy.
- Heredity and set point are the major biological factors associated with obesity.
- The development and distribution of body fat are under substantial genetic control.
- The classic types of body shapes are ectomorph, endomorph, and mesomorph. Ectomorphs have a low capacity for fat storage; endomorphs have a larger capacity for fat storage; and mesomorphs fall somewhere in between ectomorphs and endomorphs.

- Physical activity is the best way to alter the body's set point for fatness.
- Overeating and lack of physical activities are the major behavioral explanations of obesity.
- Restaurants serve food in larger portions than ever before and Americans are eating more than ever before. People eat more when they are served more food. Portion sizes and volume eating contribute significantly to the high caloric intake of Americans.
- The abundance of food high in fat and calories is a major factor in the prevalence of obesity in the United States.
- Dietary fat has less of a thermic effect than do carbohydrate and protein and therefore is more efficiently and easily stored as fat tissue.
- The general decline in physical activity is highly correlated with the rise in obesity.
- Engaging in a physically active lifestyle is the best way to prevent weight gain.
- Approximately 70 percent of the energy liberated from food is expended to support BMR.
- Physical activity improves body composition, increases BMR, improves insulin sensitivity, and increases oxygen capacity and glycogen storage in muscles.
- Weight loss requires a caloric deficit in which food intake and exercise are manipulated, so that caloric expenditure exceeds caloric intake.
- For many people, weight maintenance, or weight stability, is a better goal than weight loss. Because weight-maintenance approaches usually involve only modest changes in lifestyle,

they are sustainable and help curb the tendency toward creeping obesity.

- Complex forces influence the success of weight-loss efforts and help explain why people respond so differently to similar dieting strategies.
- Low-fat diets often result in overcompensatory eating behaviors, as a result of which the dieter ends up consuming more total calories.
- A desirable long-term goal for losing weight is 1 to 2 pounds per week until about 10 percent of excess weight is lost. A six-month maintenance period is suggested before more weight loss is attempted.
- Diet-only strategies should provide a loss of at least 1,200 calories per day for women and 1,400 for men.
- Low-carbohydrate diets are the most common diet strategy of Americans. Research from the medical community suggests that people lose weight and improve their blood fat profile by limiting their intake of carbohydrates. People who lose weight on low-carbohydrate diets do so because they consume fewer calories. Criticisms of low-carbohydrate diets are that they don't discriminate between types of fat and they limit the intake of many foods (fruits and vegetables) that are good for health.
- Foods with a low Glycemic Index (e.g., whole-wheat bread) have an advantage over foods with a high Glycemic Index (e.g., white, refined bread) because they are digested more slowly, cause less of a surge in blood sugar and insulin, and don't cause an increase in appetite.
- The optimal approach to weight loss combines mild caloric restriction with regular physical activity. Together these

two strategies should provide a caloric deficit of 500 calories per day.

- In structuring a diet to lose weight, follow the recommendations in the Mayo Clinic Healthy Weight Pyramid. Emphasize fruits and vegetables. Observe recommended servings for carbohydrates, protein sources, and fats.
- Diet drugs include fat inhibitors, appetite suppressants, and antidepressants. New drugs that influence cravings are currently being studied. Diet drugs are not intended for people who are overweight or only marginally obese. The harmful effects of long-term use of diet drugs may outweigh the health benefits of losing weight.
- The National Academy of Sciences recommends that Americans accumulate a minimum of 60 minutes of physical activity each day.
- Low-intensity exercises sustained for a prolonged period are effective in burning fat calories. However, regardless of intensity level, exercising on a consistent basis is the best strategy for managing weight.
- Surgery to reduce weight is called bariatric surgery. When the purpose of surgery is to reduce the size of the stomach, it is called gastroplasty. Surgery is recommended as a last resort for people classified as morbidly obese and for people with significant complications of obesity.
- Liposuction is a cosmetic procedure used to remove fat deposits. It yields no proven health benefits.
- Anorexia, bulimia, binge eating, and female athlete triad are four potentially destructive eating disorders and/or disordered eating patterns with complex causes.

Review Questions

1. What evidence exists to support the idea that Americans are obsessed with weight control?
2. In terms of BMIs, what are the definitions of *healthy weight*, *overweight*, and *obesity*?
3. What health problems and chronic conditions are associated with obesity?
4. What is the relationship between obesity and morbidity and mortality?
5. What are the major biological and behavioral factors that help explain obesity?
6. What evidence can you use to support the existence of an influential role of heredity in the development of obesity?
7. What does the term *set point* mean in reference to body shape and body weight? What strategy is best for altering a person's set point for fatness?
8. What dieting strategies need to be emphasized in weight-loss programs?
9. Why are more Americans overweight today than in the past, especially when considering that there has been a drop in the percent of calories from fat consumption?
10. What are the major differences between the dietary recommendations in the Food Guide Pyramid and those in the Mayo Clinic Healthy Weight Pyramid?
11. Compare and contrast dieting and exercise as strategies for (a) losing weight and (b) maintaining weight or preventing weight gain.
12. What is weight cycling?
13. Why is the thermic effect of food an important issue in weight management?
14. Explain the relationship among blood sugar, insulin response, low- and high-Glycemic-Index foods, and appetite.
15. What are the pros and cons of low-carbohydrate diets?
16. What is the National Academy of Sciences recommendation regarding exercise and physical activity? How does it compare with previous recommendations from the surgeon general?
17. What is the relationship among BMR, physical activity, and body composition?
18. What are the differences and similarities among anorexia, bulimia, binge eating, and female athlete triad?
19. What guiding principles should be observed in planning a reasonable approach to weight loss/weight management?

References

1. Veale, D. 2004. Body dysmorphic disorder. *Postgraduate Medical Journal* 80(940):67–72.

2. Tiggemann, M., and D. Hargreaves. 2003. The effect of "thin ideal" television commercials on body dissatisfaction and schema activation during early adolescence. *Journal of Youth and Adolescence* 32(5):367–74.

3. Mayo Foundation for Medical Education and Research. 1998. Body image: What do you see in the mirror? (www.mayohealth.org/mayo/9704/htm/body_ima.htm).

4. Federal Interagency Forum on Child and Family Statistics. 2004. *America's children in brief: Key national indicators of well-being.* Federal Interagency Forum on Child and Family Statistics. Washington, DC: U.S. Government Printing Office.

5. Wardlaw, G., J. Hampl, and R. DiSilvestro. 2004. *Perspectives in nutrition.* 6th ed. New York: McGraw-Hill.

6. Molla, M. T., J. H. Madans, D. K. Wagener, and E. M. Crimmins. 2003. *Summary measures of population health: Report of findings on methodologic and data issues.* Hyattsville, MD: National Center for Health Statistics.

7. American Obesity Association. 2004. AOA fact sheets (www.obesity.org/subs/fastfacts/obesity_US.shtml).

8. American Obesity Association. 2004. AOA fact sheets (www.obesity.org/subs/fastfacts/childhood/prevalence.shtml).

9. Lethbridge-Cejku, M., J. S. Schiller, and L. Bernadel. 2004. *Summary health statistics for U.S. adults: National health interview survey, 2002.* Hyattsville, MD: National Center for Health Statistics.

10. Harvard Medical School. 2003. Top 10 health stories of 2003. *Harvard Health Letter* 29(2):1.

11. Peterson, M., S. Goodwin, and D. Ellenberg. 2004. Analysis of the American Cancer Society's generation fit project. *American Journal of Health Education* 35(3):141–44.

12. U.S. Department of Health and Human Services. 2000. *Healthy people 2010.* 2d ed. With *Understanding and improving health and objectives for improving health.* 2 vols. Washington, DC: U.S. Government Printing Office.

13. Mokdad, A. H., J. S. Marks, D. F. Stroup, and J. L. Garberding. 2004. Actual causes of death in the United States, 2000. *Journal of the American Medical Association* 291(10): 1238–45.

14. Wilder, L. B., L. J. Cheskin, and S. Margolis. 2004. *The Johns Hopkins white papers: Nutrition and weight control for longevity.* New York: Medletter.

15. Welland, D. 2003. Researchers at international summit cite new links between diet and cancer. *Environmental Nutrition* 26(9):1, 4.

16. American Alliance for Health, Physical Education, Recreation and Dance. 1999. Fit or fat may not fit. *Physical Activity Today* 5(1): 1.

17. Nieman, D. C. 2003. *Exercise testing and prescription: A health-related approach.* 5th ed. New York: McGraw-Hill.

18. Wardlaw, G. M. 2003. *Contemporary nutrition: Issues and insights.* 5th ed. New York: McGraw-Hill.

19. Tufts Media. 2003. Do the extra pounds result from too much food or too little exercise? *Tufts University Health and Nutrition Letter* 21(2):3.

20. Tufts Media. 2003. You underestimate calorie intake, but by how much? *Tufts University Health and Nutrition Letter* 21(9):2.

21. Consumers Union. 2004. Cut the fat. *Consumer Reports* 69(1):12–16.

22. Environmental Nutrition. 2003. EN asks the experts how to put the brakes on runaway portion sizes. *Environmental Nutrition* 26(3):1, 4.

23. Center for Science in the Public Interest. 2001. 10 mega trends. *Nutrition Action Healthletter* 28(1):3, 6–10.

24. Liebman, B. 1998. Supersize foods, supersize people. *Nutrition Action Healthletter* 25(6):6.

25. Harvard Medical School. 2001. Weight loss and gain. *Harvard Health Letter* 26(5):1–3.

26. Harvard Medical School. 2004. Obesity in the extreme. *Harvard Health Letter* 29(5):4–5.

27. Consumers Union. 2002. The truth about dieting. *Consumer Reports* 67(6):25–31.

28. Mayo Foundation for Medical Education and Research. 2001. Healthy weight: A process of changing your lifestyle habits. *Mayo Clinic Health Letter* 19(1):1–2.

29. *Environmental Nutrition.* 1999. Yo-yo dieting danger? *Environmental Nutrition* 22(5):3.

30. Liebman, B. 1997. Fooled by low-fat. *Nutrition Action Healthletter* 24(3):2.

31. *Environmental Nutrition.* 2002. Low-fat foods find little favor among weight-loss experts. *Environmental Nutrition.* 25(8):3.

32. Liebman, B. 2000. Diet vs. diet: Battle of the bulge doctors. *Nutrition Action Healthletter* 27(4):9–13.

33. Goldblatt, B. I. 1997. Advertisers get away with incredible weight-loss claims; how not to succumb. *Environmental Nutrition* 21(1):3.

34. Harvard Medical School. 2003. Is the Atkins diet on to something? *Harvard Health Letter* 28(7):1–2.

35. Physician's Committee for Responsible Medicine. 2003. Atkins diet alert (www.pcrm.org).

36. Consumers Union. 2003. Carbohydrates without fear. *Consumer Reports on Health* 15(10):1, 4.

37. *Environmental Nutrition.* 2003. Calories do count more than carbohydrates. *Environmental Nutrition* 26(5):1.

38. Harvard Medical School. 2004. Low carb vs. low fat. *Harvard Health Letter* 29(10):4.

39. Massachusetts Medical Society. 2004. More on low-carb diets. *HealthNews* 10(7):13.

40. *Environmental Nutrition.* 2003. Atkins diet gains some credibility, but long-term safety still a concern. *Environmental Nutrition* 26(2):3.

41. Massachusetts Medical Society. 2003. Low-carb diet lowdown. *HealthNews* 9(7):1–2.

42. Harvard Medical School. 2003. Top 10 health stories of 2003. *Harvard Health Letter* 29(2):3.

43. Tufts Media. 2003. Low-carb craze, or low-carb crazy? *Tufts University Health and Nutrition Letter* 21(8):4–5.

44. Consumers Union. 2004. Low-carb diet hazard. *Consumer Reports on Health* 16(7):7.

45. Peck, P. 2004. A new "wonder" drug for weight loss? Study shows losing pounds and inches is easier with experimental diet drug. *WebMD Medical News* (www.webmd.com/content/article/93/102335.htm).

46. Columbia University Department of Surgery. 2004. Surgical options (www.columbiasurgery.org/divisions/obesity/surgical_roux.html).

47. Klein, S., L. Fontana, L. Young, A. Coggan, C. Kilo, B. Patterson, & S. Mohammed. 2004. Absence of an effect of liposuction on insulin action and risk factors for coronary heart disease. *New England Journal of Medicine* 350(25):2549–57.

48. Consumers Union. 2004. Revived hope for fighting fat. *Consumer Reports on Health* 16(9):7.

49. Consumers Union. 2004. Heart dangers in disguise. *Consumer Reports* 69(1):22–23.

50. Welland, D. 2003. Protecting yourself against misleading supplement claims. *Environmental Nutrition* 26(9):8.

51. *Environmental Nutrition*. 1997. Fasting for health offers few benefits, questionable safety. *Environmental Nutrition* 20(5):7.

52. American College of Sports Medicine. 2000. *ACSM's guidelines for exercise testing and prescription*. 6th ed. Philadelphia: Lippincott Williams and Wilkins.

53. Mayo Foundation for Medical Education and Research. 2003. Exercise and your health. *Mayo Clinic Health Letter* 21(4): 1–3.

54. Kraus, W., J. Houmard, B. Duscha, K. Knetzger, M. Wharton, S. McCartney, C. Bales, S. Henes, G. Samsa, J. Otvos, K. Kulkarni, & C. Slentz. 2002. Effects of the amount and intensity of exercise on plasma lipoproteins. *New England Journal of Medicine* 347(19): 1483–92.

55. Tufts Media. 2003. Note to women: Thinner, healthier, and longer life within easy reach. *Tufts University Health and Nutrition Letter* 21(9):4.

56. Consumers Union. 2003. Lose the remote control. *Consumer Reports on Health* 15(6):2.

57. *Environmental Nutrition*. 2004. The bottom line on boosting metabolism: Exercise works best. *Environmental Nutrition* 27(6):7.

58. Liebman, B. 1999. Ten tips for staying lean. *Nutrition Action Healthletter* 27(6):1, 3–7.

59. White, D. 1999. Inner joy is key to dutiful exercise. *The Commercial Appeal* 160(4):C1–3.

60. Tufts Media. 1998. What it takes to take off weight [and keep it off]. *Tufts University Health and Nutrition Letter* 15(11):4–5.

61. Furia, J. 2001. The female athlete triad. *Medscape Orthopaedics and Sports Medicine* (www.medscape.com/medscape/Orthosportsmed/journal).

62. American Psychiatric Association. 1994. *Diagnostic and statistical manual of mental disorders*. 4th ed. Washington, DC: American Psychiatric Association.

63. Consumers Union. 2003. Quit the clean-plate club. *Consumer Reports on Health* 15(9):20.

64. American College of Sports Medicine. 2001. *ACSM's resource manual for guidelines for exercise testing and prescription*. 4th ed. Philadelphia: Lippincott Williams and Wilkins.

65. Consumers Union. 2000. Secrets of successful losers. *Consumer Reports on Health* 12(1):1, 3–4.

66. Tufts Media. 2004. For your weight control effort, breakfast. *Tufts University Health and Nutrition Letter* 22(1):1, 7.

67. *Environmental Nutrition*. 2004. Calories eaten in the a.m. affect appetite in the p.m. *Environmental Nutrition* 27(5):3.

68. Tufts Media. 1999. Hungry an hour after eating Chinese food. *Tufts University Health and Nutrition Letter* 17(8):4–5.

69. Tufts Media. 1996. If you want to quit smoking but fear the weight gain. *Tufts University Health and Nutrition Letter* 13(11):6–7.

70. *Environmental Nutrition*. 2003. More leisurely weight loss: 20 ways to cut 100 calories a day. *Environmental Nutrition* 26(1):8.

71. Consumers Union. 2002. Dieting? Do it your way. *Consumer Reports on Health* 14(11):3.

Suggested Readings

Fletcher, A. 2003. *Thin for life: 10 keys to success from people who have lost weight and kept it off*. Boston: Houghton Mifflin.

Anne M. Fletcher, nationally known health writer and former executive editor of *Tufts University Health and Nutrition Letter*, highlights keys to success for losing weight and keeping it off. Her advice is based on observations and case histories of people who have been successful. Rather than dwelling on why people fail, the book provides insights into how people succeed. The book also includes 150 recipes for shaving calories and fat grams.

Nieman, D. C. 2003. *Exercise testing and prescription: A health-related approach*. 5th ed. New York: McGraw-Hill.

In this text, a separate chapter is devoted to the relationship of physical activity and obesity. The author provides a comprehensive review of the literature on physical activity and obesity, citing more than 300 studies. Concepts, issues, and misconceptions are thoroughly discussed and documented.

Rolls, B., and R. Barnett. 2000. *The volumetrics weight-control plan: Feel full on fewer calories*. New York: HarperCollins. Editors of the highly respected newsletter *Tufts University Health and Nutrition Letter* claim that this book is one of the three best diet books on the market. It makes no sensational promises; it contains no gimmicks; instead, it treats readers respectfully. Its premise is that people eat about the same weight of food every day, regardless of caloric intake. Lower the calorie content of your meals by choosing foods with bulk and fiber, and weight will drop without your going hungry.

Wardlaw, G., J. Hampl, and R. DiSilvestro. 2004. *Perspectives in nutrition*. 6th ed. New York: McGraw-Hill.

This is a comprehensive reference text on nutrition, with separate chapters on dieting, weight control, and eating disorders.

Wilder, L., L. Cheskin, and S. Margolis. 2004. *The Johns Hopkins white papers: Nutrition and weight control for longevity*. Palm Coast, FL: Medletter.

Designed for the lay public, this monograph presents an overview of issues related to nutrition and weight loss, compares popular weight-loss methods, describes medical conditions that may cause obesity, and outlines lifestyle treatments for weight loss. This monograph is updated annually.

☆ This Just In

Physical activity as a strategy for weight maintenance takes on added emphasis in the recently published update of *Dietary Guidelines for Americans, 2005*. New guidelines confirm that obesity is epidemic in the United States and does not discriminate among race, ethnicity, age, or gender. Eating fewer calories while increasing physical activity is the key to controlling body weight.

Three recommendations in the new dietary guidelines that relate specifically to obesity include the following:

- To reduce the risk of chronic disease in adulthood: Engage in at least 30 minutes of moderate-intensity physical activity, above usual activity, at work or home on most days of the week.

- To help manage body weight and prevent gradual, unhealthy body weight gain in adulthood: Engage in approximately 60 minutes of moderate- to vigorous-intensity activity on most days of the week while not exceeding caloric intake requirements.

- To sustain weight loss in adulthood: Participate in at least 60 to 90 minutes of daily moderate-intensity physical activity while not exceeding caloric intake requirements.

These recommendations address three issues: reduction of chronic diseases, prevention of obesity, and weight maintenance. Thirty minutes of physical activity is recommended to help reduce the risk of chronic diseases. While 30 minutes of physical activity is good for health, it is not sufficient to prevent gradual weight gain and creeping obesity. For this reason, new guidelines bump the physical activity prescription to 60 minutes. However, to sustain weight loss for previously overweight/obese people, about 60 to 90 minutes of moderate-intensity physical activity per day is recommended. This is 30 to 60 minutes longer than that of previous recommendations. The increase in time devoted to physical activity acknowledges the difficulty that previous overweight/obese people have in maintaining weight loss, and it provides a way to compensate for the typical weight gain that occurs when the body adapts to the new weight (see discussion on Set Point Theory on page 257).

SOURCE: U.S. Department of Health and Human Services and U.S. Department of Agriculture. 2005. *Dietary guidelines for Americans, 2005*. 6th ed. Washington, DC: U.S. Government Printing Office.

Name _____ **Date** _____ **Section** _____

Assessment Activity 8-4

Assessing Calorie Costs of Activities

According to the ACSM, optimal weight-loss benefits are derived from activities that burn 300 calories per activity session. The purpose of this assessment is to determine the amount of time required to expend 300 calories.

Directions: Following are listed the caloric costs for three activities (see Table 8-3). Add seven activities of your choice from Table 8-3 and complete the information required in each column to determine the amount of time required to burn 300 calories. An example is provided for a person weighing 180 pounds who walks at a rate of 4.5 MPH.

Activity	Caloric Cost/Min./Lb.	×	Weight	=	Calories/Min.	300 Calories/Min.	=	Recommended Workout Time
Example (180-lb. person):								
1. Walking	0.048	×	180	=	8.64	300 / 8.64	=	34.7 min.
Personal assessment:								
1. Walking	0.048	×		=		300 /	=	
2. Aerobic dance	0.062	×		=		300 /	=	
3. Raking	0.034	×		=		300 /	=	
4.		×		=		300 /	=	
5.		×		=		300 /	=	
6.		×		=		300 /	=	
7.		×		=		300 /	=	
8.		×		=		300 /	=	
9.		×		=		300 /	=	
10.		×		=		300 /	=	

9

Coping with and Managing Stress

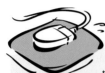

Online Learning Center

Log on to our Online Learning Center (OLC) for access to these additional resources:

- Chapter key term flashcards
- Learning objectives
- Additional goals for behavior change
- Concentration game
- Self-scoring chapter quizzes

- Additional lab activities

The OLC also offers Web links for study and exploration of wellness topics. Access these links through **www.mhhe. com/anspaugh6e**, click on Student Center, click on Chapter 9, and then click on Web Activities.

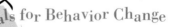

Goals for Behavior Change

- Identify your personal sources of stress.
- View stress as holding potential for personal growth.
- Develop a time management plan.
- Select strategies for managing stress.
- Put into action a stress management plan.

Key Terms

coping
distress
eustress
general adaptation
  syndrome (GAS)

psychoneuroimmunology
  (PNI)
relaxation techniques
stress
stressor

Objectives

After completing this chapter, you will be able to do the following:

- Define *stress.*
- Identify potential stressors.
- Describe the various types of stress.

- Describe the stages of the general adaptation syndrome (GAS).
- Explain the body's physiological response to stress.
- List the short- and long-term health effects of stress.
- Identify strategies that effectively deal with stress.

Stress profoundly affects people's lives. Everyone—students, businesspeople, parents, athletes—lives with stress. Stress is frequently viewed as an enemy. This is a misconception. Stress is often neither positive nor negative. How people deal with or react to what they perceive as stress is what determines its effect on their lives. As has been stated, "It is often said that stress is one of the most destructive elements in people's daily lives, but that is only a half truth. The way we react to stress appears to be more important than the stress itself."[1] The effects of stress can be either positive or negative. Positively used, stress can be a motivator for an improved quality of life. Viewed negatively, it can be destructive.

What Is Stress?

Dr. Hans Selye was the first to define the term *stress* as the "nonspecific response of the body to any demands made upon it." It can be characterized by diverse reactions, such as muscle tension, acute anxiety, increased heart rate, hypertension, shallow breathing, giddiness, and even joy. From a positive perspective, stress is a force that generates and initiates action. Using Selye's definition, stress can accompany pleasant or unpleasant events. Selye referred to stress judged as "good" as **eustress.** This form of stress is the force that initiates emotional and psychological growth. Eustress provides the experience of pleasure, adds meaning to life, and fosters an attitude that tries to find positive solutions to complex problems. Eustress can accompany a birth, graduation, the purchase of a new car, the development of a new friendship, the accomplishment of a difficult task, and success in an area that previously produced

anxiety. **Distress,** on the other hand, is stress that results in negative responses. Unchecked, negative stress can interfere with the physiological and psychological functioning of the body and may ultimately result in a disease or disability.[2]

Stress also provides humans with the ability to respond to challenges or dangers. It is vital to self-protection and serves as a motivator that enhances human ability.

A **stressor** is any physical, psychological, or environmental event or condition that initiates the stress response (Figure 9-1). See Assessment Activity 9-2 to evaluate your own stress level in the different categories listed in Figure 9-1.

What is considered a stressor for one person may not be a stressor for another. Speaking in front of a group may be stimulating for one person but terrifying for another. Some people experience extreme test anxiety and others feel confident about written assessments. Fortunately, the stress response is not a genetic trait, and because it is a response to external conditions, it is subject to personal control. A person may not avoid taking a test, but he or she can apply techniques and take precautions that lessen the effects of the stress. For example, knowing the material thoroughly and engaging in deep breathing several minutes before a test help dissipate anxiety. To maximize quality of life, people can find positive ways of dealing with stress.

A stress response can enhance and increase the level of either mental or physical performance. This response is referred to as the *inverted-U theory.*[3] Not enough stress (hypostress) may result in a poorer effort, but too much stress can inhibit effort. There appears to be an optimal level of stress that results in peak performance (Figure 9-2). Achievement of an appropriate level of stress depends on the person and the type of

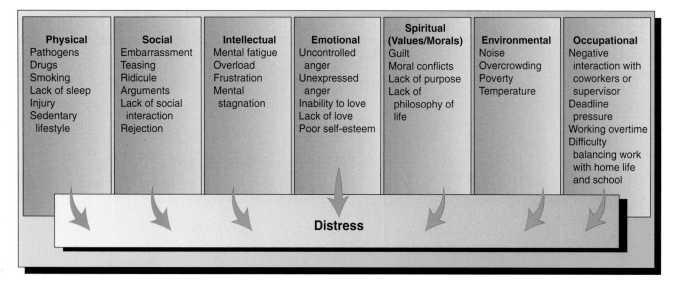

Physical	Social	Intellectual	Emotional	Spiritual (Values/Morals)	Environmental	Occupational
Pathogens	Embarrassment	Mental fatigue	Uncontrolled anger	Guilt	Noise	Negative interaction with coworkers or supervisor
Drugs	Teasing	Overload	Unexpressed anger	Moral conflicts	Overcrowding	
Smoking	Ridicule	Frustration	Inability to love	Lack of purpose	Poverty	
Lack of sleep	Arguments	Mental stagnation	Lack of love	Lack of philosophy of life	Temperature	Deadline pressure
Injury	Lack of social interaction		Poor self-esteem			Working overtime
Sedentary lifestyle	Rejection					Difficulty balancing work with home life and school

Distress

Figure 9-1 Stressors That Can Create Distress

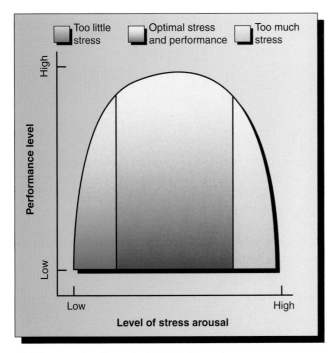

Figure 9-2 The Inverted-U Theory

task. Table 9-1 lists some of the potentially positive outcomes associated with stress. Your body is constantly attempting to maintain a physiological balance. This balance is referred to as *homeostasis*. Any event or circumstance that causes a disruption (a stressor) in your body's homeostasis requires some type of adaptive behavior. Physiologically, whether a stressor is perceived as positive or negative, the body responds with the same three-stage process. This series of changes is known as the **general adaptation syndrome (GAS)**.[4] The three phases are alarm, resistance, and exhaustion (Figure 9-3, page 298).

The *alarm* phase occurs when homeostasis is initially disrupted. The brain perceives a stressor and prepares the body to deal with it, a response sometimes referred to as the *fight or flight response*. The subconscious appraisal of the stressor results in an emotional reaction. The emotional response stimulates a physical reaction associated with stress, such as the muscles becoming tense, the

stomach tightening, the heart rate increasing, the mouth becoming dry, and the palms of the hands sweating.

The second stage is *resistance*. In this phase, the body meets the perceived challenge through increased strength, endurance, sensory capacities, and sensory acuity. Hormonal secretions regulate the body's response to a stressor. Only after meeting and satisfying the demands of a stressful situation can the internal activities of the body return to normal. Other researchers[5] argue that people have different levels of energy to deal with stressors. For short-term stressors, only a superficial level of energy is required, allowing deeper energy levels to be protected. Superficial levels of energy are readily accessible and easily renewable. Unfortunately, not all stress can be resolved with superficial energy levels. When long-term or deep levels of stress are experienced, the amount of energy available is limited. If sufficient stress is experienced for an extended period, loss of adaptation can result. Although some scientists believe that energy stores may be genetically programmed, all people can replenish their energy stores through exercise, good nutrition, adequate sleep, and other positive behaviors.

When stressors become chronic or pervasive, the third phase, *exhaustion*, is reached. In exhaustion, energy stores have been depleted and rest must occur. Although weeks to years may pass before the effects of long-term stressors occur, if a person does not learn how to deal adequately with stress, exhaustion will result. At this point, stress may affect the stomach, heart, blood pressure, muscles, and joints. Fortunately, the effects of stressors can be completely or partially reversed when adequate management techniques are initiated. The earlier these management techniques are learned and used, the fewer problems result.

Sources of Stress and Warning Signs

Most stressful situations fall into one of three categories: (1) harm and loss, (2) threat, and (3) challenge.[6] Examples of *harm-and-loss situations* are the death of a loved one, the loss of personal property, physical assault, physical injury, and the severe loss of self-esteem. *Threat*

Table 9-1 Positive Outcomes of Stress

Mental	Emotional	Physical
Enhanced creativity	Sense of control	High energy level
Enhanced thinking ability	Responsiveness to environment	Increased stamina
Greater goal orientation	Improved interpersonal relationships	Flexibility of muscles and joints
Enhanced motivation	Improved morale	Freedom from stress-related disease

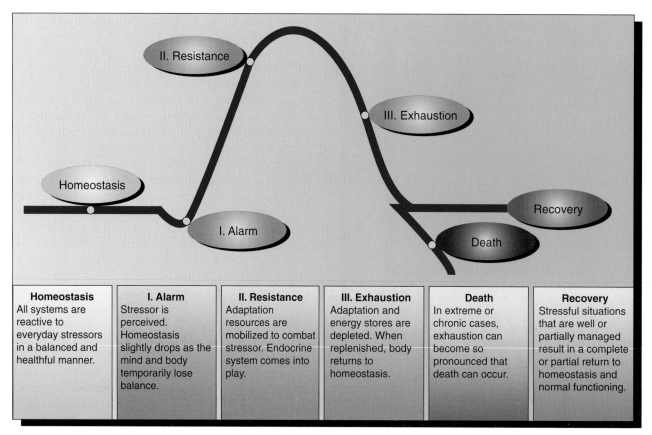

Figure 9-3 The General Adaptation Syndrome (GAS)

Homeostasis	I. Alarm	II. Resistance	III. Exhaustion	Death	Recovery
All systems are reactive to everyday stressors in a balanced and healthful manner.	Stressor is perceived. Homeostasis slightly drops as the mind and body temporarily lose balance.	Adaptation resources are mobilized to combat stressor. Endocrine system comes into play.	Adaptation and energy stores are depleted. When replenished, body returns to homeostasis.	In extreme or chronic cases, exhaustion can become so pronounced that death can occur.	Stressful situations that are well or partially managed result in a complete or partial return to homeostasis and normal functioning.

situations may be real or perceived and can range from being caught in traffic to being unable to perceive an event. Threatening events tax a person's ability to deal with everyday life. Threat stressors are any stressors that result in anger, hostility, frustration, or depression. *Challenge situations* are catalysts for either growth or pain. These stressors often involve major life changes and include such events as taking a new job, leaving home, graduating from college, and getting married. Challenge events are usually perceived as being good but involve stress because they disrupt homeostasis and require considerable psychological and physical adjustment.

Being aware of the mental and physical signals associated with stress is the beginning step in learning how to manage it. Assessment Activity 9-1 will aid you in identifying some of the major stressors. By using self-assessments to monitor for signs of stress, you can avoid excessive stress. The negative results of distress are shown in Table 9-2. Indicators of excessive distress include the following:

- Chronic fatigue, migraine headaches, sweating, lower-back pain, sleep disturbances, weakness, dizziness, diarrhea, and constipation
- Harder and/or longer work or study while accomplishing less, an inability to concentrate, general disorientation

- Denial that there is a problem or troubling event
- Increased incidence of illness, such as colds and flu, or constant worry about illness or becoming ill; overuse of over-the-counter drugs for the purpose of self-medication
- Depression, irritability, anxiety, apathy, an overwhelming urge to cry or run and hide, and feelings of unreality
- Excessive behavioral patterns, such as spending too much money, drinking, breaking the law, and developing addictions
- Accident proneness
- Signs of reclusiveness and avoidance of other people
- Emotional tension, "keyed up" feeling, easy startling, nervous laughter, anxiety, hyperkinesia, and nervous tics

Factors Generating a Stress Response

As mentioned earlier, the criteria for a stressful event and the response to that event for any person are unique to the individual. Figure 9-4 provides an overview of the complexity of the stress experience and some of the many moderating effects. For instance, a dysfunctional

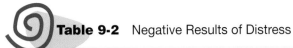

Table 9-2 Negative Results of Distress

Mental	Physical	Emotional
Short-Term Effects		
Poor memory	Flushed face	Irritability
Inability to concentrate	Cold hands	Disorganization
Low creativity	Gas	Conflicts
Poor self-control	Rapid breathing	Mood swings
Low self-esteem	Shortness of breath	Chronic sleep problems
	Dry mouth	Acid stomach
		Overindulgence in alcohol or other drugs, food
Long-Term Effects		
Bouts of depression	Hypertension	Overweight/underweight
Mild paranoia	Coronary disease	Drug abuse
Low tolerance for ambiguity	Ulcers	Excessive smoking
Forgetfulness	Migraine/tension headaches	Ineffective use of work/leisure time
Inability to make decisions/quickness to make decisions	Strokes	Overreaction to mild work pressure
	Allergies	

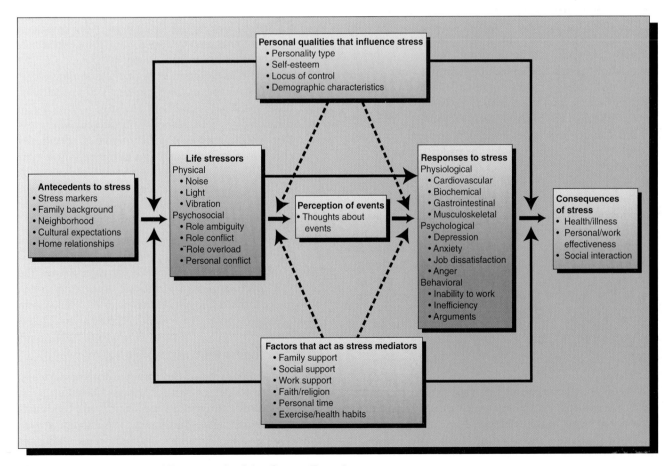

Figure 9-4 Theoretical Framework of the Stress Experience

home life (characterized by an alcoholic parent, a difficult divorce, or extreme poverty) may contribute to a personality that is more susceptible to difficult events, such as poor grades or a failed relationship. This combination of inadequate preparation for life along with an event perceived as personal failure is likely to lead to depression, anxiety, or anger. Conversely, a person whose background has fostered a deep sense of self-worth and meaningfulness will be able to better handle a difficult event and not perceive the event as a personal failure. Poor grades may be the result of poor study habits, an undiagnosed learning behavior, or inadequate sleep, and a failed relationship may be the result of a poor match, bad timing, or immaturity.

Physiological Responses to Stress

Stress abounds in life and can be experienced as the result of happy and unhappy events. Regardless of the stressor, each time a stressful event occurs, a series of neurological and hormonal messages are sent throughout the body.

The nervous system serves as a reciprocal network that sends messages between the awareness centers of the brain and the organs and muscles of the body. Part of this system is referred to as the *limbic system*. The limbic system contains centers for emotions, memory, learning relay, and hormone production and includes the pituitary gland, thalamus, and hypothalamus.

When a stressor is encountered, the body sends a message to the brain via the nervous system. The brain then synthesizes the message and determines whether it is valid. If a message is not verified by the brain as being threatening, the limbic system overrides the initial response and the body continues to function normally. If the initial response is translated as accurate and a stressor is detected, the body responds with some emotion (fear, joy, terror), and the hypothalamus begins to act.

The hypothalamus sends a hormonal message to the pituitary gland, which then releases a hormone (ACTH), which helps signal other glands in the endocrine system to secrete additional hormones, providing fuel to respond with the fight or flight response. Systolic blood pressure may rise 15 to 20 mmHg while fluid is retained. The adrenal cortex increases blood pressure to facilitate the transportation of food and oxygen to active parts of the body.[7] Blood volume is increased.

The hypothalamus also sends a message to release the hormones epinephrine and norepinephrine, which initiate a variety of physiological changes. These changes include increased heart rate, increased metabolic rate, increased oxygen consumption, and the release of hormones called *endorphins*, which decrease sensations of pain.

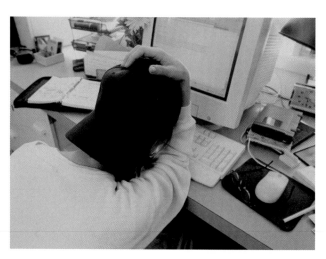

Everyday problems can trigger the stress response. What are your biggest stressors?

The autonomic nervous system is also responsible for a second major set of physiological responses:

1. The autonomic nervous system is responsible for a second major set of physiological responses. It is referred to as autonomic because this system can function without conscious thought or voluntary control. However, it is now recognized that the autonomic system can be influenced by conscious thought[8] and works closely with the central nervous system to maintain homeostasis.

2. There are two components of the autonomic nervous system, the parasympathetic and sympathetic divisions. The sympathetic division is involved in the fight or flight response. It accomplishes this through the release of catecholamines, specifically epinephrine (adrenaline) and norepinephrine (noradrenaline). The parasympathetic division helps constantly maintain homeostasis and returns the body to a normal state. Thus, you cannot be aroused and relaxed at the same time.

In reaction to a threat, the autonomic nervous system increases heart rate, strength of the skeletal muscles, mental activity, and basal metabolic rate; dilates the coronary arteries, pupils, bronchial tubes, and arterioles; and constricts the abdominal arteries. This system also returns the body to a normal, relaxed state.

Stress and the Immune System

The mind and body act on each other in remarkable ways. Our immune system is a part of the body's defense against illness and disease originating from factors and conditions both outside and inside our bodies. The immune system consists of a variety of mechanical and chemical defenses that protect against such outside invaders as microorganisms, allergens, and other substances, as well as such inside factors as mutating cells or improperly functioning tissue. The immune system is a functional system rather than an organ system and, as a result, seems to be prone to the effects of stress when fighting off the situations and conditions previously mentioned.[8]

The biological link between emotions and disease and even death is strong. Mortality is three times higher in people with few close relationships than in those with numerous such relationships, and people with strong support groups have additional protection against life stressors. Death rates are higher for cancer patients with pessimistic attitudes. Illness is more common among people who feel locked into strife-ridden marriages. AIDS patients with healthy psyches seem better able to withstand disease.[9]

In a study involving cancer patients with malignant melanoma, health education, enhanced problem-solving skills, and stress management techniques provided significant increases in natural killer cells and increased activity of these cells in patients receiving these behavioral interventions. A six-year follow-up showed a trend toward greater recurrence and a statistically significant higher mortality rate in the control group as opposed to those receiving behavioral interventions.[10]

Another study demonstrated a system of nerve fibers that transmits messages between the brain and lymphocetes that fight infection and cancer in the body. This research found that neurotransmitters, such as epinephrine and norepinephrine, can attack immune cells and influence their ability to replicate and destroy invading pathogenic agents.[11]

The immune system becomes dysfunctional and can lead to stress-related illnesses in three ways: (1) underactivity (cancer), (2) hyperactivity (asthma), and (3) misguided activity (lupus). The immune function seems to be affected by the relationship between the brain and nervous system. This relationship among brain, nervous system, and immune response has been the outgrowth from the field of study called **psychoneuroimmunology (PNI)**. This relatively new medical discipline seeks to explain the connection among the brain, the nervous system, and the body's response to infections and deviated cell division. Several studies have shown that chronic stress suppresses the body's ability to initiate an effective immune response. This suppression is attributed to an increase in corticosteroids, produced during chronic stress. This increase in corticosteroid levels delays and weakens the immune response.[12] Research has found that chronic stress suppresses the immune system, particularly when the stress is associated with social disruption (such as leaving home for the first time), psychological depression (such as feeling "down" for prolonged periods), or some negative personality attribute (lack of self-confidence).[13] It has also been found that immunosuppression is associated with loneliness and feelings of hopelessness.[14] Stress has

also been demonstrated to be associated with infertility.[15,16,17] No known specific reason exists for this correlation. Whether the stress is the result of infertility problems or another source, stress-reduction intervention results in significant improvement in conception rates.

Because stress affects the immune system, the body becomes more susceptible to a multitude of ailments, from colds to cancer. Respiratory conditions, such as asthma, may become worse. The cardiovascular system reacts by constricting the blood vessels while increasing blood volume. The result is a rise in blood pressure throughout a stress-ridden day. Multiple increases in blood pressure can eventually contribute to chronic high blood pressure. More forceful contraction of the heart elevates levels of free fatty acids, enhancing the development of clogged arteries leading to and including the heart. In extreme cases, sudden death can occur, especially for a person who has been experiencing high levels of uncontrolled stress for an extended period.

Headaches, including migraines, have long been associated with stress. Tension headaches are caused by involuntary contractions of the scalp, head, and neck muscles. Typical muscular reaction to stress is contracting or tensing. When chronic stress occurs, the body reacts by being constantly ready to respond, and the muscles become braced, always in a state of tension. More stress magnifies the tension the muscles are already undergoing. Increased muscular tension manifests in headaches, backaches, neckaches, and other pains. The smooth muscles that control internal organs also experience pains. More intense contractions can lead to stomachache, diarrhea, hypertension, heartburn, gastritis, bloating, inflammation of the pancreas, and blockage of the bile ducts.

Stress decreases saliva in the mouth, often making speaking awkward. Swallowing may become difficult, and the increase in stomach acids contributes to ulcer pain. People tend to perspire more, and electrical currents are transmitted more quickly across the skin. Skin conditions, such as acne, psoriasis, herpes, hives, and eczema, are exacerbated.

Stress also seems to affect the body's nutritional status. Individual nutritional patterns can also influence stress management efforts. For example, eating too much or too little, eating the wrong kinds of food, and overusing products such as caffeine or alcohol upset homeostasis. Diets high in fat, sugar, and processed foods place a heavy burden on various body systems. Ingesting too few calories can lead to the breakdown of lean tissue. To meet the demands of stress, you should maintain adequate nutrition through a balanced and varied diet. (Chapter 6 provides guidelines for developing a beneficial nutrition plan.) Table 9-3 on page 302 provides some insight into the interactive natures of stress, nutritional status, and immunity.

Ultimately, no body system escapes the effects of stress. The long-term presence of certain stress-associated

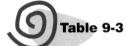

Table 9-3 Stress, Nutritional Status, and Immunity: An Interactive Effect

Although the mechanism is not completely understood, stress significantly affects nutritional status and therefore immunity. Several nutritional factors have implications for how your body responds to stress.

Energy

Stress can increase the body's basic caloric needs by as much as 200%. The stress hormones increase body heat production. When this heat is released, it is not available for cell metabolism. The caloric inefficiency induced by stress accounts for the increased need for energy intake.

Protein

Stress may increase the body's need for protein from 60% to as much as 500%. The integrity of the body's tissues, such as the skin and the tissue lining the mouth, lungs, and nose (called *mucosal tissue*), depends on adequate protein repair and maintenance of secretions of biochemicals that serve as protective agents. The formation of antibodies also requires protein.

Fats

Dietary fatty acids influence the synthesis of a group of fatty acid derivatives called *prostaglandins.* Prostaglandins stimulate or depress other cellular and immune functions in relation to stress.

Vitamins

Vitamin A maintains healthy skin and mucous membranes. Vitamin A–deficient individuals have fewer mucus-secreting cells and those they do have produce less mucus; thus, the protection provided by the mucous lining is diminished. Vitamin C has been shown to enhance the engulfing, or "eating," actions of the immune cells called *macrophages.* If vitamin C is deficient, macrophages are less mobile and less able to consume disease-causing organisms. Deficiencies of vitamin A, vitamin B_{12}, and folate can impair production of the cells that enable antibody responses. Large doses of vitamin E have been associated with suppression of B-cells, vital to the immune response. Finally, metabolic requirements for thiamin, riboflavin, and niacin are increased in response to a stressful situation.

Minerals

Deficiencies of zinc impair immune cell reproduction and responsiveness.

hormones in the brain damages receptors and cells found in the hippocampus. .(The hippocampus sends messages when stress is occurring.) Because brain cells do not regenerate, these cells are lost forever. The effects of this loss are unknown, but indications are that eventually affected people become less able to respond to stress appropriately.[18] Assessment Activity 9-3 provides

guidelines for identifying stress style and suggests relaxation activities.

Self-Esteem and Stress

How people feel about themselves and others and their perceptions of the stressors in their lives are part of the psychology of stress. Ability to deal with stress often hinges on impressions of how detrimental a stressor is and how adequately resources can deal with the situation. How much stress people feel themselves experiencing is closely associated with their sense of self-esteem. Self-esteem includes beliefs and attitudes about changes, personal talent, skills, and one's ability to deal with the changes and challenges that inevitably occur in life. It is also the basis of self-efficacy and the locus of control (see Chapter 1). The most influential factor in determining response to stress may be people's perceptions of themselves.

Attitude and Stress

The question many researchers have asked is why one person is more susceptible to stress than another. The answer is not altogether clear, but evidence is mounting that one's perception, or attitude, is a key factor in the stress equation. The realization that our attitude has such a significant impact on our health has led to a new movement in psychology termed "positive psychology." Dr Martin Seligman of the University of Pennsylvania is the founding father of positive psychology. He believes that optimism is a key in maintaining not only our mental health but our physical health as well. Other writers have examined the differences between optimism and pessimism and the impact that these attitudes have on health. What researchers have found is that the fundamental difference between a pessimist and an optimist is the degree of control one feels over the amount of control one has concerning one's life.[19] What is suggested is that we learn feelings of helplessness and this becomes a major factor in depression and stress. Not surprisingly, both depression and stress are highly correlated with pessimism. Researchers report that optimists are much better at coping with the anxiety and distress associated with everything from infertility to higher grade point averages in law students. A study by Mayo Clinic researchers compared the health of 839 men and women to scores on a personality test they had taken 30 years previously. It was found that those who had had an optimistic attitude in their younger years were 19 percent more likely to still be alive than their pessimistic counterparts.

To help develop more positive optimistic attitudes,

1. *Teach yourself a lesson.* Find something positive in a sad or stressful situation by what you have learned from the experience. Don't ignore the negatives but do learn from them without dwelling on them.

2. *Interrupt negative thoughts.* Get out of the pessimistic frame of mind. Force yourself to think positive thoughts. Think of pleasant memories. Don't allow the negative to set you off on a "pity party" or a self-flagellation.

3. *Set realistic goals.* Set achievable, realistic goals. Positive thinkers have developed the art of meeting goals (see Assessment Activity 9-6).

4. *Be good to yourself.* Treat yourself to the things you love—it is essential to building confidence and creating a sense of control over your life. Keep in mind that the purpose is to take control; don't do something because it is a habit—do it because you want to.

5. *Go digging for silver.* Seek the bright side of things. Make sure you find at least one positive thing that happens each day. Take an appreciation appraisal each day. When irritating or disappointing events occur, ask yourself, "What did I learn from this that will make me a better person?"

6. *Be glad it's not worse.* When you are low, think of someone less fortunate than you. Write down or say, "I'm glad that . . ." or "I'm lucky to. . . ." People who can find positives to reflect on report more satisfaction with their lives than those who are always pointing to the negative.

7. *Fake it.* When all else fails, keep on smiling. Project the mood you want to get back. Find something that makes you laugh. It is hard to be down if you are smiling and laughing.

Gender and Stress

Researchers have found interesting differences between men and women in their reactions to stress. Women's blood pressure goes up less than men's in reaction to stress. However women tend to react to a wider range of outside stressors than men. Women feel stress more often because they take a holistic view of everyday life. A man tends to worry if his family is sick; a woman takes on the burdens of the whole neighborhood[20] (see Wellness for a Lifetime: Women's Changing Roles). For certain, life is more stress-filled than 200 years ago. Stress and anxiety have become a core theme in our lives. The challenge we face in our quest for high-level

Wellness for a Lifetime

Women's Changing Roles

As many families now have two-career households and more women work outside the home, it is natural to wonder if the double demands of household and worksite pose a threat to women's physical and psychological health. A study done at Duke University Medical Center by Linda Luecken and her colleagues suggests that they do.

The study focused on 109 women with full-time clerical and customer-service jobs. Some had children and some did not. The results indicated that working women with children at home had higher levels of cortisol (a stress hormone thought to reflect high levels of distress), a greater lack of personal control, and more risk for cardiovascular disease than working women with no children. Both groups of women reported similar levels of work strain, but the working mothers reported higher levels of home strain, including greater demands and less control. This increased strain seemed to be caused by the reality that these women performed most of the child-rearing and household duties. Such chores as laundry, cleaning, cooking, chauffeuring,

and homework more often fell to the women in the study than to their male partners.

Luecken and her colleagues estimated that working women with children have up to 21 hours more work per week than men have. They also found that working mothers have little chance to "unwind," so they have increased sympathetic nervous system arousal both during and after work. Even if male partners help with household duties, they often finish their duties with enough time to relax. The presence of a spouse or significant other does not significantly reduce the physiological and psychological consequences of stress on the working mother. Interestingly, higher income, ethnicity, and the number of children at home does not influence the level of stress.[21]

Following are some ways working mothers might balance the demands of work and household duties:

- Set limits. Schedule and honor your time to relax. Learn to say no.

- Make lists of your priorities, from most important to least important. Get done what is really important and let the rest go.

- Remember that perfection is the enemy of happiness.

- Team up with other parents to share the load: child care, dinner clubs, or shuttling.

- Pay attention to the moments of joy that parenting and connecting with a partner and friends have to offer.[22]

wellness is not to master the threats (stressors) but to master our all-too-human responses to them.

Personality and Stress

Two physicians, Friedman and Roseman,[23] have written extensively about personality, cardiovascular disease, and stress. These researchers have described two stress-related personality types—type A and type B. Most people are neither type exclusively but fall somewhere between the two.

The type A personality is characterized by an urgent sense of time, impatience, competitiveness, aggressiveness, insecurity over status, and inability to relax. People with type A behavior characteristics are likely to be highly stressed. Type B people have a more unhurried approach to their lives. The type B personality does not become as upset at losing or not attaining a goal. Type B people also tend to set more realistic goals.[24] Researchers disagree on whether there is a possible relationship between the stress-prone type A personality and cardiovascular disease.[23]

In general, researchers believe that being a type A personality is not a problem if there is no underlying hostility. However, regardless of whether type A people are more susceptible to heart disease, they do experience more negative effects, such as tiredness and frustration, from short-term stress. [24]

"Stress survivors"—people who handle stress successfully—have several common characteristics. Psychologist Suzanna Kobasa[28] has isolated these attributes and characterized the type of person who exhibits them. A hardy personality tends to remain healthy even under extreme stress. Characteristics of a hardy personality or hardiness are challenge, commitment, and control (see Assessment Activity 9-5).

Challenge is the ability to see change for what it is— that is, not only inevitable but an opportunity for the growth and development of unique abilities. *Commitment* is delineated by a strong sense of inner purpose. It is necessary to want to succeed to achieve success. Commitment is the ability to become involved while maintaining the discernment to know when dedication and desire are harmful. *Control* is the recognition that one has power over one's life and attitudes. People who have a sense of control act in situations rather than react to them (see Wellness for a Lifetime: The Time of Our Lives).

Dealing with Stress

All events in life precipitate a reaction. How people react or respond to situations differs. **Coping** is the attempt to manage or deal with stress. Coping is independent of outcome—it does not necessarily result in success (see Wellness on the Web: What's Your Stress Index?).

Wellness for a Lifetime

The Time of Our Lives

Although middle age is often dreaded, the changes that inevitably occur as we grow older are not necessarily bad. In fact, more and more elderly adults report that the best time in their lives was not their youth but, rather, their midlife years.

One recent study of this question involved more than 3,000 people, each of whom answered more than 1,100 questions. Researchers found that more than 70 percent of the respondents viewed themselves as being in excellent health and felt their lives had purpose and meaning. In fact, 9 of 10 study participants said they had never experienced the proverbial midlife crisis. Most middle-aged people reported that they had been able to make the adjustment necessary for life to remain rewarding. Most said that they did not have arthritis, backaches, skin problems, indigestion, constipation, depression, gum disease, high blood pressure, or migraines. And contrary to popular belief, most middle-aged women reported that menopause was a fairly benign experience.

One negative finding of the study is that middle-aged adults are not working hard to maintain a high quality of life. In addition, respondents reported not having enough money and sex—probably two things lacking at any age, not just middle age. However, while sexual satisfaction was low, middle-aged adults seemed to be content overall with their marriages and relationships. Seventy-two percent said that their relationships were very good or excellent, and 90 percent felt that their relationships were unlikely to break up.

Finally, the survey found that by the time adults reached age 65, men felt an average of 12.6 years younger than their actual age and women felt 14.7 years younger than their actual age. As we grow older, our lives can become even more fulfilling, particularly if we can maintain a sense of control over our well-being by practicing healthful lifestyle habits. How can *you* ensure optimal health as you age?

SOURCE: Adapted from Johns Hopkins InteliHealth Online (www. intelihealth.com/IH?ihtIH?d=dm).

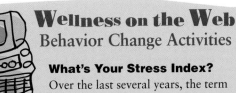

Wellness on the Web
Behavior Change Activities

What's Your Stress Index?

Over the last several years, the term *stress* has become a cultural cliché used to convey feelings of fatigue, burnout, tension, and discouragement, to name a few. There's job stress, relationship stress, technological stress—and the list goes on. Cliché or not, though, we probably can all agree that, however we experience it, stress is real—and it can be extremely challenging to understand and manage. The destruction it causes can make our daily lives miserable. It can also affect every dimension of our health, sometimes severely. Strangely, we're not always aware that we're under stress. The signs and symptoms that can alert us to problems may be hard to recognize because we've become so accustomed to them. Want to quantify your stress level? Go to www.mhhe.com/anspaugh6e, and select Student Center, Chapter 9, Wellness on the Web, and Activity 1 to complete the checklist; then evaluate your results.

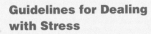

Real-World Wellness
Guidelines for Dealing with Stress

Being in school can be so overwhelming. I have many classes, extracurricular activities, and a pile of homework each night. How can I balance it all?

Following are guidelines for effectively dealing with potential harmful stress:

- *Schedule time effectively.* Practice good time management techniques by using time wisely. This means taking time out for yourself every day and scheduling work when you are usually at your peak ability (see Assessment Activity 9-7).

- *Set priorities.* Know what is important to you. Do not attempt to work on four or five projects simultaneously. Keep your efforts focused on one or two major items.

- *Establish realistic goals.* Goals must be achievable. Do not establish impossible expectations and then become frustrated when they are not accomplished as quickly as you would like. Write down long-range goals and then establish checks for keeping yourself on track and monitoring progress. Short-term goals help you see how you are moving toward your goal and provide rewards as you advance toward success.

- *See yourself as achieving the goals.* Visualize yourself as being successful. Go over in your mind what it will look and feel like to accomplish a goal.

- *Give yourself a break.* Take time every day to exercise and relax.

Dealing successfully with stress may require using a variety of techniques (see Real-World Wellness: Guidelines for Dealing with Stress). Because stress-related responses are based primarily on mental perceptions, coping strategies that achieve desirable results may need to originate in a change in attitude or outlook. If specific situations or people are perceived as disruptive, one solution is to avoid them.

Although there are no easy answers, there is always some type of answer or solution. When dealing with a stressor reaches a point where it seems there are no solutions, the tension from the situation becomes increasingly detrimental. It may then become necessary to consider changing attitudes, goals, and values.

Seeking the help of a professional counselor is frequently beneficial when attempting to resolve particularly stressful situations. Assessment Activity 9-4 identifies ways to recognize some of the positive and negative behaviors that can be used to deal with stress.

Engaging in positive self-talk and relabeling negative experiences (viewing difficulties as challenges rather than as problems, for example) are positive steps in reducing stress-related disorders. Eating well, taking time to enjoy life, laughing, exercising, and living in the present reduce stress. People can handle stress effectively when they work on developing all of their abilities to the fullest, when they develop lifestyles compatible with personal values, and when they develop realistic expectations for

themselves. Working toward these goals is the way to establish a wellness lifestyle (see Real-World Wellness: Marta's Day on page 306).

Successful coping includes being aware of incidents and situations that you might perceive as being stressful. Recognition of stressors means being aware of how your body responds to stress. Recognition requires continuous monitoring of your body and mind for evidence of excessive stress (see Real-World Wellness: Sleep and Stress Reduction on page 307).

Successful coping takes effort. One suggestion is to focus on the signals your body is sending when experiencing stress and then to think back to the event or situation that might have triggered those feelings. Another suggestion is to recreate a recent event that has been stressful. After visualizing the episode, write down six ways that the outcome could have been different—three ways it could have been worse and three ways it could have been

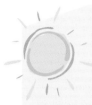

Real-World Wellness

Marta's Day

This semester I've been getting up late for class, putting off studying, and eating poorly. I'm feeling very stressed out, and my grades have begun to suffer. What can I do to get out of this downward spiral?

Following is an analysis of Marta's day, including her stress responses to events in her day and suggestions for other ways to react.

Event	Marta's Stress Response	A Better Approach
Morning: is late rising for first class; stayed up late, studying, the night before	Skips first class to study for exam; misses notes from that class and cannot contact friend to see if she can use her notes; skips breakfast	Begin studying for a test a few days before the exam; do not attempt to cram everything into one night; get a good night's rest and get up early to review your notes; eat breakfast and attend first class.
Is late for test	Stays home too long and gets caught in traffic; arrives late for the test; does not have a full hour to complete the test	Leave early to allow for traffic and parking problems; be on time to concentrate on the test and have time to relax a few minutes.
Lunch	Skips lunch—has a soft drink and potato chips	Have a nutritionally balanced meal in a relaxing atmosphere; go with a friend just to chat.
Afternoon: is late for work because had to return overdue library book	Rushes to library; has to pay fine; has to stand in line at the library for 15 minutes	Write down when books are due and return them on time; use a daily calendar to plan activities and allot time to take care of personal business.
Evening: watches TV until midnight; neglects to study for test the day after tomorrow	Is too tired and "stressed out" to study, so watches TV all evening; has a hamburger and soda for dinner	Take a short nap after work and have a nutritious meal; plan the evening so that some time is spent watching TV and some is spent studying; go to bed early, so you can get to school on time and rested.
Next morning: gets up late for class again	Begins the same cycle of feeling tired and pressured and being late	Analyze current time constraints to determine where more time needs to be allotted and how to develop a more efficient plan (see Assessment Activities 9-6 and 9-7).

better. The latter will increase awareness of how to handle similar situations better in the future. A last suggestion is to try something new. The idea is that you be challenged and meet that challenge successfully. Trying something new and meeting the challenge reinforce your sense of being able to deal with life successfully.[28]

Relaxation Techniques

The ultimate goal in stress coping and management is to reduce the negative effects of stress. Various **relaxation techniques** have proved successful. Brief descriptions of various techniques follow. If you are interested in pursuing the use of these techniques, you can find more information about them in books or on tapes. These books and tapes can be purchased at bookstores or may be found at your library.

Deep breathing

Deep breathing is the most basic technique used in relaxation and is often the foundation for other methods. The primary benefit of this technique is that it can be done anywhere and anytime. It is beneficial to

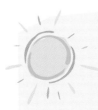

Real-World Wellness

Sleep and Stress Reduction

Sleep is one of those factors that we all seem to be aware of, yet we seem to do little to correct lifestyle habits that create sleep deprivation. Recently *U.S. News and World Report* featured a full-length article and an editorial on the results of sleep deprivation. Research has shown that sleep is essential not only to brain function but also to the function of every organ in the body. Additionally, researchers have found that sleep deprivation can result in heart attack, prediabetic state, slowed reaction time, and mania episodes in bipolar patients.[25]

The National Sleep Foundation (NSF) reports that 47 million adults aren't getting sufficient sleep. Sleepiness is especially acute among 18–29-year-olds. Forty-four percent of this age group reported experiencing tiredness a few days a month. This compares with 38 percent of 36–64-year-olds, and 23 percent of subjects age 65 and over. The NSF survey found that those who got fewer than six hours of sleep were more likely to report feeling tired than those getting eight hours of sleep (32 percent vs. 15 percent). The group that got less than six hours per night more often reported feeling stressed (32 percent vs. 16 percent), sad (14 percent vs. 7 percent), and angry (11 percent vs. 4 percent). People who reported often being sleepy during the day were compared with those reporting not feeling sleepy. Those who reported feeling sleepy were more likely to describe themselves as dissatisfied with life (21 percent vs. 7 percent of nonsleepy individuals) and angry (12 percent vs. 4 percent of nonsleepy individuals).[26]

Although it is generally recommended that adults average seven to nine hours of sleep each night, adolescents need an additional hour of sleep—nine hours per night. Even as we age we still need seven to nine hours of sleep. Sleep patterns may change, but the need for sleep doesn't. The choice is either get enough sleep or suffer the consequences.[27]

practice deep breathing several times a day. The methodology consists of completely filling the lungs when breathing, so that the abdomen expands outward. Begin by taking a deep breath and then exhaling slowly through the mouth. A hand can be placed on the stomach to ensure that it is fully expanded. If the stomach does not rise, the breath is not deep enough or the abdomen is being held too tightly. Repeat this cycle several times and then rest quietly for three to five minutes.

Progressive muscle relaxation

Progressive muscle relaxation creates awareness of the difference between muscular tension and a relaxed state. This is a three-step process, which begins with tensing of a muscle group and noticing how the tension feels. Next, make a conscious effort to relax the tension and notice that feeling. The third phase consists of concentrating on the differences between the two sensations. Beginning at either the head working down or at the feet working up, tense and relax all major muscle groups (see Real-World Wellness: Progressive Muscle Relaxation on page 308).

Autogenics

Autogenics is the use of self-suggestion to produce a relaxation response. Autogenics begins with a deep breath and a conscious effort to relax. This technique may follow a progression from head to feet or feet to head. Repeat the phrase "My arm feels heavy and warm" several times before moving on to the next muscle group. You can repeat other phrases that carry a calming message, such as "I am completely calm and relaxed." End the session by thinking, I am refreshed and alert. Autogenics takes practice, time, and commitment and should be practiced twice a day for about 10 minutes. Commercial tapes may help guide people wanting to learn autogenics.

Meditation

Meditation can be approached from a variety of perspectives. As a stress-reduction technique, its purpose is to help the practitioner temporarily tune out the world and to invoke relaxation. During a meditation session, the person meditating focuses his or her attention on a *mantra*, a particular word or sound, while attempting to eliminate all outside distractions.

Begin by taking a comfortable position on a couch or in a chair. Take several deep breaths, slowly inhaling and exhaling. Shut your eyes or softly focus them on an object so that the details are blurred. Concentrate all your thoughts on a word or phrase that you have selected to use, such as *peace* or *relax*, while continuing to breathe slowly and deeply.[29] The relaxation response can also be initiated by counting breaths backward from 100 or by imagining a white light that slowly travels throughout your body, letting in light and energy while expelling tension and fear. Many commercial meditation tapes are available.

Visualization

Visualization (imagery) is a form of relaxation that uses the imagination. Begin by finding a comfortable position; then shut your eyes and take several deep breaths.

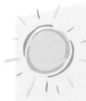

Real-World Wellness

Progressive Muscle Relaxation

When I'm uptight, my muscles get so tense that I can't relax. What can I do to loosen them again?

There are numerous progressive muscle relaxation activities. The exercises are frequently structured by a facilitator. Some exercises begin with the feet, hands, or face, but because of space constraints, only the relaxing of the face will be described here. You can add the other parts of the body by recording the entire process on audiotape and listening to the tape as often as desired—usually once a day or two or three times a week. Take your time (three to four minutes) for each area of the body.

- Assume a comfortable position and concentrate on the instructions. You may find it beneficial to lie down or sit in a comfortable chair.
- Close your eyes.
- Allow all your muscles to relax and feel loose and heavy. Take several deep breaths.
- Wrinkle your forehead and hold for six seconds.
- Notice the feelings.
  - Relax; allow the forehead to become smooth.
  - Notice the feeling of relaxation.
- Frown with your eyes, forehead, and scalp and hold for six seconds.
  - Experience the sensation of tension.
  - Relax the muscles.
  - Notice the feelings of relaxation.
- Keeping your eyes closed, clench your jaw and push your teeth together.
  - Hold for six seconds.
  - Notice the tension.
  - Relax your jaw and allow your lips to part slightly.
- Now press your tongue against the roof of your mouth and feel the tension.
  - Hold for six seconds.
  - Allow your tongue to return to its normal position, experiencing the sensation of relaxation.
- Now press your lips together as tightly as possible.
  - Hold for six seconds.
  - Relax and notice the feelings of relaxation over your lips.
- Using the same principles, gradually move through the body from the shoulders to the arms, hands, fingers, back, chest, abdomen, hips, legs, ankles, feet, and toes.

Several variations of visualization can then be used. You can imagine a tranquil scene, such as a beach on a sunny day or a valley with a stream or forest, and then place yourself in the scene. Imagine all of the scene's sights, sounds, smells, and feelings. People suffering from a terminal illness frequently imagine scenes in which their immune system attacks or destroys their disease, or they envision themselves as healthy and disease-free. People who want to make major life changes, such as losing weight or stopping smoking, can envision themselves slim or not smoking or imagine themselves in trouble situations, such as a situation in which they are tempted to overeat or smoke. Then people can envision themselves making wise choices or not engaging in undesirable behaviors. Visualization can also be used to improve athletic performance. Tapes are available that can assist people in learning how to develop this technique.

Biofeedback

Biofeedback, based on scientific principles, is designed to enhance the awareness of body functions—it is an educational tool. Sensory equipment demonstrates subtle body changes, such as increases or decreases in skin temperature, muscle contraction, and brain wave variations. This biofeedback, or feedback on biological processes, enables people to become aware of what is happening in their bodies when stressed and learn how to control tensions through awareness of relaxing sensations. After a few sessions, people should begin to recognize and thereby alter their typical body responses to situations that serve as stressors for them (see Nurturing Your Spirituality: Enjoying Healthy Pleasures).

Massage therapy

Massage therapy has become an acceptable form of stress reduction and a healing alternative. Some people consider today's American society to be in the midst of a "touch famine." Appropriate touching is lacking, even though we recognize the need for physical interaction. Babies who are not handled can die from this type of deprivation. Although adults are not likely to respond so extremely to lack of touch, the need to be touched does not disappear with age. Research findings indicate that massage can promote physical relaxation and well-being. Certified massage therapists are licensed by the American Massage Therapy Association.[31]

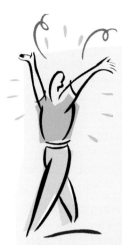

Nurturing Your Spirituality

Enjoying Healthy Pleasures

Certain lifestyle patterns have detrimental effects on our well-being and quality of life: not exercising, smoking, drinking to excess, not wearing a seat belt, and eating poorly. However, just as important as avoiding lifestyle patterns that can negatively affect quality of life is appreciating the joys, thrills, delights, and happiness that are part of our lives. The idea is to minimize the negative and maximize the positive in our lives. Pleasure has gotten a bad name and we have become almost phobic about enjoying ourselves and having fun. In their book *Healthy Pleasures*, Sobel and Ornstein[30] point out that, even though certain negative habits and addictions are unhealthy, we also must seek to feel good mentally and emotionally. We need to seek enjoyment to enhance our survival. Ornstein and Sobel emphasize that no better way exists to ensure healthy, life-saving behaviors than to make them pleasurable. From eating to reproduction to caring for others, pleasure can guide us to better health. Doing what feels good is often beneficial for health and survival.

A pleasurable experience can be as simple as taking time to enjoy a sunset, smelling the air after a rain shower, napping for half an hour in the afternoon, making a kind comment to a stranger or friend, or letting go of anger toward another human being. Seeking out pleasure may involve giving ourselves positive self-talks, looking for humor, and hanging out with happy people. Enjoying our gifts of pleasure is powerful medicine and can be contagious. It is cheap and effective, and its only side effect is a happy life. The following Web site provides a storehouse of information on the importance of adding pleasure to your life: **www.arise.org**.

Music

The power of music is undisputed. A strong beat and rhythmic music instill in almost all people of any age the desire to respond by moving or dancing. Quiet music soothes by causing people to breathe more deeply, stilling turbulent emotions, reducing metabolic response, and calming the autonomic nervous system.

Humor

Laughter is a powerful stress-reducing agent. A deep laugh temporarily raises pulse rate and blood pressure and tenses the muscles. After a good laugh, however, pulse rate and blood pressure go down and the muscles become more relaxed. Laughter works in two ways. Being able to laugh at a situation reminds you that life is seldom perfect or predictable. Laughing helps keep events in perspective. Laughing also works to reinforce a positive attitude. Laughing or even smiling can improve mood.

Tai chi

Although tai chi is an ancient form of Chinese martial arts, it differs from all other forms. Tai chi emphasizes tranquility and teaches the participant to remain calm against stressors and to harmonize with aggression and fear, rather than fight it. Further, it emphasizes internal strengths mixed with flexibility/agility rather than brute force. There are more than 100 positions/movements

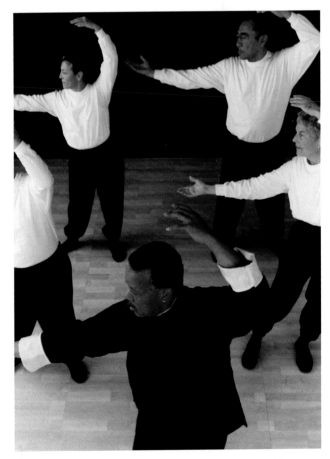

Exercise is a great way to reduce anxiety, increase positive feelings, and relieve stress.

found in tai chi's four basic philosophical concepts. The essence of each concept is

- Finding silence and solitude
- Regressing to the joys of childhood through embracing innocence, laughter, joy, and play
- Acting without forcing; moving in accordance with the flow of nature's course
- Acknowledging failure as the first step to success

Because of its philosophy, tai chi is sometimes referred to as morning meditation. There are many forms offered in the United States. Many community centers, private agencies, and universities offer various types of tai chi. The important factor is for you to find one that emphasizes the relaxation component.

Time management

A major contributor to stress is the pressure associated with time constraints. By effectively using time, you can eliminate a great deal of stress. For the college student, effective use of time is crucial, especially when working and attending school at the same time. Procrastination can add to stress and undermine academic work, personal relationships, and work efforts. Good time management, including appropriate prioritizing, scheduling, and the completion of personal responsibilities, can contribute to feelings of personal satisfaction.

Certain behaviors or habits can unnecessarily rob you of time:[32]

1. *Workaholism.* Workaholism is spending excessive amounts of time working, even though the activity may not be productive. Generally, people who engage in workaholic behavior like to work long hours and do not use time-saving techniques. They also may become overinvolved in unimportant tasks that eat away at their time, requiring them to use extra time to accomplish important tasks.
2. *Time juggling.* Time jugglers constantly overschedule themselves, often making promises to be in more than one place at a time. Because it is frequently impossible to do several things at once or be in two places at the same time, this behavior often results in the neglect of important activities.
3. *Procrastination.* Procrastinators consistently put off until later things that could just as easily be done now. Some procrastinators choose the simplest of two tasks to do now to avoid the really important ones until the last possible minute, when the pressure is on.
4. *Perfectionism.* Perfectionists go beyond trying to do their best to achieve perfection. Because standards of perfection vary from one person to the next, this behavior rarely results in a sense of accomplishment, and the inability to achieve impossible goals contributes to feelings of dissatisfaction and failure.

5. *Yesism.* Yesism is the inability to tell anyone no. Extremely nice people often suffer from this condition because they don't like to disappoint others or they fear being rejected, even if saying yes ends up costing them.

Effective time management allows us to have a sense of direction and to fulfill the requirements for using time in a productive, satisfying fashion. Following are some suggestions for appropriate use of your time:

1. *Set goals.* Spend time planning your goals. Think of short-term (one year or less) goals and long-term (one to three years) goals. Ask yourself if the goals established are essential, important, or trivial. A good question is "When does this task have to be completed?" Your goals should cause you to "stretch" but not "break" as you strive to achieve them.
2. *Prioritize.* Use the 80/20 rule, which states that 80 percent of the reward comes from 20 percent of the effort. Prioritize time to concentrate your efforts on those items that will provide the greatest reward for fulfilling your short- and long-term goals. Once your priorities have been established, start with the most important tasks to be accomplished—don't procrastinate.
3. *Develop a time framework.* To help alleviate stress, establish the amount of time to be spent on each activity. Some tasks cannot be completed in a day's time. Estimate the days or weeks required to complete the task. This is especially important in accomplishing long-term goals. Allotting blocks of time each day of each week helps alleviate the pressure of completing a difficult task in a short time. For example, if a term paper is due at the end of a semester, you can spend a certain number of hours each week working on the paper. You can establish benchmarks for the completion of the paper and devise rewards for yourself each time you achieve a benchmark.
4. *Use a to-do list.* Two suggestions for using a to-do list are to (1) develop a list of activities each day and create priorities for accomplishing the list and (2) combine your daily list with a calendar or schedule; this allows you to see a running agenda of the important tasks to be accomplished over time. The important thing is to find a method that works for you. Don't be afraid to experiment with a variety of methods to help provide focus on your priorities.
5. *Ask for help.* If responsibilities become overwhelming, ask for help. Say no when there are too many tasks to handle. Do not feel guilty about saying no; this only adds more stress. For example, if sorority or fraternity demands are too great, either

ask others to share the workload or refuse the responsibility.

6. *Be flexible.* Allow time for interruptions and distractions. Time management experts suggest planning for just 50 percent of your time. With 50 percent of your time planned, you will have the flexibility to handle interruptions and the unplanned emergency. When you expect to be interrupted, schedule routine tasks. Save larger blocks of time for your priorities.

7. *Take a break.* Every day should provide for fun, leisure, time alone, and relaxation. Make the most of every day. Schedule in time every day for yourself.

Assessment Activity 9-6 is a prioritization worksheet to help you organize your tasks. Assessment Activity 9-7 provides you with a log. Use it to record your daily activities for several days to a week. Then review it and see if you are spending your time as effectively as you thought or if you have overscheduled what you can do in 24 hours. This can provide you with a basis for devising improved time management plans.

Exercise

Because the fight or flight response stimulates the body into action, exercise is a logical method of responding to that physiological command. Exercise has been found to directly affect brain chemistry. Studies have shown an increase in endorphin levels after an easy or a strenuous run.[33] (Endorphins are natural pain killers that help alleviate sensations of pain and stimulate a positive response from the immune system.) Exercise is a positive stressor (eustressor) and, when properly used, seems to offset the adverse effects of distress.[31] Studies have demonstrated that exercise reduces the severity of the stress response, shortens the recovery time from the stressor, and diminishes vulnerability to stress-related disease. The higher the fitness level, the more beneficial the exercise in reducing stress. (The recommended types of exercise programs are discussed in Chapter 3.)

A correctly designed exercise program produces beneficial physiological responses and can induce psychological effects that reduce anxiety, promote feelings of accomplishment, and evoke muscle relaxation.

Many people consider stretching a means of invoking feelings of relaxation, and stretching is associated with reduced tension. Moderate levels of exertion are frequently considered most beneficial for most people. (A moderate-level activity is a walk at the rate of approximately 3 miles an hour.) Excessive or addictive exercise habits can have the reverse effect and contribute to feelings of tension and irritability. When engaging in exercise as a stress-reduction technique, strive to find the level that creates the greatest sense of well-being on completion.

Selecting a Stress-Reduction Technique

No single stress-reduction technique automatically reduces stress for everyone. People are comfortable with and enjoy different activities, and personal preference is what determines long-term use. When dealing with stress, you must first become aware that a stress response is occurring. People are frequently unaware that the reason they are always tired or irritable or have body aches is they are experiencing stress's negative effects. Second, find the stress-reduction techniques that work best for you. Usually, more than one approach is required, depending on the person and his or her type of stress response. Any technique that helps create a sense of relaxation, provides personal time, and allows you to gain control can lead to a happier, healthier, more enjoyable life. Third, the best form of stress management is the prevention of negative effects before they become unmanageable. Well-thought-out, prudent lifestyle decisions based on a knowledge of health behaviors and an understanding of your needs and expectations may be the best contribution you can make to your stress management plan. Finally, it is not the goal of stress-reduction strategies to overcome every stressor we face in our lives but, rather, to find effective responses to those stressors for purposes of managing our responses to them.

Spirituality

Many of the relaxation techniques briefly described in this chapter are designed to help people cope with stress. Several of these techniques include aspects of helping to find spiritual well-being. Carl Jung, a pioneer psychologist, proposed a spiritual element to human nature. Jung's work has led to the area of study called psychospirituality—the study of the relationship between mind and soul.

Although recognized as a significant component of the wellness paradigm, the spiritual aspect is not always understood. What is becoming increasingly obvious is how important our spirituality is to our total well-being.

In an attempt to grasp a difficult concept, it is essential to realize that the mind and soul are integral parts of understanding stress and finding ways to deal effectively with it. A recent trend in research has been the study of prayer, faith, and the healing/recovery of patients undergoing surgery and other medical treatments.[34]

Ray has stated that "the mind—a manifest functioning of the brain—and the other body systems interact in ways critical for health, illness, and well-being."[35]

Seaward, in his writings, points out that spiritual health is more than our religious beliefs and practices. He discusses potential characteristics, or inner resources, that help create "spiritual potential." These traits include creativity, will, intuition, faith, patience, courage, love, humility, and optimism. These traits allow for specific emotional responses that enable the expansion of human potential, thus allowing for the reduction of stress in difficult emotional or physical situations. Seaward believes that "employing faith or an optimistic attitude in the face of diversity exemplifies spiritual health."[36]

For some, the religious beliefs they hold can contribute to spirituality. For others, their spirituality may be enhanced through other efforts, such as exploring their personal value systems, working on their sense of connectedness with nature, and finding a meaningful purpose for their lives. In attempting to summarize, this achieving of spiritual wellness to aid in reducing stress requires a continuing assessment of our values, our purpose in life, and how we choose to deal with conflict.

Summary

- Stress is the nonspecific response of the body to any demands on it.
- Anything that creates stress is a stressor.
- Stressors may generate eustress (good stress) or distress (bad stress).
- The general adaptation syndrome (GAS) explains how the body responds to a stressor. The three stages of GAS are alarm, resistance, and exhaustion.
- The stress response can enhance physical and mental performance. This is referred to as the inverted-U theory.
- Whether positive or negative, a stressful event always produces a series of neurological and hormonal messages that are sent through the body.
- The responses to stress can be physiological (cardiovascular, gastrointestinal, musculoskeletal), psychological (causing depression, anxiety, anger), or behavioral (generating an inability to work, arguments).

- The immune system can be compromised as the result of prolonged stress, resulting in increases of susceptibility to comunicable diseases and chronic conditions.
- Coping is the effort(s) made to manage or deal with stress.
- Many techniques—including autogenics, deep breathing, visualization, muscle relaxation, meditation, massage, tai chi, biofeedback, exercise, yoga, music, and humor—can help reduce stress.
- Effective time management can be a key to stress reduction.
- People's perceptions of stress are associated with self-esteem, self-efficacy, and locus of control.
- People who deal effectively with stress seem to view stressful situations as opportunities for growth, have a sense of inner purpose, and view themselves as having power over their lives.

Review Questions

1. What is stress? What are stressors?
2. What are the stages the mind and body go through when exposed to a stressor?
3. What are some potential signals that a person is experiencing chronic stress, and what are the possible effects?
4. What factors influence how a person perceives and copes with stress?

5. Define *hardiness* and how it may help a person effectively deal with stress.
6. What are some guidelines for handling stress positively?
7. Discuss various stress-reduction techniques.

References

1. Siegal, B. S. 1988. *Love, medicine, and miracles.* New York: Perennial Library.
2. Selye, H. 1975. *Stress without disease.* New York: New American Library.
3. Hanson, P. G. 1986. *The joy of stress.* Kansas City, KS: Andrews, McMeel, & Parker.
4. Selye, H. 1978. *The stress of life.* Rev. Ed. New York: McGraw-Hill.
5. Girdano, D., D. E. Dusek, and G. S. Everly. 2005. *Controlling stress and tension.* San Francisco: Pearson/Benjamin Cummings.
6. Folkman, S. 1984. Personal control and stress and coping processes: A theoretical analysis. *Journal of Personal and Social Psychology* 46:839.
7. Seward, B. L. 2004. *Managing stress.* Boston: Jones and Bartlett.
8. McEwen, B. S., M. J. DeLeon, and M. J. Meaney. 1999. Corticosteroids, the aging brain and cognition. *Trends in Endocrinology and Metabolism* 10:92–96.
9. Blonna, R. 1996. *Coping with stress in a changing world.* St. Louis: Mosby.
10. Fawzy, F. I., N. Fawzy, C. Hyur, R. Elashoff, D. Guthrie, J. Ashley, and D. Morton. 1993. Malignant melanoma: Effects of an early structured psychiatric intervention, coping and affective state on recurrence and survival 6 years later. *Archives of General Psychiatry* 50:681–89.
11. Pert, C. 1999. *Molecules of emotion.* New York: Simon and Schuster.
12. Gelman, D., and M. Hager. 1988. Body and soul. *Newsweek,* 7 November.

13. Glaser, R., et al. 1987. Stress-related immune suppression: Health implications. *Brain Behavior-Immunity* 1(1):7.

14. O'Leary, A. 1990. Stress, emotion, and human immune function. *Psychology Bulletin* 108(3):363.

15. Pellitier, K., and D. Herzing. 1988. Psychoneuroimmunology: Toward a mind-body model: A critical review. *Advances* 5(1):27.

16. Domar, A., and H. Dreher. 1996. *Healing mind, healthy woman: Using the mind-body connection to manage stress and take control of your life.* New York: Henry Holt.

17. Domar, A., P. Zuttermeister, and R. Friedman. 1997. *The relationship between distress and conception in infertile women.* Paper presented at the Annual Meeting of the American Society of Reproductive Medicine, Cincinnati, Ohio.

18. Greenberg, J. 2004. *Comprehensive stress management.* New York: McGraw-Hill.

19. Newman, J. 2000. C'mon get happy. *Health* 14(6):130.

20. Adler, J. 14 June 1999. How stress attacks you. *Newsweek.*

21. Luecken, L. J., et al. 1997. Stress in employed women: Impact of marital status and children at home on neurohormonal output and home strain. *Psychosomatic Medicine* 59:352.

22. Light, K. C. 1997. Stress in employed women: A woman's work is never done if she's a working mom. *Psychosomatic Medicine* 59:360.

23. Friedman, M., and R. Roseman. 1984. *Type A behavior and your heart.* New York: Alfred A. Knopf.

24. Flannery, R. B. 1987. Toward stress-resistant persons: A stress management approach to the treatment of anxiety. *American Journal of Preventative Medicine* 3(1):25.

25. Barefoot, J. C., et al. 1987. Predicting mortality from scores on the Cook-Medley Scale: A follow-up study of 118 lawyers. *Psychosomatic Medicine* 49:210.

26. National Sleep Foundation. 2002. Epidemic of daytime sleepiness linked to increased feelings of anger, stress, and pessimism. National Sleep Foundation Website. May 31, 2004 (http://www.sleepfoundation.org).

27. Boyce, N., and S. Brink. 17 May 2004. The secrets of sleep. *U.S. News and World Report* 136(17):58–68.

28. Kobasa, S. 1984. How much stress can you survive? *American Health* 5(7):64.

29. Benson, H. 1985. *The relaxation response.* New York: Berkley.

30. Sobel, D. S., and R. Ornstein. 1989. *Healthy pleasures.* Reading, MA: Addison, Wesley.

31. Lamb, L. E. 1992. Understanding stress. *Health Letter* 39(suppl.):12.

32. Crews, D., and D. Landers. 1987. A meta-analytic review of aerobic fitness and reactivity to psychosocial stressors. *Medicine and Science of Sports Exercise* 19:5114.

33. Appenzeller, D., et al. 1980. Neurology of endurance training versus endorphins. *Neurology* 30:418.

34. Miller, W., and C. Thoresen. 2003. Spirituality, religion, and health: An emerging research field. *American Psychologist* 58(1):24–36.

35. Ray, O. 2003. How the mind hurts and heals the body. *American Psychologist* 59(1):29–40.

36. Seaward, B. 1991. Spiritual wellness. A health education model. *Journal of Health Education* 22(3):166–69.

Suggested Readings

Johnson, S. 2003. *The present.* New York: Doubleday.

This book emphasizes the importance of focusing on the present; if the desire is to make the future, then we must maintain our attention to the moment, live with a purpose, and plan the future. It is easy to read and can be read in a single sitting.

Levin, J. 2001. *God, faith and health.* New York: John Wiley & Sons.

The author's research has established a convincing link between faith or spirituality and achieving and maintaining good health. Dr. Levin provides compelling evidence of the connection between health and a wide array of beliefs/practices, including prayer, religious service attendance, meditation, and faith in God.

Maskach, C., and M. Leiter. 1997. *The truth about burnout: How organizations cause personal stress and what to do about it.* San Francisco: Jossey-Bass.

The authors encourage employees and managers to view the problems of burnout as an opportunity to address the major contributing pressures, such as exhaustion, cynicism, and ineffectiveness at work. The book is based on the real-world experiences of the authors working with companies to prevent and deal with burnout.

Orloff, J. 2004. *Positive energy.* New York: Harmony Books.

The author provides 10 detailed prescriptions for harnessing one's "positive energy" to replace fatigue with physical and emotional vigor. The book contains many techniques/tactics to actively involve the reader in energetic transformation.

Schiraldi, G. R. 1997. *Conquer anxiety, worry and nervous fatigue: A guide to greater peace.* Ellicott City, MD: Chevron.

The purpose of this book is to help readers learn to recognize and understand the symptoms of worry and anxiety. It provides a guide to stress management strategies, including relaxation, rational thinking, the confiding of past trauma, solution-focused problem solving, meditation, proper sleep, nutrition, exercise, time management, assertiveness training, self-esteem, and the strengthening of spiritual commitment.

Williams, V., and R. Williams. 1998. *Lifeskills.* New York: Times Books.

This review of the research on relationships and health goes on to describe a systematic self-help program to build better relationships to strengthen physical well-being. Eight basic life skills are described.

Name _____ Date _____ Section _____

Assessment Activity 9-1

Life Stressors

The following stress scale was developed by researchers Miller and Rahe. It includes positive and negative events, because both require adaptation. Research has confirmed that stress can have a significant impact on physical and emotional health. The total score on this self-test offers you insight into your risk for illness as a result of recent life events. Stressful changes won't necessarily harm you; the potential for damage rests in how you handle stress.

Directions: To determine the possible impact of various recent changes in your life, circle the "stress points" listed that you experienced during the past year.

Health
An injury or illness that
- kept you in bed a week or more or sent you to the hospital — 74
- did not require long bed rest or hospitalization — 44

Major dental work — 26
Major change in eating habits — 27
Major change in sleeping habits — 26
Major change in your usual type or amount of recreation — 28

Work
Change to a new type of work — 51
Change in your work hours or conditions — 35
Change in your responsibilities at work
- to more responsibilities — 29
- to fewer responsibilities — 21

Home
Major change in living conditions — 26
Change in residence
- within the same town/city — 25
- to a different town/city/state — 47

Change in family get-togethers — 25
Major change in health or behavior of family member — 55
Marriage — 50
Pregnancy — 67
Miscarriage or abortion — 65
Addition of a new family member
- through birth of a child — 66
- through adoption of a child — 65
- through a relative moving in — 59

Spouse beginning or ending work — 46
Changes at work involving
- promotion — 31
- demotion — 42
- transfer — 32

Troubles at work
- with your boss — 29
- with coworkers — 35
- with persons under your supervision — 35
- involving other issues or people — 28

Major business adjustment — 60
Retirement — 52
Loss of job
- due to being laid off from work — 68
- due to being fired from work — 79

Correspondence course to help you in your work — 18

Personal and Social
Change in personal habits — 26
Beginning or ending school or college — 38
Change of school or college — 35
Change in political beliefs — 24
Change in religious beliefs — 29
Change in social activities — 27
Vacation trip — 24
New close personal relationship — 37
Engagement to marry — 45
Girlfriend or boyfriend problems — 39
Sexual difficulties — 44
Child leaving home
- to attend college — 41
- to marry — 41
- for other reasons — 45

Change in the marital status of your parents
- through divorce — 59
- through remarriage — 50

Change in arguments with spouse — 50
In-law problems — 38
Separation from spouse
- due to work — 53
- due to marital problems — 76

Divorce — 96
Birth of grandchild — 43
Death of spouse — 119
Death of
- child — 123
- brother or sister — 102
- parent — 100

Financial
Major change in finances
- through increased income — 38
- through decreased income — 60
- through investment or credit difficulties — 56

Loss or damage of personal property — 43
Moderate purchase — 20

Name _____ **Date** _____ **Section** _____

Assessment Activity 9-2

How Stressed Are You?

Directions: The stress categories and stressors originally listed in Figure 9-1 on page 296 are also listed here. Underneath the stressors in each stress category is a blank. You can use this blank to rank yourself on each category and then to give yourself an overall stress rating. To rate yourself in each category, select a number from 1 to 10. A 1 indicates that you are currently experiencing no stress in that area of your life. A 10 indicates that the amount of stress you are experiencing in that area is overwhelming. This is a subjective rating and should be based on how you feel right now. After completing the assessment, note the areas currently creating difficulty for you and try to plan ways to reduce your overwhelming emotions in the next few days. Recheck your scores over the next few months to see how they change. If you chronically experience overwhelming stress in any area, you might want to seek the advice of a professional, such as a counselor or clergy.

Physical	**Social**	**Intellectual**	**Emotional**	**Spiritual**	**Environmental**
Pathogens	Embarrassment	Mental fatigue	Uncontrolled anger	Guilt	Noise
Drugs	Teasing	Overload	Unexpressed anger	Moral conflicts	Overcrowding
Smoking	Ridicule	Frustration	Inability to love	Lack of purpose	Poverty
Lack of sleep	Arguments	Mental stagnation	Lack of love	Lack of philosophy of life	Extreme temperatures
Injury	Lack of social interaction		Poor self-esteem		
Sedentary lifestyle	Rejection				

_____ _____ _____ _____ _____ _____

Overall stress: _____

Questions to Consider

1. Is the stress created from personal pressure or outside factors?
2. What changes could you make to reduce or eliminate the identified stressor(s)?
3. With whom could you discuss your feelings concerning the identified stressor(s)?

Name _____   Date _____   Section _____

Assessment Activity 9-3

Stress Style: Mind, Body, Mixed?

Directions: Imagine yourself in a stressful situation. When you are feeling anxious, what sensations do you typically experience? Check all that apply.

_____   1. My heart beats faster.

_____   2. I find it difficult to concentrate because of distracting thoughts.

_____   3. I worry too much about things that don't really matter.

_____   4. I feel jittery.

_____   5. I get diarrhea.

_____   6. I imagine terrifying scenes.

_____   7. I cannot keep anxiety-provoking pictures and images out of my mind.

_____   8. My stomach gets tense.

_____   9. I pace up and down nervously.

_____   10. I am bothered by unimportant thoughts running through my mind.

_____   11. I become immobilized.

_____   12. I feel I am losing out on things because I cannot make decisions fast enough.

_____   13. I perspire.

_____   14. I cannot stop thinking worrisome thoughts.

There are three basic ways of reacting to stress—physically, mentally, or with a combination of the two. Physical stress type people feel tension in the body—jitters, butterflies, the sweats. Mental types experience stress mainly in the mind—worries and preoccupying thoughts. Mixed types react with both responses in about equal measure.

Give yourself a *Mind* point if you answered yes to each of the following questions: 2, 3, 6, 7, 10, 12, 14. Give yourself a *Body* point for each of these: 1, 4, 5, 8, 9, 11, 13. If you have more *Mind* than *Body* points,

consider yourself a mental stress type. If you have more *Body* than *Mind* points, your stress style is physical. Do you have about the same number of each? You are a mixed reactor.

Choosing a Relaxer

Mind

If you experience stress as an invasion of worrisome thoughts, the most direct intervention is anything that will engage your mind completely and redirect it—meditation, for example. Some people find the sheer exertion of heavy physical exercise unhooks the mind wonderfully and is fine therapy. Suggestions are

Meditation	Autogenic suggestion
Reading	Crossword puzzles
TV, movies	Games such as chess or cards
Any absorbing hobby	Vigorous exercise
Knitting, sewing, carpentry, or other handicrafts	

Body

If stress registers mainly in your body, you will need a remedy that will break up the physical tension pattern. This may be a vigorous body workout, but a slow-paced or even lazy muscle relaxer may be equally effective. Here are some suggestions to get you started:

Aerobics	Progressive relaxation
Swimming	Body scan
Biking	Rowing
Walking	Yoga
Massage	Soaking in a hot bath, sauna

Mind/body

If you are a mixed type, you may want to try a physical activity that also demands mental rigor:

Competitive sports, (racquetball, tennis, squash, volleyball, etc.)	Meditation Any combination from the *Mind* and *Body* lists

Name _____ **Date** _____ **Section** _____

Assessment Activity 9-4

Identification of Coping Styles

Directions: There are a variety of ways to deal with stress. Following is a list of positive coping behaviors. Indicate how much you currently use them to deal with stress.

	Often	Rarely	Not at All
Listen to music			
Go shopping with a friend			
Watch television/go to a movie			
Read a newspaper, magazine, or book			
Sit alone in the peaceful outdoors			
Write prose or poetry			
Attend an athletic event, a play, a lecture, a symphony, and so on			
Go for a walk or drive			
Exercise (swim, bike, jog)			
Get deeply involved in some other activity			
Play with a pet			
Take a nap			
Get outdoors, enjoy nature			
Write in a journal			
Practice deep breathing, meditation, autogenics, muscle relaxation			
Straighten up your desk or work area			
Take a bath or shower			
Do physical labor (garden, paint)			
Make home repairs, refinish furniture			
Buy something—records, books			
Play a game (chess, backgammon, video games)			
Pray, go to church			
Discuss situations with a spouse or close friend			
Other: _____ _____ _____			

Name _____ Date _____ Section _____

Assessment Activity 9-5

How Hardy Are You?

Directions: Following are 12 items similar to those that appear on a hardiness questionnaire. Evaluating an individual's hardiness requires more than one quick test, but this simple exercise can be a good indication of your hardiness. Write down how much you agree or disagree with the following statements, using this scale:

0 = Strongly disagree
1 = Mildly disagree
2 = Mildly agree
3 = Strongly agree

_____ A. Trying my best at work makes a difference.
_____ B. Trusting to fate is sometimes all I can do in a relationship.
_____ C. I often wake up eager to start on the day's projects.
_____ D. Thinking of myself as a free person leads to great frustration and difficulty.
_____ E. I could sacrifice financial security in my work if something really challenging came along.
_____ F. It bothers me when I have to deviate from the routine or schedule I have set for myself.
_____ G. An average citizen can have an impact on politics.

_____ H. Without the right breaks, it is hard to be successful in my field.
_____ I. I know why I am doing what I'm doing at work.
_____ J. Getting close to people puts me at risk of being obligated to them.
_____ K. Encountering new situations is an important priority in my life.
_____ L. I really don't mind when I have nothing to do.

Scoring: These questions measure control, commitment, and challenge. For half of these questions, a high score (agreement) indicates hardiness; for the other half, a low score (disagreement) does.

To get your scores on control, commitment, and challenge, first write in the number of your answer—0, 1, 2, or 3—above the letter of each question on the score sheet. Then add and subtract as shown. (To get your score on control, for example, add your answers to questions A and G; add your answers to B and H; and then subtract the second number from the first.)

Add your scores on control, commitment, and challenge to get a score for total hardiness. A total score of 10–18 = hardy personality; 0–9 = moderate hardiness; below 0 = low hardiness.

$$(\underline{\quad}_{(A)} + \underline{\quad}_{(G)}) - (\underline{\quad}_{(B)} + \underline{\quad}_{(H)}) = \underline{\quad} = \text{Control score}$$

$$(\underline{\quad}_{(C)} + \underline{\quad}_{(I)}) - (\underline{\quad}_{(D)} + \underline{\quad}_{(J)}) = \underline{\quad} = \text{Commitment score} \Bigg\} = \underline{\quad} = \text{Total hardiness score}$$

$$(\underline{\quad}_{(E)} + \underline{\quad}_{(K)}) - (\underline{\quad}_{(F)} + \underline{\quad}_{(L)}) = \underline{\quad} = \text{Challenge score}$$

Paths to Hardiness: Three techniques are suggested for becoming happier, healthier, and hardier:

- *Focusing:* Recognize signals from the body that something is wrong. Focusing increases the sense of control over plans and puts people in a psychologically better position to change.
- *Reconstructing stressful situations:* Think about a stress episode and then write down three ways the

situation could have turned out better and three ways it could have been worse. Doing this helps you feel better about the way situations turn out and appreciate other coping strategies.

- *Compensating through self-improvement:* It is important to distinguish between what can be controlled and what cannot. A way to regain control is by taking on a new challenge or task to master.

Name _____ **Date** _____ **Section** _____

Assessment Activity 9-6

Goals and Priorities

Directions: What follows is an activity designed to help establish your short-term (less than a year, a month, a week) goals and long-term (one year or more) goals. Try to set goals that are specific, realistic, measurable, and achievable. Your goals should require effort on your part but should not cause you to burn out or fail. Your goals should give you a sense of direction. Once your short- and long-term goals have been established, determine what priorities you need to accomplish. Remember the 80/20 rule (see discussion in this chapter). Use a to-do list and establish your priorities for each day of the week. You may wish to prioritize your lists by number, letter, or color—whatever works best for you. Keep in mind the tips for time management. Be sure to schedule time for yourself regularly. It is vital to your stress management.

Goals
Long-Term (One Year or More)

1. _____

2. _____

3. _____

Etc. _____

Short-Term (Semester/Month)

1. _____

2. _____

3. _____

Etc. _____

Priorities for Next Week

1. _____

2. _____

3. _____

Etc. _____

Day _____ to-Do List

    Must Do

    Important to Do

    Things I Would Like to Get Done

Day _____ to-Do List

    Must Do

    Important to Do

    Things I Would Like to Get Done

Name _____ Date _____ Section _____

Assessment Activity 9-7

Analyzing Your Use of Time

Managing your time effectively can significantly contribute to your feeling of being in control of your life. A by-product of this sense of control is reduced stress and tension; with effective time management, you will be able to meet daily demands with less effort. The basis of change is recognizing that there needs to be a change and then determining the areas in your life that require change, so a good way to begin meeting your time management needs is to analyze how you are currently managing your time.

Directions: Make several copies of this log and keep track of your time for a week. Include all your activities—including classes, meals, driving time, and conversations with friends. At the end of the day and week, rate each hour as to how important the activities that occurred during that time were. Taking time to relax, talk to friends, and be alone is considered important to total well-being and should not be discounted.

Daily Log

Time	Activities	Where	Essential, Important, or Trivial
6:00–7:00 a.m.			
7:00–8:00			
8:00–9:00			
9:00–10:00			
10:00–11:00			
11:00–12:00 p.m.			
12:00 p.m.–1:00 p.m.			
1:00–2:00			
2:00–3:00			
3:00–4:00			
4:00–5:00			
5:00–6:00			
6:00–7:00			
7:00–8:00			
8:00–9:00			
9:00–10:00			
10:00–11:00			
11:00 p.m.–12.00 a.m.			
12:00 a.m.–1:00 a.m.			
1:00–2:00			
2:00–3:00			
3:00–4:00			
4:00–5:00			
5:00–6:00			

10

Taking Charge
of Your Personal Safety

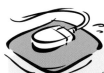

Online Learning Center

Log on to our Online Learning Center (OLC) for access to these additional resources:

- Chapter key term flashcards
- Learning objectives
- Additional goals for behavior change
- Concentration game
- Self-scoring chapter quizzes

- Additional lab activities

The OLC also offers Web links for study and exploration of wellness topics. Access these links through **www.mhhe.com/anspaugh6e**, click on Student Center, click on Chapter 10, and then click on Web Activities.

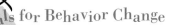

Goals for Behavior Change

- Identify and change three risky behaviors you now engage in.
- Make at least two alterations to your home environment to protect yourself and your family.
- Assess your safety precautions when participating in sports and recreational activities.
- Develop a personal safety plan for helping prevent unintentional injury.

Key Terms

acquaintance rape
carbon monoxide
date rape

homicide
rape trauma syndrome
road rage

Objectives

After completing this chapter, you will be able to do the following:

- Identify potential dangers associated with unintentional and intentional injuries.
- List protective measures for maintaining a safe home environment.

- Discuss the steps necessary to participate safely in recreational activities.
- Describe guidelines for the safe operation of a vehicle.

his chapter follows the stress chapter for good reason. As we rush through our daily lives, one of the consequences of our high-stress, tension-filled lifestyles is accidents. Many of us experience close calls or minor mishaps during the periods when we are experiencing stress. Too often during these periods, we do not pay close attention, are careless in our behavior, or engage in behavior that puts us at greater risk for accidents or personal harm.

Statistics indicate that accidents are the leading cause of death for people between 1 and 45 years. Even if HIV does become the leading killer for certain subgroups within this age range, accidents will still be the number two killer. College students and other young adults tend to give too little thought to their personal safety. As they participate in their daily academic and recreational activities, they encounter many potential dangers. No longer can the college campus be considered a safe haven from the violence and crime that are such significant parts of our society. Plenty of evidence indicates that people in a university environment are at significant risk for violence. Because you feel safe does not necessarily mean you are. This chapter explores those areas where the decisions you make can greatly influence your safety.

The first section of this chapter examines violence and intentional injury including acquaintance/date rape, homicide, relationship violence, and hate-related crime. Included in this first section are topics related to personal safety—for example, how to be safe at the ATM, in your car, and in your apartment. The second section deals with recreation and outdoor safety. Topics discussed range from bicycling safety to avoiding road rage. The third section deals with unintentional injury, which can occur in the home during recreational activities or while driving.

Violence and Intentional Injury

As we go about our daily activities, we are constantly conscious of violence. Acts of violence include assault, homicide (murder), sexual assault, domestic violence, suicide, and various forms of abuse. Each year in the United States, intentional violence accounts for 50,000 deaths and more than 2 million nonfatal injuries.[1] Violence has the potential to touch the lives of the college student, regardless of school, gender, or ethnicity (see Assessment Activity 10-1).

Acquaintance and Date Rape

The terms *acquaintance* and *date rape* have been brought to the national consciousness over the last 15 years. **Acquaintance rape** is forced sexual intercourse between

people who know one another well. **Date rape** is a form of acquaintance rape that involves forced sexual intercourse between people in a dating situation. Statistics indicate that 60 percent of rapes are committed by people the victims know or are dating.[1] Researchers reported that 24 percent of college women claimed to be victims of attempted rape, and 17 percent claimed to have been forced to have sex against their will.[2]

In the college setting, poor communication is associated with behavior that results in attempts at seduction. One survey of 600 college men and women found there was substantial agreement among both genders that aggression and coercion usually occurred when one partner felt "led on" and the other did not make it clear how far she or he was willing to go.[3] One solution is for couples to learn that no really means no, regardless of the tone or hesitancy with which it is stated (see Just the Facts: Guidelines for Avoiding Acquaintance and Date Rape).

Researchers also point to a special problem on some college campuses on which there are strong fraternity or sorority organizations. Just because some athletic and other campus groups have condoned inappropriate actions on the part of their group members does not mean that all student social organizations are suspect. However, given the drinking, potential for intimacy, sexual teasing, and competitiveness characteristic of the house party, such gatherings sponsored by social organizations may provide social settings that encourage aggressive sexual behavior.[4] Many sorority and fraternity organizations have classes that educate members in an effort to improve mutual understanding and avoid date coercion or rape.

An important strategy in avoiding date and acquaintance rape is to not use alcohol or other drugs. Statistics indicate that 75 percent of male students and 55 percent of female students involved in rape have been drinking or using drugs when rape occurs.[4] For a discussion of Rohypnol, the so-called date rape drug, see Just the Facts: Rohypnol—Setup for Rape. Also see Chapter 11.

When a traumatic, often violent experience occurs, such as acquaintance or date rape, the victim usually experiences a great amount of enduring and substantial psychological damage. Date rape victims are particularly vulnerable because they are the victims of misplaced trust. Once the trust in a relationship is broken because of forced sex, developing new relationships becomes much more difficult for the victim.[4]

Regardless of how psychologically strong they are, most rape victims are likely to experience shock, anxiety, depression, shame, and a host of other psychosomatic symptoms. The psychological reactions following a rape are referred to as **rape trauma syndrome.** The syndrome is characterized by fear, nightmares, fatigue, crying spells, and digestive upset. Sexual function and desire may be

～Just the Facts～

Guidelines for Avoiding Acquaintance and Date Rape

Men should observe these guidelines:

- *Know your sexual desires and limits.* Be aware of the effects of social pressure. It's okay not to "score."

- *Being turned down when you ask for sex is not a rejection of you personally.* If someone says no to sex with you, it does not mean you are being rejected personally; what is being expressed is the desire not to engage in a single sex act. Personal actions are within your control.

- *Accept the woman's decision.* Don't read other meanings into the situation; *no* means exactly that!

- *Don't assume that the way a woman dresses or flirts indicates she wants to have sexual intercourse.*

- *Don't assume that previous permission for sexual contact applies to the current situation.*

- *Avoid excessive use of alcohol and other drugs.* Alcohol and other drugs interfere with clear thinking, perception, and effective communication.

Women should observe these guidelines:

- *Know your sexual desires and limits.* Believe in your right to set limits.

- *Communicate your limits clearly.* If you are offended, say so in a firm manner and do so immediately. Say no when you mean no.

- *Be assertive.* Men sometimes interpret passivity as permission. Be direct and firm with anyone pressuring you sexually.

- *Be aware that your nonverbal actions send a message.* If you dress in a sexy manner and flirt, men sometimes assume you want to have sex. You should be able to dress as you please and flirt without its meaning anything. However, be aware of the possibility for someone to misunderstand and misinterpret your actions.

- *Pay attention to your surroundings.* Do not put yourself in vulnerable situations.

- *Trust your intuitions.* If you feel you are being pressured, you are!

- *Avoid excessive use of alcohol and other drugs.* Alcohol and other drugs interfere with clear thinking, perception, and effective communication.

～Just the Facts～

Rohypnol—Setup for Rape

The drug Rohypnol (flunitrazepam) is a type of sleeping pill; it is illegal in the United States and Canada. Following is some key information about the drug:[5]

- It is produced legally in Mexico by Hoffmann-LaRoche.

- It is the most widely prescribed sedative or hypnotic in Europe.

- Manufactured illegal versions are available—the branded product seems to be preferred by illicit users.

- In the United States, it appears to be most frequently used in conjunction with alcohol, creating an enhancing (synergistic) effect.

- It is odorless and tasteless when mixed with alcohol.

- The drug seems to produce amnesia and a loss of inhibition.

- Several arrests have been made in conjunction with alleged date rape involving the use of Rohypnol. Allegations are that the drug was added to women's drinks without their knowledge.

- Adverse effects can include loss of memory, impaired judgment, dizziness, and prolonged periods of blackout. Although a sedative, Rohypnol can produce aggressive behavior.

- Use appears to be spreading among high school and college groups.

- Street names include rophies, roofies, ruffies, R2, roofenol, Roche, roachies, larocha, rope, and rib.

impaired. The victim of violent sex may want her partner to be warm, tender, affectionate, and understanding, but she may not desire sexual intercourse for a long time after the rape. Sometimes lengthy counseling is necessary to help the rape victim reestablish a trusting attitude toward her relationships and sexuality.[4]

Another common psychological effect of rape is self-blame (the victim blames herself for what has occurred). The victim tends to review every aspect of the attack to understand what she could have done differently to prevent the rape. Although victims are blameless, self-accusation is common.[4] Self-blame is particularly prevalent in acquaintance or date rape because victims believe such rapes occurred because they created situations that permitted sexual coercion. Victims also tend to view their friends as being successful in the dating situation; it is common for victims to believe they are the only ones who have "failed." Rape victims tend to perceive themselves as having permitted a social occasion to turn into a

ꞈꞈ Just the Facts ꞈꞈ

What to Do If You Are Raped

If you are raped, you should do the following:

- Call the police and tell them you were raped. Provide your location.

- Don't wash or douche before the medical exam. Take a change of clothes, but do not change until you have been examined.

- At the medical facility, you will have a complete examination. Point out any bruises, cuts, scratches, and so on.

- Tell the authorities exactly what happened. Be honest and thorough.

- Be sure you are checked for pregnancy and STDs.

- Contact the campus agency that can help with rape counseling or contact the nearest rape crisis center for counseling.

ꞈꞈ Just the Facts ꞈꞈ

United States Crime Clock

- Every 2.7 seconds, some type of crime occurs.

- Every 22.1 seconds, one violent crime is committed in the United States.

  - Every 35.3 seconds, one aggravated assault
  - Every 1.2 minutes, one robbery
  - Every 5.5 minutes, one forcible rape
  - Every 32.4 minutes, one murder

- Every 3.0 seconds, one property crime is committed in the United States.

  - Every 4.5 seconds, one larceny-theft
  - Every 14.7 seconds, one burglary
  - Every 25.3 seconds, one motor vehicle theft

SOURCE: Federal Bureau of Investigation. 2002. *Uniform crime reports.* Washington, DC.

painful event. Victims need the understanding of friends, family, significant others, and possibly professional counselors to help them work through these feelings.[6] Just the Facts: What to Do If You Are Raped describes the steps a rape victim should follow or be encouraged to follow as soon as possible after the assault.

The best protection against date or acquaintance rape is preparation and constant awareness that the potential always exists for unwanted sexual advances and potentially traumatic sexual experiences. Planning what to do if faced with unwanted advances and acting assertively may prevent or terminate many potentially devastating situations.

Homicide

Murder, or **homicide,** is a crime that has been on the decline for the last several years. However in 2002 (the latest statistics available), the estimated number of murders rose by 1 percent over the 2001 volume.[6] (See Just the Facts: United States Crime Clock.) FBI statistics indicate that the number of murders in 2002 was estimated at 16,204.[7]

The murder victims in 2002 consisted of 10,054 individuals. Of that number, 6,757 were white, 6,730 black, and 567 of another race or the race was unknown. The largest group of murder victims was black males (5,544) followed by white males (4,853) and white females (1,905). Almost 3,500 of the murder victims were age 22 and under. Of this age group, almost 50 percent were black males. The murder weapon most frequently used

was some type of firearm (8,890), and the second most frequently used weapon was a knife or cutting instrument (1,831).[7] The circumstances under which the murders occurred were robbery (1,092), drug-related (894), juvenile groups (911), romantic triangle (130), and rape (43).

Most of us never think we might be involved in a situation where murder might occur. One only need to think of the Ted Bundys of the world, or the disappearances of college students that occur each year. The implication for students is, first, do not put yourself in harm's way. Examples of such behavior would be making drug purchases, not locking apartment doors, using an ATM machine late at night, and allowing firearms around when alcohol is present. Several of these issues will be discussed in the remaining parts of this chapter.

Relationship Violence

There are several types of violence. The first type of violence this chapter will focus on is domestic violence and the effects on any children involved in a domestic situation. The second type of violence/abuse is that found in the dating situation.

Today's families take many shapes, including single parents, blended families, and two-career families. More and more children are being left unattended while parents are either working or commuting home. Parents frequently feel overworked and children may feel neglected. The mix of related and unrelated people living in the same home can create new problems.

It is estimated that more than 4.0 million women are the victims of some form of violence each year.[8] Domestic violence is also called spouse abuse, intimate partner abuse, battering, and partner violence. Whatever term is used, it is when an individual is in some way hurt by a person whom he or she knows. These hurts are not limited to physical harm but also include sexual and psychological abuse.[9] Authorities estimate that only about half of crimes of violence against a partner are reported. It is easy to be critical of people who do not report these crimes, but there are compelling reasons for their silence: Many women do not report abuse for fear of being killed or further injured and concern for the lives of any children who are part of the household. Many abused women may have little or no financial support other than the abuser, so they feel trapped. See Nurturing Your Spirituality: Learning to Communicate for some insight into the basis for some domestic violence.

Anyone, regardless of age, gender, race, or economic, educational, or religious background, can be abused. Men can be victims of abuse. However, most victims of abuse are women and are much more likely to be seriously injured. Certain groups of women seem to be at higher risk. They include women who[9]

- Are single, separated, or divorced
- Are between the ages of 17 and 28

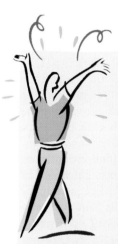

Nurturing Your Spirituality

Learning to Communicate

Much of what occurs in relationships can be traced to how couples learn to communicate. As couples fall in love, it is important that, as they experience the wonderful, sometimes overwhelming emotions of being in love with another person, they become aware of how their communication patterns are developing. Each person brings to a relationship a different history and different perceptions and expectations. Dating couples who find that their methods of communication (or lack thereof) lead to periods of intense angry or physical confrontation, such as pushing or hitting one another, should seek to find more effective ways to communicate or, perhaps better yet, end the relationship.

Growing relationships should involve a maturing of love, care, trust, and concern. Such growth can occur only if people learn to communicate effectively and in a nonthreatening manner. Although everyone wants to avoid physically and emotionally abusive situations, learning how to understand and communicate with a person whom you care deeply about is not just something that happens. Couples must work at developing communication. The starting point is how each person views the other: No one "belongs" to someone else; no one is anybody else's property. People make choices to be with and share their lives with others and actively attempt to do so by behaving with kindness and thoughtfulness and by exhibiting a desire to grow with their partners along the journey of life. For continued personal growth, we must find ways to communicate effectively with our partners.

The starting point for good communication is mutual *trust* between partners. Honest communication requires some vulnerability. An untrustworthy partner may misuse personal, private information by mocking it, revealing it to others, or using it to justify behavior. When both partners respect and treasure verbal intimacy, trust is created.

Partners should agree on the ground rules for approaching conversations in which there is potential for disagreement. Each partner should listen carefully to what the other is saying—not to try to win the conversation but to understand. Each person should be allowed to speak about his or her perceptions and feelings without interruption or fear of verbal or physical abuse. Each person should ask clarifying questions and attempt to repeat what the other has expressed. Anger does not lead to effective communication, and people should know when to take a time-out and move away from each other for a few minutes to allow their anger to subside.

When communicating, it is important to use *I* messages whenever possible. *I* messages convey what the speaker is feeling, not what the speaker thinks his or her partner is feeling or doing. For example, "You make me feel angry" is not an *I* message, but "*I* feel angry when you mention my family" is an *I* message. Through *I* messages, the speaker takes responsibility for his or her feelings and does not attribute them to a partner.

When communicating, it is also important to demonstrate an interest in listening and understanding. This entails maintaining eye contact and nodding or saying yes.

Finding ways to resolve conflict can improve the quality and extend the longevity of relationships. Remaining silent only fosters anger and indifference. Failing to discuss issues in a relationship merely builds walls, one brick at a time. The feelings of frustration and anger may eventually manifest in extreme verbal or physical abuse, or they may lead to indifference and loss of love.

- Abuse alcohol or other drugs or whose partners do
- Are pregnant
- Have partners who are excessively jealous or possessive

An abuser can be anyone. The abuser may be a husband, wife, boyfriend, girlfriend, or roommate. Many abusers were exposed to family violence as children. Adults who grew up in a violent home are more likely to become abusers or victims of domestic abuse. They see abuse as a normal way of life. A third of women who are physically abused grew up in a home where their mother was abused. Almost 20 percent were abused themselves. Adults who were abused as children are more likely not to see their abuser's behavior as damaging, since they were raised in that fashion.[10]

The results of domestic abuse are not limited to physical or emotional scars. Some of the long-term effects of the abuse include

- Self-neglect or self-injury
- Depression, anxiety, panic attacks, and sleep disorders
- Alcohol and other drug abuse
- Aggression toward themselves and others
- Chronic pain
- Eating disorders
- Sexual dysfunctions
- Suicide attempts

As disgusting as domestic violence is, the impact this has on children is perhaps even more saddening. Children who either hear abuse from another room or witness actual abuse are clearly traumatized. Children in domestic abuse situations are in a situation that is detrimental to their emotional development and physical well-being. Children of domestic abuse are more likely to suffer sleeplessness, bed wetting, anxiety, and temper tantrums; do poorly in the academic setting; are more likely to attempt suicide; and have a higher chance of abusing alcohol or other drugs. In addition, children from abusive situations are more likely to become abusers and to abuse their own children.[8] These facts remain true whether the child was in an abusive situation or was actually abused.

There is no reason any person should have to suffer the indignity of abuse. Every person has the right to the highest quality life possible, and no one has a right to inflict physical or psychological pain on anyone else. Anyone aware of an abusive situation has the moral and ethical responsibility to report the suspected abuse to authorities, so that action can be taken to protect the innocent victim and to help ensure either the punishment or rehabilitation of the abuser.

It is unfortunate that people sometimes become involved in a dating situation in which abuse occurs. Dating should be a time of having fun, getting to know a prospective mate, learning to trust and respect another, providing support, being honest, and growing more comfortable in social settings with other people. Some people may not even recognize when they have become involved in an abusive situation. Like domestic violence, dating violence can come in many forms. Abuse can be physical, sexual, psychological/emotional, verbal, or what the American Bar Association calls "abuse of male privilege."[10] Table 10-1 lists the types of occurrences under each type of abuse.

Abusers in the dating situation use their abusive behaviors and comments to maintain control and power over the dating partner. The American Bar Association has developed a series of questions to ask

Table 10-1 Examples of Abuse in the Dating Situation

Physical	Sexual	Psychological/Emotional	Verbal	Abuse of Male Privilege
Punching	Unwanted touching	Humiliation	Name-calling	Making all decisions
Slapping	Sexual relations	Intimidation	Ridiculing	Expecting to be waited on
Kicking	without consent	Extreme jealousy	Insults	or pampered
Pulling of hair	Calling sexual names	Put-downs	Yelling	Treating another like
Choking	Threatening to get another	Untrustworthiness	Public humiliation	property
Striking with	sex partner	Blaming of partner for own		Expecting partner to be
an object	Striking with an object	faults		available at all times
Biting	Making fun of	Emotional withholding		
Scratching	sexual activity	Stalking		
Burning				
Physical				
confinement				

SOURCE: Adapted from the American Bar Association. Domestic Violence. Source available online at **www.abanet.org/domviol/typeofabuse.html**.

oneself when evaluating if one is in an abusive dating situation:[10]

- Are you discouraged from pursuing your interests?
- Does he or she act extremely jealously when you talk to other people?
- Does he or she embarrass you in front of friends or make you feel stupid by calling you names?
- Has he or she forced you to do anything sexually that you didn't want to?
- Does he or she threaten you?
- Does he or she make all the decisions in the relationship?
- Does he or she control you by being bossy or giving orders?
- Does he or she make your family uneasy and concerned for your safety?
- Does he or she say it is your fault when he or she hurts you?
- Have you apologized for your partner's behavior when he or she has done something wrong to you?
- Have you been worried about upsetting your partner?

If any of these signs are present, you should examine carefully the quality of the relationship and if it is really beneficial to continue in the relationship. Remember, if marriage occurs, those little things that you think will change usually become even more of a problem—including abuse. In a healthy relationship, both partners respect each other, encourage and support the other's goals, encourage each other to have friends outside the relationship, communicate openly and honestly, trust each other, feel safe, and share in decision making (see Wellness on the Web: Home Sweet (Safe) Home).

Hate Crimes

Hate crimes are crimes directed at people or groups because of perpetrators' hatred of their race, nationality, ethnicity, religion, or sexual orientation. In 2002, 8,832 hate-motivated criminal incidents were reported to the FBI. Of these offenses, 48.8 percent were motivated by racial bias; 19.1 percent by religious bias; 19.1 percent by sexual-orientation bias; and 14.8 percent by ethnicity or country of origin.[11] In 2002, the majority of hate crime incidents (29.5 percent) occurred in or on residential properties. Twenty percent of incidents were perpetrated on highways, on roads, in alleys, and on streets. Nine percent of hate crimes occurred at schools or colleges.[7] Perhaps the 9 percent occurring at schools or colleges is one of the most alarming statistics, because colleges are institutions in our society that we might expect to celebrate diversity. Hate crimes can occur anywhere, but educated college students and faculty should understand the importance of tolerance and acceptance

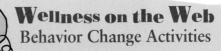

Wellness on the Web
Behavior Change Activities

Home Sweet (Safe) Home
We like to believe our home is a safe haven—but to a large degree, safety is something we must create for ourselves. Whether you live in a dormitory or an off-campus apartment, your personal safety depends on being alert to potential hazards and knowing what you can do to prevent or minimize them. Go to your textbook Web site at www.mhhe.com/anspaugh6e, click on Student Center, Chapter 10, Wellness on the Web, and then Activity 1 to learn more about the dangers related to living on or near campus and what you can do to lower your risk. Select areas where you may be most vulnerable and write down things you can do now that will reduce your risk.

What's Your Domestic Violence IQ?
Domestic violence shouldn't happen to anybody, ever. But it does—and when it does, help is available. Maybe you've lived with abuse, maybe experienced it just once; maybe you work or live next to someone who is being abused. Today, family patterns are much more complex than years ago. Sociologists indicate that families, and the individuals in those families, are under more stress than ever. To test your knowledge of this problem, go to the Web site listed previously; click on Activity 2 and select "True or False." Answer the questions related to domestic violence. How much did you know?

of individual differences. No person should have to suffer a diminished quality of life because of another's hatred of his or her race, religion, sexual orientation, ethnic background, nationality, or political beliefs.

Safety at the Automated Teller Machine

Many people use automated teller machines (ATMs) to carry out various banking transactions. These machines provide a convenient way to make deposits or withdrawals in a variety of locations and at almost any time, when banks are closed, during holidays, evenings, and weekends. Over the last few years, many violent crimes have been committed at ATM sites. If you must make an ATM transaction, keep the following rules in mind at all times:

- Use the ATM during daylight hours if possible. If you must use an ATM at night, take someone with you and use a machine only in a well-lighted area.
- Before using the machine, check to make sure no one is acting suspiciously or hanging around the area.

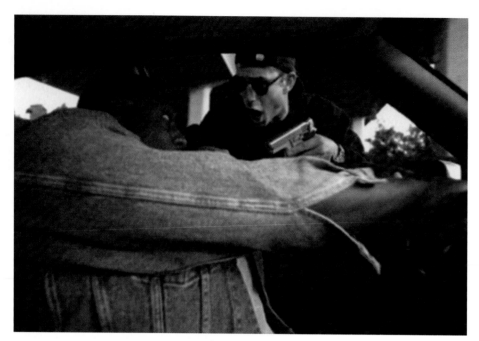

Carjacking is an increasingly frequent crime.

Trust your instincts if you feel uneasy. Seek a machine in another area if you sense something is not right where you are.
- Make sure no one attempts to crowd you while you are using the ATM. Take all receipts with you—do not discard your receipt nearby.
- Do not write down your personal identification number (PIN) or carry it in your billfold or purse.
- If you drive to an ATM, park in a highly visible location and under a light at night. Always lock your car and hold your keys in your hand.
- Do not assume that a drive-up ATM is free of assault potential. Always be alert to your surroundings.

Carjacking

One of the crimes that seems to be becoming more prevalent is carjacking, a crime in which someone attempts to steal a car while the driver or owner is present. Of carjackings, 45 percent occur on the street and another 30 percent occur in parking lots or garages. A gun is used in 70 percent of carjackings, which makes this crime potentially violent.[13] To protect yourself against such crime and to help reduce the risk for potential assault, do the following:

- Keep the doors of your car locked at all times, even when you are in it.
- Always park in a well-lighted, busy area. Avoid parking in underground or enclosed parking because the security may be poor.
- Always check the backseat before entering your car.

- When walking to your car at night, have a friend or a security guard accompany you. Take your friend to his or her car.
- If you become lost, go to a police station or well-lighted service station for directions. Do not ask bystanders or other motorists for directions.
- If you break down on the road, raise the hood, put a white cloth on the antenna, turn on your flashers, and stay in the car. If approached, lower the window slightly and ask the person to call the police if you don't have a cell phone. Do not get out of the car or accept a ride.
- If you are bumped from behind and the circumstances seem to be suspicious, stay in the car and drive to a police station or well-lighted service station and ask for help.
- Never pick up a hitchhiker.

Apartment/Dormitory Safety

We like to think that our homes are places where we can be safe. However, within the confines of the home, dormitory, or apartment many potential hazards exist. By conducting a personal survey and remaining alert to these dangers, you can minimize many risks. Following are some suggestions for safe living in one's home (see Just the Facts: Being Safe in Our New World):

- Install smoke detectors and make sure they are in working order.
- If you are going to live above the fifth floor, make sure your fire department has the equipment necessary to reach above that level.

⌇⌇⌇⌇⌇⌇⌇⌇⌇ Just the Facts ⌇⌇⌇⌇⌇⌇⌇⌇⌇

Being Safe in Our New World

Since the September 11, 2001, terrorism attacks on the World Trade Center in New York City and the Pentagon in Washington, DC, many of our thoughts concerning personal safety have changed drastically. For the first time, we realize that there are dangers here in the United States; we are not immune to foreign invasion; and extremist groups can create havoc on our society psychologically, emotionally, and physically. The way we knew life prior to September 11th has probably changed forever.

The question many of us are asking is "What are we in danger of next?" Certainly, the possibility of further attacks such as those on the World Trade Center exist. We know that the threat of bioterrorism is ever present in forms of anthrax (cutaneous, intestinal, and inhalation). Other potential threats include smallpox, the plague, botulism, and viral hemorrhagic fevers, such as the Ebola virus, and chemical weapons, such as sarin, mustard gas, chlorine, phosgene, and hydrogen cyanide.

What can we do? One certainty is that fear is contagious. As a nation, we must not panic but instead must use common sense, be alert to suspicious activity, and report it to authorities. Further, we need to be alert to suspicious packages and letters. They may have characteristics such as excessive postage, incorrect titles, discoloration, odors, no return address, or excessive tape or string. If a suspicious letter or package is encountered, place it on a stable surface, leave and secure the area, wash your hands, and seek instructions from law enforcement. If you come in contact with any type of gas or chemical weapon, cover your mouth and nose and leave the area immediately. Use water to quickly rinse your eyes and skin exposed to the agent; then remove any contaminated clothing. Whatever the situation, don't panic. Certainly, we need to live our lives as normally as possible, but we must stay alert to questionable or suspicious situations and maintain a heightened sense of awareness to potential dangers.

There are several useful Web sites that can provide continually updated information. Some examples are The Center for Disease Control and Prevention available at **www.bt.cdc.gov/**, the Federal Emergency Management Agency at **www.fema.gov/library/terrorf.htm**, the FAA Fly Smart Guide at **www.faa.gov/apa/traveler.htm**, and the National Transportation Safety Board at **www.ntsb.gov/aviation/aviation.htm**.

- Properly maintain all electrical and heating equipment.
- Plan and practice escape in case of an emergency.
- Plan alternative methods of escape in case your first-choice plan fails.
- Know how to get emergency help. Most areas of the country have 911 service, but many universities have special telephone numbers other than 911. Know your number.
- Never smoke in bed or leave lighted cigarettes unattended.
- Inspect living areas for surfaces, objects, or room design that can lead to slipping or tripping.
- Make sure all rugs have skid-proof backing.
- Never overload electrical outlets.
- Do not place extension cords under rugs or where people walk.
- Never use a portable heater in an unvented area or near flammable materials.
- Keep outside doors locked at all times. Install chain locks on all doors.
- Check carefully before allowing anyone to enter.
- Look through the peephole or ask who is there before opening the door.

- Require people who claim to be maintenance workers to show identification before you allow them to enter.
- Place metal poles in the tracks of sliding doors, so that they cannot be opened unless you remove the poles.
- Be especially careful in parking garages, laundry rooms, and hallways and when entering and leaving living quarters.
- Always tell someone where you are going, and whenever possible have a friend accompany you.
- See Just the Facts: Firearms in the Home for firearm safety guidelines on page 338.

This list is not all-inclusive, but it includes items for which you need to take responsibility. Discuss the rules for safe living with your housemates to help ensure each person's safety (see Assessment Activity 10-2). It is very important that you carry some type of insurance to protect personal property (see Real-World Wellness: Apartment and Dormitory Insurance on page 338).

Fire Detection Devices

There are two types of devices that warn of fire: (1) heat detectors, which activate when the temperature reaches a certain point, and (2) smoke detectors, which sense the

Real-World Wellness

Apartment and Dormitory Insurance

I currently live in the dormitory but hope to move into a nonuniversity apartment. Do I need a rental policy? What about remaining in the dorm—do I need insurance there?

While living in the dormitory, your possessions are generally covered under your parents' homeowners coverage. To be absolutely certain, you should check with your family insurance agent to confirm the type and amount of coverage. If you are not a dependent of your parents, you should check with an insurance agent to determine what coverage is available.

If you decide to move to an apartment, check with an insurance agent. Each insurance company offers slight variations, but in general good apartment/renters' insurance protects your personal property against loss or damage in the dwelling caused by fire and lighting, windstorms and hail, explosion, riot and civil commotion, aircraft, vehicles, smoke, vandalism, theft, falling objects, weight of ice or snow, glass breakage, accidental overflow of water, and accidental electrical damage to appliances. For additional costs, some insurance companies will cover computers, guns, tools, jewelry, cameras/camcorders, or money/coins/gold. Some companies will provide personal liability, which covers claims against bodily injury, sickness, disease, and accidental death of others.

The important thing is to check with an insurance specialist to determine your personal needs either when living in a dorm or when moving into an apartment.

first traces of smoke and set off an alarm before toxic levels of smoke and gas are reached. Heat detectors are not recommended for the home. Smoke detectors are either photoelectric or ionization chamber detectors. Both types are effective and reliable. Both types come in battery-operated models and models that depend on household electrical current. It is advisable to have a smoke detector for each level of an apartment or a home. In placing the detector, be aware that it should (1) be on the ceiling or a sidewall 6 to 12 inches from the ceiling, (2) not be placed in the corner of a room because air does not circulate well in the corners, and (3) be at least 3 feet from registers and air vents, so that drafts will not affect proper functioning.[12]

It is estimated that between 40 and 55 percent of fire deaths could be prevented by properly installed and well-functioning smoke detectors.

Just the Facts

Firearms in the Home

Many homes in the United States have firearms. If you choose to have a rifle, shotgun, or handgun, follow these guidelines for safely maintaining it:

- Keep all firearms unloaded within the home.
- Make sure firearms are locked and secured in a rack or case and have a trigger lock.
- Check to be sure a firearm is not loaded before storing it.
- Keep firearms in good working order.
- Keep your finger off the trigger when handling any firearm.
- Always point the muzzle in a safe direction (never point it at anything you do not intend to shoot).
- Store ammunition in a place separate from firearms.
- Lock the ammunition in a secure place.
- Educate all members of the household about gun safety.
- Enroll in a gun safety course if you are a new owner of a firearm.

Carbon Monoxide Detection

Carbon monoxide is a colorless, odorless, tasteless gas that results from incomplete combustion of carbon-containing fuels. Anywhere fuels that contain carbon are burned, there is the potential danger of death from carbon monoxide (CO) poisoning. A report by the National Center for Environmental Health (NCEH) illustrates the significance of this problem. According to the NCEH, each year more than 300 people die from exposure in the home.[13] Motor vehicle exhausts are the leading cause of CO deaths, but deaths also result from poorly vented cooking stoves, furnaces, and ventilating systems. Death occurs when the oxygen normally found in the red blood cells is replaced by CO. Thus, to prevent CO accidents, several precautions ought to be observed: (1) Never operate a motor vehicle in an enclosed area; (2) never use charcoal in an enclosed area, such as an apartment, a garage, or the bed of a pickup with a camper top; and (3) make sure furnaces and all ductwork are inspected annually. Very small amounts of CO are potentially harmful, and anyone renting an apartment or living in a house should be aware of this danger. There are several clues you can look for to detect CO in your home. Consistently stuffy, stale, or smelly air; high humidity; moisture on the windows; no draft in the chimney; soot gathering around the outside of a furnace or fireplace; and the smell of exhaust fumes all point to the presence of CO.

Battery-operated and wired CO detectors are available. Although these detectors are usually more expensive than smoke detectors, it is recommended that all homes and apartments have at least one. Placement should be in approximately the same location as fire detectors. If a second CO detector is used, it should be placed near the heating source.

Ten percent blood level is considered the vital cutoff for exposure to carbon monoxide. CO affects children and people with smaller bodies more quickly. A healthy person can withstand a 60 to 80 percent CO blood level. Someone with heart disease may die at CO levels as low as 35 percent.[13]

Recreational and Outdoor Safety

One of the joys of life is participating in recreational or sporting activities. To reduce stress, improve cardiovascular conditioning, and promote personal spirituality, some people find that there is nothing more satisfying than being outdoors. Regardless of the season, there are risks if personal alertness is not maintained (see Assessment Activity 10-3). Heat- or cold-related emergencies are always a potential problem. Chapter 3 discusses the prevention of these types of emergencies.

In addition to the emergencies created by extreme heat or cold, many other injuries can result from involvement in recreational activities. Some of the more common injuries are blisters, bruises, sprains, muscle cramps, nosebleeds, wounds, and sunburns. Table 10-2 provides information on how to deal with these injuries.

The list of outdoor recreational activities is almost inexhaustible, as is the potential for the unexpected to happen. As you prepare to engage in outdoor or recreational activities, be familiar with the safety rules of your endeavor, have safe and appropriate equipment for the activity, and maintain an attitude of alertness to potentially dangerous situations. Although not all-inclusive, the following rules will help keep you safe in a variety of recreational settings:

- Seek training and instruction from certified or respected instructors.
- Purchase appropriate safety equipment for the activity. Make sure your eyes and head are properly protected.
- Make sure all equipment is in proper operating order.
- Obey the laws related to your recreational pursuit.
- Begin any activity slowly and do not attempt advanced skills or actions until you are experienced enough to meet the necessary skill level.

Table 10-2 Recreational Injuries and Conditions

Injury	Signs and Symptoms	Prevention	Treatment
Blisters	Fluid under skin	Wear shoes that fit and gloves on your hands.	Avoid breaking them; if painful, clean area, puncture, squeeze, leave skin, cover with sterile dressing.
Contusions (bruises)	Swelling, pain, discoloration	Wear protective equipment.	Rest; apply cold compression; bandage.
Sprains	Pain, tearing sensation, tenderness, loss of function, swelling	Warm up before activity; strengthen your muscles.	Apply RICE—rest, ice, compression, elevation.
Muscle cramps	Painful muscle contractions (legs most often affected)	Condition for the activity; warm up before the activity; strengthen your muscles.	Stretch affected muscles.
Nosebleeds	Bleeding from nostrils	Protect your face; moisten your nose linings in dry air or high altitude.	Pinch your nose with your fingers for five minutes; apply ice.
Wounds (skin)	Cut, bleeding skin	Wear protective equipment and clothing; inspect equipment before use.	Apply direct pressure, elevate, clean with soap and water, apply a sterile dressing.
Sunburns	Redness, pain, chills, blisters	Use sunscreen with a protection factor of at least 15; avoid sun exposure during peak hours.	Apply cool compresses; after pain has stopped, use a cream to keep skin moist; don't treat with oil-based products.

- Stay aware of weather conditions. Always prepare for the worst possible weather.
- Never use alcohol when engaged in a dangerous recreational endeavor or during extremely hot or cold conditions. Alcohol increases the likelihood of emergency situations.
- Take a first-aid course that will prepare you to deal with a variety of unexpected situations.[12]

Bicycling

The National Safety Council estimates that 57 million Americans ride bikes. Biking can be a highly enjoyable and, with proper precautions and common sense, safe activity. Safe biking begins with the rider. Defensive riding is the key to protecting against injury or even death. The National Safety Council reported that, in 1995, 900 bicyclists were killed and more than 70,000 cyclists suffered disabling injuries. To ensure safe biking, taking precautions in traffic and wearing protective equipment are essential. Follow these guidelines for safe riding:[15]

- Always wear a helmet with a stiff outer shell designed to distribute impact and protect against sharp objects. Wear protective gloves. Wear sunglasses to reduce glare.
- Obey traffic rules. Cyclists must follow the same rules as motorists.
- Ride in single file with traffic, not against it. Watch for opening car doors, sewer gratings, soft shoulders, broken glass, and other debris.
- Use hand signals, so that drivers will know your intention to make a turn, change lanes, or stop.
- When riding at night, wear reflective clothing. During the day, wear bright, visible clothing.
- Make sure your bicycle has the proper safety equipment: a red rear reflector; a white front reflector; a red or colorless spoke reflector on the rear wheel; an amber or colorless reflector on the front wheel; pedal reflectors; a horn or bell; and a rearview mirror. A bright headlight is recommended for night riding.
- Keep a safe distance from others and never hitch a ride on another vehicle.
- Be especially careful on wet surfaces, because stopping is much more difficult when brake pads and rims are wet. Be careful when applying the front brakes in wet conditions, because it is easy to be thrown over the front handlebars.

Skateboarding

More than 15,600 people require hospital emergency room treatment each year from injuries associated with skateboarding. Common skateboarding injuries range from fractures to death as a result of falls or collision with motor vehicles. Wrist injuries (fractures or sprain) are the primary injuries associated with skateboarding.

Irregular surfaces account for more than half of the skateboarding injuries involving falls. To make skateboarding as safe as possible, observe the following guidelines:[16]

- Wear protective equipment, including slip-resistant shoes, a helmet, and specially designed padding. This may not protect from fractures, but it will protect against the number and severity of cuts and scrapes.
- Use a helmet that fits properly and has a chin strap. The helmet should have a hard outer shell with ample padding to help absorb any blows to the head. Because there are no government standards, all equipment should be selected carefully.
- Wear wrist braces, knee and elbow protectors, and skateboarding gloves. You might also consider padded shorts and shirts.
- Learn how to fall. Although it is difficult to do, try to relax your body as you are falling. Attempt to roll rather than absorb the force with your arms.
- Check your skateboard each time before beginning to ride. Check the wheels and the board for cracks, loose screws, and nuts.
- Never ride in the street.
- Obey the city laws. Pay attention to traffic and avoid areas where skating is prohibited.

In-Line Skating

One of the most popular forms of recreational activity is in-line skating. The concept of in-line skating originated with hockey players who wanted to extend their off-season training options. In-line skating is now used by everyone from hockey players to skiers to fitness and recreation enthusiasts. In-line skating burns as many calories as cycling or running. In addition, it is low-impact, causing less stress to the lower-body joints than caused by other sports. In-line skates protect ankles well because they are heavy, are made of thick plastic, and rise above the ankle.[16] Be sure to follow these safety tips:[17]

- Select good skates. If the plastic of the boot can be squeezed, the material is not strong enough to support your ankle.
- When buying skates, try them on with thick socks to ensure proper fit and comfort.
- Wear safety equipment, including a helmet, knee and elbow pads, and wrist braces.
- Know how to fall. See the skateboarding guidelines in the previous section for recommendations for falling.
- Learn how to skate on a smooth surface while learning how to stop and slow down. Achieve a basic skating proficiency before tackling more challenging surfaces.

- Be conscious of other skaters, joggers, walkers, and bicyclists.
- Watch for changes in skating surfaces and conditions such as potholes, sewer grates, gravel, broken pavement, or obstacles. Do not skate on wet or oily surfaces.
- Check your skates regularly to make sure they are in good condition. Replace worn wheels and brake rubbers.
- Warm up before beginning to skate.

Boating and Using Personal Watercraft

Everyone who plans to operate a boat should take a course on boat or personal watercraft (PWC) safety. Most boating deaths are caused by drowning and are preventable through the use of a personal flotation device (PFD), according to the U.S. Coast Guard. Most major accidents and deaths while boating are caused by "operator error." The four major factors associated with operator error are the following:[4]

1. Inattention: looking away from the direction in which the boat is moving
2. Carelessness: boating in bad weather or rough water conditions
3. Intoxication
4. Speeding[18]

Operator safety awareness is key to saving lives and preventing injury. It is the responsibility of the operator to know and practice Coast Guard safety recommendations and to ensure that every passenger has, and preferably is

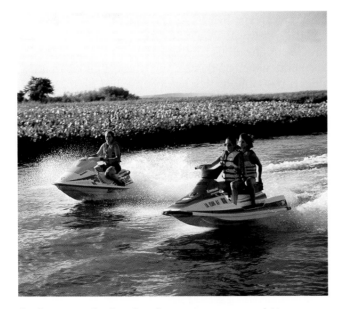

Outdoor recreation is safer when you use proper safety equipment, observe appropriate safety rules, and learn as much as you can about each activity you engage in.

wearing, a PFD. The National Safety Council, the Coast Guard, and most boat dealers have information about the various types of PFDs.

The number of people using PWCs is also growing. This growth in use has resulted in an increase in injuries and fatalities. In 2002, there were 71 fatalities and 1,362 PWC-related injuries.[18] These small boats (sometimes referred to as *jet skis* or *wave riders*) range in size from one-person to four-person machines. They tend to be quick and maneuverable. The key to the safe operation of PWCs is understanding their nature and practicing safe operation through proper adherence to the safety rules. The Underwriters Laboratories and the National Safety Council make the following recommendations to PWC operators:[18]

- Remember that a PWC is jet-propelled. This means that, when the throttle is released, the ability to steer the craft is lost. Operators must know the characteristics of their boats and the space and time needed to safely slow their boats.
- Never get on a PWC without first putting on a vest-type PFD. This vest should be worn even when launching the PWC from a trailer.
- Take a safe-boating class.
- Use extra precautions when operating a PWC. Know the state laws regarding age limits for operation, other regulations, and PFD requirements.
- Never loan your PWC to an inexperienced operator.
- Never rent a PWC without learning and practicing, with supervision, the operation of the craft.
- Don't jump the wakes of other boats. Maintain a safe distance from other boats and PWCs.
- Don't operate a PWC after drinking alcoholic beverages or while intoxicated.

Snowmobiling

A highly enjoyable cold-weather recreational activity is snowmobiling. The Snowmobile Safety and Certification Committee (SSCC) is a nonprofit organization sponsored by the manufacturers of various types of snowmobiles. Through the efforts of this group, standards have been developed for brakes, controls, seats, lights, shields, guards, handgrips, fuel systems, and sound levels. Anyone considering buying or renting a snowmobile should look for Certification 1 of the SSCC on the right side of the machine.

The SSCC also promotes safe operation. Following are some of their guidelines for safe operation of a snowmobile:[19]

- Always perform an inspection of the machine before attempting to start it (check the brakes, throttle, steering controls, fittings, screws, and nuts).
- Make sure no one is standing in front of the machine when you turn on the ignition.

- Before operating a snowmobile, receive basic instruction in how to start it, steer it, turn it, and stop it and in how to shift your weight when on the machine.
- Ride only on easy trails at first. Don't attempt difficult trails or off-trail riding until your experience level permits it.
- Ride with an experienced operator until you are accomplished at riding safely.
- Wear protective clothing that provides protection from the cold and wear safety equipment, such as a helmet with a full-face shield. A full-face shield helps provide warmth as well as protection from branches or other debris.
- Never drink alcohol and operate a snowmobile at the same time. A study in Wisconsin found that more than 60 percent of those fatally injured in snowmobile accidents had elevated blood alcohol concentrations.[20]

Vehicle Safety

Human error accounts for nearly 85 percent of vehicle accidents.[14] Experts use the term *improper driving* for speeding, failure to yield right-of-way, driving left of center, incorrect passing, and following too closely. Figure 10-1 provides information on the types of accidents and ages of victims.

One major cause of accidents is speed. In 13.6 percent of fatal motor vehicle accidents, speed is the major factor. Another persistent hazard is the use of alcohol and other drugs. Estimates are that two of five Americans will be involved in an alcohol-related crash at some point in their lives. In 1999, alcohol was involved in 38 percent of fatal crashes.[14] The role that other drugs play in accidents is not clear, but a study by the National Highway Traffic Safety Administration reported that drugs other than alcohol were found in the blood samples of 18 percent of people killed in vehicle accidents.[14] In most cases, these other drugs were used in combination with alcohol.

Alcohol and high speeds are not the only factors that affect driving. Drowsiness is another important factor. See Real-World Wellness: Driving Drowsy for ways to minimize your risk of injury while driving your vehicle.

One of the most important factors in vehicle safety is the use of restraint systems (seat belts and air bags). The National Highway Traffic Safety Administration now requires all 1998 passenger cars and all 1999 multipurpose vehicles (jeeps, SUVs) to have dual airbags. It is estimated that at least 5,000 deaths and 70,000 critical injuries could be prevented if people would wear their seat belts.[21]

For restraint systems to improve safety, they must be used properly. Children and infants should be placed in the back seat in car seats designed for their age and size. Deaths of young children have been caused by deployed air bags. Some companies have reduced the force of air bags' deployment and/or have provided drivers with the ability to disengage the passenger-side air bag. Many states have passed laws requiring that all children riding in cars be in a restraint system. All drivers transporting children should become familiar with the related state laws and be sure to use the type of car seat and restraint system recommended, according to age and size, for their child passengers. The use of restraint systems is not a luxury for adults, either. Proper restraint use is imperative to significantly improve the chances of surviving an automobile accident.

In the last few years, two other factors in vehicle safety have received a great deal of public attention. The first is the use of cell phones while driving. While cell phones are convenient and can add a measure of safety for people traveling on highways and in areas of high risk, too often cell phones are a distraction that can cause accidents. The National Safety Council recommends that drivers who do use cell phones when driving should be sure to use a phone that allows the driver to keep both hands on the steering wheel, a phone that features a microphone that can be installed on the sun visor, out of the driver's line of vision. Some companies, such as Exxon Mobil, have enacted a ban on cell phone

Type of accident	Collision with railroad train	Collision with pedalcycle	Pedestrian accidents	Collision between motor vehicles	All motor vehicle accidents
Death total	400	700	5700	21,300	43,200
Change from 1996	0%	0%	-2%	+9%	.05%
Death rate	0.1	0.3	2.1	8.0	16.1

Figure 10-1 Accident Types, 1997

SOURCE: From The National Safety Council, *Accident facts, 1998*. Itasca, IL: National Safety Council.

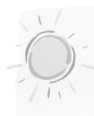

Real-World Wellness

Driving Drowsy

Sometimes, when I'm driving, I seem to get really tired. What can I do to help myself remain awake and alert when driving?

A number of conditions lead to driver drowsiness. First, today's cars and trucks have interiors with comfortable seats, are quiet and carpeted, and have temperature-regulated environments. Many vehicles also have cruise control, which can allow a driver's concentration to drift. Second, highways are constructed to eliminate sharp curves, hills, and bumps, which contributes to drowsiness while driving. Third, the repetitive patterns of oncoming light and of white and yellow lines during night driving can cause a trancelike state known as *highway hypnosis*. To prevent becoming drowsy and falling asleep behind the wheel of a vehicle, the National Safety Council offers the following tips:[21]

- Before starting a trip, get enough sleep—at least seven to eight hours—the night before.

- Don't start a trip late in the day. Driving long distances is hard work and you need to be fresh and alert.

- If possible, don't drive alone. Passengers can take turns driving and help keep each driver awake. Never allow all passengers to sleep in the vehicle at the same time.

- Avoid long drives at night because night driving increases the risk for highway hypnosis.

- Make sure the vehicle environment is cool in both the summer and winter. Turn the radio volume up and switch stations frequently; avoid soft, sleep-inducing music.

- Stay involved in the driving process—don't use cruise control. Don't allow yourself to become too comfortable. Drive with your shoulders back, your buttocks against the seat back, and your legs flexed at about a 45° angle.

- Never use alcohol when driving.

- Take frequent breaks—stop for light meals, stop at a gas station, walk in a safe area for a few minutes.

- If you feel yourself drifting off and no one else can share the driving, stop at a safe place, such as a truck stop, well-lit gas station, or rest area, and sleep for a short time; even 20 minutes will help. Always keep the doors locked.

- If you feel yourself getting drowsy, getting off the road may determine not only whether you stay awake but also whether you stay alive!

use while on company business.[22] Following are guidelines for car phone users:

- Safe driving should be the priority, not talking on the phone.
- Do not attempt to use the phone in heavy traffic conditions that require complete concentration.
- Program frequently called telephone numbers into speed dial to minimize the loss of concentration on driving required by dialing a bunch of numbers.
- Do not attempt to dial a number when the vehicle is moving. Wait for a stoplight or pull into a safe area.
- Do not attempt to take written notes while the vehicle is moving. If you need to write something down, pull off the road to a safe location.
- When using the phone, drive in the slow traffic lane in case you have to pull over.

The second factor of concern is overaggressive driving. The United States seems to have become a nation of rude, unthinking, aggressive drivers, manifested in what has become known as **road rage** (see Assessment Activity 10-4). According to one report, in 10 years, aggressive driving killed an average of 1,500 people each year; injured another 800,000; and cost the country roughly $24 billion in medical costs, property damage, and lost time from work.[24] This study, conducted by the National Highway Traffic Safety Administration, used information from 400 police departments nationwide at which some 500,000 accidents were analyzed from 1988 through 1997. The investigators believe the actual numbers were underreported because many aggressive driving crashes do not cause injuries, and in many such crashes there is not enough evidence to justify a citation. Also, aggressive driving does not always result in an accident.[22]

Men have typically been considered more aggressive drivers than have women. The National Highway Traffic Safety Administration (NHTSA) reports that aggressive drivers are more likely to be high-risk drivers, to drive impaired, to speed, and/or to drive unbuckled. Further, the aggressive drivers see their vehicles as providing a cover of anonymity; therefore, they drive more aggressively. Their behavior is characterized by running stop signs, disobeying red lights, speeding, tailgating, weaving in and out of traffic, blowing the horn, flashing their lights, and making threatening hand/facial gestures.[23] Women are now viewed as being as aggressive as their male counterparts and are increasingly displaying the aggressive driving characteristics once associated primarily with men. As a nation of road ragers, we have come to use our cars as weapons, along with tire irons, golf clubs, guns, pepper spray, and even crossbows.[24]

What we must remember, in our overaggressive commutes to our daily destinations, is to give our fellow drivers a break. It is not our responsibility to teach

Just the Facts

Safe Air Travel—Post-9/11

Since the events of September 11, all of us should be prepared to take reasonable measures to protect our safety. AirSafe.com offers the following advice.[25]

1. *Be aware of your surroundings.* Take notice of any activities or situations that do not appear to be normal.
2. *Report unusual activity.* Inform authorities immediately if anything either in the airport or on the aircraft looks out of place or inappropriate.
3. *Make no assumptions about who may pose a threat.* Any person intent on violent acts against air transport can be of any age, gender, or nationality. Don't assume anything simply because of outward appearances.
4. *Stay away from suspicious circumstances.* Move away immediately from any unaccompanied packages, suspicious behavior, or unusual commotion. Notify authorities and warn others in the immediate area.
5. *Listen to the flight attendants.* If there is any kind of emergency, look to the flight attendants for guidance.
6. *Be familiar with your aircraft.* When first seated, review the written safety instructions; count the number of rows to the nearest exit. Check to see if there are seatback telephones available.
7. *Have a plan for the emergency use of a wireless device.* In case of an in-flight emergency, assess the situation before using any communication device. If the situation requires, use your personal wireless phone to contact someone who can help, such as the FBI. A second choice is to contact a loved one and ask him or her to call authorities.

others how to drive. To respond with less anger to our fellow drivers, we may have to leave a few minutes early to reach our destinations; listen to quiet, relaxing music while driving; and even pretend that the person in the next car (the one possibly driving dangerously or carelessly or too slowly or stupidly) is a loved one. Each of us must assume the personal responsibility to drive in a courteous manner. Be willing to give up the right-of-way and don't take another's foolish, inconsiderate behavior personally. Some guidelines that may help prevent road rage are provided in Just the Facts: Preventing Road Rage.

Motorcycle Safety

Motorcycles and mopeds offer several advantages over other modes of transportation. Their cost of operation is low, they consume less fuel, they take up less room on already overcrowded roads, and they provide their drivers with an often exhilarating feeling of freedom. Unfortunately, they are also two of the most dangerous transportation modes. The only protection most riders have is a helmet, and some states do not require that riders wear one. Over the last five years an average of 2,260 motorcyclists have been killed each year and more than 3 million more have been injured. Of fatal motorcycle crashes, 60 percent involve collisions with other vehicles. It has been reported that 65 percent of motorcycle-vehicle collisions are caused by the actions of vehicle operators and not motorcyclists.[26] The weather, malfunctioning equipment, and the surface of the road play a role in 10 percent of accidents. In addition, most cyclists do not receive formal training in safe riding. This becomes evident in analysis of the evasive actions of motorcycle riders. When avoidance actions are taken, 77 percent of those actions are improper.[26] Skidding from overbraking is the most common problem, and failure to use both brakes when attempting to avoid a collision is the second. A constant problem is the use of alcohol. Approximately 55 percent of motorcycle accidents involve the use of alcohol by the

Just the Facts

Preventing Road Rage

Following are some guidelines for reducing the incidence of road rage:[24]

- Give the other person a break.
- Do not tailgate.
- Do not let the car phone distract you.
- Do not switch lanes without signaling.
- If you are moving more slowly than most of the traffic, use the right lane.
- Do not drive in the passing lane when not attempting to pass another vehicle.
- Do not park in handicap parking if you are not disabled.
- Do not let your doors hit another person's car in a parking lot.
- Do not make obscene gestures to another motorist.
- Do not make faces at other drivers.
- Do not roll down the window and scream at other drivers.
- When confronted with an aggressive driver, slow down and back off.

cyclist.[11] Finally, motorcycles present a visibility problem: Even with their headlights on, many cyclists are not seen or are overlooked by vehicle drivers.

Following are some rules of the road that make motorcycle and moped riding safer:

- Always wear a helmet. Even though some states do not require you to, you significantly improve your chances of surviving an accident on a motorcycle or moped if you wear an approved helmet.
- Helmets should meet the federal safety standards set by the Department of Transportation, indicated by the word *DOT* appearing on the helmet. Some helmets read "Approved by the Snell Memorial Foundation," which means they have passed tests even more stringent than the federal standards.
- Wear gloves, boots, and heavy clothing to protect your body if you slide on the pavement, sidewalk, or gravel.
- Seek proper training in how to ride your vehicle; take a course in safe riding.
- Do not ride after drinking alcohol or taking medications that can diminish alertness or performance.
- Ride defensively. Motorcycles are harder to see and some motorists take advantage of their superior vehicle size and weight.
- Avoid riding in the rain or other wet conditions.

Pedestrian Safety

In their haste to get from one class to another, college students are notorious jaywalkers. The majority of the time, nothing of consequence happens. However, nearly 60 percent of pedestrian accidents involve attempts to cross a street either at an intersection or between intersections. Usually, such accidents are the pedestrians' fault. Pedestrians make poor choices on when and where to cross streets, or they do not adequately observe traffic before attempting to cross. The student who darts suddenly from between two parked cars puts the motorist at a distinct disadvantage for seeing him or her and for stopping the vehicle. An invention of modern society, the stereo headset, causes users to be unaware of traffic noise and other sounds that would alert them to possible hazards or dangers.

The implication of statistics about accidents involving pedestrians is to be extremely careful when crossing a street. Remaining alert at all times, not wearing stereo headsets, crossing only at designated crosswalks, and not entering the street from between parked vehicles are important safety precautions. When walking or jogging at night, wear light-colored clothing. Even better, wear a jacket or other apparel with reflective strips to make you visible to oncoming motorists. Statistics indicate that alcohol is a factor in 50 percent of fatal pedestrian accidents involving adults. In this

study, these adults had blood alcohol content (BAC) levels at or above 0.10 (the legal level of intoxication in most states).[27]

~~~ Just the Facts ~~~

Dealing with Disaster—Tips for Students

Since the terrorist attack in New York and Washington on September 11, many people across the nation have had great concern for what the future may hold. If another such attack should occur, all of us may experience difficulty dealing with the event(s). Not all of us will react exactly the same, but some common responses to a terrorist attack or any other disaster are

- Disbelief and shock
- Fear and anxiety about the future
- Disorientation
- Inability to focus on schoolwork and extracurricular activities
- Apathy and emotional numbing
- Irritability and anger
- Extreme mood swings
- Feelings of powerlessness
- Eating pattern changes—overeating or loss of appetite
- Crying for "no apparent reason"
- Headaches and stomach problems
- Difficulty sleeping
- Excessive use of alcohol and other drugs

To cope with any disaster, the following suggestions are provided by the National Mental Health Association:

1. *Talk about it.* Share your feelings. Talking about a situation helps relieve stress and helps you realize that others have similar feelings.
2. *Take care of yourself.* Get plenty of rest and exercise. Do those things that are relaxing to you. Eat nutritiously and limit your viewing of media reports and images of the tragedy.
3. *Stay connected.* Call friends and family. Go home for the weekend, if possible. If you cannot visit in person, keep in touch by phone or e-mail.
4. *Do something positive.* Get involved with campus activities in response to the disaster, such as a candlelight vigil, benefit, or discussion group.
5. *Ask for help.* If you feel overwhelmed or have lingering thoughts concerning the events, talk with a friend or seek help from the college counseling center.

Summary

- Accidents are the leading cause of death for people 1 to 25 years of age.
- Awareness of potentially hazardous situations is imperative for accident prevention.
- Acts of violence can occur anywhere and anytime. Acts of violence include assault, homicide, sexual assault, domestic violence, suicide, and abuse.
- Acquaintance rape is forced sexual intercourse between people who know one another well. Date rape is a form of acquaintance rape.
- Most rape victims suffer psychological effects, such as shock, anxiety, depression, and shame.
- Rape trauma syndrome is characterized by fear, nightmares, fatigue, crying spells, and digestive disturbances.
- Homicide has been declining for the last several years.
- Domestic violence can take the form of partner abuse or child abuse (physical and sexual).
- Hate crimes are crimes directed at people or groups solely because of the perpetrators' hatred of victims' sexual orientation, race, ethnicity, nationality, or religion. Nine percent of hate crimes occur at schools or on college campuses.
- Try limiting the use of ATM machines to daylight hours. Never use an ATM machine at night alone.
- To help protect against carjacking, always lock the doors, park in a well-lighted area, and check the back seat before entering the vehicle.
- A personal survey should be conducted to determine potential hazards, danger, and risks in the home, apartment, or dormitory.
- Heat detectors and smoke detectors are the two types of devices for warning of fire. Heat detectors are not recommended for the home.
- Knowing and obeying the rules for safe participation in recreational activities is the first step to fully enjoying a wide variety of activities.

- Common recreational injuries include blisters, bruises, sprains, muscles cramps, nosebleeds, wounds, and sunburns. A first-aid course that teaches how to mange emergencies is helpful for safe participation in recreational activities.
- Over 57 million Americans ride bikes. Defensive riding is the key to protecting against injury and death.
- Many people require hospital emergency room treatment each year for skateboarding accidents. Protective gear is essential. Wrist fractures and sprains are the number one injury to skateboarders.
- In-line skating is a popular recreational activity. Wearing protective gear and knowing how to fall are imperative.
- Anyone planning to operate a powerboat or personal watercraft (PWC) should be familiar with safe boating practices and the rules of boating.
- Being familiar with how to operate watercraft and wearing a personal flotation device (PFD) are essential to boating safety. Alcohol should be avoided when operating watercraft.
- Snowmobiling is an enjoyable activity in cold climates. Knowing how to operate the machines safely and wearing proper protective clothing are essential. Alcohol and the operation of a snowmobile should not be mixed.
- Most vehicle accidents are caused by human error.
- Alcohol is involved in 39 percent of fatal crashes.
- All occupants of a vehicle must use a restraint system (seat belts).
- Car phones can contribute to inattention and accidents during driving.
- The United States is a nation of road ragers who commit acts of belligerence, hostility, and physical violence.
- Helmets are essential for riders of motorcycles and mopeds.
- Nearly 60 percent of pedestrian accidents involve jaywalking.
- A pedestrian should always remain alert, never wear stereo headsets, and cross only at designated crosswalks.

Review Questions

1. Identify measures to protect against rape.
2. How can rape trauma syndrome affect a victim?
3. What guidelines should men and women consider following to prevent rape?
4. Discuss wellness in relationship to homicide, abuse, and hate crimes.
5. Discuss some of the guidelines to follow to maintain a safe home environment.
6. List measures that help protect against crimes of violence, such as carjacking and ATM robberies.

7. What precautions should be taken to prevent fires and to protect oneself if a fire should occur?
8. What are guidelines for safely participating in any recreational activity?
9. What steps need to be taken to prevent hate crimes on colleges campuses?
10. What does the term *improper driving* connote, and what are some guidelines for safer driving?
11. Discuss measures for avoiding or dealing with road rage.
12. What would be suggestions for safely riding a motorcycle?

References

1. Federal Bureau of Investigation. 2004. Crime in the United States 2002. (http://www. fbi.gov).

2. Ledserman, D. 1995. Colleges report rise in violent crime. *Chronicle of Higher Education* 45:A32.

3. Copenhaver, S., and E. Gaverhola. 1991. Sexual victimization among sorority women: Exploring the link

between violence and institutional practices. *Sex Roles* 24:3142.

4. Payne, W. A., and D. B. Hahn. 2002. *Understanding your health.* 7th ed. New York: McGraw-Hill.

5. Higher Education Center. 2004. Sexual assault and alcohol and other drug use (www.edc.org/hec/pubs/factsheets/fact_sheet.html).

6. Kelly, G. 2004. *Sexuality today.* New York: McGraw-Hill.

7. U.S. Department of Justice. 2002. Federal Bureau of Investigation crime statistics for 1997 (www.fbi.gov/ucr/urr97prs.htp).

8. American Medical Association. 2004. Medical library. Domestic violence (http://www.medem.com).

9. Mayo Clinic. 2004. Domestic abuse: Help is available (www.mayoclinic.com).

10. American Bar Association. 2004. What is a healthy relationship? (http://www.abanet.org).

11. Federal Bureau of Investigation. 2002. Uniform crime reports. Hate crime statistics, 2002. Washington, DC: U.S. Government Printing Office.

12. Bever, D. L. 1996. *Safety: A personal focus.* 4th ed. St. Louis: Mosby.

13. National Center for Environmental Health. 2004. Carbon monoxide questions & answers (www.epa/iaq/pubs/coftsht.html).

14. The National Safety Council. 2003. *Accident facts: 2003 edition.* Chicago: The National Safety Council.

15. The National Safety Council. 2004. *Safe bicycling fact sheet.* Itasca, IL: The National Safety Council.

16. The National Safety Council. 2004. *Skateboarding fact sheet.* Itasca, IL: The National Safety Council.

17. The National Safety Council. 2004. *In-line skating fact sheet.* Itasca, IL: The National Safety Council.

18. Commander Bob. 2004. Personal watercraft (www.commanderbob.com/cbpwc.html).

19. International Snowmobile Industry Association. 2004. *Snowmobile fact book.* Annandale, VA: International Snowmobile Industry Association.

20. Peter, R., and F. Wenzel. 1986. A ten-year survey of snowmobile injuries and

fatalities in Wisconsin. *The Physician and Sport Medicine* 14(1):140

21. The National Safety Council. 1998. Driver fatigue fact sheet. Itasca, IL: The National Safety Council.

22. The National Safety Council. 2004. National Safety Council praises Exxon Mobil for enacting cell phone policy (www.NSC.org/News/nr061804.htm).

23. American College of Emergency Physicians. 2004. Aggressive driving fact sheet (www.acet.org).

24. Bowles, S., and P. Overberg. 23 November, 1998. Aggressive driving: A road well-traveled. *USA Today.*

25. Air Safe. 2004. Tips for travel under increased hijack threats (http://www.airsafe.com/events/war/safetips.htm).

26. National Highway Traffic Safety Administration. 2004. Motorcycle safety program (www.nhsta.dot.gov/people/injury/pedbimot/motorcycle/motorcycle03/khtaknowledge.htm).

27. National Highway Traffic Safety Administration. 2004. *Traffic safety facts 2001.* Washington, DC: National Center for Statistics and Analysis.

Suggested Readings

Dreissman, B. 1997. *The complete winter sports safety manual: Staying safe and warm snowshoeing, skiing, snowboarding, snowmobiling and camping.* Helena, MI: Falcon.
This book provides the information needed to stay safe while participating in winter sports, including information about emergency equipment and emergency field procedures.

Gillis, J., A. B. Cheng, K. Fierst, and A. B. Curran. 1998. *The car book 1998: The definitive buyer's guide to car safety, fuel economy, maintenance, and much more.* New York: Harper-Perennial Library.
Easy-to-read ratings concerning crash tests, fuel economy, preventive maintenance, insurance costs, and consumer satisfaction are provided for all vehicles.

Gutman, B. 1996. *Be aware of danger (focus on safety).* Breckenridge, CO: Twenty-First Century Books.

This book focuses on helping children deal safely with strangers and dangerous situations in school and on the streets. It is an excellent resource for parents who have children ages 9 through 12.

Marques, L., L. Carter, and M. Nelson. 1998. *Child safety made easy.* Concord, CA: Screamin' Mimi.
This humorous, easy-to-read publication explores poignant issues about safety for children and families. It gives excellent safety tips for people caring for newborns and children up to 5 years of age.

Rawls, N., and S. Kovach. 2002. *Be alert, be aware, have a plan: The complete guide to personal safety.* New York: Lyons Press.
This book provides advice on how to protect oneself and one's family in any situation. The text provides excellent information on protecting children,

dealing with stalkers, violence in the workplace, and traveling safely.

Robinson, F. 2003. *It didn't happen.* Boston: Custom Multimedia Creations.
This book is based on a true story involving a young woman who graduated from college with honors and became a rising star in her profession. After her involvement with a coworker who gave her liquid ecstasy (GHB), her association with the coworker and exposure to ecstasy almost ruined her life and left her with amnesia. It took her almost 10 years to find the answers to what had happened to her.

Tilton, B. 1995. *Camping healthy hygiene for the outdoors.* Merrillville, IN: Ics Books.
This publication provides tips on how to camp safely and protect yourself from disease and illness at the campsite.

Name _____ Date _____ Section _____

Assessment Activity 10-1

Encounters of the Dangerous Kind

Unfortunately, our everyday lives seem to be associated with many aspects of violence. This activity is designed to help you determine how at risk you are for such violence as carjacking, ATM robbery, gang violence, domestic violence, rape, and even homicide. This survey will ask you to think about some issues and situations that can have dangerous, life-threatening consequences.

Directions: Indicate whether each statement is always, sometimes, or never true for you.

General Safety Considerations	Always	Sometimes	Never
I am aware of my surroundings.	___	___	___
I tell someone where I am going when leaving my home.	___	___	___
I am careful about providing personal information and daily schedule information to people I do not know.	___	___	___
I vary my daily routine and walking patterns.	___	___	___
If I walk at night, I walk with others.	___	___	___

Carjacking

	Always	Sometimes	Never
I look in the back seat before entering my car.	___	___	___
I survey the location before parking, stopping, or getting into or out of my car.	___	___	___
I keep my car doors locked.	___	___	___
I have a plan of action if my car should break down.	___	___	___
I check my mirrors and scan ahead for potential dangers.	___	___	___
I avoid driving alone at night.	___	___	___

General Safety Considerations	Always	Sometimes	Never
I avoid dangerous areas that have a reputation for being high-risk areas.	___	___	___
If hit from behind, I travel to the nearest police station, motioning to the person who hit me to follow.	___	___	___
If I notice anyone loitering near my car, I do not go near it but go to a safe place and call the police.	___	___	___

ATM Safety

	Always	Sometimes	Never
I avoid using an ATM at night.	___	___	___
I attempt to take someone with me when going to use an ATM.	___	___	___
I look for suspicious people or activity before entering an ATM area.	___	___	___
If I drive to an ATM, I park under a light in a highly visible area.	___	___	___
I remember my PIN number.			
I take all receipts with me.			
Even if using a drive-up ATM, I survey the area carefully.	___	___	___

Violence, Rape, and Homicide

	Always	Sometimes	Never
I avoid dangerous areas of my city or campus.	___	___	___
I watch my alcohol intake carefully when at parties.	___	___	___
I do not drink alcohol on a first date.	___	___	___
I avoid arguments or potentially violent situations after drinking alcohol.	___	___	___
I refuse to be with anyone who seems to be violent.	___	___	___

I do not strike or allow myself to be struck by another person. _____ _____ _____

I do not allow myself to be around anyone who has a gun and is drinking alcohol or using other drugs. _____ _____ _____

I break off a verbally or physically abusive relationship. _____ _____ _____

Scoring: In each section of the survey, give yourself 3 points for each time you checked the "always" column and 2 points for each check in the "sometimes" column.

Give yourself 0 points for any checks in the "never" column. Although not scientific, the following point scheme may help you assess your total risks. Even though your score may reflect a high level of safety, make sure to examine each section for too many "sometimes" or "never" answers, which could indicate you are at serious risk.

87–81:	You are probably safe if you continue to observe current precautions.
80–70:	You may have some areas to reexamine and change.
69 and below:	You may engage in some behaviors that require significant change.

11

Taking Responsibility for Drug Use

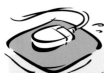

Online Learning Center

Log on to our Online Learning Center (OLC) for access to these additional resources:

- Chapter key term flashcards
- Learning objectives
- Additional goals for behavior change
- Concentration game
- Self-scoring chapter quizzes

- Additional lab activities

The OLC also offers Web links for study and exploration of wellness topics. Access these links through **www.mhhe. com/anspaugh6e**, click on Student Center, click on Chapter 11, and then click on Web Activities.

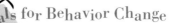

Goals for Behavior Change

- Make more informed decisions about alcohol, tobacco products, and other drugs.
- Assess your personal attitudes about drugs and drug use behavior.
- Discontinue any risky behaviors related to drug use.
- Develop a personal plan for your use of alcohol.

Key Terms

addictive behavior
alcohol
binge drinking
caffeine
cocaine
depressants
designer drugs
drug
inhalants
mainstream smoke

marijuana
narcotics
nicotine
passive smoking
psychoactives
reward deficiency syndrome
sidestream smoke
stimulants

Objectives

After completing this chapter, you should be able to do the following:

- Identify reasons people use drugs.
- Define specific terms associated with drugs and drug use.

- Explain how drugs are classified.
- Describe the dangers associated with the use of various drugs.

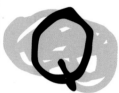

uality of life is a frequently used term that refers to the "how" of life—how well you live, how healthy you are, how much you are able to accomplish your goals, and how happy you are. The primary determinants of quality of life are the decisions you make that affect your life either positively or negatively. As suggested by this book, a high quality of life balances the physical, mental, emotional, social, and spiritual needs of a person for optimal health, satisfaction, and enjoyment. Achieving this goal means making intelligent choices—ones that contribute to your well-being—both for the moment and for your future. To make informed choices, you must have accurate information and you must understand that your actions have consequences. The decisions you make are cumulative. As time goes on and as you age, the consequences of previous decisions, actions, habits, and modes of behavior increasingly affect the way your body and your mind function. The emphasis of much of this book is on personal behaviors, such as exercise, weight maintenance, proper nutrition, and the prevention of disease through lifestyle. Other factors and decisions also influence your quality of life.

This chapter deals with drugs. Drug use or nonuse can strongly affect your health and quality of life. Drugs used for treatment, cure, prevention, or relief of pain or disease are categorized as medicines. Many people are alive because of the therapeutic effect of drugs used to prevent or manage disease and maintain health. However, not all drugs are used as medicines. When usage involves reasons other than medicinal, even if usage is considered recreational, the potential exists for tragic consequences. Understanding potential problems can help you make wiser decisions about drug use.

Reasons for Drug Use

A **drug** is any substance that kills organisms (such as bacteria and fungi) in the body or that affects body function or structure.[1] (Other terms that may be important for understanding drugs are listed in Just the Facts: Understanding Drug Terminology.) People use drugs for many reasons. Some need drugs for health reasons—to maintain a normal life or to alleviate symptoms or complications of diseases or other conditions. Others indulge in drugs to alter their moods. Researchers have identified several reasons people use drugs:[1]

- *Medicinal purposes:* Medicines are used for a wide range of purposes—from reducing symptoms of the cold and flu or treating headaches to lowering blood pressure or cholesterol to extend life and maintain quality of life. People who suffer from chemical imbalances, such as with bipolar disorder or depression, would be unable to live normal lives without

the availability of certain drugs. Methylphenidate (Ritalin), commonly used illegally as a stimulant, is also used to treat adults and children who have attention-deficit disorder. When used in this capacity, Ritalin frequently helps such people focus on and complete tasks—something difficult for these people to do without medical intervention. Medicines, although dangerous even under a physician's supervision if misused or prescribed incorrectly, are invaluable to many for maintenance of an active, positive lifestyle.

- *Recreational/social facilitation:* People frequently use drugs with the belief that they will lessen the tension associated with social encounters. Marijuana and **alcohol** are particularly popular in social situations. Potential dangers of using drugs for this purpose include mental dependency on the drug and an inability to cope with social events without using the drug.

- *Sensation seeking:* Some people enjoy taking risks. For them, drugs fulfill the need for excitement and adventure. Others turn to drugs out of boredom or a feeling of inadequacy in their lives. Unfortunately, when they become tolerant to the drug or they do not find the type of "high" they were looking for, users frequently turn to increasingly dangerous drugs or to increased doses to provide equivalent or more exciting thrills.

- *Religious or spiritual factors:* Throughout history, people have used drugs to enhance their spirituality or to achieve spiritual states or awarenesses. Too often in these situations, the drug becomes the object of worship. Though many people have tried, the spiritual realm has not been achieved through the use of mind-altering drugs.

- *Altered states:* Drugs are sometimes used to increase the intensity of a mood or create a state of euphoria. Some people attempt to enhance physical performance or stimulate artistic creativity. Evidence indicates that perceptions of improved abilities induced by drugs are false.

- *Rebellion and alienation:* The use of drugs can be a deliberate act of rebellion against social values, especially the values of parents or society. Many people who experience extreme pressures and have difficulty coping turn to drugs as an escape. These people include college-age students facing academic pressure and increased personal freedom.

- *Peer pressure and group entry:* People who have a great desire to feel accepted socially often use drugs to demonstrate their sameness with other members of their group. People claim to use drugs to feel accepted, to imitate people they admire, and to attempt to create an identity or project a specific image. Self-esteem seems to be a vital component. People with high self-esteem see themselves as competent, successful,

~~~~~~~~~~~~~~~~ Just the Facts ~~~~~~~~~~~~~~~~

Understanding Drug Terminology

Following are possibly unfamiliar terms that are useful for understanding the effects of substances:

- *Addiction:* Compulsive, uncontrollable, chronic dependence on a drug or drugs to the degree that severe emotional, mental, or physiological reactions occur; a desire to use drug(s) contrary to legal and/or social prohibitions

- *Alcohol:* Generally refers to grain alcohol or ethanol as opposed to other forms of alcohol which are too toxic for ingestion

- *Antagonistic:* Opposing or counteracting

- **Binge drinking:** Consuming five or more drinks in a row for males and four in a row for women

- **Designer drugs:** Illegally manufactured psychoactive drugs similar to controlled drugs on the FDA's schedule

- *Drug:* Any substance, except food, that upon entering the body alters its function

- *Drug abuse:* The excessive and pathological use of a drug that has dangerous side effects

- *Drug misuse:* The use of a drug for purposes other than intended

- *Effective dose:* The amount that produces the desired effect

- *Habit:* As pertains to drug use, a patterned, regular, and possibly involuntary involvement with a particular drug

- *Lethal dose:* The amount capable of causing death

- *Medicines:* Drugs used to prevent illness or to treat the symptoms of an illness

- *Narcotic:* A morphinelike substance that relieves pain and induces a stuporous state.

- *Over-the-counter (OTC) drugs:* Nonprescription drugs

- *Physical dependence:* A physiological need for a drug

- *Polyabuse:* The use of multiple drugs

- *Potentiating:* An exaggerated drug response obtained when two drugs are taken together; a much greater effect is obtained than when either drug is taken separately

- *Prescription drugs:* Drugs obtained only by order of a physician or dentist

- *Psychoactive:* Affecting mood and/or behavior

- *Psychological dependence:* An emotional or a mental need to use a drug

- *Synergistic:* A combined effect greater than the sum of the individual effects when two or more drugs are used at the same time; the combination produces an exaggerated effect or a prolonged drug action

- *Therapeutic index:* The difference between the minimum amount of a drug needed for a therapeutic effect and the minimum amount that has a toxic concentration or effect

- *Toxic dose:* The amount that produces a poisonous effect

---

self-sufficient, accepting, outgoing, and well rounded. People with low self-esteem tend to feel isolated and unloved and have a reduced capacity for joy or self-fulfillment. To overcome these sensations and perceptions, many people turn to drugs.

- *Curiosity:* Many people first experiment with drugs out of curiosity—the desire to see what using the drug feels like or what the attraction is for chronic users. Although curiosity is normal and healthy in many circumstances, the primary problem associated with experimentation with drugs out of curiosity is the inability to know how a drug will affect any one person. Whereas one person may consider the effects of a drug pleasurable, someone else may have a different, even fatal, reaction. Most people try alcohol during their lives. For most people, this creates no problem; they can choose to use it or not use it. For some people, however, one act of curiosity about alcohol can result in the disease of alcoholism.

The reasons any person uses drugs are usually not easily categorized. (List yours in Assessment Activity 11-2.) Most drug use situations depend on personality, experience, perceptions of the environment, and expectations (see Just the Facts: What's the Cause of Addiction? on page 360).

What Causes Addiction—a Model

There are a variety of models used to explain why addiction develops. The disease model of addiction, also known as chemical dependency, has been favored for many years. According to this model, alcoholics are medical patients who need treatment rather than condemnation. Today most experts purport to rely on the *biopsychosocial model of addiction.* According to this theory, addiction is due to the interaction of different individual and social pathologies, as well as biochemical and genetic factors. The primary factors addressed in the biopsychosocial

∿Just the Facts∿

What's the Cause of Addiction?

Addiction has been defined as "a condition characterized by the compulsive abuse of a drug or drugs."[1] In other words, addiction is a pathological relationship with a substance that has life-damaging potential. Following are some theories about addiction:

- The spectrum of addictions ranges from alcohol and tobacco to behavior such as eating and working.

- The causes of addiction are complex and interrelated. A number of interacting variables may contribute to the development of addiction.

- Variables that may contribute to addiction include genetics, family influences, friends, life events, social and cultural values, availability, and personality.

- Studies indicate that some inherited traits may lead to alcoholism.[4] For instance, alcoholics may have an inherited inability to determine their levels of intoxication when drinking alcoholic beverages.

- Studies have found that addictive, impulsive, and compulsive disorders may have a common genetic origin.[6] These disorders may result from the failure of cells to signal molecules in the brain's reward system, so that the brain is unaware of certain sensations of pleasure or success. This failure is viewed as a type of sensory deprivation of the brain's pleasure mechanisms. The manifestation of this disorder is referred to as **reward deficiency syndrome.**

- Personality type, temperament, and attitudes may also contribute to drug use and addiction.

- Personality traits associated with drug abuse include rebelliousness, resistance to authority, independence, and low self-esteem. In addition, people who abuse drugs seem to have a high tolerance for deviance in others, place a low value on education and religion, display low levels of competence in task performance, have low degrees of obedience, and have an underdeveloped sense of diligence.[11]

- Because innumerable circumstances, factors, and conditions influence personality and predisposition to addiction, it has not yet been determined whether predetermination of addiction is chemical, genetic, or psychological.

model include biological, environmental, psychological, and social interaction elements. This model incorporates the majority of theories that have been used in an attempt to explain addiction and is considered the most compre-

hensive and holistic body of theory and practice today. This more holistic approach allows for the frequent outcome of most treatment, which is relapse, and addresses this issue through psychological vulnerability assessments while incorporating other factors to explain why one person becomes alcoholic and another one doesn't—even if both are from the same genetic and social family. The following are the basic tenets of the theory.

Studies investigating genetic influences toward addiction indicate a strong tendency to run in families. In several studies, children of parents who were drug-addicted were much more likely to engage in drug-taking behaviors than were the children of nonaddicted parents.[4,5] The correlation remained consistent even if the children did not live with their addicted parents.

Oakley Ray states that "no genetic physiological or biochemical marker has been found that strongly predicts alcoholism or any other addiction."[2] However, researchers who believe in biological causes of addiction have found that addicted people metabolize mood-altering substances differently than nonaddicted individuals. Some studies have found that adult children of alcoholics have abnormal concentrations of neurotransmitters that affect mood (endorphins, enkephalins, norepinephrine, and serotonin). Theoretically, abnormal levels of these hormones cause mood disorders, which lead individuals to seek mood-altering drugs.[3]

Humans are strongly influenced by the cultural expectations and social mores of their environment. Language, clothing, and acceptable behavior are all modeled by family, friends, and the media. In cultures where drinking is a part of life and intoxication is viewed with strong disapproval, there is less drunkenness and addiction. When special events or activities are viewed as impossible to have fun without excessive consumption of alcohol, addiction is more evident—more overlooked and more acceptable. In the United States, television, movies, and music all glamorize the liberal consumption of alcohol and other drugs. This opens the door for abuse and addiction without the stigma. Add the fast pace of life found in large cities, as well as the sense of isolation and availability of addictive substances, and the chance of addiction's occurring increases.

Psychological makeup has been considered a contributing factor for a long time. People have even spoken of the "addictive personality," indicating that certain behaviors tend to be found in people who become addicted to alcohol or other drugs. Individuals who become addicted tend to have lower self-esteem and seek positive reinforcement from others. They may also be having more trouble managing life events (fewer coping skills) in a positive way and want someone else to solve their problems rather than reacting more aggressively to situations.

Social learning theory states that people learn by watching others and that much **addictive behavior**

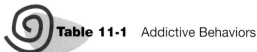

Table 11-1 Addictive Behaviors

Compulsion	Excessive preoccupation/obsession with a behavior or preoccupation with the need to perform it
Loss of control	Loss of the ability to control an action or a behavior; inability to block the impulse to engage in a behavior
Escalation	More of an activity is needed in order to produce a desired effect. This requires more time and frequently more monies directed toward the behavior.
Denial	Inability or refusal to see or comprehend that a behavior is destructive or the extent of its destructiveness
Negative consequences	Serious negative consequences, including academic, family/personal relationships, health, legal, and financial

(behavior that is excessive, compulsive, and psychologically and physically destructive) is learned. The tendency for addictions to run in families could be due to the behavior children learn about how to spend their spare time or what to do when faced with a difficult or traumatic situation. If the family of origin tends to drink or use other drugs, then the child learns the same behavior.

In general, children who feel unloved or insecure or who feel as if they cannot "be themselves" or are abused are more likely to engage in addictive behaviors. Throughout life, when people are faced with traumatic or extremely difficult situations, such as the loss of a spouse, addictive behaviors are more likely to surface.

Habit and addiction are not the same. Addiction is defined by continued involvement in a behavior in spite of ongoing negative consequences. Examples of addictive behaviors are listed in Table 11-1.

Drug Classification

Drugs can be classified in a number of ways. For example, they can be classified according to legality (legal or illegal), whether their effects are primarily physiological or psychological, or whether their use has more medicinal benefits or a greater potential for abuse. The last system is based on the Controlled Substance Act of 1970, which classifies **narcotics** and other dangerous drugs. The system contains five classifications called *schedules*. Schedule I drugs have no medical use and a high potential for abuse (such as heroin and LSD); schedule II through V drugs have approved medicinal uses with varying potentials for abuse and significant psychological and physical dependence. Excluded from this classification system are two of the most deadly drugs found in modern society: alcohol and tobacco products.

Drugs are also classified according to the physiological effect they have. Categories include stimulants, depressants, hallucinogens, narcotics, and inhalants. Two other types are also important. Designer drugs are manufactured to mimic the effects of drugs found in the previously mentioned categories, and marijuana, or cannabis, is difficult to classify but is usually included as a hallucinogen. Depending on the dose, marijuana can mimic a variety of substances found in other categories. The following is a list of drug categories and the effects they have on the body:

- *Stimulants:* **Stimulants** speed up the central nervous system, producing an increase in alertness and excitability. Examples are amphetamines, **cocaine,** crack cocaine, methamphetamines, and drugs such as Ritalin and phentermine (Ionamin).
- *Depressants:* Also known as *sedatives* and *tranquilizers,* **depressants** slow down the central nervous system, causing a feeling of relaxation. Examples of the depressant drugs are barbiturates; methaqualone (Quaaludes, or "quad"); and tranquilizers such as diazepam (Valium), chlordiazepoxide HCl (Librium), and meprobamate (Miltown).
- *Psychoactives:* **Psychoactives** can alter feelings, moods, and/or perceptions. Marijuana is classified as a psychoactive drug but can exhibit effects similar to those of stimulants, depressants, and narcotics. Some examples of psychoactive drugs are lysergic acid diethylamide (LSD), mescaline, peyote, phencyclidine (PCP), and psilocybin.
- *Narcotics:* Narcotics are powerful painkillers. They also produce pleasurable feelings and induce sleep. The narcotic drugs include codeine, heroin, methadone, morphine, opium, and substances such as oxycodone (Percodan), propoxyphene (Darvon), pentazocine (Talwin), and difenoxin (Lomotil).
- *Inhalants:* **Inhalants** are volatile nondrugs that cause druglike effects if inhaled. Examples are glue and gasoline. Some, such as nitrous oxide and amyl nitrate, have medical uses.
- *Designer drugs:* **Designer drugs** are drug analogs (newly synthesized products that are already outlawed or for which no law yet exists) of amphetamines, methamphetamines, narcotics, and hallucinogens

Just the Facts

What Products Contain Caffeine and How Much?

Item	Milligrams of Caffeine	
	Typical	Range*
Coffee (8-oz. cup)		
Brewed, drip method	85	65–120
Instant	75	60–85
Decaffeinated	3	2–4
Espresso (1-oz. cup)	40	30–50
Teas (8-oz. cup)		
Brewed, major U.S. brands	40	20–90
Brewed, imported brands	60	25–110
Instant	28	24–31
Iced (8-oz. glass)	25	9–50
Some soft drinks (8 oz.)	24	20–40
Cocoa beverage (8 oz.)	6	3–32
Chocolate milk beverage (8 oz.)	5	2–7
Milk chocolate (1 oz.)	6	1–15
Dark chocolate, semi-sweet (1 oz.)	20	5–35
Baker's chocolate (1 oz.)	26	26
Chocolate-flavored syrup (1 oz.)	4	4

* Due to brewing method, plant variety, brand, and so on.

manufactured in illegal laboratories to mimic controlled substances. They are often more powerful and less predictable than the drugs they imitate. The number and variations of designer drugs available are increasing rapidly.

Currently, three main types of illegal synthetic analog drugs are available: (1) analogs of phencyclidine (PCP); (2) analogs of synthetic narcotic analgesics, such as Demerol; and (3) analogs of amphetamines and methamphetamines. Perhaps one of the best-known analogs in the third category is MDMA, known as *ecstasy* or *Adam*. It is widely used in the college setting as a euphoriant.[7]

Commonly Abused Substances

This section briefly examines some of the most well-known and frequently used drugs—caffeine, alcohol, tobacco products, designer drugs, club drugs, cocaine, and marijuana. This section is not intended to be all-inclusive.

There is a wide range of other substances that are potentially dangerous if misused or abused. Because these drugs are so frequently used, it is important for you to understand their positive and negative effects, so that you can make decisions based on information rather than myth.

Caffeine

Caffeine is probably the most commonly used drug in American society. Each day, millions of Americans drink, chew, or ingest approximately 4 mg of caffeine for every 2.2 pounds of body weight. The average American adult consumes 200 mg of caffeine daily.[8] Caffeine is a stimulant that speeds heart rate, temporarily increases blood pressure, and disrupts sleep. It also relieves drowsiness, helps in the performance of repetitive tasks, and improves work ability.[9] Negative effects include insomnia, anxiety, heart dysrhythmias, gastrointestinal complaints, dizziness, and headaches.

The active ingredient in caffeine belongs to a group of drugs with similar structures known as *xanthines*.

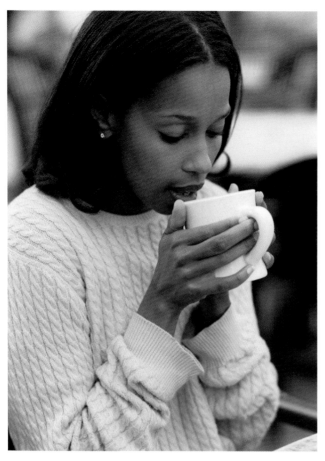

Today, millions of Americans ingest caffeine in some form.

Xanthines include a substance found in cocoa beans, which are used to make chocolate, and in tea leaves. In the past, caffeine consumption was thought to cause birth defects, breast-feeding problems, cardiovascular disease, cancer, and fibrocystic breast disease. Current research has found no substantial association with these conditions.[8] However, pregnant and nursing women should consume no more than two cups of coffee a day and should consume tea and caffeinated soft drinks only in moderation (less than 300 mg per day).[8] Furthermore, women who suffer from premenstrual tension (PMS) should eliminate caffeine. Research has indicated that women who drink one-half to four cups (25 to 200 mg) of caffeinated tea a day are twice as likely to suffer PMS symptoms as are women who drink none at all.[8]

The majority of adults can consume relatively low doses of caffeine (the equivalent of two to three cups of coffee per day) safely. Approximately 10 percent of the adult population experiences *caffeinism*, a condition in which frequent high-dose use causes psychological and physical problems. Doses as low as 250 mg per day can produce restlessness, nervousness, excitement, insomnia, flushed face, diuresis, muscle twitching, rambling thoughts and speech, and stomach complaints. Doses greater than 1 gram per day can cause muscle twitching, rambling thoughts and speech, heart dysrhythmias, and motor agitation. Higher doses can cause ringing in the ears and flashes of light.[7] (See Just the Facts: What Products Contain Caffeine and How Much for caffeine amount found in various products.)

It is easy to consume a great deal of caffeine. By becoming familiar with the amount of caffeine in a product and restricting your consumption to less than 400 mg of caffeine per day, you can benefit from the effects of the drug without suffering any negative effects.[8]

Alcohol

Alcohol use is pervasive. Alcohol is a drug generally deemed socially acceptable. Nevertheless, no other drug causes so much physical, social, and emotional damage to people and their families. People drink alcoholic beverages in many situations and for many reasons. They drink when they are among friends and when they are upset or depressed. People drink to spark romantic feelings, to put themselves at ease in social situations, and to celebrate special occasions. In addition, people drink because their role models drink and because the advertising industry has convinced them that alcohol contributes to self-enhancement. Unfortunately, the devastation associated with alcohol is often not mentioned. Table 11-2 (page 364) summarizes the short- and long-term effects of the drug. Because society has labeled alcohol appropriate and even necessary for some occasions, abstinence may seem unrealistic for many people.

As with many drugs, there are times and places where medicinal and health reasons are cited for alcohol use. Current research suggests that moderate amounts of alcohol may help reduce the risk for heart disease. The possible benefits and pleasures of the use of alcoholic beverages do not eradicate the dangers that result from misuse or abuse, however (see Assessment Activity 11-1). Nearly half of annual traffic deaths are caused by accidents involving alcohol consumption. This figure does not include permanent physical injuries and emotional damages caused by alcohol-induced traffic accidents and deaths, nor does it include the increased number of violent acts associated with alcohol intoxication. Drinking of alcohol, if it occurs, ought to be approached responsibly, with recognition of the potential for harm to self and others. Real-World Wellness: Responsible Drinking on page 365 provides suggestions for responsible drinking.

Although there are several types of alcohol, the intoxicating agent in all alcohol drinks is ethyl alcohol, a colorless liquid with a sharp, burning taste (see Just the Facts: How Much Alcohol Is in Beer, Wine, and Other Drinks? on page 365). The percentage of alcohol in a beverage is measured by its proof, twice the percentage of alcohol. A

Table 11-2 Effects of Alcohol Use

Short-Term or Immediate			Long-Term	
Number of Drinks*	Blood Alcohol Concentration (BAC)	Effect(s)	System/Organ	Health Risks
1–2	0.00–0.05	Usually relaxation and euphoria; decrease in alertness	Breast	50% higher risk for cancer in women who drink any alcohol; 100% increase for women having three or more drinks per day
2–3	0.05–0.10	Exaggerated feelings and behavior; emotional instability; increased reaction time and diminished motor coordination; impaired driving; a legally drunk designation in most states	Cardiovascular	High blood pressure; irregular heartbeat; chest pain/angina; myocardial infarctions; damage to coronary arteries
4–5	0.10–0.15	Loss of peripheral vision; highly impaired driving ability; unsteady walking/standing	General gastrointestinal	Risk for mouth, tongue, throat, esophageal, stomach, and liver cancer; pancreatitis; malnutrition; digestive impairment
5–10	0.15–0.30	Significant impairment of sensory perceptions; slurred speech; decreased sensitivity to pain; difficult and staggering walk	Immune system	Lower resistance to infectious diseases
			Liver	Hepatitis; cirrhosis
			Pancreas	Interference with insulin production
10+	> 0.30	Stupor or unconsciousness; anesthetization; possible death at levels greater than 0.35	Small intestine	Interference with or prevention of absorption of proteins, iron, calcium, thiamine, and vitamin B_{12}
			Stomach	Bleeding from irritation, ulcers
			Muscular system	Destruction of muscle fibers
			Nervous system	Destruction of brain cells; interference with neurotransmitters; slowing of reaction time
			Reproductive system	Impotence; decreased testosterone production; fetal alcohol syndrome; miscarriage

* 1 drink = 12 oz. beer, 6 oz. wine, 1 oz. hard liquor.

beverage that is 40 percent alcohol has a proof of 80. The blood alcohol concentration (BAC) is the percentage of alcohol content in the blood. This percentage determines the alcohol's effect on a person (Table 11-2). The more quickly the alcohol is absorbed, the quicker the BAC increases.

Alcohol enters the bloodstream quickly from the stomach and even more quickly from the small intestine. In the stomach, food inhibits absorption of alcohol. Food does not affect absorption in the small intestine.[10]

Following are some other factors that affect the rate of absorption and effect of alcohol:

- *Rate of consumption:* How quickly is the beverage consumed? Large amounts of alcohol quickly consumed expose the brain to higher peak concentrations, altering perceptions and response times.

- *Type of beverage:* Beer and wine contain substances that slow the rate of absorption; thus, the effects are experienced more slowly than are the effects of drinking distilled spirits, even when the same amount of alcohol is consumed. Carbonated beverages added to liquor speed absorption, but diluting them with water slows the process.

- *Body weights:* Body weight and body composition do not influence the rate of absorption, but they do influence the effects of alcohol. More weight and/or more muscle mass (muscle with more fluid volume than fat) results in a greater distribution of the alcohol, lowering its concentration in the body and weakening its effects.

- *Tolerance to alcohol:* Some people seem to remain sober, while others react quickly to the same amount

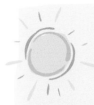

Real-World Wellness

Responsible Drinking

I enjoy an occasional drink, and I often invite friends to my home to celebrate holidays and special events. How can I make sure I'm drinking and hosting parties responsibly?

Following are suggestions to help each person be a responsible drinker and host:

- Drink slowly; never consume more than one drink per hour.
- Eat while drinking, but do not eat salty food.
- When mixing drinks, measure the amount of alcohol; never just pour.
- Serve and choose nonalcoholic drinks as an alternative.
- As host, always serve the guests or hire a bartender. Do not have an open bar or serve someone who is intoxicated.
- Stop using or serving alcohol one hour before a party is over.
- Don't drink and drive. Have a nondrinker drive or call a cab.

Just the Facts

How Much Alcohol Is in Beer, Wine, and Other Drinks?

Did you know that all of the following contain the same amount of alcohol? Each contains the equivalent of 3 ounces of pure alcohol. A 160-pound person who consumed these amounts within a two-hour period would be considered legally intoxicated in most states:

- Six 12-oz. glasses of beer
- 15 ounces of fortified wine (about two glasses)
- 24 ounces of table wine (about four glasses)
- Six servings of liquor (1.3 oz. of 80 proof)
- One measure of vermouth
- One jigger ($1\frac{1}{2}$ oz.) of whiskey

of alcohol. One drink for a novice may have the same effect as three drinks for a more experienced drinker. This indicates that the experienced drinker's body has adapted to the alcohol at the cellular level and is encouraging increased consumption. Tolerance consists of an increase in the rate of alcohol absorption metabolism as well as a reduced response to the drug. It is the reduced response that is frequently associated with physical and psychological dependence. Increased tolerance to alcohol can also result in a decreased response to other drugs, specifically other central nervous system depressants.

Alcoholism is a disease in which a person loses control over drinking. According to a definition approved by the National Council on Alcoholism and Drug Dependence and the American Society of Addiction Medicine, alcoholism is a "primary, chronic disease with genetic, psychosocial, and environmental factors influencing its development and manifestations. The disease is often progressive and fatal."[11] An alcoholic is a person who suffers from the disease of alcoholism. For alcoholics, alcohol increasingly becomes the focus of life, and family, social, work, or school responsibilities become less important and are eventually disrupted by the desire and need for alcohol. Some alcoholics make this transition rapidly, whereas others maintain the

appearance of being social drinkers for many years. Unfortunately, predetermining who will have trouble with alcohol is impossible. Alcoholism crosses all social and economic barriers and can affect everyone from clergy, medical doctors, high school students, and college students to professors.

Women who are alcoholics face unique problems, and women who use alcohol or tobacco during pregnancy put their children at risk of developing certain health problems. The rate of alcoholism is increasing among younger women (see Wellness for a Lifetime: Alcohol and Tobacco Use Among Young Women on page 366).

There is no single accepted reason any person becomes an alcoholic. Most researchers think that a variety of events, genetic tendencies, and situations working together result in alcoholism for some people. The medical model of alcoholism includes biological, or genetic, explanations of abuse. It views alcohol abuse as uncontrollable because of physiological differences between alcoholics and nonalcoholics. Research seems to link alcoholism to an inherited susceptibility, or predisposition, for the disease:[4] Children of alcoholic parents are four times more likely to become alcoholics even when raised by nonalcoholics.

Treatment for alcoholism is often long-term (see Just the Facts: The 12-Step Program on page 367). The course of treatment usually occurs in three stages: (1) detoxification (eliminating the alcohol from the body), (2) medical care (attending to any health-related problems), and (3) the changing of long-term behavior (helping the recovering alcoholic overcome long-established drinking patterns and destructive behaviors). Several sources provide long-term medical and

Wellness for a Lifetime

Alcohol and Tobacco Use Among Young Women

At one time, it was thought that alcohol-related problems occurred more often in men than women. Now mounting evidence indicates that women—especially young women—are drinking more. This fact is reflected in the increased number of admissions of younger women to treatment centers.[12] Women who are alcoholics often drink for reasons different from those that prompt men to abuse alcohol, and some of the consequences of drinking are different between the genders. Smoking, too, poses special risks for women, especially those who are pregnant. Here are some of these gender differences:

- More women than men who abuse alcohol can identify a specific triggering event that prompted them to start drinking, such as a death, a divorce, a job change, or the departure of a child from home.

- Women tend to begin abusing alcohol later in life than men do and to progress more quickly in their abuse pattern.

- Women are prescribed more mood-altering drugs than men are and are thus at greater risk for drug interactions and cross-tolerance.

- Alcoholic women are less likely than men are to have a family support system to aid them in their recovery attempts.

- Women alcoholics tend not to receive as much social support as men do during their treatment for and recovery from alcoholism.

- Women tend to have more financial problems than men do, which makes entry into a treatment program more difficult.[13]

Here are some alcohol- and tobacco-related effects of concern to parents and couples considering pregnancy:

- The children of pregnant women who drink are at a high risk for fetal alcohol syndrome (FAS), which causes a variety of birth defects, including abnormal eye alignment, nose and jaw irregularities, cleft palate, joint defects, heart defects, and inadequate brain development. FAS has been reported in children of women who drank as little as 30 milliliters of alcohol per day (about two mixed drinks, three bottles of beer, or two glasses of wine). Thus it is recommended that women abstain from drinking any alcohol during pregnancy.

- Babies born to mothers who smoke have a lower average birth weight and length and have a smaller head circumference.[13]

- Infants born to mothers who smoke are more likely than children born to nonsmokers to die from sudden infant death syndrome (SIDS).[13]

- Smoking during pregnancy may cause hyperactivity in children.

Finally, men and women who smoke should know the following:

- Smoking by both men and women is associated with premature facial wrinkling.

- Osteoporosis (loss of calcium from the bone) is associated with smoking.

psychological support to people with alcohol or other drug problems.

Alcoholics remain alcoholics for life, regardless of whether they drink. Recovering alcoholics must therefore be careful about any products they consume, including medicines and mouthwashes, which sometimes contain alcohol. Currently, an estimated 10 million adults and 3 million adolescents under the age of 18 are alcoholics.[11]

Alcohol use has been demonstrated to have a strong association with crime and violence. Data clearly indicate that homicide is more likely to occur in a situation in which drinking has occurred.[14] In the same study, all incidents of spouse and child abuse were correlated with drinking. A Canadian study found that at least 42 percent of violent crimes involved alcohol.[2] In addition, 75 percent of suicide attempts involved alcohol use.[1]

As explained in Chapter 10, alcohol and driving can be a lethal combination. Alcohol is linked to at least half of all highway fatalities, and this figure includes only crashes involving drivers classified as legally intoxicated. Finally, in single-vehicle fatal wrecks occurring on weekend nights, the driver is legally intoxicated almost 70 percent of the time.[2]

Binge drinking among college students

Binge drinking is defined as consuming five or more drinks in a single session for men and four or more for women at least once within the previous two weeks.

∿Just the Facts∿

The 12-Step Program

Twelve-step programs remain the basis of most addiction recovery programs. The first step in all 12-step programs is the individual's admitting that he or she is powerless over alcohol, and step 2 is seeking a higher power to help him or her get the strength he or she needs to change. The 12-step program states that successful treatment and change require six principles of change:[2]

1. Believing you can change is the key to change.
2. The type of treatment is less critical than individual commitment to change.
3. Brief treatments can change behaviors as successfully as longer interventions.
4. Life skills can be the key to licking addiction.
5. Repeated efforts are critical in change.
6. Improvement without abstinence counts.

While Alcoholics Anonymous says abstinence is vital, this approach says getting better counts and that most people will not succeed the first time they try to quit. What do you think?

According to a national survey conducted by the Harvard School of Public Health, nearly half of college students surveyed drank four or five drinks in the previous two weeks prior to the survey.[15] Another study reported that 39 percent of college women binge drank within a two-week period prior to the survey.[16] In a multicampus survey, white non-Hispanic students reported the highest percentage of binge drinking in a two-week period (43.8 percent), followed by Native American (40.6 percent), Hispanic (31.3 percent), Asian (22.7 percent), and black non-Hispanic (22.5 percent) students.[16]

(For a discussion of how much alcohol is contained in various types of alcoholic drinks, review Just the Facts: How Much Alcohol Is in Beer, Wine, and Other Drinks?) This information is alarming in light of the number of deaths in the last few years caused by binge drinking during fraternity or campus rituals. Problems associated with student binge drinking include residence hall damage, fights, sexual assault, and drunken driving. The greater a student's alcohol use, the poorer his or her academic performance.[17] The most distressing fact is that binge drinking too often causes unnecessary deaths of drinkers, their friends, and other innocent victims.

Many colleges and universities have begun programs that emphasize responsible, rather than total, abstinence. Guidelines published for reducing the risk associated with heavy or binge drinking are

Wellness on the Web
Behavior Change Activities

When "Social Drinking" Becomes Antisocial

Despite the proven health risks, the ruined lives, and the rising toll of fatal drunken-driving accidents, alcohol use continues to be pervasive in our society. Alcohol is a drug that many people deem socially acceptable. Slick TV and magazine advertisements glamorize drinking and portray it as the pastime of attractive, healthy, affluent people. The grim reality is that no other drug causes so much physical, social, and emotional damage to both individuals and families. People drink alcoholic beverages in many situations and for many reasons, and many people don't know why they drink. To test your knowledge of alcohol use, go to www.mhhe.com/anspaugh6e, click on Student Center, Chapter 11, Wellness on the Web, and then Activity 1, and complete the alcohol quiz. How much did you know about alcohol and our society?

Kicking the Habit

If you've ever tried to quit smoking, you know how hard it can be. That's because nicotine is a highly addictive drug. For some people, it can be as addictive as heroin or cocaine. Within seconds of your taking a puff of smoke, nicotine travels to your brain. It tells your brain to release chemicals that make you want to smoke more. Although quitting is difficult, the health benefits you gain far outweigh the temporary discomfort of withdrawal. Most people make two to three tries, or more, before finally being able to quit. Studies show that, each time you try to quit, you'll become more determined and learn more about what helps and what hurts. Regardless of age, health, or lifestyle, anyone can quit smoking. The decision to quit and your chances of success are strongly influenced by how much you want to stop smoking. Go to the Web site listed previously and click on Activity 2 to learn about the steps the Centers for Disease Control recommends to help you quit—and win.

1. *Pace your drinking.* Allow time between drinks and sip the drink.
2. *Do not drink every day.* Tolerance is developed and a person must increase the amount of alcohol consumed before effects are noticed. BAC is still rising even though effects are unnoticed.
3. *You decide when to drink.* Do not allow others or situations to determine your drinking. Drink on your terms.

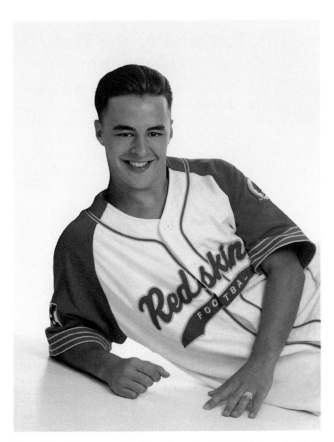

Jason Alan Bitter was killed on November 19, 1994, by a drunken driver who crossed the center line. The offender's BAC was .36, more than three times the legal limit in Missouri. Dina Khoury-Hager was also killed in the crash. Both were 17 years old and would have graduated from college in 1999.

4. *Consider alternating nonalcoholic drinks with those containing alcohol.* Drink a soft drink without alcohol every other drink or drink plain orange juice every other drink.

5. *Don't drink on an empty stomach.* Food with fats and/or protein slow the absorption of the alcohol.

6. *Measure the alcohol.* Pay attention to the size of containers. Do not provide kegs of beer or use larger wine, beer, or shot glasses. Do not participate in "chugging" contests or other drinking games.

7. *Don't drink for more than one hour.* Decide what nonalcoholic drink you are going to drink after the hour.

8. *Learn how to calculate your BAC.* Know how many drinks are allowed within your hour period.

9. *If you are a female, drink less.* Women become more intoxicated than men after drinking the same amount of alcohol, even when differences in body weight are take into account. Women have proportionately less water in their bodies than men; thus, women become more highly concentrated in BAC.

10. *Avoid taking over-the-counter (OTC) or prescription medications.* More than 100 medications interact with alcohol. If you are taking any OTC or prescription drugs, ask your doctor or pharmacist whether you can safely drink alcoholic beverages.

Fortunately, most college students moderate their drinking after their college years. However, about 12 percent are unable to control their drinking and continue to abuse alcohol. You should weigh carefully the potential harmful consequences of alcohol use and abuse before partaking in binge or heavy drinking. Is it worth the price?

Tobacco Products

All tobacco products, including cigarettes, cigars, pipes, and smokeless tobacco (snuff and chewing tobacco), contain the drug **nicotine**. Nicotine is an addictive substance and an alkaloid poison. It affects the body by increasing heart and respiratory rates, elevating blood pressure, increasing cardiac output and oxygen consumption, and constricting the bronchi (the two main branches of the trachea that lead to the lungs). A person inhales nicotine when smoking a tobacco product. Nicotine in smokeless tobacco is absorbed through membranes of the mouth and cheek.

Smoking is directly or indirectly responsible for the conditions and diseases listed in Just the Facts: Risks of Smoking. Some components of cigarette smoke are known as *carcinogens* (substances that cause cancer or foster the growth of cancer cells). Nicotine, tar, and carbon monoxide are found in cigarette smoke. The tar in tobacco is a black, sticky, dark fluid composed of thousands of chemicals. Many of the chemicals found in tar are cancer-causing. Carbon monoxide is a deadly gas emitted in the exhaust of cars and in burning tobacco. The carbon monoxide level in cigarette smoke is 400 times greater than what is considered safe in industrial settings. Carbon monoxide binds to hemoglobin more readily than oxygen, interfering with the ability of blood to transport oxygen to the body. Carbon monoxide impairs the nervous system and increases the risk for heart attacks and strokes. See Just the Facts: Risks of Smoking.

The addictive nature of nicotine has come under substantial public scrutiny. Some experts consider nicotine to be as addictive as cocaine and other drugs. Tobacco is considered the leading preventable contributor to disease and early death in the United States (from heart disease and cancer, specifically) and is listed as a primary risk factor for heart disease by the American Heart Association. Cigarettes are responsible for 442,000 deaths annually.[18] Because of the health risks and because of what is seen by many as an effort on the part of tobacco companies to intentionally increase nicotine addiction to increase the sales of cigarettes, some people suggest that tobacco should be made an illegal drug.

Just the Facts

Risks of Smoking

Following is some information about the risks of smoking.

 Conditions and Diseases That Can Be Caused by Smoking and Tobacco Products

Risks	Results
Coronary heart disease	An estimated 442,000 die each year of smoking-related illnesses. The largest portion of these deaths is related to cardiovascular disease (AHA).
Peripheral arterial disease	Smokers are 2 to 3 times more likely to suffer from abdominal aortic aneurysm than are nonsmokers. Smokers have more atherosclerotic occlusions.
Lung cancer	Smoking cigarettes is the major cause of lung cancers in men and women. Rates are currently increasing faster among women than men.
Cancer of the larynx	Laryngeal cancer is 2.0 to 27.4 times more likely in smokers than in nonsmokers.
Oral cancers	The use of smokeless tobacco and snuff is associated with an increased risk for oral cancer. Pipes and cigars are also major risk factors. The use of alcohol seems to enhance the possibility of developing oral cancer.
Cancer of the esophagus	Smoking cigarettes, pipes, and cigars increases by as much as 9 times the risk of dying from esophageal cancer. Alcohol use in combination with smoking adds to that risk.
Bladder cancer	The percentage of bladder cancer attributed to smoking is estimated at 40 to 60 percent in men and 25 to 35 percent in women.
Cancer of the pancreas	Smokers have twice the risk of nonsmokers for cancer of the pancreas.
Chronic obstructive pulmonary (lung) disease (COPD)	Between 80 and 90 percent of more than 60,000 deaths per year from COPD (chronic obstructive pulmonary disease) are caused by smoking.
Peptic ulcers	Cigarette smokers develop peptic ulcers much more frequently than do nonsmokers. Ulcers are also more difficult to cure in smokers.
Complications in pregnancy, illnesses in children	Smoking mothers have more stillbirths and babies with low birth weight. The hospital admission rate for pneumonia and bronchitis is 28 percent higher for children of smoking mothers than for children of nonsmoking mothers. Asthma is more common among children of smoking mothers. Parental smoking is a risk factor associated with persistent middle-ear infection in young children.

SOURCE: American Cancer Society. 2004. Surveillance Research. Atlanta: American Cancer Society.

Secondhand and sidestream smoke

Passive smoking is the inhalation of what is known as *secondhand cigarette smoke* from the environment by a nonsmoker. Smokers inhale what is known as **mainstream smoke;** passive smokers most frequently inhale **sidestream smoke,** which results from burning tobacco products (the end of the lighted tip of a cigarette, cigar, or pipe).[18] Because it is not filtered by either a cigarette filter or the smoker's lungs, sidestream smoke contains higher concentrations of carbon dioxide and carbon monoxide. For each pack of cigarettes smoked indoors by a smoker, a nonsmoker in the vicinity passively smokes the equivalent of three to five cigarettes.[18] Research shows that nonsmokers living with smokers have a 20 percent higher mortality rate than do the nonsmoking partners of nonsmokers. Nonsmoking wives of smokers have been found to be at greater risk for lung cancer than the wives of nonsmoking husbands. Other studies have reported that nonsmokers living with smokers have a greater risk of developing respiratory problems and that nonsmoking women living with smokers have a greater risk for cervical cancer.[19] The bottom line about passive smoking is that there is no safe level of exposure to tobacco smoke.

Cigars and pipes

In the hope of avoiding the dangers associated with cigarette smoking, some smokers have turned from cigarettes to cigars or pipes. Since pipe and cigar smokers don't inhale, they do seem less likely to develop lung and heart disease. However, pipe and cigar smokers have a much higher risk of developing mouth, larynx, and esophageal cancers because they hold the nicotine and tars from their tobacco products in their mouths instead of inhaling them. Furthermore, when a cigarette smoker switches to cigars or a pipe, he or she tends to continue to inhale and, thus, to remain at the same risk for lung and heart disease while the risk of other cancers increases.[20]

Smokeless tobacco products

Smokeless tobacco products consist of snuff and chewing tobacco. Snuff is a finely shredded or powdered tobacco sniffed by the user, allowing nicotine to be absorbed through the mucous membranes of the nose and mouth. Chewing tobacco consists of loose-leaf tobacco mixed with molasses or other flavors and pressed into what are called *plugs* or twisted into ropelike strands. This material is then placed between the gums and cheek or lower lip, where the nicotine is absorbed. In 1994, it was estimated that more than 6 million men and 730,000 women used smokeless tobacco products.

Smokeless tobacco is not a safe alternative to cigarettes. It contributes to the development of periodontal (gum) disease, which can result in bleeding gums, loss of teeth, staining of teeth, and tooth decay. Periodontal disease is less significant than the oral cancers that may

be caused by frequent contact of the cells of the gums and cheek with the carcinogenic agents in the tobacco. Two early danger signs of such cancers are leukoplakia (white spots) and erythroplakia (red spots), which indicate precancerous conditions; they should be evaluated by a physician immediately. If treatment is delayed, cancer can quickly spread to the jaw, neck, brain, and digestive and urinary systems.[1]

Clove cigarettes

Some people smoke clove cigarettes as an alternative to regular cigarettes. Clove cigarettes usually consist of 60 percent tobacco and 40 percent clove buds. Clove cigarettes generate even more nicotine, tar, and carbon monoxide than do regular cigarettes, so the dangers are even greater. Some users have developed serious lung and respiratory illnesses.[21]

Advantages of quitting

Smoking is an extremely strong addiction. To quit completely, many people require the help of trained professionals (see Real-World Wellness: Charting a Plan to Quit Smoking or Stop Using Tobacco Products and Real-World Wellness: Choosing a Smoking Cessation Aid). Although quitting is difficult, the health benefits gained far outweigh the problems. When people stop smoking, their risk of developing heart disease and some kinds of cancer (if not already present in the body) eventually

---

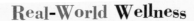

Real-World **Wellness**

Charting a Plan to Quit Smoking or Stop Using Tobacco Products

I've tried several times to quit smoking, but I'm still lighting up. This time I want to be prepared. Is there a plan I can follow that will help me quit for good?

The *Mayo Clinic Health Letter* offers the following suggestions:[22]

- *Set a date.* Make the date reasonably soon. Make a list of reasons you want to quit.

- *Start stopping before you reach the date.* Taper off the number of cigarettes you are currently smoking. Choose a milder brand.

- *Make your plans known.* Tell a friend, your family, and colleagues of your plans. Ask for their support.

- *Take it one day at a time.* Get up every morning and decide not to smoke that day. Focus your attention on that day only.

- *Change your routine.* Avoid or change situations in which you have previously smoked.

- *Alter your surroundings.* Start new activities, such as exercising or needlepoint.

- *Time the urge.* Identify when your urge to smoke is the strongest. Being prepared will help you resist.

- *Use substitutes.* Substitutes can include gum, celery, carrots, and pickles.

- *Prepare a daydream.* Have a pleasant daydream ready to help fight off the desire to smoke. This can be an image of yourself without a cigarette in a situation you find highly desirable.

- *Use relaxation techniques.* Deep breathing or progressive muscle relaxation can help.

- *Stay busy.* Find ways to keep yourself and your mind occupied, so you do not miss smoking or having a cigarette in your hand.

- *Practice positive thinking.* Tell yourself, "I can make it." Remember that you *can* do it.

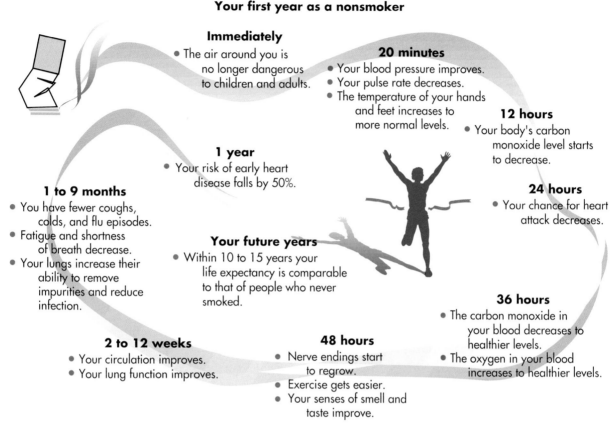

Your first year as a nonsmoker

Immediately
- The air around you is no longer dangerous to children and adults.

20 minutes
- Your blood pressure improves.
- Your pulse rate decreases.
- The temperature of your hands and feet increases to more normal levels.

12 hours
- Your body's carbon monoxide level starts to decrease.

1 year
- Your risk of early heart disease falls by 50%.

24 hours
- Your chance for heart attack decreases.

1 to 9 months
- You have fewer coughs, colds, and flu episodes.
- Fatigue and shortness of breath decrease.
- Your lungs increase their ability to remove impurities and reduce infection.

Your future years
- Within 10 to 15 years your life expectancy is comparable to that of people who never smoked.

36 hours
- The carbon monoxide in your blood decreases to healthier levels.
- The oxygen in your blood increases to healthier levels.

2 to 12 weeks
- Your circulation improves.
- Your lung function improves.

48 hours
- Nerve endings start to regrow.
- Exercise gets easier.
- Your senses of smell and taste improve.

Figure 11-1 Health Benefits of Quitting Smoking

Quitting smoking results in benefits that begin immediately and become more significant the longer a person stays smoke-free.

decreases to that of nonsmokers; in other words, some of the effects of smoking are reversible (see Figure 11-1). Real-World Wellness: Choosing a Smoking Cessation Aid (page 372) includes products that can help control cravings and stop smoking.

Illegal Drugs

Designer Drugs/Club Drugs

Designer drugs resemble those controlled by the Federal Drug Administration (FDA); that is, they act like known drugs but have a different chemical composition. Probably the two best-known designer drugs currently being used are *China white*, an analog of heroin, and *ecstasy*. Ecstasy is an analog of the amphetamines and hallucinogens under FDA control since 1985. Designer drugs appear so rapidly that it is difficult or impossible to restrict sales. Poor quality control and combinations with other, often poisonous, substances can result in neurological damage or death. Brain damage is often caused by a single dose.

Club drugs are among a group of drugs used by teens and young adults who are part of a bar, rave, or trance scene. Raves and trances are generally night-long dances, often held in warehouses. Not everyone attending these events uses drugs, but those who do are attracted to the low cost, the seemingly increased stamina, and the intoxicating highs said to increase the rave or trance experience.[26]

The drugs of concern are MDMA (ecstasy), Rohypnol, GHB, and Ketamine. Researchers are finding that critical parts of the brain are showing changes from the use of these drugs. When used in higher doses, most of these drugs can cause a sharp increase in body temperature, which leads to muscle breakdown, cardiovascular incidents, and kidney failure.[23]

MDMA (ecstasy)

MDMA is a chemical substance that combines methamphetamines with hallucinogenic (LSD-like) properties. Ecstasy is the street name for MDMA. Other names include Adam, X-TC, hug, beans, love bug, clarity, and lover's speed. Ecstasy is a combination of several illicit drugs. Because so many different recipes are used to make ecstasy, the risk for death and permanent brain damage is heightened. The drug works

Real-World Wellness

Choosing a Smoking Cessation Aid

I've been smoking since my freshman year in high school, and I'm about to graduate from college and enter the workforce. I'd like to quit, but I'm confused about all the smoking cessation products available. How do I choose the one that's best for me?

Several tools are available to help smokers wean themselves off cigarettes. These smoking cessation aids can be purchased over the counter (OTC) or with a doctor's prescription. The dosages for both versions can vary widely. For this reason, it is probably better to seek a prescription version, which will be targeted more specifically to your needs. Read the following information about three commonly used methods, and then talk to your doctor to choose the one best suited to your needs.

- *Nicotine-containing gum:* Nicotine gum requires immediate smoking cessation. The dosage is 2 to 4 mg of nicotine per piece of gum. When used under a physician's guidance, the success rate is about 40 percent. Chewing the gum may cause mouth ulcers and nausea in some people, and the product should not be used by pregnant or nursing women. Initial doses of the chewing gum cost about $50, with weekly refills costing about $30.

- *Transdermal patches:* The patch is designed to aid smoking cessation by relieving nicotine withdrawal cravings. Two types are available: a step-down version and a single-dose version. The single-dose version provides the same milligrams of nicotine in each dose (15 mg). The step-down version provides different levels of nicotine for various periods after cessation, theoretically reducing the amount of nicotine available as the person is weaned away from the drug. The step-down method is designed to ease withdrawal by making the symptoms less severe and withdrawal more gradual. The patches contain 15 to 21 mg of nicotine a day for the first weeks. After 4 to 12 weeks, the dosage is reduced

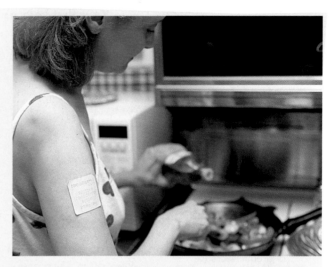

Many people have used nicotine patches to help them quit smoking. If you're a smoker, have you considered trying the patch?

to 10 to 14 mg a day. A final set of patches used for 2 to 4 weeks contains 5 to 7 mg of nicotine. Single-dose patches eliminate the step-down effect. Used alone, both versions of the patch seem to be less than 25 percent effective. When used with the prescription medication mecamylamine, however, the effectiveness rate rises to 40 percent. The patch can cause skin irritation, redness, and irregular heart rate in some users. The cost is about the same as for nicotine-containing gum.

- *Nicotrol™ inhaler.* A federal advisory panel to the FDA has endorsed a prescription inhalation device that is an alternative to chewing gum and transdermal patches. The Nicotrol inhaler is meant to simulate cigarette smoking. The device has a mouthpiece with a nicotine plug attached to it. Seventy to 80 puffs on the inhaler provide the amount of nicotine in 10 puffs on a regular cigarette. Having the inhaler to handle may help smokers who miss having something to do with their hands while providing a low level of nicotine to ease cravings.

---

primarily by affecting nerve cells that produce serotonin, one of several chemicals transmitting signals from one nerve to the next. Ecstasy causes nerve cells to release all the stored serotonin at once and then keeps it from being reabsorbed, further increasing the concentration in the synapse. The result can lead to long-term or permanent damage to those areas of the brain critical to thought, memory, and pleasure.[24] The aftermath of use can include a depressive hangover, sometimes called "Terrible Tuesday." Other psychological effects are confusion; sleep problems; severe anxiety; paranoid thinking; enhanced mental and emotional clarity;

sensations of floating; and violent, irrational behavior. Some reported physical effects of the drug include muscle tension, involuntary teeth clenching, blurred vision, hypertension, loss of control over voluntary body movements, tremors, kidney failure, heart attack, stroke, seizures, and malignant hyperthermia (increased body temperature).[24]

Rohypnol

Rohypnol, a trade name for flunitrazepam, has been a serious concern for several years because of its abuse in date rape (see Chapter 10). When mixed with alcohol, Rohypnol incapacitates its victims and prevents them from resisting sexual assault. Slang names for the drug include rophies, roofies, roach, and rope. The drugs (alcohol and Rohypnol) produce a form of amnesia, in which individuals may not remember events they experienced while under the effects of the drugs. Further, Rohypnol may be lethal when mixed with alcohol or other depressants.[25]

GHB

GHB (gammahydroxbutrate) has been abused in the United States for euphoric, sedative, and anabolic (bodybuilding) effects. It is a central nervous system depressant that was widely available over the counter in health food stores during the 1980s and until 1992. It was purchased mostly by bodybuilders to aid in muscle building and fat reduction. Street names include liquid ecstasy, soap, easy lay, and Georgia home boy. GHB is difficult to distinguish from water. Coma and seizures can occur with abuse and, when it is combined with methamphetamines, there appears to be an increased risk for seizure, nausea, and difficulty breathing. Withdrawal effects include insomnia, anxiety, tremors, and sweating. The drug is sold over the Internet and is available in some workout gyms, rave night clubs, gay male parties, and college campuses, as well as on the street. The duration of the drug is short, but it may cause unconsciousness when mixed with alcohol.[25]

Ketamine

Ketamine is an anesthetic approved for both human and animal use in medical settings. Over 90 percent of the drugs sold legally is used for practice of veterinary medicine. Ketamine can be injected or snorted. On the street, it is known as special K or vitamin K. At high doses, Ketamine can cause delirium, amnesia-impaired motor function, high blood pressure, depression, and potentially fatal respiratory problems. Certain doses can cause dreamlike states and hallucinations. Because of the last characteristics, it has become common in club and rave scenes and has been used as a date rape drug.[23]

How to protect yourself from being a victim of designer drugs/club drugs

If you go to parties or clubs and drink alcohol, you are at increased risk for becoming a victim of date rape drugs. GHB has been used most in California, Texas, Georgia, and Florida. Rohypnol has been used extensively across the South, but it has been most used in Texas, where it is popular among high school students, and Florida, especially around Miami. The good news

about Rohypnol is that it has been reformulated to be more detectable. In light-colored drinks, Rohypnol will turn the drink bright blue; in darker beverages, the drink will appear cloudy. It also dissolves more slowly than before and forms small, chunky pieces.

There are behaviors you can use to help defend yourself. If you are at a party or club, never leave your drink unattended. Cover it with your hand in between sips (not gulps) to discourage anyone from tampering with it. Even if you are not drinking an alcoholic drink, use caution. Go out with friends you can trust and watch out for each other. Double date instead of going alone. At a party, accept a drink only in a closed can or container. Never drink from punch bowls or drink anything that tastes or smells strange. If drinking a mixed drink, make sure you watch the bartender prepare it. Always be aware of your surroundings (don't get so incapacitated that you cannot do this; that is, drink moderately, so you can keep your wits about you) and trust your instincts. If you feel ill, do not wait to get help but seek out a safe person you can trust (*never* a stranger or someone whom you do not know very well).

Cocaine

At one time, cocaine was considered the drug of upper-class America. Unfortunately, the use of cocaine and its derivative, crack, is now epidemic. It is estimated that 25 to 30 million people have experimented with cocaine in the United States. Approximately 5 million people use the drug regularly. Among young adults, 9.8 percent have tried crack and 40 percent have tried cocaine.[26]

A powerful stimulant, cocaine is derived from the leaves of the South American coca shrub and ground into a crystalline powder. The most common methods of using the drug are snorting it, liquefying it and then injecting it, and freebasing (smoking). When snorted, the white powder is sniffed up through the nose. The most potent and expensive method of cocaine use is freebasing. The drug is usually smoked in a water pipe because this provides faster absorption into the bloodstream.

Crack is relatively easy to make and fairly inexpensive to buy. At $10 to $15 a dose, crack is the form of cocaine most prevalent on the streets. When snorted, crack reaches the brain in about five minutes. When injected or smoked, it takes only a few seconds for the drug to take effect.

The use of cocaine produces feelings of well-being, euphoria, and extreme exhilaration. Mental alertness seems to increase. Blood vessels constrict, causing heart rate and blood pressure to rise. Cocaine is rapidly metabolized by the liver. Snorting cocaine results in a 5- to 15-minute "high," and the effects of crack last 20 to 30 minutes. Psychological and physical dependency on crack develops rapidly because of the brief period of stimulation. The feelings of exhilaration experienced while under the influence of the drug are quickly followed by depression.

The physical consequences of cocaine use are extreme and highly dangerous. Cocaine use can cause headaches, exhaustion, shaking, blurred vision, nausea, impaired judgment, hyperactivity, loss of appetite, loss of sexual desire, and paranoia that can lead to violence. Snorting cocaine can destroy the septum in the nose. Freebasing may damage the liver and the lungs; fluid buildup in the lungs caused by freebasing has resulted in death. Cocaine can initiate strokes, bleeding in the brain, heart attacks, irregular heartbeat, and sudden death.[26]

Cocaine addiction is extremely difficult to overcome. Addiction researchers currently believe a broad-based treatment program, including medical, psychiatric, pharmacological, and psychosocial elements, is the most successful.

Marijuana

In the 1960s, **marijuana** became a cultural phenomenon, the symbol of one generation's disregard for or anger with another. The marijuana found on the streets at that time, however, lacked the potency of current crops. The crossbreeding of more potent varieties, improved cultivation, and the use of different parts of the plant all contribute to increased levels of delta-9-tetrahydrocannabinol (THC), the major psychoactive drug found in marijuana. Some marijuana currently grown in the United States rivals the previously stronger varieties of Mexico, Jamaica, and other areas. The THC percentage of *Cannabis sativa* (the Indian hemp plant from which marijuana is derived) in plants grown in the United States can range from 2 percent to as high as 7 percent. A variety of marijuana know as *sinsemilla*, made from the buds of flowering tops of female plants, can have a potency as high as 24 percent.[2] The higher the percentage of THC, the more potent the drug. Marijuana is composed of the dried leaves and flowering tops of the cannabis plant. Hashish, which has stronger effects, is processed from the resin of the plant. The resin is either dried and pressed into cakes or sold in liquid form called *hash oil*. Marijuana is used more extensively than hashish in the United States.

It is estimated that each year there are 2.6 million new marijuana users. In 2002, 14 million Americans age 12 and older used marijuana at least once in the month prior to being surveyed. This translates into 3.1 million people using marijuana on a daily basis over a 12-month period. In 2002, marijuana was the third most commonly abused drug mentioned in hospital emergency department visits in the United States.[27]

More than 400 known chemicals constitute marijuana. More than 60 of these are *cannabinoids*, chemicals found only in cannabis. THC is the cannabinoid that appears to be most responsible for the sensations experienced by marijuana users. Cannabinoids are different from other drugs in that they are fat-soluble rather than water-soluble; they have a decided affinity for binding to fat in the human body. Although other drugs enter and then leave the body within relatively short periods, marijuana tends to attach to fatty organs, such as the gonads and brain, and remain.[2] A single ingestion of THC may require up to 30 days to be eliminated from the body.

Marijuana can be eaten in baked goods, such as brownies, but the effects tend to be less predictable. Because it better controls the amount ingested, smoking is generally a more efficient and powerful technique for achieving the desired effect. When inhaled, THC reaches the brain in as little as 14 seconds. Hashish is so concentrated that a single drop can equal the effects of an entire marijuana joint (cigarette). Cannabis products are difficult to classify but are considered hallucinogens.

Small doses or the short-term use of marijuana creates sensations of euphoria and relaxation often accompanied by hunger or sleepiness. Time seems to slow, and the senses appear heightened. Memory of recent events, physical coordination, and perceptions may be impaired. Students, for example, may have difficulty remembering events that occurred when they were high. Even with small amounts of marijuana, driving ability can be affected. Physiologically, heart rate speeds up and certain blood vessels become dilated, which may create problems for people with any types of heart problems. Some users experience anxiety, panic, and paranoia. In rare cases or with stronger doses, people may suffer from a sense of depersonalization, image distortion, and hallucinations. Chronic use seems to lead to behavior changes in some people that may be permanent. Lack of motivation or interest in activities unrelated to drug use is one result. Use by teenagers leads to impaired thinking, poor reading comprehension, and reduced verbal and mathematical skills.

All the long-term effects of marijuana use have not been determined. This is partly because of the lesser potency of marijuana used previously. In addition, people vary greatly in their responses to the drug. Chronic users may experience psychological dependence and need increased doses as tolerance develops. Very heavy users experience withdrawal symptoms of restlessness, irritability, tremors, nausea, vomiting, diarrhea, and sleep disturbances.[2]

Physically, marijuana appears to be more carcinogenic than tobacco. Known carcinogens occur in larger amounts in marijuana, and when marijuana is smoked, the smoke is held in the lungs. Cannabis smoke contains more tar than does tobacco smoke. Marijuana use quickly affects pulmonary function adversely, and long-term use causes cellular changes in the lungs. People who have angina pectoris (chest pains associated with heart disease) may be significantly at risk because more oxygen is required during marijuana use. Marijuana binds readily to hemoglobin, reducing the amount of oxygen carried to the heart and other tissues. One study has indicated that a user's risk for heart attack more than quadruples in the first hour after smoking marijuana.[28]

Many people consider cannabis an aphrodisiac. Over time it has the opposite effect, depressing the sex drive and causing impotence. Regular male users show a decrease in sperm count and reduced motility of sperm. Proportionately, more sperm appear abnormally shaped, a phenomenon associated with lessened fertility. In women, THC blocks ovulation. Pregnant women who smoke marijuana frequently use other drugs, all of which have a detrimental effect on the fetus. Marijuana also depresses the immune system.[2]

Therapeutic use is still being explored. At this time, the most promising application seems to be as an antinausea drug for chemotherapy patients. Glaucoma patients may have access to and may use marijuana to reduce intraocular pressure (pressure within the eye).

Marijuana is an illegal drug. Many people who use marijuana eventually experiment with or use other harder drugs. Some researchers consider marijuana thus to be a *gateway drug*. As with alcohol and all other drugs, the way a person reacts to marijuana or is most adversely affected by it cannot be predicted. People do not begin use with the intention of having a drug become the focus of their lives, but some ultimately allow the drug to control them. Marijuana is a drug that has that potential.

Other Drugs of Concern

The drugs discussed in the following sections have been abused for many years. Unfortunately, some that had become less popular seem to be reappearing, along with a dangerous new generation of illicit drugs. All illegal drugs have quality-control problems: Because there is no federal regulation of these drugs and because people involved in the transportation and distribution of illegal drugs are not always concerned about purity or quality, dangerous and even poisonous substances may be added to drugs. Also, it is frequently impossible to determine the potency of a drug. A very pure form of a drug can easily be lethal for a person who has been using a less potent form.

Heroin

Heroin is a narcotic synthesized from morphine. This drug induces a strong sensation of euphoria but quickly leads to physical and psychological dependency. The physical tolerance for heroin develops rapidly. Because heroin is usually injected, addicts often share needles, which increases the risk of contracting diseases, such as AIDS and hepatitis. Experts fear the younger generation may become addicted to heroin through a substance called *moonrock*—a mixture of heroin and cocaine that can be injected, smoked, or snorted. Heroin is used in this way to reduce the paranoia and depression that follow a cocaine high. Heroin use is considered to be on the rise. Recent studies have suggested a shift from injecting heroin to snorting or smoking. This trend seems to have resulted from the misconception that these forms are safer.[29]

In recent years, heroin use has increased significantly, especially among well-educated people, often women, employed in white-collar and other professional jobs.[29] Heroin use has also reportedly increased among junior high and high school groups. One reason for this trend may be the availability of more potent forms of heroin, which allow the user to experience a more pronounced effect by snorting it instead of injecting it, which people may be reluctant to do in part because of fear of HIV transmission. In addition, many users believe that smoking or snorting heroin, unlike injecting it, is nonaddicting.[29] Heroin may appeal to children because it is cheap and can be purchased fairly easily on the street. Users may not realize they are becoming addicted because they may function normally for some time after starting to use the drug before their behavior changes significantly enough for friends and family to become aware of their use. Heroin is undeniably rearing its ugly head again in the form of increased use, and it has reached the country's youth regardless of educational attainment, social class, and ethnic and racial background.

Methamphetamine (Crank)

Methamphetamine is a potent stimulant that can cause uncontrollable manic behavior or paranoid thinking. The most current use of this drug is as crystal methamphetamine, or *ice*. Although crystal methamphetamine has been touted as a safe alternative to cocaine, evidence indicates otherwise. Recent headlines told about a father who, under the influence of methamphetamine, decapitated his son. Overdoses are often fatal, and the drug is extremely addictive. In many areas of the United States, the use of ice is a widespread problem. In many rural areas, the drug is manufactured because of the ease of preparation. Forty-six percent of crank labs in 2002 were reported in middle America.[30]

Lysergic Acid Diethylamide (LSD)

LSD is a hallucinogenic drug that has become more popular, especially among the upper class. The substance induces altered perceptions of shapes, images, time, self, and sound. Tolerance to the drug develops quickly with daily use.[12] Flashbacks can occur in some people.

Phencyclidine (PCP)

PCP was originally intended for use as a surgical anesthetic for humans. However, the drug was determined unsuitable for this purpose because of its unusual and undesirable effects on patients.[2] Also called *angel dust, ozone, wack,* and *rocket fuel,* PCP provokes a variety of unpredictable responses in users. These reactions include feelings of unreality, depersonalization, confusion, depression, anxiety, aggressive and violent behavior, acute or permanent psychosis, and coma. Users often fail to experience sensations of pain and report feeling uncoordi-

nated in their movements. Classified as a hallucinogen, PCP has been used as an additive to cocaine, a combination that multiplies the toxic effects of both drugs.

Over-the-Counter Drugs

An area of drug use that is sometimes overlooked and assumed to be safe is the use of over-the-counter drugs (OTCs). The power of OTCs is often underestimated. As with all drugs, the ultimate responsibility for the correct use of OTC drugs rests with each person. Because OTCs are readily available, abuse is a possibility. OTCs may potentiate the effects of prescription drugs, herbs, vitamins, alcohol, or other OTCs, especially when not taken according to directions. OTCs can cause physiological damage to various body structures, with symptoms

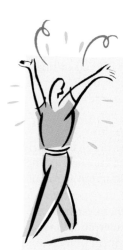

Nurturing Your Spirituality

Finding Alternatives to Drug Use

The best treatment for any alcohol or other drug abuse problem is to prevent it. Adolescents and college-age students need attractive alternatives to drugs, such as participation in organizations or groups that fulfill in safe, constructive ways their need for camaraderie, acceptance, and group involvement. These organizations or groups can be developed around athletics, recreational activities, career development, or service opportunities. Involvement in enjoyable and meaningful activities tends to discourage drug use by providing a strong reinforcement system that helps people feel good about themselves and their abilities. All people, young and older, need a positive group atmosphere that fosters self-esteem, develops participants' ability to help others, and provides role models who pursue selfless, achievement-oriented goals.

At the college and university level, students aged 25 and younger may be faced with an autonomy never before experienced when they leave home to go to school. They are faced with the fact that no one is standing over them to ensure their attendance at and productivity in school, at work, or in other areas. Their decision-making power is increased as well as is the pressure to conform to peer standards, many of which they are encountering for the first time. This newfound freedom sometimes requires a continuation of prevention education and activities that direct them toward positive activities and behaviors. University administrators should seek to make such programs highly visible within the institutions they serve. It

is helpful for everyone connected with a college or university to demonstrate positive behaviors concerning the prevention of drug and alcohol abuse on campus. This may require that the president not serve alcoholic beverages at receptions and that faculty actively discourage binge drinking and other dangerous forms of drinking and be willing to engage in activities outside the classroom that involve positive alternatives to alcohol and other drug use. Another important component of any alternative program is a strong peer education network, in which student leaders promote a healthy campus life by discouraging alcohol and other drug abuse and related problems, such as property destruction, violence, and sexual assault.

Other prevention-oriented programs are recreational activities, such as hiking, camping, and canoeing, and leadership challenge courses, such as rope courses and outward-bound experiences. The programs should offer diverse opportunities that appeal to a wide variety of student interests. Art exhibits; musical events; movie or book clubs; and community service programs, such as Humanity for Mankind, can all offer further opportunities for students to engage in personally and socially beneficial activities. Having mentors assigned to incoming first-year students and holding group discussions of various problems associated with collegiate life, perhaps with mandatory attendance by first-year students, may also be helpful. In addition, the college or university should emphasize to students that the purpose of higher education is to gain the experience and expertise to better serve one's family, community, and country. To truly accept responsibility for their lives, all people need to understand and accept responsibility for their behavior and recognize that alcohol and other drug use never offers a long-term solution to personal, emotional, or spiritual difficulties.

ranging from disorientation to kidney or liver damage. Following are some guidelines for safe use of OTCs:[7]

- Always know what you are taking and the product's active ingredients.
- Know the drug's effects (including its undesired ones) and possible side effects. Be sure you understand how the drug is supposed to work.
- Read and heed warnings and cautions concerning the use of the product.
- Don't use any OTC product continuously for more than two weeks. If the problem for which you are taking the drug persists, consult your physician.
- Be particularly cautious if you are also taking any prescription drugs, because serious interactions can occur.

- If you have any questions about an OTC product, consult a pharmacist.
- If you don't need a drug, don't use it.

A Final Thought

To develop a high level of wellness, you must address the issue of drug use. Drugs prescribed as medicine can promote quality of life, but unwise use severely diminishes quality of life. Alcohol continues to be the most abused drug among college students. Perhaps as people become more aware of the dangers associated with alcohol and drug use, a smaller percentage of college students will use them (see Nurturing Your Spirituality: Finding Alternatives to Drug Use).

Summary

- People use drugs for a variety of reasons, including for recreational or social enjoyment, to seek novel sensations, to enhance religious or spiritual experiences, to alter consciousness, to rebel or alienate oneself from society, and to submit to peer pressure.
- Drugs are commonly classified in a variety of ways, including according to their physiological effects.
- Caffeine is probably the most commonly used drug in the United States. It is a stimulant that speeds heart rate, increases blood pressure, and can cause insomnia.
- Alcohol is a socially acceptable drug that is a major source of physical and emotional damage and death.
- The blood alcohol concentration (BAC) of ethyl alcohol is affected by the rate of consumption, the type of alcoholic beverage being consumed, and the drinker's body weight and tolerance to alcohol.
- Binge drinking often occurs on college campuses and can lead to property destruction, sexual assault, and even death.
- Alcoholism is a disease in which a person loses control over drinking.
- Determining who will become an alcoholic is impossible because alcoholism crosses all social, economic, gender, educational, and racial lines.
- Nicotine is an addictive drug contained in tobacco. The tars found in tobacco are carcinogenic agents.
- No tobacco product is safe. Cigarettes, cigars, pipes, and smokeless products all pose threats to health.
- Carbon monoxide, formed when tobacco is smoked, interferes with the body's ability to transport oxygen and increases the risk for heart attack and stroke.

- Sidestream smoke has a higher concentration of tar and nicotine than the smoke inhaled by the smoker.
- Clove cigarettes contain even more nicotine and carbon monoxide than do regular cigarettes.
- Cocaine use has become epidemic in the United States. Cocaine can be snorted, injected, or freebased (smoked).
- The primary psychoactive ingredient in marijuana is delta-9-tetrahydrocannabinol.
- Carcinogens can be found in more potent levels in marijuana than in tobacco.
- Hashish is more potent than regular marijuana. Sinsemilla is a form of marijuana that can have a potency as high as 24 percent.
- Short-term effects of marijuana use include euphoria and perceptual impairment. Some people experience anxiety, a sense of depersonalization, and hallucinations.
- Some drugs, such as heroin, methamphetamine (crank), and LSD, have been abused in our society for many years.
- The newest form of methamphetamine is ice, which is smokable and more addictive, potent, and destructive than crack cocaine.
- Heroin use has been increasing among college and high school students.
- Designer drugs are analogs of controlled substances and are more powerful and less pure and have less predictable effects than do controlled substances.
- OTC drugs must be used carefully to avoid psychological and physiological problems.

Review Questions

1. What are some reasons people choose to use drugs?
2. Discuss the ways in which drugs can be classified.
3. What are the positive and negative effects of caffeine use?
4. What factors affect a drinker's blood alcohol concentration (BAC)?
5. How can a person practice responsible drinking?

6. What are some potential effects of long-term alcohol use?
7. Discuss the risks of using any tobacco product.
8. Discuss the specific benefits of quitting smoking.
9. Why is heroin use increasing among high school and college students?

10. What makes cocaine such a dangerous drug?
11. What factors should you consider before using any OTC product?

References

1. Pinger, R., W. Payne, D. Hahn, and E. Hahn. 1998. *Drugs: Issues for today.* Dubuque, IA: WCB/McGraw-Hill.
2. Ray, O., and C. Ksit. 2002. *Drugs, society, and human behaviors.* New York: McGraw-Hill.
3. Blum, K., and J. Payne. 1991. *Alcohol and the addictive brain.* New York: Free Press.
4. National Institute on Drug Abuse. 2001. Genetic factors in drug abuse and dependence. In *The biobehavioral etiology of drug abuse.* Edited by H. W. Gordon and M. D. Glantz. Research Monograph. 159. Duarte, CA.
5. Morse, R. M., and D. K. Flavin. 1992. The definition of alcoholism. *Journal of the American Medical Association.* 268:1012–14.
6. Blum, K., G. Cull, E. Braverman, and D. Comings. 1996. Reward deficiency syndrome. *American Scientist* 84:132–45.
7. Hanson, G., and P. J. Venturelli. 2002. *Drugs and society.* 7th ed. Boston: Jones and Bartlett.
8. Family Haven. 2004. Caffeine and health: Clarifying the controversies (www.familyhaven.com/health/ir-caffh.html).
9. Consumers Union. 1997. What caffeine can do for you—and to you. *Consumer Reports on Health.* 9 September: 97–101.
10. Carroll, C. R. 2001. *Drugs in modern society.* 5th ed. Dubuque, IA: Wm. C. Brown.
11. Morse, R. M., and D. K. Flavin. 1992. The definition of alcoholism. *Journal of*

the American Medical Association 268:1012–1014.
12. Ikonomidocou, C., et al. 2000. Ethanol-induced apopototic neuro degeneration and the fetal alcohol syndrome. *Science* 287:1056–60.
13. American Academy of Pediatrics. 1998. *AAP releases new findings on teen and underage drinking.* Washington, DC: American Academy of Pediatrics.
14. National Clearinghouse for Alcohol and Drug Information. 2004. *Mind over matter—the brain's response to hallucinogens.* Rockville, MD: U.S. Government Printing Office.
15. Wechsler, H., et al. 1998. Changes in binge drinking and related problems among American college students between 1995 and 1997. *Journal of American College Health* 45:57–68.
16. National Institute on Alcohol Abuse and Alcoholism. 2003. Underage drinking: A major public health challenge. *Alcohol Alert* vol. 59.
17. Lyall, K. 1999. *Binge drinking in college: A definitive study in binge drinking on American college campuses: A new look at an old problem.* Report supported by the Robert Wood Johnson Foundation. Princeton, NJ: The Robert Wood Foundation.
18. Mayo Clinic. 2003. Secondhand smoke: Protect yourself from the dangers (www.mayoclinic.com/invoke.cfm).
19. Heart Center. 2004. Smoking-related diseases (www.heartcenteronline.com).
20. American Heart Association. 2001. Biostatistical fact sheet—risk factors of

cigarette and tobacco smoke (www.americanheart.org/statistics/biostat/bioci.htm).
21. Action on Smoking and Health. 2001. Herbal cigarettes not safe (www.no.smoking.org/jan02/01-03.01-2.html).
22. Mayo Clinic. 2004. Stop smoking: Kick the habit for a long and healthy life. (www.mayoclinic.com).
23. National Institute on Drug Abuse. 2004. Club drugs (www.nida.nih.gov/Infofax/clubdrugs.html).
24. National Institute on Drug Abuse. 2004. MDMA (ecstasy). (www.nida.nih.gov/Infofax/ecstasy.html).
25. National Institute on Drug Abuse. 2004. Rohypnol and GHB (www.nida.nig.gov/Infofax/RohypnolGHB.html).
26. National Institute on Drug Abuse. 2004. Crack and cocaine (www.nida.nig.gov/Infofax/cocaine.html).
27. Substance Abuse and Mental Health Service Administration. 2003. *National survey on drug abuse—Annual report.* Washington, DC: U.S. Government Printing Office.
28. Mittlemon, M., et al. 2001. Triggering myocardial infarction by marijuana. *Circulation* 103:2805–2809.
29. National Institute on Alcohol Abuse and Alcoholism. 2004. Heroin (www.nida.nig.gov/Infofax/heroin.html).
30. National Institute on Alcohol Abuse and Alcoholism. 2004. Methamphetamine (www.nida.nig.gov/Infofax/methamphetamine.html).

Suggested Readings

DeSena, J., J. Schaler, and J. Gerstein. 2003. *Overcoming your alcohol, drug and recovery habits: An empowering alternative to AA and 12-step treatment.* Tucson, AZ: Sharp Press.
This text is a self-help guide for those who have gone through Alcoholics

Anonymous, Narcotics Anonymous, and other formal 12-step addiction treatments to overcome self-destructive beliefs and attitudes.
Gately, I. 2003. *Tobacco: A cultural history of how an exotic plant seduced civilization.* New York: Grove Press.

This text provides an excellent look at the complex history of tobacco from the time of Columbus to the present day. It is provocative and interesting reading.
Nakken, C. 1996. *The addictive personality: Understanding the addictive process*

and compulsive behavior. Center City, MN: Hazelden.

This book examines genetic factors tied to addiction, cultural influences on addictive behavior, the progressive nature of the disease, and the steps necessary for a successful recovery.

Ruden, R. 2002. *The craving brain: A bold new approach to breaking free from drug addiction, overeating, alcoholism, and gambling.* 2d ed. New York: Perennial.

This book offers an interesting comment concerning addiction. The author states that the roots of addiction are found in our genes and builds a solid foundation for his beliefs.

Whelan, E. M. 1997. *Cigarettes: What the warning label doesn't tell you: The first comprehensive guide to the health consequences of smoking.* Amherst, NY: Prometheus Books.

Noted experts detail all the known health risks of smoking, explaining clearly how cigarette smoking can damage the body.

Name _____ Date _____ Section _____

Assessment Activity 11-2

What Are Your Reasons for Drug Use?

Directions: In the following table are listed various drugs and products that can affect your life either positively or negatively. Think about how you view each product and what the long-term and short-term conse-quences of use might be. You might wish to consult other sources to help you determine possible effects. In the last column, explain briefly why you choose to use or to refrain from using the drug or product.

Drug	Possible Negative Effects	Possible Positive Effects	Reasons for Using or Not Using
Caffeinated drinks (tea, coffee, cola)			
Alcohol			
Cigarettes			
Pipe or cigar			
Cocaine (any form)			
Marijuana (any form)			
Designer drugs (any form)			
Heroin			
Over-the-counter medications			

Points to Ponder

1. Which drugs do you view positively?
2. Are you unsure of your feelings about any sub-stance? If so, why?
3. What potential is there for abuse or misuse of any of the drugs (even those you have positive feel-ings about)? If so, what is the potential source of problems?

Name _____ Date _____ Section _____

Assessment Activity 11-5

Drug Diary

For each day for two weeks, record every drug you take on the following forms. Include any prescription and over-the-counter drugs as well as alcohol, nicotine, caffeine, and street (illicit) drugs. Record the exact type and amount of the drug taken and the setting in which you took the drug. Also make note of your mood (angry, happy, depressed, bored, etc.) at the time you used the drug. Finally, make note of your stress level at the time using the following level designations: 1. very relaxed; 2. low stress; 3. moderate stress; 4. very stressed. In order for this exercise to be a useful tool, you must be honest.

An example of a completed daily record follows:

DATE: Friday, December 4, 2004

	Type	Amount	Setting/Mood	Stress
Prescription	Birth control pill	1	Home	1
Over-the-counter	Tylenol	2	School/headache	3
Caffeine	Coffee Pepsi	1 cup 16 oz.	Home School—lunch	2 2
Nicotine	——			
Alcohol	Beer	4	Party	2
Steroids	——			
Street drugs	——			

DATE:

	Type	Amount	Setting/Mood	Stress
Prescription				
Over-the-counter				
Caffeine				
Nicotine				
Alcohol				
Steroids				
Street drugs				

DATE:

	Type	Amount	Setting/Mood	Stress
Prescription				
Over-the-counter				
Caffeine				
Nicotine				
Alcohol				
Steroids				
Street drugs				

12

Preventing Sexually Transmitted Diseases

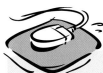

Online Learning Center

Log on to our Online Learning Center (OLC) for access to these additional resources:

- Chapter key term flashcards
- Learning objectives
- Additional goals for behavior change
- Concentration game
- Self-scoring chapter quizzes

- Additional lab activities

The OLC also offers Web links for study and exploration of wellness topics. Access these links through **www.mhhe.com/ anspaugh6e**, click on Student Center, click on Chapter 12, and then click on Web Activities.

Goals for Behavior Change

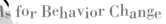

- Make choices regarding your personal sexual behavior.
- Practice safer sex if you have chosen to be sexually active.
- Take responsibility for the potential consequences of your sexual behavior.
- Learn how to talk with your partner about your sexual history.

Key Terms

abstinence
acquired immunodeficiency
  syndrome (AIDS)
chlamydia
cunnilingus
fellatio
genital warts
gonorrhea
hepatitis B

herpes
human immunodeficiency
  virus (HIV)
safer sex
sexually transmitted
  diseases (STDs)
syphilis
viral hepatitis

Objectives

After completing this chapter, you will be able to do the following:

- Discuss the difference between being HIV positive and having AIDS.
- Identify the signs and symptoms of various STDs.

- Evaluate the risks of having multiple sex partners.
- Discuss the meaning of having a monogamous relationship.
- Identify safer sex practices.

exuality is a lifelong part of a person's life, affecting and being affected by relationships, anatomy, behaviors, thoughts, and values. Sexual behavior is only one aspect of sexuality.

Decisions concerning sexual behavior have many far-reaching consequences. These choices can enhance or severely diminish feelings of well-being. Sex can be wonderful and fulfilling but may also cause serious problems. This chapter examines some of the **sexually transmitted diseases (STDs)** that can result when people engage in behavior that puts them at risk. The chapter also identifies how to avoid contracting and spreading STDs. The chapter examines viral, bacterial, and other common STDs and infections.

Safer Sex

This book discusses the various components of optimal wellness. Sexual behavior can have a strong positive or negative impact on physical and emotional health (see Assessment Activity 12-2). Making decisions concerning sexual behavior is not easy (see Nurturing Your Spirituality: Making Decisions About Sex). If people (whether heterosexual or homosexual) choose to have multiple sexual partners, they must realize that, each time a sexual act occurs, the potential sexual histories of two people are brought together. Even though it may be the first experience for one, the other partner may have had sex

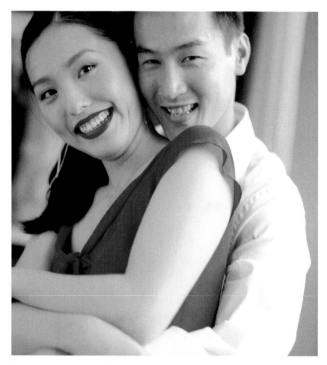

Decisions concerning sexual behavior can enhance wellness.

with three other people. In this case, the person for whom it is the first experience is essentially exposed to the sexual histories of four others. The diseases or infections of any of those four people may be brought to the present relationship (see Assessment Activity 12-1).

Unfortunately, people are not always honest about their past relationships. For many reasons, they may not tell the truth about the number of past partners or about the frequency of condom use. The potential for dishonesty in others makes the prevention of STDs a personal responsibility for everyone.

Some people choose abstinence. **Abstinence** means voluntarily refraining from all sexual acts—which includes practicing sexual activities that involve vaginal, anal, or oral stimulation or penetration. People choose abstinence for a number of reasons, most frequently moral or religious. Abstinence is the only way that STDs can be avoided and the possibility of pregnancy eliminated. This is an area that must be discussed with one's partner. It is difficult to accomplish abstinence if both partners are not in agreement.

A second frequent choice is to have sexual contact within a monogamous (involving only one long-term partner) relationship. Monogamy obviously is dependent on both partners' willingness to maintain a monogamous relationship. Monogamy may be a choice for two people who have never had sexual intercourse with anyone else or for two people who have had sex partners in the past but have decided to limit their future sexual practices to those they share with each other. Having sex with only one uninfected and faithful partner is as equally effective in preventing STDs (not pregnancy) as abstinence—if it is practiced consistently by both partners. However, even with monogamy, precautions are necessary to prevent unwanted pregnancies.

People embarking on a monogamous relationship who have had partners in the past need to discuss their sexual histories as well as their commitment to the present relationship. This commitment may involve a willingness to be tested for possible STDs (see Real-World Wellness: Communicating with Your Partner About STDs on page 394). Some STDs take time to manifest, so testing for them may have to be done several times over a period of years. Assuming that the people involved are committed to monogamy and are honest about their sexual histories, monogamy can protect against the spread of STDs.

In modern society, many relationships are not of long duration, and the practice of *serial monogamy* is common. Serial monogamy is monogamy for as long as a relationship is intact; for the duration of their relationship, two partners have sex only with each other. Because relationships may be of relatively brief duration (ranging from weeks to years) and each partner

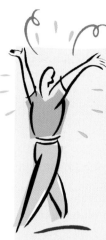

Nurturing Your Spirituality

Making Decisions About Sex

Everyone must decide at some point whether to engage in sexual activity. For some people, the decision is ongoing. Even after having a sexual experience, a person must decide whether to have sex with the first partner again, to have sex with another person, or not to have sex. Having sex *is* always a choice, unless rape or abuse is involved.

People sometimes change their minds about wanting to have sex. A person may have sex with someone once or many times and then decide to refrain from having sex with that person again. Some people decide to wait to have sex until they are married or until their financial, social, or emotional circumstances change. Some decide to change their sexual behavior to be more closely aligned with moral, ethical, or religious beliefs.

Why do people change their minds about sex? The decision to refrain from further sexual intercourse is sometimes referred to as *secondary virginity.* Couples choosing to engage in sex must make sure that their choice fits with their value systems and understand that they are emotionally, socially, and financially responsible for the results of their decisions. Before initiating sexual intercourse, couples should discuss the following:

- Their thoughts and feelings about sexual activity

- Whether sexual intercourse fits their moral and ethical codes

- Willingness to practice safer sex to protect themselves as well as to deal with the potential pregnancy created as the result of their decision

What considerations are important when deciding whether to have sex? Reasons for having or not having sex are varied. Some couples may believe their feelings are strong enough for one another that sex would seal their commitment to the relationship. Others may decide that if two people love one another it is OK to have sex. Some

people engage in sexual activity because they see it as a way to be popular or as evidence that they are attractive. Some people have sex because they think everyone else is and that not to have sex would make them outsiders. (Not everyone is having sex! Many people, young and old, choose to abstain until marriage or some other long-term commitment.)

Some people choose to refrain from having sex until marriage because they view sex outside marriage as morally wrong. Another reason for abstinence is a desire to get to know one's partner well (which takes time) before sex. Having sex may alter expectations and the nature of a relationship; some people do not have sex because they don't want their relationship to change. If the physical component of a relationship is emphasized over other aspects, partners may find it difficult to get to know each other well. Many people choose to abstain because they do not want to risk unwanted pregnancy; STDs; or the financial, emotional, and social responsibility of having sex. Some say that not having sex allows them to know themselves better and to figure out what they are looking for in a potential mate. Still others say that not having sex reduces the stress in their lives, freeing them from worries about problem pregnancies and STDs.

How do you decide whether to have sex? It is vitally important to know what your values are and to do only what furthers your total wellness. If you are choosing to have sex because of peer pressure or fear of being alone, then you are not acting out of a wellness perspective. If you are having sex for what you consider to be valid reasons and you are truly comfortable with your decision, then having sex may be an overall positive experience for you. Young adults often fail to realize that, during the next few years, they will be going through many changes as they move from home and from school out into the work world. These changes will alter their self-perceptions and their values. Making the wrong decision now may put that future in jeopardy. Taking time to consider behaviors carefully is crucial, because the regret of an unwanted pregnancy or a lifelong STD can be life altering or even fatal.

What factors will affect your decision to have or not have sex?

may then seek new partners, the risk with serial monogamy for contracting and spreading an STD is significant.

A third choice is to have sex with more than one partner but to practice **safer sex.** There is no such thing as *safe* sex with multiple partners, but steps can be taken to help ensure *safer* sex. Regardless if you are heterosexual or homosexual, or male or female, you can follow certain practices to limit your exposure to STDs. The

starting point for safer sex is using some of the guidelines outlined in Real-World Wellness: Communicating with Your Partner About STDs on page 394. Anyone who is sexually active with multiple partners should be checked every three to six months for possible STDs. It is often the case that people, especially women, who are not disease-free are asymptomatic (have no symptoms);[1] no persons should let their lack of symptoms lull them into assuming they are disease-free.

Real-World Wellness

Communicating with Your Partner About STDs

My partner and I have been very close to having sex on several occasions. I am very worried about contracting an STD. I really don't know much about my partner's sexual history. How do I open the discussion or ask the questions concerning safer sex practices? How do I find out if there is anything I should be aware of in this person's past?

The decision about whether to have sex is extremely important. Considerations include the possibility of contracting an STD, the potential for an unwanted pregnancy, and the psychological and emotional ramifications of intimate contact, should the relationship end. Sex represents a psychological, physical, emotional, and financial commitment to another person. Don't be reluctant to bring up the topic of safer sex. The ability to discuss important issues is a sign of personal and social maturity. The following are some suggestions on ways to introduce the topic. What others can you suggest?

- "I feel that we both are thinking about sex, but before I make a final decision, I have some concerns I'd like to discuss with you."

- "I've always practiced safer sex in the past and, if we're going to have sex, I think it's important for us to use condoms."

- "What type of protection do *you* have if we decide to have sex? This is the type of protection *I* have."

- "I know if you really care about me you'll be willing to use a condom."

- "Before this relationship goes any further, I want to ask you about your sexual history and our plans for practicing safer sex."

- "I really like you and I hope we can have a more intimate relationship at some point. But I think there are some important things we should talk about first."

- "You're so sexy that sometimes I just get carried away when I'm close to you. Why don't we have a quiet dinner together to discuss our sexual past and what we want from this relationship?"

You can probably think of even better ways to approach a conversation concerning sex. What is important to remember is that sex can be a wonderful emotional and physical experience, but it's not worth dying for.

Following are some practices for people who are straight or gay that represent either safer sex, possible safe practices, or unsafe practices:

Safer Practices

- Hugging
- Kissing (not deep or French kissing)
- Petting
- Watching erotic videos, reading erotic books, and so on
- Masturbation (solo or mutual unless there are sores, lesions, and/or abrasions on the genitalia or hands)

Possibly Safer Practices

- Deep, French kissing, unless there are sores in the mouth
- Vaginal intercourse with a latex condom with nonoxynol-9
- **Fellatio** (oral stimulation of the penis) with a latex or polyurethane condom
- **Cunnilingus** (oral stimulation of the clitoris and vaginal opening) with a latex dental dam, unless a female partner is menstruating or has a vaginal infection
- Anal intercourse with a latex condom with nonoxynol-9, but there is a great amount of disagreement concerning the safety of this practice even with a condom—this is the most risky sexual behavior

Unsafe Practices

- Vaginal or anal intercourse without a latex condom with nonoxynol-9
- Fellatio or cunnilingus without a condom or latex dental dam
- Oral-anal contact
- Contact with blood, including menstrual blood
- Taking semen in the mouth
- Sharing a vibrator or other sex toys without washing them between uses

See Just the Facts: Effective Condom Use.

Sexually Transmitted Diseases (STDs)

Each year in the United States it is estimated that more than 13 million people contract an STD.[2,3] Approximately 25 percent of new cases occur among teenagers. Two-thirds of STD cases occur in people under the age of 25.[4] Another particularly disturbing fact is that young women under 24 years of age may be at more risk for STDs than are older women because the cells of the cervix in young women are immature and more easily infected.[5] An important component of these statistics is that a large number of STD cases go unreported because many are asymptomatic (particularly in women) or because they are treated by a private physician and never reported.

∿Just the Facts∿

Effective Condom Use

Condoms can be effective in protecting against STDs if used properly:

- Use one every time you have sexual intercourse or oral sex involving a penis.
- Use only latex or polyurethane condoms.
- When having vaginal or anal intercourse, make sure the condom has nonoxynol-9.
- Put the condom on before any contact with the vagina.
- When the condom is on the penis, there should be about ½ inch of space left at the condom tip to hold the ejaculate.
- Withdraw the penis soon after ejaculation. Hold the base of the condom firmly against the penis as it is withdrawn, so the condom does not come off.
- Use foam, spermicide, or a female condom in combination with a condom.
- Check for possible breaks immediately after the use of any condom.
- Always use a water-based lubricant, such as K-Y jelly. Vaseline or other oil-based lubricants can cause the condom to break down and become ineffective.
- Never reuse a condom.

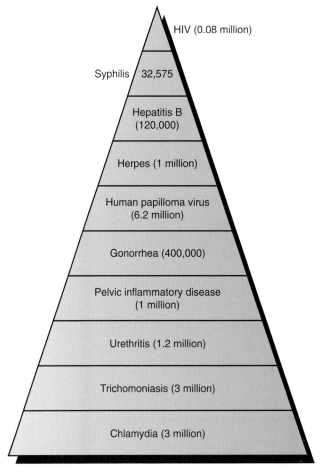

Figure 12-1 Annual STD Incidence—New Cases

SOURCE: National Center for Health Statistics. 2004. Available online at **www.cdc.gov/nchs/fastets/stds.htm.**

Consequently, the estimated 13 million may reflect a vast underreporting of the number of cases. The estimates for annual STD incidence are shown in Figure 12-1.

Viral Diseases

Human Immunodeficiency Virus and Acquired Immunodeficiency Syndrome

Damage to the immune system as a result of infection with **human immunodeficiency virus (HIV)** leads to a complex of rare diseases called **acquired immunodeficiency syndrome (AIDS).** The Centers for Disease Control (CDC) lists two conditions to be used in diagnosing AIDS. These are an HIV seroconversion (the development of evidence of antibody response to a disease) and a blood T-cell count below 200 cells per millimeter, regardless of other specific symptoms that may or may not be present.[5] A normal range of T-cells is 800 to 1,000. In the presence of these two conditions, some other conditions may be used to diagnose AIDS. These conditions

fall into several categories and are presented in Just the Facts: Conditions Used to Diagnose AIDS (page 396).

People infected with HIV may experience a variety of symptoms or may appear to be quite healthy. A small percentage of HIV-positive people seem to have been able to suppress and survive HIV infection for more than 20 years without developing AIDS. The reason for this is not understood by experts. It has been suggested that suppressor compounds formed by the immune system cells may be responsible. However, even people with no obvious symptoms can transmit HIV to others. The indicators of possible HIV infection include persistent diarrhea, dry cough, and shortness of breath; fatigue; skin rash; swollen lymph nodes (neck, armpits, groin); candidiasis (infection of the skin or mucous membranes, usually localized in skin, nails, mouth, vagina, or lungs); unexplained fever or chills; night sweats (over several weeks); and unexplained weight loss of 10 pounds or 10 percent of body weight in less than two months. Women may experience these symptoms as well as abnormal Pap smears, persistent

Just the Facts

Conditions Used to Diagnose AIDS

The following are some conditions besides HIV seroconversion and low T-cell counts used to diagnose AIDS:

Opportunistic Infections (Infections That Take Advantage of a Weakened Immune System)

- Pneumocystis carinii pneumonia (PCP)—a type of lung disease caused by a protozoan or fungus, usually not harmful to humans

- Tuberculosis—either *Mycobacterium avium-intracellulare* (MAI) or *Mycobacterium tuberculosis* (TB), with MAI being the most common among AIDS patients

- Bacterial pneumonia—caused by several common bacteria

- Toxoplasmosis—a disease of the brain and central nervous system

Cancers

- Kaposi's sarcoma, a cancer that causes red or purple blotches on the skin

- Lymphomas, cancers of the lymphatic system

- Invasive cervical cancer—more common in women who are HIV positive

Other Conditions

- Wasting syndrome, which involves persistent diarrhea, severe weight loss, and weakness

- AIDS dementia, impairment of mental function, mood changes, and impaired movement as a result of HIV infection of the brain

Other Infections

- Candidiasis (also called *thrush*), a fungal infection that affects the vagina, mouth, throat, and lungs

- Herpes, a common viral STD

- Cytomegalovirus, a virus that, in AIDS patients, can lead to brain infection, infection of the retina, pneumonia, or hepatitis

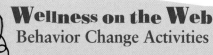

Wellness on the Web
Behavior Change Activities

What Do You Know About STDs?

More than 20 sexually transmitted diseases (STDs) have been identified, and all are preventable. But STDs are thriving, and it's largely because of ignorance and inaction. People who have multiple sex partners are at the highest risk of contracting STDs. The only sure way of preventing STDs is to abstain from sex or for two uninfected people to participate in a mutually monogamous relationship. Another effective but not foolproof way to reduce the risk for infection is the proper use of condoms.

Education about STDs is another form of prevention. How much do you know about STDs? To learn about STDs, including their symptoms and common treatment practices, visit **www.mhhe.com/anspaugh6e**, Student Center, Chapter 12, Wellness on the Web, Activity 1.

Breaking the Silence: Talking About Sex

Safer sex sounds like a great idea, but it can be difficult to achieve because few people want to discuss it. In this case, silence definitely is *not* golden. Having sex should be viewed as a major decision that may have lifelong consequences. The choice to engage in safer sexual behavior rests with each individual. One of the best ways to protect yourself is to know as much as possible. To find the answers to a number of questions about sex frequently asked by adults go to **www.mhhe.com/anspaugh6e**, Student Center, Chapter 12, Wellness on the Web, Activity 2 and select from the categories of questions listed. You are sure to find some questions whose answers you will find helpful.

vaginal candidiasis, and abdominal cramping as a result of pelvic inflammatory disease (PID). These infections are a result of HIV infection and are caused by immunodeficiency, but they are not AIDS (see Wellness for a Lifetime: HIV and AIDS Pose Special Risks to Women and Their Children).

The reason some people develop AIDS rapidly and others do not is not known. Factors that may contribute to the advancement of the condition are weakening of the immune system through other infections, alcohol or other drug abuse, poor nutrition, and stress.[2] The longer the virus is in the system, the greater the chances of developing AIDS. In one study spanning six years, 30 percent of the participants with the virus developed AIDS, 49 percent displayed symptomatic HIV infections, and 21 percent remained free of symptoms. All these people could continue to spread the disease.[6] Another problem is the rapid development and emergence of new drug-resistant strains of HIV.[2]

Two types of HIV have been identified.[7] Almost all cases of HIV in the United States are a virus known as HIV-1. Another type of virus, HIV-2, is found mainly in West Africa and appears to take longer than HIV-1 to damage the immune system. The virus replicates inside

Wellness for a Lifetime

HIV and AIDS Pose Special Risks to Women and Their Children

In 2002, women represented 25 percent of all AIDS cases reported.[8] Most women are infected through the use of injected drugs or through sex with infected partners. Activities that put women at high risk include being a partner of an injected-drug user or of a gay or bisexual man and having multiple sex partners. Although lesbians with HIV are in a small minority, they can and do contract HIV in the same ways as heterosexual women. Lesbians who share sex toys without first washing and cleaning them are at greater risk for HIV than are those who practice safer sex.

Heterosexual women are at greater risk of contracting HIV from an infected man than are non-HIV-positive men from HIV-positive women. Women are more susceptible to HIV infection because they have more surface area of contact in the vagina and the tissue there is softer and more easily scratched or torn. Further, semen is often ejaculated directly into the uterine and cervical canal. Semen normally contains 10 to 100 times more migratory lymphocytes than does cervical mucus, thus placing more virus in the area for potential infection.[8]

Women tend to be diagnosed at a later stage in the HIV process than are men and they have almost a 30 percent greater chance than men do of dying before they have an AIDS-defining condition.[1] Because female physiology is different from male physiology, women need to participate in clinical trials to ensure that new experimental drugs and therapies work for them as effectively as they do for men. There are several studies underway that investigate gender-specific differences in disease progression, complications, and treatment.

A pregnant woman has about a 30 percent chance of passing the virus to her newborn. The Centers for Disease Control and Prevention has recommended HIV testing for all pregnant women. HIV transmission from mother to infant can be reduced from almost 26 percent to slightly more than 8 percent when both the HIV-positive mother (predelivery) and infant (postdelivery) are given doses of a drug called AZT. An HIV-positive mother can infect her newborn by breast-feeding. The exact risk for this form of transmission is not known, but the risk can be completely avoided through the use of formula as opposed to breast milk.

human cells and is transmitted by blood, blood products, semen, vaginal secretions, and breast milk. HIV is an extremely fragile virus in that it does not survive in air and can be destroyed readily by soap and water, household bleach, and chlorine used in swimming pools. Just the Facts: How HIV Is and Is Not Transmitted on page 398 explores transmission in greater detail.

The HIV virus attacks the helper T-lymphocytes, specifically the T-4 cells, possibly the most critical element in the body's immune system. HIV attaches to the part of the T-cell that recognizes viral infections and blocks its ability to react to them. Over time, HIV may even multiply and destroy T-cells, leaving the body more defenseless against invasion by opportunistic organisms that can lead to illness and eventually death.[4,9]

In the United States, whether through homosexual or heterosexual contact, anal intercourse is still the most prevalent means of spreading HIV infection. This may be because this activity increases the likelihood of making small tears that facilitate the spread of the virus from semen to blood. Vaginal and oral sex are also considered highly dangerous.[10] Sharing needles among drug users and having sex with an IV drug user are high-risk activities. Sex with a prostitute is a significant risk factor.

Anyone who has had multiple sexual partners during the last 5 to 10 years is at risk because there is no way of knowing the sexual histories of all the sex partners of one's multiple sex partners. People who are not sexually active are not at risk. People in monogamous relationships in which neither partner has an STD or has used IV drugs are considered safe. It is estimated that HIV infections among nondrug-using heterosexuals in the United States doubled during the 1990s.[11]

AIDS is a preventable disease, and education is still the best defense. People who have sex outside a monogamous relationship and those who share needles from intravenous drugs are still at extremely high risk for infection.

HIV is spread through intimate sexual contact; through transfusion of blood from an infected individual; and from an infected mother to her fetus during the prenatal period, the birth process, or breast-feeding (see Just the Facts: Preventing the Spread of AIDS, page 398). In no case has HIV been spread through casual contact—this includes close contact between family members or friends and infected adults or children. Very few health care professionals working with AIDS patients have contracted the disease, and their infection was caused by rare

~~~~~~~~~~ Just the Facts ~~~~~~~~~~

How HIV Is and Is Not Transmitted

Following are possible means of transmission of HIV and some activities that, contrary to misinformed opinion, do not transmit HIV.

How HIV Is Transmitted

Sexual Activity

- Homosexual, between men
- Heterosexual, from men to women and women to men

Blood

- Through needle sharing among intravenous drug users
- Through transfusions of blood and blood products
- To health care workers through a needle stick, an open wound, or mucous membrane exposure
- Through injection with an unsterilized needle (including needles used in acupuncture, medical injections, ear piercing, and tattooing)

Childbirth

- Intrauterine (within the uterus)
- Peripartum (during labor and delivery)

How HIV Is Not Transmitted

- Through food and water
- Through sharing of eating and drinking utensils
- Through shaking or holding hands
- Through use of the telephone
- Via a toilet seat
- Via insects
- In whirlpools or saunas
- Through coughing or sneezing
- Via domestic pets
- Through an exchange of clothing
- From swimming in a pool
- Through bed linens

~~~ Just the Facts ~~~

Preventing the Spread of AIDS[6]

The spread of AIDS can be stopped by preventing the transmission of the HIV virus from one person to another. This means eliminating direct sexual contact with infected people and not using contaminated needles. Recommendations to reduce the possibility of becoming infected include the following:

- Practice abstinence or mutual monogamy.
- Always use protection (that is, latex condoms and spermicide, such as nonoxynol-9) if having sex with multiple partners or with people who have multiple partners.
- Do not have unprotected sex with people with AIDS, those who engage in high-risk behavior, or those who have had a positive test for the AIDS virus.
- Avoid sexual activities that might cut or tear the rectum, vagina, or penis.
- Do not have sex with prostitutes.
- Do not use IV drugs or share needles. Refrain from having sex with IV drug users.

mishandling of blood. The AIDS virus is not transmitted from toilet seats, foods, beverages, or social kissing. The virus is found in small amounts in tears and saliva, although transmission through these mediums is undocumented.

Probably no other infectious disease has taken or is taking such a devastating toll on Americans. It is estimated that, through 2002, 877,273 adult and adolescent AIDS cases have been diagnosed. Of this number, 718,002 were males and 159,271 were female. In 2002, 9,300 AIDS cases were estimated in children under the age of 13.[11] Further, the CDC reported 41,287 cases of AIDS among people 13 through 24 years of age.[11] By 2002, an estimated 501,669 people with AIDS in the United States had died.[11]

Testing for HIV

Two tests are currently being used to detect HIV. The ELISA is the antibody test initially used. If the ELISA result indicates that the patient has HIV, another test—the Western blot technique—is administered for confirmation. A person may not have abnormal results on the ELISA if the virus has not been present long enough for antibodies to develop. Antibodies may develop within 2 months or may take up to 36 months to develop.[12] Usually, Western blot results are clearly either HIV positive or negative. If there is an inconclusive Western blot test, the person should be retested in 6 months. A third test, the single-use diagnostic system (SUDS), is currently being readied for determining if HIV infection has occurred. Home tests are now available for over-the-counter use. The home tests are much less invasive, since a finger lancet is used to collect a few drops of blood. The sample is placed on blotter paper and mailed to a laboratory, which then performs the test to determine if the sample is positive or negative. The person then telephones the lab for the results. The results are discussed with a counselor if the HIV test is positive. Any positive HIV home test should be followed up with one of the aforementioned tests for HIV. Remember, anyone who tests positive is infected with HIV and can transmit the infection. Although not always reliable, two other tests are now available for use in diagnosis.[14]

Treatment of HIV and AIDS

At present, no cure exists for HIV and AIDS, which results in a multitude of infections leading to death. It is essential that treatment begin as soon as possible after the diagnosis. Currently, 20 drugs have been approved for treating HIV-infected individuals. They fall into the following categories:[13]

- *Reverse transcriptase (RT) inhibitors.* RT inhibitors interfere with HIV's ability to make copies of itself. There are two main types of RT inhibitors and they work differently. *Nucleoside* and *nucleotide* provide faulty DNA building blocks, halting the DNA chain that the virus uses to make copies of itself. Nonnucleoside RT inhibitors bind RT so the virus cannot carry out its copying function.
- *Protease inhibitors (PI).* Protease inhibitors interfere with the protease enzyme that HIV uses to reproduce copies of itself.
- *Fusion inhibitors.* This is the newest class of antiretroviral drugs, which are substances used to kill or inhibit the multiplication of retroviruses such as HIV. They act by interfering with the virus's ability to fuse or invade cells.

Table 12-1 on page 400 lists the current drugs available for treatment.

Early, aggressive treatment with a combination of a protease inhibitor and two nucleoside analogs (AZT and ddI), sometimes called a *cocktail,* has cut the death rate by 70 percent and has inhibited opportunistic infections by 73 percent.[13] However, dangerous side effects seem to accompany this type of therapy, including diabetes, abnormally high cholesterol and triglyceride levels, shrinking limbs, and the bizarre appearance of disfiguring deposits of fat on parts of the body.[13]

Just the Facts

AIDS and HIV Sources of Information

Contact the following organizations for information about HIV and AIDS:

CDC National AIDS Hotline
(800) 342-2437
Free information on HIV and AIDS available in several languages

CDC National AIDS Clearinghouse
(800) 458-5231
www.cdcnpin.org
Information on services and education services; copies of Public Health Service publications available

Linea Nacional de SIDA
(800) 344-7432
Twenty-four-hour hot line that provides information and referrals in Spanish for HIV and AIDS

HIV Insite Gateway to AIDS Knowledge
www.ashastd.org/nah/sida
Information concerning prevention, education, treatment, and clinical trials

Local health departments also offer valuable information concerning HIV and AIDS.

Even with this dramatic improvement, the AIDS crisis is far from over. Although some patients appear virus-free, it has been demonstrated that discontinuing therapy will increase the amount of HIV found in the blood. Even with all the advancements, the best protection for those choosing to be sexually active is education and the practice of safer sex.

There are currently no HIV vaccines to prevent infection or disease. There is a great deal of research being done on the possible development of vaccines, but, unfortunately, there is not a great deal of hope in the immediate future. The task is made difficult because of the HIV's ability to mutate and thus avoid developing immune system recognition. In fact, many HIV-positive individuals may carry several versions of the virus.[14]

AIDS is the most deadly of all STDs, but it is preventable. With education, wisdom, and reduction in high-risk behaviors, AIDS can be prevented (see Just the Facts: Preventing the Spread of AIDS). Information on AIDS can be obtained through various sources (see Just the Facts: AIDS and HIV Sources of Information).

Herpes

Herpes is caused by the herpes simplex virus (HSV). Five different strains of the herpes virus infect human beings.

Table 12-1   Drugs Approved for Treating HIV Infections

Nucleoside/Nucleotide RT Inhibitors	Nonnucleoside RT Inhibitors	Protease Inhibitors	Fusion Inhibitors
Abacavir	Delavirdine	Ritonavir	Pentafuside
ddC	Nevirapine	Saquinavir	
ddI	Efavirenz	Indinavir	
D4T		Amprenavir	
3TC		Nelfinavir	
ZDV ATZ		Lopinavir	
Tenofovir		Atazanavir	
		Entricitabine	
		Fosamprenavir calcium	

SOURCE: United States Department of Health and Human Services. 2004. Antiretroviral drugs. Available online at AIDS info. http://www.aidsinfo.nih.gov/drugs/

The most common strains are herpes simplex-1 (HSV-1) and herpes simplex-2 (HSV-2). Type 1 is usually confined to congenital areas in the form of cold sores or fever blisters. It is a common form of herpes but is not categorized as an STD. Type 2 generally causes lesions on and around the genital areas and is an STD. However, through either direct or indirect contact, type 1 can affect the genital area and type 2 can produce sores in the mouth. The common sites for type 1 and type 2 can thus be reversed. Estimates indicate that 60 million people in the United States are infected with genital herpes.[15]

Type 2 herpes usually appears as a single blister or a series of painful blisters on the penis or inside the vagina or cervix. The blisters may also be present on the buttocks and thighs and in the groin area. Following a short prodromal (time interval between the earliest symptoms and appearance of actual disease) of tingling, discomfort, or itching, small red lesions appear. This phase is followed by the formation of a small blister filled with clear fluid. This fluid is highly contagious. The infection usually lasts one to three weeks and then abates, but it does not leave the body. The virus retreats to the nerve endings, where it remains dormant. Herpes can become active again without any warning; that is, the disease may be recurrent. Menstruation, stress, trauma to the skin (such as too much sunlight), lack of sleep, and poor nutrition seem to trigger recurrences. Recurrences are generally less severe and of shorter duration than the initial episode.[16]

Genital herpes is acquired by sexual contact. It was once believed that herpes could be transmitted only when the virus was active and causing symptoms, such as the presence of blisters or sores. It is now known that the virus can be spread even when there are no symptoms.[17] Research does indicate that the risk for transmission is greatest among couples during the first three months of a sexual relationship. Estimates are that half of couples transmit within this period, indicating the possibility that partners develop a natural immunity to the virus over time.[17]

Men do not seem to experience any major long-term complications from herpes. Women, however, may be faced with the possibility of cancer of the cervix and infection of their newborns during the birth process. Any woman with a history of herpes should have an annual Pap smear test. Physicians attending the pregnancy of a woman with a history of herpes should be informed, so that the course of the pregnancy can be monitored. If herpes becomes active or the physician feels the baby would be at risk through a vaginal birth, caesarean section delivery (surgical removal of the fetus through the abdominal wall) is often used. Additional hazards of herpes infection are herpes encephalitis, in which the virus invades the brain, and herpes keratitis, or eye infection. These two conditions are rare and can be treated effectively with antiviral drugs.

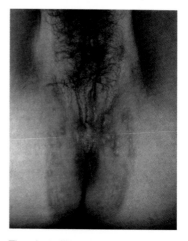

The photo illustrates an example of a severe herpes infection.

Three antiviral prescription drugs are available for treating herpes. Acyclovir (brand name Zovirax, now available as a generic) promotes healing and helps suppress future outbreaks. Two newer drugs, valacyclovir and famciclovir, are similar to acyclovir but are designed to make higher levels of the drug's active ingredient available to the body. Some physicians prescribe a course of suppressive therapy with one of these drugs, which keeps herpes from recurring in up to 90 percent of patients. Patients must start taking the drugs at the first hint of symptoms. This therapy works only as long as the drug is taken, and if the drug is stopped there may be recurrences.[17] Warm compresses, sitz baths, and aspirin may help relieve discomfort.

Hepatitis B

Hepatitis is an inflammation of the liver caused by one or more viruses. There are six distinct types of **viral hepatitis**: hepatitis A (formerly *infectious hepatitis*), hepatitis B (formerly *serum hepatitis*), hepatitis C (non-A, non-B hepatitis), hepatitis E (another form of non-A, non-B), hepatitis D *(delta hepatitis),* and hepatitis G.

Hepatitis B is considered the most serious of the six types of hepatitis. It has an incubation period of between 45 and 160 days. The symptoms of hepatitis B include vomiting, abdominal pain, loss of appetite, and jaundice (an excess of a bile pigment in the blood that causes the skin to look yellow). Some infected people do not develop the worst symptoms of the disease but experience mild, flulike illness without jaundice. However, the CDC estimates that approximately 25 percent of carriers suffer chronic symptoms, and these people are at the greatest risk for one of the most serious consequences of infection, cirrhosis of the liver. Cirrhosis is a degenerative disease in which liver cells are damaged and scarred, with the eventual outcome of death or the necessity of liver transplantation. All carriers of hepatitis B are at greater risk of developing primary liver cancer than are noncarriers. At one time, hepatitis B was spread primarily through tattoo needles, the sharing of needles by drug users, and transfusions of contaminated blood. Today, it is more commonly spread through body secretions, including sweat, breast milk, and semen. A vaccine has been developed to immunize against the disease.

The symptoms of all forms of viral hepatitis are similar. They include fatigue, loss of appetite, mild fever, nausea, vomiting, diarrhea, aching muscles and joints, and tenderness in the upper right abdomen. A few people may have jaundiced (yellowed) skin and eyes, itching skin, darkened urine, and light-colored feces. Still others may exhibit no symptoms except those usually associated with the flu. This group does not usually seek treatment but still can transmit the infection to others.

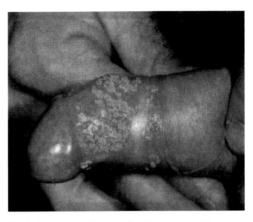

Genital warts are the result of human papilloma virus.

Viral hepatitis is a type of liver injury. Most patients with hepatitis recover without serious problems. However, serious scarring of the liver or even death may occur. In some cases of hepatitis B, the person with the disease becomes a chronic carrier or can develop chronic progressive hepatitis, which eventually leads to liver failure.

Genital Warts

Warts on the genitalia, around the anus, in the vagina, and on the cervix are called **genital warts,** or *condyloma.* These warts are caused by the human papilloma virus (HPV). There are more than 30 forms of HPV. Experts postulate that this condition is the third most prevalent STD. It is also estimated that 5.5 million people are infected annually. Approximately 1 in 10 Americans may be carrying the virus.[18] Twenty million people in the United States are already infected. Genital warts most commonly involve people between the ages of 15 and 24.

Genital warts are cauliflower-like. In moist areas, they are soft and either pink or red. On dry skin, they are usually yellow-gray and hard. The warts are transmitted sexually and generally appear one to six months after exposure. There are 30 distinct varieties of HPV, some of which have been specifically linked to cervical cancer and cancers of the rectum, vulva, skin, and penis. The warts appear most often on the shaft of the penis, the vulva, the vaginal wall, the cervix, and the perineum. They may also be found in the anal area of both sexes and are associated with anal intercourse with an infected partner. Cryosurgery (freezing) is the treatment of choice, although electrocautery (burning) and use of the topical agent podophyllin also are successful methods of treatment. Podophyllin should not be used during pregnancy or on warts in the cervical area. If the infected person has had a variety of partners, the genitalia of all partners should be examined, so that treatment can be initiated if appropriate.

Bacterial Diseases

Chlamydia

Chlamydia is the most common STD in the United States, with an estimated 2.8 million new cases each year.[20] The causative agent is the bacterium *Chlamydia trachomatis*. Chlamydia is frequently found with other STDs, such as herpes, and it may be contracted through oral, anal, and vaginal intercourse. Approximately 75 percent of women and 50 percent of men have no symptoms. Most people infected with chlamydia are not aware of their infections and therefore do not seek medical help.

In men the infection is usually manifested by inflammation of the urethra (urethritis). Infected men generally experience a burning sensation during urination and possibly a mild discharge.

Symptoms in women include vaginal discharge, intermittent vaginal bleeding, and ill-defined discomfort or pain on urination. Infected mothers may pass the infection to their babies during the birth process. This may result in conjunctivitis in the baby or a more serious condition known as *chlamydial pneumonia*.

When left untreated, chlamydia can lead to arthritis and can damage the heart valves, blood vessels, and heart muscle. In men the condition can also lead to sterility. In women the disease can infect the uterus, fallopian tubes, and upper reproductive areas, producing the chronic condition pelvic inflammatory disease, or PID. This scarring of the fallopian tubes by PID causes sterility and an increased risk for ectopic pregnancy (a condition in which the embryo is implanted outside the uterus). Women infected with chlamydia have a three- to fivefold increased risk of acquiring HIV, if exposed.

Most of the time, chlamydia is treated with an antibiotic, such as azithromycin, which requires taking for only one day. Doxycycline is taken for seven days but is widely prescribed. Other drugs used include tetracycline, erythromycin, and ofloxacin. These drugs are taken orally for one to three weeks. Taking the full course of medication is extremely important because relapse can occur. All sexual partners should be treated, or the disease can be passed among them.[19]

Gonorrhea

Nearly 400,000 cases of **gonorrhea** are reported each year, making it the second most prevalent STD. Gonorrhea is caused by the bacterium *Neisseria gonorrhoeae*, which attacks the mucous membranes of the penis, vagina, rectum, throat, and eyes. The disease is spread by vaginal, oral, and rectal contact.

Gonorrhea produces symptoms in 80 percent of men. The symptoms appear 2 to 10 days (an average 3 to 5 days) after contact with the bacteria and include a thick, milky discharge from the penis and a painful,

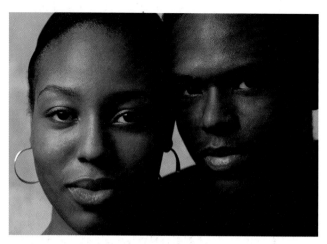
Practicing safer sex helps diminish the risk of contracting an STD.

burning sensation on urination. These signs should cause men to seek medical treatment immediately. Untreated gonorrhea can result in sterility.

The symptoms in women are discharge and burning on urination, but they may be so mild that they are unnoticed. The bacteria can survive in the vagina and other areas of the female reproductive system for years. During this time, women can infect any sex partners and their fetuses if they become pregnant. The baby's contact with the bacteria during childbirth can lead to an eye infection, resulting in blindness. Untreated gonorrhea can lead to PID, the leading cause of sterility in women. In both men and women, rectal and oral gonorrhea may go unnoticed. The disease can develop into a serious infection, resulting in arthritis; meningitis; skin lesions; and liver, heart, brain, and spinal cord problems.

Gonorrhea is diagnosed either by obtaining a smear from the penis or cervix or by doing a urine test. Physicians commonly treat for chlamydia as well when gonorrhea has been diagnosed. This dual therapy can be most cost-effective because the cost of treatment is less than the cost of testing. Most gonococci in the United States can be cured with doxycycline and dzithromycin; therefore, cotreatment might hinder the development of antibiotic-resistant strains of gonorrhea.[19] Over the last two decades, four types of antibiotic-resistant strains have developed and new antibiotic or combination drugs must be used to cure the infection.[19] Gonorrhea can be completely cured, although there is no immunity to the disease. If a person has multiple sex partners, medical help and advice must be sought regularly.

Syphilis

Syphilis is caused by a corkscrew-shaped bacterial spirochete called *Treponema pallidum*. Kissing, oral-genital contact, and intercourse are the most common forms of transmission. The spirochete dies quickly when exposed

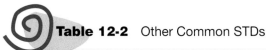

Table 12-2 Other Common STDs

STD	Causative Agent	Symptoms	Treatment
Candidiasis (yeast infection)	A fungus (*Candida albicans*) that can be transmitted through sexual coitus or an imbalance of the acidity of the vagina	White, "cheesy" discharge; irritation of vaginal and vulva tissue	Vaginal cream or suppositories, such as miconazole (Monistat)
Chancroid	A bacterium (*Haemophilus ducreyi*) that can be contracted through a lesion or its discharge	Cluster of small bumps or blisters on the genitals or around the anus that rupture and ulcerate	Antibiotics, such as erythromycin
Granuloma inguinale	A bacterium (*Calymmatobacterium granulomatis*) that can be contracted through contact with a lesion or its discharge	Painless red bumps or sores in the groin that ulcerate and spread	Antibiotics, such as tetracycline or doxycycline
Nongonococcal urethritis (NGU)	A bacterium (mostly *Chlamydia trachomatis*) that can be transmitted during coitus	Inflammation of the urethra; for men, discharge and irritation during urination; for women, possible mild discharge of pus from the vagina or no symptoms	Antibiotics, such as tetracycline, doxycycline, or erythromycin
Pediculosis (crabs)	*Phthirus pubis* (pubic lice)	Intense itching in the genital area	Shampoos, such as those with lindane solution (Kwell)
Pelvic inflammatory disease (PID) (women only)	Untreated chlamydia or gonorrhea; may lead to infertility or arthritis	Low abdominal pain, bleeding between menstrual periods, persistent low fever	Penicillin or other antibiotics
Trichomoniasis (trich)	A protozoan parasite (*Trichomonas vaginalis*) contracted through sexual intercourse; can be spread by towels, toilet seats, or bathtubs used by an infected person	White to yellow discharge with an unpleasant odor	Anti-infectives, such as metronidazole (Flagyl)

to air, so primary entry to the body is through a break in the skin. Once in the bloodstream, it exists in a variety of organs and mimics the symptoms of many major chronic diseases. Because of this ability to mimic other diseases, it is referred to as *the great imitator*.

One interesting fact concerning syphilis is that some HIV infections seem to be exacerbated by it. The lesions caused by syphilis seem to help the HIV virus seep into or out of the body. Not everyone who has sex with a person who is HIV positive becomes infected, but if either partner also has primary or secondary syphilis, the risk of transmission increases sixfold.[20] There are four stages of syphilis.

Primary syphilis

The initial sign of primary syphilis is a lesion called a *chancre*, located at the site of entry of the pathogen. The incubation period ranges from 10 to 90 days (an average of 21 days) before symptoms appear. The chancre varies from the size of a pinhead to the size of a dime. Even though the chancre may look painful, it is not and may

go unnoticed. If the lesion occurs on the labia, vagina, or rectum, it can easily remain undetected. The chancre disappears within 10 days to 3 months. In 90 percent of women and 50 percent of men, the chancre is difficult to identify.[21]

Secondary syphilis

From 4 to 12 weeks after the chancre disappears, the symptoms of secondary syphilis may appear. Symptoms include headaches, swollen glands, low-grade fevers, skin rash, white patches on the mucous membranes of the mouth and throat, hair loss, arthritis pain, and large sores around the mouth and genitals. These sores contain the bacteria responsible for syphilis, and contact with them can spread the disease. Symptoms may be mild or severe, and in rare instances no symptoms appear. If left untreated, symptoms usually run their course, lasting anywhere from a few days to several weeks. The pathogen remains active in the body even with the absence of symptoms and will reappear later—perhaps as long as 20 years after the initial infection.

Latent syphilis

During latent syphilis, there are few or no clinical signs that the disease exists, although the spirochetes are invading the various organs and systems of the body, including the brain, heart, and central nervous system. The spirochetes multiply relentlessly and begin to destroy the tissues, bones, and organs. At this stage, a person is not contagious.

Tertiary syphilis

From 15 to 20 years after the onset of latent syphilis, the disease progresses to its most devastating stage. Tertiary syphilis can cause heart damage, central nervous system damage, blindness, deafness, paralysis, and psychosis. Death from the effects of this stage of syphilis is probable.

Penicillin is the preferred drug for treating syphilis. People who are penicillin-sensitive are placed on other antibiotics, such as tetracycline or erythromycin. For an individual who has had syphilis less than a year, a single dose will cure the disease. Larger doses are needed for those who have had the disease longer than a year.[21,22] Antibiotics can kill the pathogen at any stage, but any damage incurred cannot be reversed. People with syphilis commonly have other STDs, such as gonorrhea and chlamydia, thereby requiring greater doses of antibiotics.

Other Common STDs

In addition to the STDs mentioned, there are several others that have potential for harm. Table 12-2 on page 403 lists several other common STDs.

Summary

- The only way to completely avoid acquiring an STD is to abstain from sex or to have sex in a purely monogamous relationship.
- Practicing safer sex helps reduce the possibility of contracting an STD. The use of condoms is associated with decreased risk.
- The human immunodeficiency virus (HIV) attacking the immune system causes a complex of rare diseases called acquired immunodeficiency syndrome (AIDS).
- Although no cure exists for AIDS, some of the latest combinations of drugs seem to be prolonging life and reducing the HIV content in the body.
- Genital herpes is a viral disease characterized by lesions around the genital area. The disease can recur at any time and represents a serious threat to women by increasing their risk for cancer of the cervix. Three drugs are used to treat the disease (acyclovir, valacyclovir, and famciclovir).

- Viral hepatitis is an injury to the liver. There are several types of hepatitis. Hepatitis B is perhaps the most serious.
- Genital warts, or condyloma, are caused by the human papilloma virus (HPV) and have been linked to some cancers.
- Chlamydia is caused by a bacterium that produces the most common STD in the United States. Untreated, it can cause arthritis, sterility, damage to the heart and blood vessels, and ectopic pregnancies.
- Gonorrhea is the second leading STD. It can lead to sterility in both men and women. The symptoms are often unnoticed by women.
- Syphilis is a bacterial disease that has four stages. The stages are primary, secondary, latent, and tertiary.
- Several other STDs that have damaging potential are candidiasis, chancroid, granuloma inguinale, nongonococcal urethritis (NGU), pediculosis, pelvic inflammatory disease (PID), and trichomoniasis.

Review Questions

1. How can people accept responsibility for their sexual behavior?
2. What makes HIV an extremely dangerous infection?
3. What precautions can you take to protect against the spread of AIDS?
4. What are the various kinds of viral hepatitis and how are they spread?
5. Discuss why HPV is more dangerous for women than for men.

6. Why does chlamydia represent a serious problem?
7. Why is gonorrhea a more serious problem today than it was just a few years ago?
8. List and explain the four stages of syphilis.
9. Discuss some other common STDs.
10. If one STD is present, why may it be necessary to get treatment for more than one?

References

1. Strong, B., C. DeVault, and S. B. Werner. 1999. *Human sexuality—Diversity in contemporary America.* 3d ed. Mountain View, CA: Mayfield.

2. Centers for Disease Control and Prevention. 2004. 2002 report (www.wonder.cdc.gov/wonder/STDSTDD007.PCW.html).

3. Sexuality Information and Educational Council of the United States. 2002. Sexually transmitted diseases in the United States (www.siecus.org/pub/fact/fact0008.html).

4. National Institute of Allergy and Infectious Diseases. 2004. How HIV causes AIDS (www.niaid.nih.gov/factsheets/howhiv.htm).

5. Pallella, F. L., et al. 1998. HIV outpatient study investigation. Declining morbidity and mortality among patients with advanced human immunodeficiency virus infections. *New England Journal of Medicine* 338(13):853.

6. Cox, F. D. 1999. *The AIDS booklet.* 5th ed. Boston: WCB/McGraw-Hill.

7. Stine, G. J. 1993. *Acquired immune deficiency syndrome—Biological, medical, social, and legal issues.* Englewood Cliffs, NJ: Prentice-Hall.

8. National Institute of Allergy and Infectious Diseases. 2004. HIV infections in women (www.niaid.nih.gov/factsheet/aidsstat.htm).

9. Nevid, J. S. 1995. *Choices: Sex in the age of STDs.* Boston: Allyn and Bacon.

10. Notes from the Twelfth World AIDS Conference, Geneva, Switzerland. 26 June–12 July 1998. (www.mhhe.com/hper/health/personalhealth/aidsnotes.mhtml).

11. Centers for Disease Control and Prevention. 2004. HIV/AIDS surveillance report 2002. *Mortality and Morbidity Weekly Report* 14:1–40.

12. Hirsch, M. 2000. Antiretroviral drug resistance testing in adult HIV-1 infection: Recommendations of an international AIDS society–USA panel. *Journal of the American Medical Association* 283(18):2417–26.

13. National Institute of Allergy and Infectious Diseases. 2004. Treatment of HIV infection (www.niaid.nih.gov/factsheets/treat-hiv.htm).

14. National Institute of Allergy and Infectious Diseases. 2004. HIV vaccines—Questions and answers (www.niaid.hig.gov/factsheets/treat-hiv.htm/publications/vaccine/faqhivadvoctes.htm).

15. National Institute of Allergy and Infectious Diseases. 2004. Sexually transmitted infections (www.naid.nih.gov).

16. National Women's Health Resource Center. 2004. Health topics—Genital herpes (www.healthywomen.org).

17. National Women's Health Resource Center. 2004. Treatment of genital herpes (www.healthywomen.org).

18. National Institute of Allergy and Infectious Diseases. 2004. Human papillomavirus and genital warts (www.naid.nig.gov).

19. Centers for Disease Control and Prevention. 2004. Guidelines for treatment of sexually transmitted diseases (www.cdc.gov/wonder/STD/STD98TG).

20. Editors. 22 December 1998. Syphilis eradication: So near, so elusive. *USA Today,* 6D.

21. National Institute of Allergy and Infectious Diseases. 2004. Syphilis (www.niaid.nih.gov/factsheets/sTdsyph.htm).

22. Centers for Disease Control and Prevention. 2004. Syphilis fact sheet (www.cdc.gov/nchstp/dstd/fact_sheets).

Suggested Readings

Centers for Disease Control and Prevention. 1998. *1998 guidelines for treatment of sexually transmitted diseases.* New York: International Medical Publications.

This replaces the 1993 *Guidelines for Treatment.* It was developed by CDC staff members after consultation with a group of experts on the treatment of STDs.

Nevsid, J. S., and F. Gotfried. 1993. *201 things you should know about AIDS and other sexually transmitted diseases.* Boston: Allyn and Bacon.

This book provides information on all the common STDs, offers guidelines for prevention, and lists available treatments.

Shilts, R. 1987. *And the band played on: Politics, people, and the AIDS epidemic.* New York: St. Martin's Press.

This classic book, written by a gay man with AIDS, expresses the author's views about the political aspects of AIDS and the difficulties in receiving treatment.

13

Reducing Your Risk
for Cancer

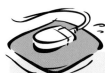

Online Learning Center

Log on to our Online Learning Center (OLC) for access to these additional resources:

- Chapter key term flashcards
- Learning objectives
- Additional goals for behavior change
- Concentration game
- Self-scoring chapter quizzes

- Additional lab activities

The OLC also offers Web links for study and exploration of wellness topics. Access these links through **www.mhhe. com/anspaugh6e,** click on Student Center, click on Chapter 13, and then click on Web Activities.

Goals for Behavior Change

- Identify and change two behaviors that put you at risk for cancer.
- Begin an exercise program for preventing cancer as well as promoting overall wellness.
- Regularly perform the self-examinations for cancer described in this chapter.
- Consult your physician to arrange any appropriate medical screening tests, such as a mammogram or a PSA test.

Key Terms

basal cell carcinoma
benign
cancer
carcinogens
carcinoma
leukemia

lymphoma
metastasis
oncogene
sarcoma
squamous cell carcinoma

Objectives

After completing this chapter, you will be able to do the following:

- Define *cancer.*
- Identify the various types of cancer.

- List the signs and symptoms of the various types of cancer.
- Identify ways of protecting against various cancers.
- Discuss treatments for cancer.

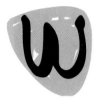

ith the possible exception of AIDS, there is probably no disease that strikes more fear in people than cancer. The term **cancer** refers to a group of diseases characterized by uncontrolled, disorderly cell growth. It is the second leading cause of death.

In 2004, almost 563,700 Americans were expected to die of cancer, over 1,500 people a day.[1] Since 1999 cancer has been the leading cause of death in the United States for people under 85 years of age.[36]

Death rates for many major cancers have leveled off or declined over the past 50 years. Still, one of four Americans will eventually develop one or more of the 100 different forms of cancer; 40 percent of people who get cancer will be alive 5 years after diagnosis and considered cured. Others, however, who survive for 5 years may still show evidence of cancer.[2] *Cured* means that a patient has no evidence of disease and has the same life expectancy of a person who never had cancer. Although

it strikes more frequently with advancing age, cancer causes the deaths of more children than any other disease (see Wellness for a Lifetime: Children and Cancer). The chances of developing cancer can be reduced by assuming control of your daily behaviors and activities (see Just the Facts: Tips for Cancer Prevention; see also Assessment Activity 13-2).

Cell growth is controlled by deoxyribonucleic acid (DNA) and ribonucleic acid (RNA) in the nucleus of each cell in the body. If the nuclei lose the ability to regulate and control this growth, cellular metabolism and reproduction are disrupted and a mutant cell is produced that varies in form, quality, and function from the original. When a mass of these cells develops, it is considered a neoplasm, or tumor. It may be malignant (cancerous) or **benign** (noncancerous). A benign tumor will not spread throughout the body. It is enclosed by a membrane, which prevents it from invading other tissues. A benign tumor is not life-threatening unless it is in an area that

Wellness for a Lifetime

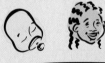

Children and Cancer

Despite its rarity, cancer is the chief cause of death by disease in children under the age of 15. Cancer is a devastating event, particularly when the diagnosis occurs in children. The overwhelming emotional and psychological trauma associated with cancer affects not only the child but also brothers, sisters, parents, and other relatives. If there is any good news to report, it is that mortality rates have declined 57 percent since the 1970s. St. Jude Children's Research Hospital, the only cancer research center in the world devoted solely to children, reports that, since 1962, the survival rates for various childhood cancers have risen

significantly. For example, children with acute lymphocytic leukemia (cancer of the blood) now have a survival rate of 80 percent, compared with the 1962 rate of 4 percent. Children now have the following survival rates (see list):

Even though the survival rates are significantly better today than they were in 1962, the families of children diagnosed with cancer still need support. St. Jude provides not only medical treatment for the child but also social support, psychological counseling, and education about the cancer for all the members of the family. Its mission is to serve as an advocate for the family as well as for the child affected, regardless of the prognosis.

As researchers move slowly toward providing cures and increasing life expectancy of children affected by cancer, we can all hope that, one day, we will know of children dying from cancer only through reading about them in textbooks. For more information about childhood cancers, visit the following Web site: www.stjude.org.

	Now	1962
• Hodgkin's lymphoma (cancer of the lymph nodes):	90%	50%
• Non-Hodgkin's lymphoma (malignant tumor):	80%	7%
• Retinoblastoma (cancer affecting the eyes):	90%	75%
• Neuroblastoma (cancer of the nervous system):	56%	10%
• Wilms' tumor (cancer of the kidney):	90%	50%
• Osteosarcoma (bone cancer):	70%	20%
• Rhabdomyosarcoma (cancer affecting the muscles):	75%	30%

Just the Facts

Tips for Cancer Prevention

More than 200 studies demonstrate a strong association between diets high in vegetables and fruits (five to nine servings a day).[3] Observe the following guidelines to improve your chances of avoiding cancer:

What to Do

- Eat more broccoli, cauliflower, and brussels sprouts. Eat more cabbage-type vegetables, such as cabbages and kale. These vegetables protect against cancers of the colon, rectum, stomach, and lung.

- Add more high-fiber foods to your diet. Eat more peaches, strawberries, potatoes, spinach, tomatoes, wheat and bran cereals, rice, popcorn, and whole-wheat bread. Fiber protects against cancer of the colon.

- Choose foods containing vitamin A. Eat more carrots, peaches, apricots, squash, and broccoli. Fresh foods are the best sources and are far better than vitamin pills. Vitamin A protects against cancers of the esophagus, larynx, and lung.

- Choose foods containing vitamin C. Eat more grapefruit, cantaloupe, oranges, strawberries, red peppers, green peppers, broccoli, and tomatoes. These help fight cancers of the esophagus and stomach.

- Practice weight control. Exercise and eat foods low in calories. A good exercise for most people is walking. Obese people have a high chance of getting cancers of the uterus, gallbladder, breast, and colon. Check with your doctor before you start an exercise program or a special diet.

- If female, perform monthly breast exams, and get annual mammograms after age 40. Males should get annual digital and prostate-specific antigen (PSA) exams after age

50 (40, if African American or with a family history). Males over age 16 should perform monthly testicle exams. Males and females over age 50 should get annual colon cancer checks.[3]

What to Avoid

- Avoid fat. Eat lean meat, fish, and low-fat dairy products. Cut extra fat off meats and skin poultry before cooking. Avoid pastries and candies. A high-fat diet increases the chance of getting cancer of the breast, colon, and prostate. Calories loaded with fat cause weight gain.

- Avoid salty foods. Stay away from nitrite-cured and smoked foods. Bacon, ham, hot dogs, and salt-cured fish are examples. People who eat these foods have a greater chance of getting cancer of the esophagus and stomach.

- Avoid smoking. Smoking is the main cause of lung cancer. Pregnant women who smoke harm their babies. Parents who smoke at home cause breathing and allergy problems for their children. Chewing tobacco can cause cancers of the mouth and throat. Pick a day to quit and call the American Cancer Society for help.

- Avoid alcohol in excess. If you drink a great deal, you may get cancer of the liver. It is worse to smoke and drink. This increases the chances of getting cancers of the mouth, throat, larynx, and esophagus.

- Avoid too much sun. The sun causes skin cancer and other damage to skin. Use a sunscreen. Wear long sleeves and a hat between 11 a.m. and 3 p.m. Do not use indoor sunlamps, visit tanning parlors, or take tanning pills. Be alert for changes in a mole or sore that does not heal. If changes occur, go to a doctor.

---

interferes with normal functioning. A malignant tumor is the most dangerous tumor because it has a tendency to spread from its original location to other parts of the body, which can make it life-threatening. Cancer cells can crowd out normal cells, invade surrounding tissue, and move through the lymphatic or circulatory system to infiltrate other areas of the body. (The lymphatic system is a network of nodes and vessels that drains fluid from tissues and returns it to the bloodstream. It is also part of the body's immune system.) The process by which cancerous cells spread from their original site (primary site) to another location (secondary site) is called **metastasis.** The ability of cancerous cells to metastasize makes early detection critical. Table 13-1 on page 414 describes the types of cancer and where they are most often found.

Causes and Prevention

Cancer is caused by both external factors (chemicals, diet, radiation, viruses, pollutants, etc.) and internal factors (hormones, immune conditioning, and inherited mutations). Any combination of these factors may initiate or promote carcinogenesis—the development of cancer cells. Ten or more years often pass between exposures or mutations and the detection of cancer.[3]

Although the causes of cancer are not clearly understood, correlations have been found between cancer and everything from genetic factors to exposure to the sun's radiation. Many **carcinogens** (cancer-causing agents) trigger the development of cancer. (Table 13-2 on page 414 contains a list of substances known to be carcinogenic.)

Table 13-1   Types of Cancer and Most Common Sites

Type	Most Common Site	Method of Spread
Carcinoma	Tissues covering body surfaces and lining the body cavities are the most common locations. Sites include the breast, lungs, intestines, skin, stomach, uterus, and testes.	Lymphatic and circulatory systems
Sarcoma	The connective system is most commonly affected. Sites include bones, muscle, and other connective tissue.	Circulatory system
Lymphoma	The condition develops in the lymphatic system, infectious regions of the neck, armpits, groin, and chest. Hodgkin's disease is an example.	Lymphatic system
Leukemia	The blood-forming tissues, bone marrow, and spleen are particularly affected.	Circulatory system

An inherited tendency for cancer has been theorized for years. Everyone seems to have genes that may cause cancer, but not everyone gets cancer. In most cases, environmental factors activate the cancer. A good example of the interplay between genetic and environmental factors is found in cigarette smoking. Approximately 87 percent of lung cancers occur in cigarette smokers,[4] but only 15 percent of smokers develop lung cancer. Why not the other 85 percent? The 15 percent who develop cancer are thought to be susceptible to the disease on the basis of their genes. If they had not activated the cancer genes by smoking, they probably would not have contracted the disease.

A gene that causes cancer is called an **oncogene.** Within a tiny segment of DNA is an area that can be

Table 13-2   Factors That Can Cause Cancer

Carcinogen	Site of Cancer	Comments
Alcohol	Liver, larynx, pharynx, breast, esophagus	Heavy drinking increases the risk for cancer, especially when accompanied by cigarette smoking or use of chewing tobacco.
Smoking	Lungs, mouth, pharynx, larynx, bladder, esophagus	Smoking accounts for about 30 percent of cancer deaths. It is considered the number one carcinogen in the United States and the most preventable cause of death. It is responsible for 87 percent of lung cancer deaths.
Ultraviolet radiation	Skin	Almost all skin cancers are sun-related.
Ionizing radiation	Blood-forming tissues, lungs	Excessive exposure to radiation increases cancer risk. Excessive radon exposure increases the risk for lung cancer.
Smokeless tobacco	Mouth, larynx, pharynx, esophagus	Oral cancer increases with the use of chewing tobacco and snuff.
Estrogen	Endometrium (uterus), liver, breast	Oral contraceptives increase the risk for liver cancer. Estrogen treatment to control menopausal symptoms increases the risk for cancer and heart disease.
Industrial agents		Industrial chemicals and agents, such as nickel, chromate, asbestos, and vinyl chloride, increase the risk for various cancers.
Dietary fat		High consumption of dietary fat is related to cancers of the colon, prostate, and pancreas; replacing fat with complex carbohydrates provides protection against several cancers (see Chapter 6).

SOURCE: American Cancer Society. 2004. *Cancer prevention and early detection facts and figures 2004.* Atlanta: American Cancer Society.

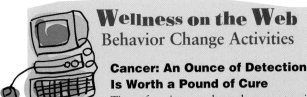

Wellness on the Web
Behavior Change Activities

Cancer: An Ounce of Detection Is Worth a Pound of Cure

Time after time, we hear the same tragic story from cancer patients: "I knew I had a lump, but I was afraid it would be cancer, so I didn't go to the doctor," or "By the time I realized something was wrong, the cancer had metastasized." The very word *cancer* strikes fear into the hearts of the bravest—yet reliable studies show that, the earlier cancer is diagnosed, the better the chances of survival. Both health care providers and the public look to the American Cancer Society (ACS) for guidelines to help detect cancer at the earliest possible stage. The ACS publicizes its recommendations (and most doctors follow them) about Pap smears and mammograms for women, prostate examinations for men, and colorectal examinations for anyone over age 50. These procedures offer hope of detecting cancer early, when it's most treatable. Go to www.mhhe.com/anspaugh6e, Student Center, and Wellness on the Web. Then select Activity 1 and read through the list of recommended early detection tests.

What Causes Cancer?

What is cancer, and how does it originate? Thanks to sophisticated research, medical science is coming closer than ever to solving these riddles and opening the door to possible cures. In the meantime, we're learning a great deal about the risk factors that increase a person's chance of developing cancer. Different cancers have different risk factors. According to the American Cancer Society, existing scientific evidence suggests that about one-third of the cancer deaths that occur in the United States each year are caused by cigarette smoking, and another third are the result of dietary factors. This means that, for the majority of Americans who don't use tobacco, dietary choices and physical activity become the most important modifiable determinants of cancer risk. To learn more about individual risk factors, go to the Web site listed previously, select Activity 2, and read through the list of risks for different types of cancers. Were you surprised by anything you learned?

activated to form an oncogene. All cells have normal regulatory genes, called *proto-oncogenes*. A variety of genetic mutations, viral infections, or other carcinogens cause these normal genes to lose their ability to replicate themselves in a normal genetic fashion. If the gene that is miscopied is one that controls specialization, replication,

repair, or tumor suppression, the result is a cancer-producing gene. Unless it is activated, however, it will never cause cancer. If an oncogene is formed, it acts with other oncogenes to produce abnormal cells that can replicate and spread.

Suppressor genes also play a role in cancer. Suppressor genes, which exist in normal cells, control cell growth. If suppressor genes mutate, cells are permitted to grow unrestrained.

Another explanation of cancer is an error in cell duplication on the basis of chance alone. Several trillion new cells are formed each year, and perfect duplication does not occur with each new cell formation. When an abnormal cell develops, the immune system recognizes it as a rogue cell and attacks it. Every cancer cell needs to be killed because almost all cancers arise from a single cancer cell. Cancer develops as a result of the immune system's failure to clear the body of cancer cells. This is one reason the immune system is receiving considerable attention from cancer researchers.

The development of cancer is a process that generally takes years. By stopping this process at any step, the deadly potential of cancer is ended. After the cancer process is initiated, due to environmental or genetic causes, several things must happen. The cancer cells have to grow and reproduce; the immune system must fail to recognize the cancer and leave it alone; and the new tumor must eventually find a way to "feed" itself by forming new blood vessels to supply itself with blood (a process called angiogenesis).[2]

Much research appears to link psychological states with the prevalence of disease in certain people. People with positive, involved attitudes who view life's challenges as opportunities for personal growth seem to have fewer diseases and recover from them more often. People who feel lonely and depressed and lack appropriate social support are more cancer-prone than are their mentally healthy counterparts.[3]

Emotional factors, such as stress, lack of social support, and the inability to express and cope with the range of emotions brought on by a frightening diagnosis of cancer, have been linked to the progression of cancer. Several studies have reported that patients who participate in support groups while receiving standard medical care live significantly longer than do those receiving medical care alone. Conversely, cancer patients who are socially isolated have poorer survival rates than do those with more social connections.[3] This doesn't suggest that stress and social isolation cause cancer. It does suggest a significant correlation between emotion and the progression of cancer once the disease is established. Many experts believe that a person's emotional state may somehow bolster the body's natural cancer-fighting power.

Although some of these concepts are controversial, it is generally accepted that substances such as tobacco,

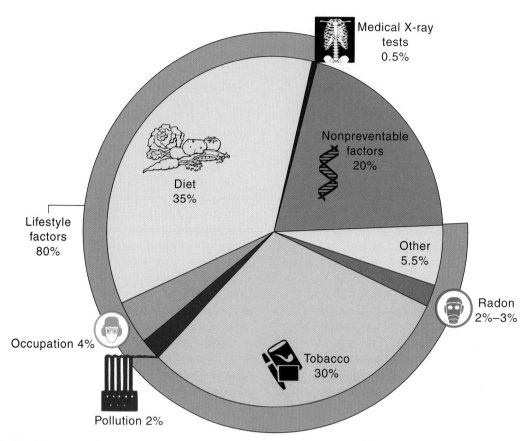

Figure 13-1 Percent of Cancer Deaths Caused by Preventable Factors[5]

tobacco smoke, alcohol, asbestos, herbicides, and pesticides are carcinogens. Scientists believe that more than 80 percent of cancers are associated with lifestyle factors that are easily controlled—diet, smoking, and exposure to the sun.[5] Almost two-thirds of cancer deaths are attributed to diet and tobacco (Figure 13-1). According to a 20-year study of 115,195 healthy women ages 30 to 55, one-third of cancer deaths are caused by excessive weight.[6] (Chapter 6 provides guidelines for cancer prevention as related to diet; Chapter 8 provides guidelines for weight maintenance.)

One of the major carcinogens may be sun radiation—more specifically, excessive exposure to the ultraviolet (UV) rays of the sun. People who spend hours in the sun without protection have an increased risk for skin cancers. UV light peaks from 10 a.m. to 2 p.m. (11 a.m. to 3 p.m. during daylight savings time). Avoiding sun exposure during these hours can cut UV light exposure by up to 60 percent. Most major newspapers now include the UV index as a routine part of the weather report. Using tanning beds also increases the risk for skin cancer.

Finally, the herpes viruses have been connected with cancer of the cervix. Viruses may be involved in the development of some forms of leukemia, Hodgkin's

disease, and Burkett's lymphoma. The exact role of viruses in causing cancer is not known, but they may provide an opportunistic environment for cancer development. Other researchers have suggested that it is a combination of factors, in which the virus may play a part, rather than the virus itself that causes cancer.

Cancer Sites

The American Cancer Society reports each year on the incidence and number of deaths from cancer for a variety of sites (Figure 13-2). Skin cancer is the most common cancer. More than 1 million people are diagnosed annually with **basal** and **squamous cell carcinoma**. Almost all of these are considered sun-related cases.[1] Fortunately, the majority of skin cancers are highly curable. For both genders, the cancer that kills most often is lung cancer. Excluding basal cell and squamous cell carcinomas, the breasts are the most prevalent cancer site for women, and the prostate is the leading cancer site for men. Sixty-two percent of cancer deaths among males are from five primary sites—bronchus, prostate, colon, rectum, and pancreas. Sixty-two percent of female cancer deaths occur from five sites—lung, breast, colon,

Cancer cases by site and sex

Male	Female
Prostate 230,110	Breast 215,990
Lung and bronchus 93,110	Lung and bronchus 80,660
Colon and rectum 73,620	Colon and rectum 73,320
Urinary bladder 44,640	Uterine Corpus 40,320
Melanoma of the skin 29,900	Ovary 25,580
Non-Hodgkin's lymphoma 28,850	Non-Hodgkin's lymphoma 25,520
Kidney 22,080	Melanoma of the skin 25,200
Leukemia 19,020	Thyroid 17,640
Oral cavity 18,550	Pancreas 16,120
Pancreas 15,740	Urinary bladder 15,600
All Sites 699,560	All Sites 668,470

Cancer deaths by site and sex

Male	Female
Lung and bronchus 91,930	Lung and bronchus 68,510
Prostate 29,500	Breast 40,110
Colon and rectum 28,320	Colon and rectum 28,410
Pancreas 15,440	Ovary 16,090
Leukemia 12,990	Pancreas 15,830
Non-Hodgkin's lymphoma 10,390	Leukemia 10,310
Esophagus 10,250	Non-Hodgkin's lymphoma 9,020
Liver 9,450	Uterine Corpus 7,090
Urinary bladder 8,780	Multiple myeloma 5,640
Kidney 7,870	Brain 5,490
All Sites 290,890	All Sites 272,810

Figure 13-2 Cancer Incidence and Death by Site and Sex—2004 Estimates
The figure excludes basal and squamous cell skin cancer and in situ carcinomas except urinary bladder.

SOURCE: American Cancer Society, Surveillance Research, 2004.

ovary, and pancreas.[1] For any cancer, early detection is imperative (see Assessment Activity 13-1). If cancer is diagnosed while it is still localized, the cure or survival rate may be 90 percent or higher for some cancers, such as skin, colon, and rectum cancers.[2]

Exercise and Cancer Prevention

Researchers are continuing to investigate the role of exercise in the prevention of some types of cancer, including of the colon, breast, and reproductive system. In 1996, regular physical activity was added to the list of cancer-prevention measures developed by the American Cancer Society. Mounting research indicates that lack of exercise is a contributing factor to the development of cancer. A panel of cancer experts concluded that as many as 30 to 40 percent of cancers worldwide

could be prevented if people exercised, maintained proper weight, and followed a proper diet.[7,8,9] Another study found that, over an eight-year period, physically unfit men had four times the overall cancer death rate of the most fit men. For women, an even greater difference exists in the death rate between the fit and unfit.[7] Many researchers have followed various groups for long periods to determine whether those who exercise seem to have some measure of protection against cancer.[10] The most impressive results have shown exercise providing protection against colon, breast, and prostate cancers.

Exercise and Colon Cancer

In a review of many studies, it was found that people who tend to sit the majority of the workday or remain inactive in their leisure time have a 30 to 100 percent greater chance of contracting colon cancer.[7] One study of 17,607 college graduates, ages 30 to 79 years, confirmed a lower risk for colon and lung cancer among physically active men.[11] A study done at Harvard University reported that, among 48,000 men, colon cancer risk decreased 50 percent in the most physically active group. This protective effect seemed to occur when the men exercised on average about one to two hours a day.[11] Another study of nearly 90,000 nurses also confirmed the protective effect of physical activity for women against colon cancer.

There are several possible explanations of why exercise is beneficial in protecting against colon cancer. One theory is that exercise increases peristalsis of the large intestine, thus decreasing transit time and the time during which potential carcinogens can be in contact with the cell lining of the colon. Another theory is that exercisers tend to be of more normal weight and are less likely to be obese than nonexercisers. Both obesity and lack of exercise increase levels of insulin, which in turn increase the growth rate of cells lining the colon, thereby increasing the likelihood of developing cancer.[10] Another interesting aspect of the Harvard study was the discovery that exercisers ate an average of 29 grams of fiber daily, whereas nonexercisers ate only 12 grams. The increased fiber increases peristalsis. Another study of men and women who exercised the equivalent of jogging five or more hours a week lowered their risk of colorectal cancer by 40 to 50 percent.[11]

Exercise and Breast Cancer

In a study of 545 premenopausal women, it was found that women exercising 3.7 hours per week reduced their risk for breast cancer by more than 50 percent.[12] A study of Norwegian women who engaged in regular exercise demonstrated a 37 percent reduction in breast cancer risk.[13] If the women were both lean and exercisers, their risk was reduced by 72 percent. Another researcher reported that as little as 30 minutes a day reduces the risk for breast cancer.[14]

Some researchers feel that exercise helps reduce the amount of body fat and protects against obesity. As mentioned in the case of colon cancer, obesity is associated with higher blood insulin levels, which promote the growth of breast cancer cells. Thus, exercising women may be protected from breast cancer because of the indirect effects of exercising on exposure to their own hormones.[13]

Exercise and Prostate Cancer

In a study on over 17,000 college alumni, prostate cancer was found to be reduced by 47 percent in highly active men, compared to sedentary men 70 years old and older.[20] At the Cooper Clinic in Dallas, it was found that men in the highest fitness group had a 74 percent smaller risk than those in the lowest fitness group of developing prostate cancer.[15] The same study found that men expending more than 1,000 calories a week in exercise had less than half the risk for prostate cancer of their sedentary counterparts.

The protective nature of exercise against the development of prostate cancer seems to be the result of repeated bouts of exercise that lower blood levels of testosterone. Men who exercise a great deal tend to expose their prostate to less testosterone, thus reducing their risk for cancer.[16]

Cancers of Concern to Everyone

Lung Cancer

Although breast cancer and prostate cancer receive the majority of attention in the United States, lung cancer is the leading cause of cancer death in the United States[1] and throughout the world.[17] This is largely because lung cancer is more difficult to detect and thereby more deadly than other, even more frequently occurring types of cancer. Lung cancer is one of the most preventable forms of cancer, because the vast majority of cases are directly associated with lifestyle—smoking cigarettes. All cancers caused by cigarette smoking are 100 percent preventable.

The incidence of lung cancer is highest among people who started smoking cigarettes at an early age and who smoke the most cigarettes daily. Tobacco products cause more than 80 percent of lung cancer.[17] The single best prevention of lung cancer is never to smoke. Passive, or involuntary, smoke also contributes significantly to lung cancer. A person who lives or works with smokers significantly increases his or her risk of developing lung cancer, even if choosing to not smoke. Symptoms of lung cancer typically include a persistent cough, blood in the sputum, chest pain, recurring pneumonia, and bronchitis.

The bad news about lung cancer is that early diagnosis tends to be rare. Regular X rays of the lungs and checkups for blood in the sputum seem to be ineffective means of early detection, perhaps because of the altered appearance and function of lung cells from smoking. By the time most lung cancers are detected, either the cancer is not treatable because of widespread metastasis or the treatment is limited to ensuring a short-term extension of life. New studies are under way to determine if a particular type of CT scan may find lung cancers early. Five-year survival rates following diagnosis of lung cancer are between 7 and 12 percent, which is low.

The colorless, odorless gas radon has been somewhat inconsistently associated with increased risk for lung cancer.[3] People living in areas designated high in radon should have their homes measured. Asbestos inhalation has also been associated with lung cancer. Marijuana cigarettes have more tar than regular cigarettes. Many of the cancer-causing substances in tobacco are also found in marijuana. However, because marijuana is an illegal substance, it is difficult to gather data on its effects on the body.[20]

Although the absolute best ways to prevent lung cancer are not smoking, not living with a smoker, not working in a smoking environment, ensuring that radon levels in the home are safe, and avoiding asbestos, substantial evidence exists for the role of diet in lung cancer prevention.[18,19,20] A diet high in whole fruits and vegetables seems to protect against lung cancer. Smokers who regularly consume much produce (fruits and vegetables) seem to have reduced incidence. While regular consumption of whole fruits and vegetables does not ensure that a smoker (or anyone else) will not get cancer, especially lung cancer, there is convincing evidence that a healthy diet provides some protection.

Colorectal Cancer

Colon cancer and cancer of the rectum rank as the third leading causes of cancer deaths in the United States for both men and women.[1] When detected early, 90 percent of localized colorectal cancers can be cured. Once the cancer has spread, however, this chance drops to only 10 percent.

A family history of colon cancer doubles the risk, but family history only accounts for 10 to 15 percent of colon cancers.[21] People with a family history need to be extra vigilant, participating in regular screenings, but so do people with family histories of benign polyps (growths) in the colon. Frequent constipation has been implicated as a risk factor; experiencing constipation even once a month may double one's risk.[11] Any change or increases in constipation or chronic constipation suggest the need for follow-up screening for abnormal growths. Consuming large numbers of calories may increase colon cancer risk.[3] Symptoms of colorectal cancer include a change in bowel habits, chronic abdominal discomfort, sudden weight loss, lack of appetite, or rectal bleeding. Long-term survival rates are much higher when potential cancers are detected before symptoms develop. Detection of colorectal cancer can frequently be accomplished via screenings, although many people avoid the screenings because they find them somewhat distasteful.

Identification of polyps is a primary screening method. The occurrence of polyps in the colon and rectum does not mean a person will develop cancer. In cases in which the polyps do become cancerous, the length of time from initiation to cancer may be 5 to 10 years.[20] The type of screening test used depends on the age of the person as well as family and personal history. Anyone over age 50, even without a family history of the disease, should be tested.

Anyone can undertake prevention of colorectal cancer. Diet is believed to be the primary cause for its development. The National Cancer Institute, the American Cancer Society, and the American Institute for Cancer Research recommend a diet high in vegetables (especially cruciferous vegetables) and fiber and low in fat.[1,11,18] Regular physical activity and maintenance of recommended body weight are also probably preventive. Long-term (15 years or more) ingestion of the B vitamin folate may reduce the risk for colon cancer. Recent studies suggest that 81 mg of aspirin (the lowest observable amount that produced desirable results) may also have a protective effect against colon cancer.[3] Although aspirin is a drug with side effects, some potentially life-threatening, it may also be beneficial for people at elevated risk who can tolerate it. However, aspirin as a preventive should never be taken without prior consultation with a physician. People who smoke have a 30 to 40 percent greater probability of developing colorectal cancer than do nonsmokers.[20]

Stomach, Liver, and Pancreatic Cancer

Stomach cancer

Stomach cancer, except for cancer of the upper part of the stomach (which may be associated with obesity), has steadily declined in the United States and other developed countries. This decrease seems to be strongly linked to the availability of refrigeration, eliminating the need for salt as a preservative. Refrigeration also provides year-round availability of fresh fruits and vegetables, linked to decreased risk. The popular interest in green tea consumption may prove beneficial in reducing the risk for stomach cancer. Diets high in salt, smoked food, and pickled vegetables probably increase the risk for stomach cancer. However, the survival rate for all people with stomach cancer is about 22 percent. The reason for this is that diagnosis usually occurs at an advanced stage of the disease. Smokers have double the rate of stomach cancer of nonsmokers. The major nonlifestyle cause of stomach cancer is infection with the *Helicobacter pylori* bacteria.[21]

Most types of stomach cancer can be prevented by diet. Although the numbers of cases are declining, stomach cancer still ranks among the top 10 cancer killers in the United States. Symptoms are nonspecific, and diagnosis at early stages is not usual.

Liver cancer

Liver cancer is relatively uncommon in the United States and other developed countries. No effective treatment exists for it; the five-year survival rate is only 6 percent. Many liver cancers are lifestyle-related. The primary risk factor for liver cancer is infection with hepatitis B or hepatitis C viruses. The major method of transmission for these viruses is the sharing of needles or sexual contact.[23,24] Research suggests that hepatitis B can also be transmitted by sharing a rolled paper used for snorting cocaine or other drugs.[24] Regular, heavy (more than moderate) consumption of alcohol, leading to cirrhosis and a condition known as *alcoholic hepatitis,* is closely associated with the development of liver cancer.[22] Ingestion of aflatoxins (a type of food mold) from contaminated food has been demonstrated to produce liver cancer, particularly among people in developing countries[22] but tends to be rare in the United States.

Pancreatic cancer

Pancreatic cancer, lesser known than the cancers mentioned previously, ranks among the leading five causes of cancer death in the United States. Pancreatic cancer does not seem to get the publicity of many other types of cancer, yet it is extremely deadly and very difficult to diagnose. In 2004, 31,860 new cases were diagnosed, and 31,270 people died from it.[1] No effective method exists to screen or diagnose this cancer. Recent research suggests that two new imaging tests can help find precancerous changes called dysplasia.[23] Occasionally, depending on where the tumor originates, jaundice may occur while the tumor is in an early stage. Even so, the five-year survival rate is only 4 percent. Little is known about pancreatic cancer except that smoking increases the risk. Because the pancreas is related to digestion and absorption, speculation is that diet affects the development and course of this cancer, but no specifics are known at this time.

Leukemia and Lymphoma

Leukemia and lymphoma (Hodgkin's disease and non-Hodgkin's lymphoma) are two of the most frequent childhood cancers, but they strike more adults than children every year. Leukemia occurs in adults nearly 12 times more often than in children. The causes of leukemia are largely unidentified, although people with genetic abnormalities, such as Down syndrome, experience it more frequently. Excessive exposure to certain chemicals, such as benzene, or infection with the retrovirus HTLV-I also places people at elevated risk. The symptoms resemble those of many other conditions, so they are frequently overlooked initially. They include fatigue, paleness, weight loss, repeated infections, easy bruising, and nosebleeds or other hemorrhages. Children usually experience the onset of these symptoms abruptly, but adults with chronic leukemia progress slowly and exhibit few symptoms.

Early, appropriate diagnosis is the key to long-term survival for leukemia. Depending on the type of leukemia and stage of diagnosis, five-year survival rates may be as high as 57 percent for adults and 80 percent for children.[1]

Lymphoma is a condition in which a tumor composed of lymphoid tissue occurs. The two most general categories of lymphoma are Hodgkin's disease and non-Hodgkin's lymphoma, which includes all types of lymphoma other than Hodgkin's. Hodgkin's disease rates have declined, especially in the elderly, but cases of non-Hodgkin's lymphoma have nearly doubled since the 1970s. Studies suggest that eating large amounts of red meat (beef, pork, or lamb) increase the risk.[22] Other causes involve reduced immune function and exposure to infectious agents via organ transplants or viruses such as HIV (human immunodeficiency virus) or Epstein-Barr. Herbicides and other chemicals may influence the development of the disease. Lifestyle habits, such as smoking and excessive drinking of alcohol, may increase risk. These lifestyle factors are not strongly linked to the development but being obese may increase the risk for non-Hodgkin's lymphoma.

The symptoms of lymphoma include enlarged lymph nodes, itching, fever, night sweats, anemia, and weight loss. The fever may come and go over periods of weeks or months. Survival rates vary greatly, according to the type of disease and stage at diagnosis but can be as high as 51 to 81 percent after five years.[1]

Skin Cancer

The most frequently occurring types of cancer are skin cancers. Skin cancers fall into three main categories: basal cell carcinoma, squamous cell carcinoma, and melanoma. Of the three categories, melanoma is by far the most deadly.

Basal cell carcinoma

Basal cell carcinoma is the most common skin cancer and, along with squamous cell, is responsible for approximately 1.0 million cases of skin cancer a year.[1] Basal cell carcinoma occurs in the outermost skin layers and tends to spread by widening rather than by growing deeper into the skin. The cancer develops into a central sore, which crusts over and bleeds but does not go away.[24] Basal cell carcinoma grows slowly and rarely spreads to other parts of the body.

Squamous cell carcinoma

The second most common type of skin cancer is squamous cell. Squamous cell carcinoma grows faster than basal cell cancer but still grows fairly slowly and can metastasize to other parts of the body. Typically, a squamous cell skin lesion is a firm, red, painless nodule.[24] Both basal cell and squamous cell carcinomas are usually the result of overexposure to sunlight. They occur on a part of the body that has been exposed to the sun.

Malignant melanoma

Although it is the least common type of skin cancer, about 75 percent of skin cancer deaths are due to malignant melanoma. The American Cancer Society estimated that 54,200 new melanomas would be diagnosed in 2004. All skin cancers, but especially malignant melanoma, have increased in number in recent years, so that the current lifetime risk of developing malignant melanoma is about 1 in 82. Although the use of sunscreens with an SPF of 15 or higher seems to reduce the number of basal and squamous cell skin cancers, it does not appear to decrease the risk for melanoma. Genetics is a strong factor in getting malignant melanoma, but it does not explain the explosive increase in the disease that has occurred in the last few decades. Melanoma often grows on parts of the body that are rarely exposed to the sun (such as the buttocks or feet) and does not increase in incidence among people whose occupations require them to spend long hours in the sun (such as farmers).[27] Melanoma appears to be more highly associated with intermittent sun exposure and blistering sunburns occurring early in life (before age 15).

All adults are susceptible, but particularly those with the following risk factors:

- A family history of melanoma
- A personal history of one or more severe sunburns as a child
- Fair skin and many freckles, blonde or red hair, and light eyes
- Occupational exposure to industrial radiation or certain chemicals
- Consumption of medications that increase sensitivity to ultraviolet light

People with these factors should check their entire bodies regularly for any change in the size or color of a mole or other spot; any scaling, oozing, or bleeding from a bump or nodule; pigmentation spreading beyond its border; and a change in sensation, itchiness, tenderness, or pain. Any skin growth that bleeds or crusts should be seen by a physician (Figure 13-3).[25]

Knowing the ABCDs of skin cancer can help people identify melanoma during the early stages when it is still highly treatable (with a 95 percent five-year survival rate):

- *Asymmetry:* If you drew an imaginary line through the center of the mole or pigmented area, the two halves would be shaped differently.

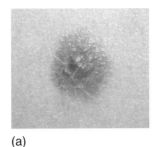
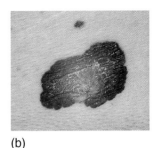

(a)   (b)

Figure 13-3 Comparison of Nonmalignant and Malignant Skin Growths

(a) A normal mole. Note its symmetrical shape, regular borders, even color, and relatively small size (about a half centimeter). (b) A malignant melanoma. Note its asymmetrical shape, irregular borders, uneven color, and relatively large size (about 2 centimeters).

- *Border:* Most normal moles are regularly shaped and their outside borders are regularly shaped. If a border appears to have scalloped edges or to be poorly defined in areas or uneven, it is not normal.
- *Color:* A mole should be one color. Variation in color—differing shades of black, brown, tan, red or some combination of colors—or an intensely black color indicates a problem and need for further investigation.
- *Diameter:* A mole or pigmented area greater than 6 mm (the size of a pencil eraser) should be looked at by a specialist.

As with all cancers, the first line of defense is prevention. Because most skin cancers are directly related to overexposure to the sun's ultraviolet rays, take caution to limit this exposure. Although the use of sunscreen (with an SPF of 15 or higher) may not prevent malignant melanoma, it does decrease the incidence of basal and squamous cell skin cancers. Newer sunscreens block a wider range of ultraviolet rays and may prove to reduce even melanoma over time.[26] Children particularly should always wear sunscreen when playing outside to prevent the blistering sunburn associated with melanoma later in life. The sun's rays are the strongest between 10 a.m. and 2 p.m. (even on cloudy days) and direct exposure at that time should be avoided, even with a sunscreen. Protective clothing, such as hats, long-sleeve shirts, long pants, and ultraviolet-protecting sunglasses (too much sun can lead to cataracts or melanoma in the eyes), should be worn. Avoid tanning booths and sunlamps (see Real-World Wellness: Are Tanning Devices Hazardous to Your Health? on page 422). No matter how dark a person's skin is, he or she becomes darker when exposed to the sun. Although the risk is greatly reduced for darker-skinned people, anyone can get skin cancer.

Real-World Wellness

Are Tanning Devices Hazardous to Your Health?

I want to be tan this summer and thought I would get a head start by using a tanning bed. Is it safe for me to do so?

Sunlight produces two types of ultraviolet radiation: ultraviolet A (UVA) and ultraviolet B (UVB). UVB is 1,000 times more likely to cause burns than is UVA. Because it penetrates the skin more deeply, UVA radiation causes the skin to tan or burn more slowly. A small amount of UVB radiation, however, can cause skin damage.

Most tanning devices (for example, sunlamps) give off either mostly UVA or UVB radiation. Newer UVA sunlamps give off as much as 10 times more UVA than is received from the sun or given by older UVB sunlamps. Although exposure to UVA sunlamps is less likely to cause burns of the skin and eyes, UVA radiation in high doses may increase the risks for skin cancer and premature skin aging. Studies also suggest that skin cancer is exacerbated when people combine tanning in the sun with tanning by sunlamps. Here are some facts concerning tans and tanning devices:

- *Skin cancer* risks increase each time the skin is exposed to UV radiation.
- *Burns* of the skin and eyes may occur.
- *Photosensitivity* means being extra sensitive to UV radiation as a result of using or consuming various substances that may cause allergic reactions, severe skin burns, itchy and scaly skin, and rash. Examples of

photosensitizing products are soaps, shampoos, makeup, birth control pills, antibiotics, antihistamines, diuretics, and tranquilizers.

- *Cataracts,* an eye condition in which the lens becomes cloudy, may develop as a result of unprotected exposure to UVA and UVB radiation. For this reason, it is required that tanning devices have labels warning users to wear protective eyewear.
- *Premature skin aging,* in which the skin becomes dry, wrinkled, and leathery, is one of the most noticeable signs of repeated UV exposure.
- *Blood vessel damage and reduced immunity* may result from exposure to UV radiation.
- People who have red or blond hair and blue eyes, are fair-skinned, have freckles, and sunburn easily are at highest risk for skin damage. If you burn and do not tan in sunlight, you will probably burn and will not tan using sunlamps.
- A UVA tan offers some protection against further UV damage—about the same as an SPF of 2 or 3. Even with a dark tan, UV damage continues to accumulate.
- Sunscreens are not recommended for tanning indoors except to protect parts of your body you do not want to tan (for example, the lips). Sunscreens do not prevent UVA allergic-type reactions of photosensitive people.
- Always wear special goggles that block UV radiation, avoid using photosensitizing products, avoid tanning if your skin never tans, and follow the manufacturer's recommended time of exposure for your skin type.

Oral Cancer

Oral cancers are cancers of any part of the oral cavity, including the lip, tongue, mouth, and throat. Oral cancer occurs more than twice as often in males than in females. This is because the risk factors of cigar and pipe smoking and the use of smokeless tobacco are practiced much more frequently by men than by women. Cigarette smoking and excessive consumption of alcohol (both on the rise among women) are also considered risk factors. Wiser lifestyle choices (choosing not to use tobacco products and reducing the consumption of alcohol) could practically eliminate oral cancers.

Cancers That Can Affect Women

Breast cancer

Some women are at increased risk for breast cancer. Breast cancer is often fatal (in approximately 25 percent of cases). On the brighter side, advances in breast cancer

research have escalated (see Just the Facts: Drugs and Breast Cancer Treatment). Women's groups have done a good job of getting the word out about early detection and have supported efforts for improved treatment for all age groups except in women over fifty. These efforts have led to a decline in cancer deaths, but the surgeries and other treatments associated with breast cancer can still be devastating. Although breast cancer is relatively rare in men, about 1,460 men were diagnosed with it in 2004.

One in nine women who live to age 85 will develop breast cancer. Being over the age of 60 automatically places a woman in a high-risk category. Mutation in the genes known as *BRCA1, BRCA2* (also referred to as p53 suppressor genes) accounts for the development of breast cancer in some women. The BRCA gene is a tumor suppressor gene. When it is mutated, it no longer functions to suppress abnormal growth. Most DNA mutations related to breast cancer occur in single breast cells during a woman's life rather than having been

∿∿ Just the Facts ∿∿

Drugs and Breast Cancer Treatment

The drug tamoxifen has received a great deal of coverage in the press about its use as an anticancer drug. As with all drugs, tamoxifen has side effects. These side effects can be deadly, and use of the drug should be carefully considered. Tamoxifen has also been used as a cancer preventive among women at high risk (which can include any woman over 60 years of age, as well as younger women with several factors, including breast cancer in first-degree relatives). Other drugs that seem to reduce the rate of invasive breast cancer are raloxifene (a drug used to prevent bone loss); taxol, as a treatment in even late-stage cancer; and herceptin, which seems to delay progression of late-stage cancer.[30] Good news emerges almost daily about treatment for breast cancer. Early detection can result in a complete recovery.

inherited.[27] A woman with a mother or sister who has had breast cancer has double the risk of getting breast cancer. This risk is particularly high if the cancer occurred in the relative before menopause, if it involved both breasts, or if it affected more than one first-degree relative (for example, a mother and sister or two sisters) or other close relatives in several generations.

Still, most cases of breast cancer cannot be explained because most women have at least one risk factor. Other risk factors include early menarche (before age 12), late menopause (after age 55), recent use of oral contraceptives or postmenopausal estrogens, and never having had children or having given birth to a first child after age 30.[28] The role of lifestyle factors remains somewhat nebulous. Although breast cancer is worldwide, a strong cultural relationship exists between diet, especially high fat intake, and cancer. The reasons for this relationship have not been established.[3] Other factors related to the incidence of breast cancer are alcohol intake (women who have two to five drinks daily have about 1½ times the risk of women who are nondrinkers); weight gain, particularly following menopause; and physical inactivity.[28] No studies have conclusively linked cigarette smoking to breast cancer. Research is building that suggests smoking does increase the risk. What is known is that smoking affects overall health and increases the risk of developing many other types of cancer.

Early detection is the best means of reducing mortality (see Just the Facts: Cancer-Related Checkup Guidelines on page 424). The five-year survival rate for localized cancers is 96 percent. Localized spread of the cancer lowers that survival rate to 76 percent, and

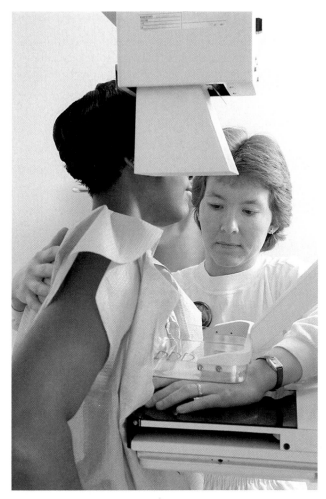

Mammography is important in the early detection of breast cancer.

distant metastasis yields only a 21 percent five-year survival rate.[28] Eighty percent of breast cancers are found by the affected women through self-examination. Monthly self-examination remains the primary way to find small, localized cancers, especially in young women (see Just the Facts: Breast Self-Examination on page 425). Mammograms are useful tools but are more useful for detection in older women whose breast tissue is less dense. Even the best mammogram misses 10 percent of tumors, because breast tissue extends beyond the area X-rayed in a mammogram. Examinations by qualified physicians are helpful in detecting breast cancer, but most examinations occur only on an annual or biannual basis. The time lapse between such exams provides aggressive, fast-growing tumors with time to spread to surrounding tissue or lymph nodes.

Symptoms include a tumor that may feel like a piece of gravel or hard nodule. The tumor will not enlarge and shrink in size from month to month. Other symptoms include thickening, swelling, dimpling, scaling, pain, and tenderness of the nipple or discharge

Cancer-Related Checkup Guidelines

Listed here are checkup guidelines to help healthy people with early cancer detection. These are guidelines and not rules. They apply only if none of the following seven warning signs is present:

C hange in bowel or bladder habits
A sore that does not heal
U nusual bleeding or discharge
T hickening or lump in breast or elsewhere
I ndigestion or difficulty swallowing
O bvious change in wart or moles
N agging cough or hoarseness

 Summary of American Cancer Society Recommendations for the Early Detection of Cancer in Asymptomatic People

Site	Recommendation
Breast	• Yearly mammograms are recommended starting at age 40. The age at which screening should be stopped should be individualized by considering the potential risks and benefits of screening in the context of overall health status and longevity. • Clinical breast exam should be part of a periodic health exam, about every three years for women in their 20s and 30s, and every year for women 40 and older. • Women should know how their breasts normally feel and report any breast change promptly to their health care providers. Breast self-exam is an option for women starting in their 20s. • Women at increased risk (e.g., family history, genetic tendency, past breast cancer) should talk with their doctors about the benefits and limitations of starting mammography screening earlier, having additional tests (i.e., breast ultrasound and MRI), or having more frequent exams.
Colon & rectum	Beginning at age 50, men and women should follow one of the examination schedules below: • A fecal occult blood test (FOBT) or fecal immunochemical test (FIT) every year • A flexible sigmoidoscopy (FSIG) every five years • Annual FOBT or FIT and flexible sigmoidoscopy every five years* • A double-contrast barium enema every five years • A colonoscopy every 10 years
Prostate	The PSA test and the digital rectal examination should be offered annually, beginning at age 50, to men who have a life expectancy of at least 10 years. Men at high risk (African American men and men with a strong family history of one or more first-degree relatives diagnosed with prostate cancer at an early age) should begin testing at age 45. For both men at average risk and high risk, information should be provided about what is known and what is uncertain about the benefits and limitations of early detection and treatment of prostate cancer so that they can make an informed decision about testing.
Uterus	**Cervix:** Screening should begin approximately three years after a woman begins having vaginal intercourse, but no later than 21 years of age. Screening should be done every year with regular Pap tests or every two years using liquid-based tests. At or after age 30, women who have had three normal test results in a row may get screened every two to three years. Alternatively, cervical cancer screening with HPV DNA testing and conventional or liquid-based cytology could be performed every three years. However, doctors may suggest a woman get screened more often if she has certain risk factors, such as HIV infection or a weak immune system. Women 70 years and older who have had three or more consecutive normal Pap tests in the last 10 years may choose to stop cervical cancer screening. Screening after total hysterectomy (with removal of the cervix) is not necessary unless the surgery was done as a treatment for cervical cancer. **Endometrium:** The American Cancer Society recommends that at the time of menopause all women should be informed about the risks and symptoms of endometrial cancer, and strongly encouraged to report any unexpected bleeding or spotting to their physicians. Annual screening for endometrial cancer with endometrial biopsy beginning at age 35 should be offered to women with or at risk for hereditary nonpolyposis colon cancer (HNPCC).
Cancer-related checkup	For individuals undergoing periodic health examinations, a cancer-related checkup should include health counseling, and depending on a person's age and gender, might include examinations for cancers of the thyroid, oral cavity, skin, lymph nodes, testes, and ovaries, as well as for some nonmalignant diseases.

*Combined testing is preferred over either annual FOBT or FIT, or FSIG every five years, alone. People who are at moderate or high risk for colorectal cancer should talk with a doctor about a different testing schedule.

SOURCE: © 2004. American Cancer Society, Inc.

Just the Facts

Breast Self-Examination

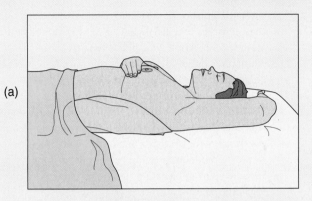
(a)

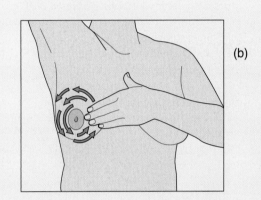
(b)

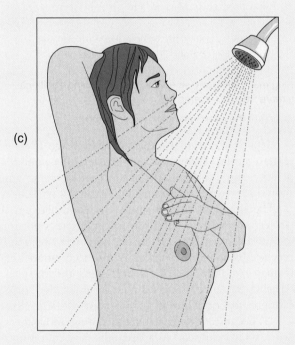
(c)

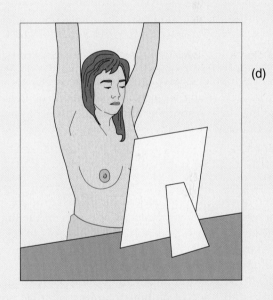
(d)

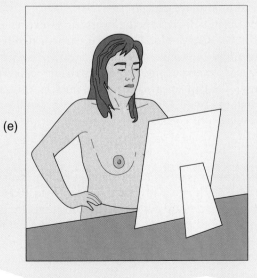
(e)

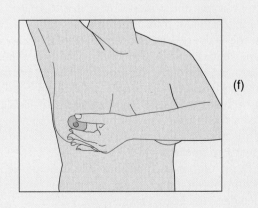
(f)

continued

Just the Facts

continued

Following are the proper techniques for examining the breasts.

1. Lying in bed, place a pillow under one shoulder to elevate and flatten the breast. Examine each breast using the opposite hand, first with your arm under your head and again with your arm at your side (a).
2. Make small, circular motions with the flat pads (not the tips) of your fingers (b).
3. Examine your breasts in concentric circles from the rims inward toward the nipples. Feel for knots, lumps, thickenings, indentations, and swellings. Be sure to include the armpit (b).
4. Wet, soapy skin makes it easier to feel lumps. Keep one hand overhead and examine each breast with the opposite hand while you are in the shower (c).
5. In front of a large mirror, stand with your arms relaxed at your sides. Examine your breasts for swelling, dimpling, bulges, retractions, irritations, and sores or changes in mole or nipple color, texture, or orientation.

Repeat with the arms extended and again with your arms clasped behind your head (d).

6. Repeat the inspection in step 5 while contracting your chest muscles: first clasp your hands in front of your forehead, squeezing your palms together; then place your palms flat on the sides of your hips, pressing downward. This highlights the bulges and indentations, which may signal the growth of tumors (e).
7. Bend forward from the hips, resting your hands on your knees or two chairbacks. Use a mirror to examine your breasts for normal irregularities and abnormal variances; both are pronounced in this position.
8. Squeeze your nipples to inspect for secretions and discharge (f).
9. Report any suspicious findings to your doctor without delay.
10. Supplement your self-examination with a breast examination by your doctor as part of a regular physical examination and cancer checkup.

---

from the nipple. Breast cancer can occur at any age, even in very young women. Anyone (male or female) detecting these symptoms should consult a physician without delay.

Uterine cancer

Uterine cancers can occur either in the cervix (cervical cancer, or cancer in the neck of the uterus) or in the endometrium (endometrial cancer, or cancer of the lining of the uterus). Cervical cancer is closely linked to sexual behavior, especially through transmission of the human papillomavirus. Because of its close association with sexual activity (sex at an early age, multiple partners, a partner who has had multiple partners, multiple pregnancies, and a history of sexually transmitted diseases, such as herpes and genital warts), many experts considered it a sexually transmitted disease. However, this is not the only reason people develop this cancer. As women have participated more frequently in annual Pap smears and preventive reproductive health, the number of deaths from cervical cancer has declined significantly (70 percent decrease).[1] Smoking seems to increase the risk for the disease. Prevention involves following safer sex practices (see Chapter 12), not smoking, and having regular Pap smears.

The symptoms include abnormal vaginal bleeding or spotting or discharge. Late symptoms include pain. When diagnosed early, invasive cervical cancer is one of the most treatable cancers, with a five-year survival rate

of 91 percent. Regular Pap smears after age 18 or after sexual activity if initiated (no matter how young) can detect early, abnormal cells or localized cancers. Women should have regular Pap smears for the rest of their lives.

The lining of the uterus is the endometrium. Endometrial cancers occur in the upper, broader portion of the uterus, as opposed to in the narrower opening (the cervix). Endometrial cancer is more common among women over the age of 50, following menopause. Increasing evidence points to high levels of the hormone estrogen as contributing to the course of the disease. This is because estrogen causes the lining of the uterus to grow, which can lead to a premalignant condition that can lead to invasive cancer.

Risk factors include being overweight (extreme obesity), diabetes, high blood pressure, early menarche (before age 12), late menopause (after age 52), never giving birth, and receiving unopposed estrogen replacement therapy. The Pap smear detects endometrial cancer less than half the time. Those with risk factors should check with their gynecologists.[28]

Ovarian cancer

Ovarian cancer is difficult to diagnose, having few symptoms until reaching an advanced stage. Five to 10 percent of ovarian cancers are inherited, meaning that family history and mutations in the same genes that are related to breast cancer (*BRCA1* and *BRCA2*) serve as potential markers. Symptoms are frequently vague and include cramping, discomfort, distention of the abdomen resulting from fluid buildup, diarrhea or constipation, gas, and a feeling of incomplete emptying of the bladder. Full-term pregnancies and breast-feeding, as well as the use of oral contraceptives, seem to reduce the risk. A high-fat diet seems to increase the risk. Fertility drugs that stimulate ovulation may be associated with increased risk.

Although considered a relatively rare cancer, late diagnosis can be deadly. If found in stage I, the cure rate is about 90 percent. The average age of women diagnosed with ovarian cancer is 61.[29]

Cancers That Can Affect Men

Testicular cancer

About 5,000 men and boys, usually ages 15 to 34, are diagnosed with testicular cancer per year. These are usually treatable. Testicular cancer is painless and asymptomatic, but it is detectable by self-examination. Every boy old enough to be in high school and every man should do a monthly self-exam until reaching the age of 40 (see Just the Facts: Testicular Self-Examination). Signs of possible testicular cancer include any lump, enlargement, or hardening of either testis. Any changes should be followed up with an examination by a physician. Undetected, the disease can spread to the lymph nodes and beyond. Early detection results in a high cure rate.[1,30]

Prostate cancer

Most men who live long enough will have some evidence of prostate cancer. The second leading cause of cancer death among men, prostate cancer has a 100 percent cure rate when diagnosed while localized (58 percent of prostate cancers). Improvement in diagnosis has resulted from a blood test for prostate-specific antigen (PSA test). The PSA test, in combination with a digital (manual) rectal exam (DRE), has made prostate cancer much easier to detect at earlier stages. There has been some research that the PSA test could still miss some prostate cancer, however.

Men at elevated risk include African Americans (who have incidence and death rates twice as high as those of white men), increasing age (PSAs and DREs should be annual events in men over age 50; prostate cancer is rare in young men), and men with family histories of prostate cancer. Dietary fat intake may also be a factor. African-American men and those with family histories should begin annual checkups at age 40.

The symptoms for prostate cancer tend to be nonspecific and similar to those of a condition known as *benign prostate hypertrophy*. They include weak or interrupted urine flow; inability to urinate; difficulty starting or stopping urine flow; frequent need to urinate, especially at night; pain or burning on urination; and continuing pain in the lower back, pelvis, or upper thighs.

Treatment

The best treatment for cancer is prevention by leading a wellness lifestyle. Even with a family history, it is impossible to determine at this time who will get cancer. Taking appropriate lifestyle measures may make the difference. Eating a healthy diet high in fruit, vegetable, and grain products; exercising regularly; avoiding tobacco products and excessive alcohol consumption; performing self-exams accurately and regularly; and getting screenings as recommended can save lives. Screenings that result in

Just the Facts

Testicular Self-Examination

Cancer of the testes (the male reproductive glands) is one of the most common cancers in men 15 to 34 years of age. It accounts for 12 percent of cancer deaths in this group. The best hope for early detection of testicular cancer is a simple, three-minute monthly self-examination. The best time is after a warm bath or shower, when the scrotal skin is most relaxed.

Roll each testicle gently between the thumb and fingers of both hands. If you find any hard lumps, or nodules, see your doctor promptly. The lumps, or nodules, may not be malignant, but only a doctor can make the diagnosis.

After a thorough physical examination, your doctor may perform X-ray studies for the most accurate diagnosis.

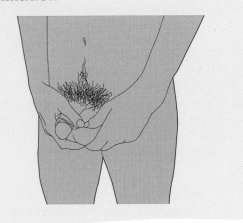

accurate diagnoses are vital. When detected while still local, prostate and thyroid cancers are considered 100 percent "curable" (the patient is still living with no signs of cancer at five years). The cure rate for melanoma and ovarian cancer, when diagnosed early is 95 percent; breast cancer is 96 percent; and testicular cancer is 99 percent.[1]

Traditional cancer treatment has involved the use of surgery, radiation, chemotherapy, or some combination of these three. Today, these more traditional approaches are being combined with new, experimental approaches. At the same time, traditional methods are being continuously refined, and every year, more experimental methods are being used. New treatments for cancer are being tested every day.

Surgery

Cancers are often treated surgically. A surgeon removes the malignant tissue and some additional normal tissue. Current surgical techniques focus on removing less surrounding normal tissue than before and combining surgery with chemotherapy and/or radiotherapy. Surgery is used most often with breast, skin, gastrointestinal tract, female reproductive organ, prostate, and testicular cancers.

Chemotherapy

Chemotherapy is the use of drugs and hormones to treat cancers. Eight years ago, 124 drugs were being tested as potential anticancer agents. Today there are 402 or more.[33] Some of the most important advances in the treatment of cancer have been in the area of chemotherapy. Most chemotherapeutic agents work by destroying the cancer cells' ability to carry out cell division and replication. Unfortunately, chemotherapy influences all cell division, even in healthy cells that need to divide to function normally. As a result, people having chemotherapy often have side effects, some of which can be dangerous. These side effects include suppression of the immune system, diarrhea, and hair loss.

Newer drug therapies take a different approach. New types of drugs include antigrowth drugs that block the body's signals that promote cancer cell growth (called antigrowth drugs); drugs that cause the cancer cells to self-destruct; antiangiogenesis drugs that cut off the cancer cell's blood supply; and drugs that "coordinate" radiation dosages with monoclonal antibodies (molecules specifically engineered to fit into the receptacles on certain cells) that target specific cancer cells. These drugs have much fewer and less severe side effects than traditional chemotherapies.

Antiangiogenesis Therapy

Antiangiogenesis therapy is the use of drugs to stop cancerous growths from developing new blood vessels. This type of therapy is one of the most promising treatments to come out of research in recent years. Since all parts of the body and every cell within those structures, including cancerous tumors, require a regular supply of blood to survive, antiangiogenic drugs prevent the formation of new blood vessels in the cancerous growths. Currently, there are more than 50 compounds that interfere with the reproduction of the blood vessels. Significant advantages of these drugs is that they have only mild side effects, as opposed to the devastating side effects of other treatments. The downside is that many of the early clinical treatments have been disappointing. What has been learned is that there are many factors that influence blood vessel growth. When combined with chemotherapy, an increase in length of life has been achieved, but, unfortunately, the present group of antiangiogenic drugs cannot bring about a cure.[31]

Radiotherapy

Radiotherapy is the use of radiation to destroy cancer cells or their reproductive mechanisms, so that they cannot replicate. As a result of radiation, side effects, such as diarrhea, itching, and difficulty swallowing, can occur. However, as the ability to plan more carefully the preciseness of focus, length of exposure, and time of treatment has improved, the damage to noncancerous cells and the potential side effects have decreased.

Bone Marrow and Peripheral Blood Stem Cell Transplants

Bone marrow is the spongy tissue that makes blood cells. Part of this process is making disease-fighting cells that are part of the immune system. Our blood cells start out as immature cells called *stem cells*. Stem cells are found primarily in bone marrow, where they produce blood cells.

There are three basic types of stem cell transplants. Where the stems are taken (the source) from determines the type. The three types are[32]

1. *Syngeneic SCT.* This is a very rare type of transplant because the donor is an identical twin.
2. *Allogeneic SCT.* This type of transplant comes from another individual whose tissue best matches the patient. The donor may or may not be a family member. There is a national registry where potential donors can be identified.
3. *Autologous SCT.* The patients act as their own donor. The stem cells are taken (called harvesting) from either the patient's bone marrow or his or her circulatory blood. After treating the stem cells with an extremely high dose of chemotherapy or radiation, they are frozen. This is called purging and is done to reduce the number of cancer cells.

Unfortunately, the purging may kill many of the stem cells. This type of transplant is used to treat lymphomas and myeloma.

Until the new bone marrow starts making new white blood cells (approximately six weeks), the patient is prone to infections, nosebleeds, bleeding gums, bruising, and pneumonia. The worse case is that the transplant can fail to function.

Immunotherapy

Immunotherapy is the use of a variety of substances to trigger a person's immune response, which then attacks malignant cells or keeps them from becoming active. The substances being used in this therapy are manufactured through genetic engineering. Among these technologies are interferon, interleukin-2 (proteins produced by the body to protect against viral invasions of healthy cells), tumor necrosis factor (TNF), and bone marrow growth regulators. Interferon is used for treating a rare blood cancer called *hairy cell leukemia*. Interleukin-2 is under study for the treatment of kidney cancer and melanoma. Vaccines against several types of cancer are also being developed. In early clinical trials, the vaccines have shown promise, but none have been approved for use against cancer.

Complementary Therapies

New technologies enhance the diagnosis and treatment of cancer. Magnetic resonance imaging (MRI) and computerized tomography (CT) scanning help detect and map hidden tumors. Bone marrow transplantation is now a treatment option for select patients with leukemia and lymphoma.

Other approaches that have been used or are under investigation as alternatives to conventional treatment or as methods to use in conjunction with traditional

Just the Facts

How 1 + 1 = 3: The Power of Synergy

Although research shows that people who eat diets high in vegetables and fruits have lower risks of developing certain cancers than people who eat less healthily, high-fat/high-meat diets, these results have not been replicated when people take supplements. The beta-carotene in a pill is not the same as the beta-carotene in a carrot because the results are not equivalent. One theory uses the word *synergy* to explain the difference. When beta-carotene, vitamin A, or vitamin C is ingested in food sources, such as fruits and vegetables, more than the vitamin is affecting the body. The phytochemicals and vitamins interact in such a way that their effect is "synergized," or magnified, so that greater results are achieved. Taking a pill is never a substitute for eating healthy food. Vitamins do not have the same ingredients in the same combinations as food, nor do they have the fiber! Don't try to take pills to make you more healthy. Eat healthily. It's as simple as five to nine fruits and vegetables every day![33]

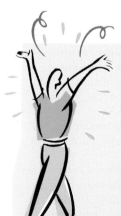

Nurturing Your Spirituality

Living Well with Cancer

Chemotherapy and other drug treatments offer potentially life-saving solutions for cancer patients. But does the cure lie solely in the doctor's office? Perhaps not. Research indicates that spiritual practices may increase a cancer patient's chance of survival and enhance his or her quality of life.

Scientists are studying how the mind affects the neurological and immune systems.[34] This discipline, known as *psychoneuroimmunology*, is of great interest to cancer researchers. For example, participation in support groups has been shown to increase the life expectancy of people with cancer. The results of a study reported by Johns Hopkins University are striking: "Women with breast cancer who took part in a support group lived an average of eighteen months longer (a doubling of the survival time following diagnosis) than those who did not participate. In addition, all the long-term survivors belonged to the therapy group."[35]

Although support groups do not improve physical health, they seem to provide a camaraderie that contributes to overall wellness. Belonging to groups such as prayer circles also plays a beneficial role in recovery. Support groups offer patients a sense of connectedness that promotes wellness. Conversely, social isolation—lack of a support network of friends and family—seems to increase the likelihood of death.[32] Although the extent of its influence is unknown, the nurturing of cancer patients' spiritual side as well as care for their physical health seems to help in the effort to maintain wellness.

therapies are acupressure, acupuncture, herbs, vitamins (for prevention and free radical removal), biofeedback (monitoring body functions to control body functions), homeopathy (use of extremely small doses of toxic substances), reflexology (massaging of certain areas of the feet), therapeutic touch (redirecting the "life forces" of the body), and visualization (envisioning a cure happening) (see Just the Facts: How 1 + 1 = 3: The Power of Synergy on page 429). Some of these alternative methods have been proven to help in the treatment process. Others seem to do nothing. Others are still being investigated (see Nurturing Your Spirituality: Living Well with Cancer on page 429). Some may become part of more traditional treatments. None of these approaches are substitutes for the medical approaches to treatment.

Today, more than ever, there is hope for anyone with cancer. Cancer trials are ongoing and new drugs are constantly being developed. Even the most deadly cancers have new treatments being tested. As more is learned about cancer, more will be done to stop its deadly attack on the human body.

Summary

- *Cancer* refers to a group of disorders characterized by uncontrolled, disorderly cell growth.
- Cancer is the second leading cause of death, and one in four Americans will eventually develop one or more of the 100 different forms.
- There are two types of tumors, or neoplasms. A malignant (cancerous) tumor can spread or metastasize (move from one location to another), while the second type of tumor, called benign, cannot.
- Cancer is caused by either external factors (chemicals, diet, radiation, viruses, pollutants) or internal factors (hormones, immune, inherited).
- A carcinogen is anything that triggers the development of cancer.
- A gene that enables cancer to develop is called an oncogene.
- Exercise has been found to help prevent colon, breast, and prostate cancers.
- Lung cancer is the leading cause of cancer death in the United States and throughout the world.
- Lung cancer is almost 100 percent preventable if people never smoke.
- Passive smoke (smoke from other people's tobacco products) is dangerous to the nonsmoker by increasing the risk of developing cancer.
- Colon and rectum cancer, when detected early, are very curable. Colon cancer is associated with family history, constipation, and high calorie consumption. Diet is believed to be the primary cause.
- Stomach cancer is relatively uncommon in the United States, although it is still ranked among the top 10 cancer killers. It is best prevented by a healthy diet.
- Liver and pancreatic cancers are relatively uncommon. Both are difficult to treat. The five-year survival rate for pancreatic cancer is only 4 percent.
- Leukemia is cancer of the blood-forming mechanisms, involving the white blood cells. It strikes both children and adults.
- Lymphoma is cancer of the lymphoid tissue. The two types of lymphoma are Hodgkin's disease and non-Hodgkin's lymphoma. Non-Hodgkin's includes all lymphomas except Hodgkin's.
- The three types of skin cancer are basal cell, squamous cell, and melanoma. Basal and squamous cell cancers are treatable. Melanoma, although most deadly, is treatable if detected early. Exposure to the sun's ultraviolet light is most responsible for causing the three types of skin cancer.
- The ABCDs of skin cancer are helpful in identifying melanoma: A = Asymmetry; B = Borders uneven; C = Color (different shades of brown or black); D = Diameter greater than 6 mm.
- Oral cancer affects the lip, tongue, mouth, and throat. Risk factors are cigar and pipe smoking and the use of smokeless tobacco.
- Statistics show that one in nine women who live to age 85 will develop breast cancer.
- A woman with a mother or sister with breast cancer has double the risk for breast cancer. Early detection is the best means of reducing mortality.
- Breast self-examination and mammograms are useful tools for preventing breast cancer.
- Uterine cancers can occur either in the cervix or in the endometrium. Cervical cancer is closely associated with sexual behavior, especially through transmission of the human papillomavirus. Smoking seems to increase the risk.
- Risk factors for uterine cancers include obesity, diabetes, high blood pressure, early menarche, late menopause, never giving birth, and unopposed estrogen replacement therapy.
- Ovarian cancer is difficult to detect. Its symptoms are frequently vague and include cramping, discomfort, distention of the abdomen, diarrhea or constipation, gas, and the feeling of incomplete emptying of the bladder.
- Testicular cancer is painless and asymptomatic but is detectable by self-examination. Early detection results in a high cure rate.
- Prostate cancer is the second leading cause of cancer death among men. The PSA and a digital rectal exam have made prostate cancer much easier to detect at earlier stages. These should be done annually after age 50. Symptoms include weak urine flow, inability to urinate, frequent need to urinate, painful or burning urination, and continuing pain in the lower back or upper thighs.
- Cancer is treated through the use of surgery, chemotherapy, radiotherapy, immunotherapy, antiangiogenesis, and stem cell transplantation.

Review Questions

1. Describe the process by which cancer cells develop.
2. What characteristics differentiate cancer cells from other cells?
3. Discuss lifestyle factors that may contribute to the development of cancer.
4. What factors other than lifestyle factors contribute to the development of cancer?
5. Explain the concept of oncogenes.
6. What role does exercise play in the prevention of colon, breast, and prostate cancers? What mechanisms seem to be aiding in the prevention of these cancers?
7. Differentiate among the three types of skin cancer.
8. What are the leading sites of cancer in females? In males?
9. Describe the conventional methods of treating cancer.
10. What are some measures an individual can take to prevent cancer?

References

1. American Cancer Society. 2004. Cancer prevention and early detection facts and figures 2004. Atlanta: American Cancer Society.
2. American Cancer Society. 2004. What is cancer? (http://www.cancer.org).
3. Margolis, S., and J. M. Samet. 1998. The Johns Hopkins White Papers: Early Detection and Prevention of Cancer. Baltimore, MD: The Johns Hopkins Medical Institutions.
4. International Agency for Research on Cancer. 2002. Tobacco smoke and involuntary smoking. IARC Monograph 83. Lyon France: IARC Press.
5. American Institute for Cancer Research. 2001. JAMA findings on diet and breast cancer misunderstood, experts say. *AICR Science News* 20:1–2.
6. American Cancer Society. 2004. Leaflet. Jesse Harris Cancer Answer Week leaflet.
7. Lee, I., and R. Paffenbarger. 1994. Physical activity and its relation to cancer risk: A prospective study of college alumni. *Medicine and Science in Sports and Exercise* 29:831.
8. American Institute of Cancer. 2004. Growing evidence clarifies numerous cancer fighting benefits of exercise (http://www.charitywork).
9. Wannamethee, S., A. Shaper, and M. Walker. 2001. Physical activity and risk of cancer in middle-aged men. *British Journal of Cancer* 85(9):1311–1316.
10. Nieman, D. 1999. Exercise testing and prescription—A health-related approach. 4th ed. Mountain View, CA: Mayfield Publishing Co.
11. Editors. July 25, 1998. Risks for colon cancer. *Health News* 7.
12. Patel, A., E. Calle, and L. Bernstein. 2003. Recreational physical activity and risk of postmenopausal breast cancer in large cohort of U.S. women. *Cancer Causes and Control* 14(6):519–29.
13. Bernstein, L., et al. 1994. Physical activity and the risk of breast cancer in young women. *Journal of the National Cancer Institute* 86:11403.
14. Dr. Anne McTiernan. 2004. Preventing breast cancer: A little exercise goes a long way. Special to ABCNEWS.com (http://abcnews.go.com/sections/living/DailyNews/exercise_breast_cancer020423.html).
15. Oliveria, S., H. Kohl, D. Trichopoulos, and S. Blair. 1996. The association between cardiorespiratory fitness and prostate cancer. *Medicine and Science in Sports and Exercise* 28:97.
16. Hackney, A. 1996. The male reproductive system and endurance exercise. *Medicine and Science in Sports and Exercise* 28:180.
17. American Cancer Society. 2004. What causes cancer? Cancer reference information (http://www.cancer.org).
18. World Cancer Research Fund/American Institute for Cancer Research. 1997. Food, nutrition and the prevention of cancer: A global perspective. Washington, DC: American Institute for Cancer Research.
19. Consumer Reports on Health. 1998. Fruits and vegetables: Nature's best protection. *Consumer Reports* 10(6):1.
20. American Cancer Society. 2004. What causes colorectal cancer? (http://www.cancer.org).
21. American Cancer Society. 2004. What are the risk factors for stomach cancer? Reference information (http://www.cancer.org).
22. American Cancer Society. 2004. Can liver cancer be prevented? Reference information (http://www.cancer.org).
23. American Cancer Society. 2004. What's new in pancreatic cancer research and treatment? Reference information (http://www.cancer.org).
24. Anderson, K. N., and L. E. Anderson. 1990. *Mosby's pocket dictionary of medicine, nursing, and allied health.* St. Louis: Mosby.
25. Editors. 1997. Health news: Evaluating melanoma risk. *The New England Journal of Medicine* 3(8):1–2.
26. University of California at Berkeley. 1998. Casting a shadow on sunscreens. *University of California at Berkeley Wellness Letter* 14(9):2.
27. American Cancer Society. 2004. Do we know what causes breast cancer? Reference information (http://www.cancer.org).
28. American Cancer Society. 2004. What are the risk factors for breast cancer? (http://www.cancer.org).
29. Harvard University. 1998. Ovarian cancer. *Harvard Women's Health Watch* 6(2):4–5.
30. Pitre, H. Prostate cancer update: An interview with Dr. Alan Koletsk. Patient Resource Center (www.salick.com/resource/features/prostateupdate.html).
31. American Cancer Society. 2004. Recent and current research in antiangiogenesis therapy (http://www.cancer.org).
32. American Cancer Society. 2004. What are the types of stem cell transplants? Available online at: http://www.cancer.org.
33. American Institute for Cancer Research. 2001. The anti-cancer power of synergy. Newsletter 72(Summer): 1–3.
34. Mayo Health Clinic. 1999. Mind over malignancy? Attitude and cancer survival (www.mayohealth.org/mayo9703/htm/mindover.htm).
35. Johns Hopkins University. 1999. Overview of NIH Office of Alternative Medicine Fields of Practice: Mind/Body Control (www.intelihealth.com).
36. American Cancer Society. 2005. Death rates dropping. ACS News. (January 2005) (http://www.cancer.org).

Suggested Readings

Dyer, D. 2004. *A dietitian's cancer story: Information and inspiration for recovery and healing from a three-time cancer survivor.* Washington, DC: American Cancer Society.

This book is used by thousands of cancer survivors as they search for strategies for improving their quality of life.

Kirkendoo, A. 2004. *The end of cancer.* Miami, FL: Lysmata.

This book is not about a magic bullet but, rather, a new way of thinking about and attacking cancer. The author brings together highly specialized topics in the areas of cancer research and molds items into a unified theory that makes a great deal of sense.

Link, J., M. James, C. Waisman, and C. Forstoff. 2003. *The breast cancer survival manual: A step-by-step guide for women with newly diagnosed breast cancer.* 3d ed. New York: Owl Books.

This is a comprehensive book on everything concerning the topic of breast cancer, including how breast cancer is characterized, the factors affecting prognosis, diet, exercise, and how to manage the psychological component of the disease.

14

Managing Common Conditions

Online Learning Center

Log on to our Online Learning Center (OLC) for access to these additional resources:

- Chapter key term flashcards
- Learning objectives
- Additional goals for behavior change
- Concentration game
- Self-scoring chapter quizzes

- Additional lab activities

The OLC also offers Web links for study and exploration of wellness topics. Access these links through **www.mhhe. com/anspaugh6e**, click on Student Center, click on Chapter 14, and then click on Web Activities.

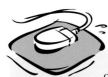

Goals for Behavior Change

- Identify your personal risk factors for the conditions discussed in this chapter.
- Select strategies for the prevention of these conditions.
- Initiate a prevention plan for any of the conditions identified as a potential personal risk.

Key Terms

allergens
arthritis
asthma
diabetes mellitus
headaches

influenza
osteoarthritis
osteoporosis
rheumatoid arthritis

Objectives

After completing this chapter, you will be able to do the following:

- Differentiate between Type 1 and Type 2 diabetes mellitus.
- Identify the common forms of arthritis.
- Describe the effects of calcium hormone therapy and exercise on osteoporosis.

- Discuss preventive measures and treatments that help reduce the severity and length of asthma attacks.
- Differentiate between the common cold and influenza.
- Distinguish among the different types of headache.
- Identify environmental factors that trigger headaches.

his chapter focuses on conditions that are detrimentally affected by lifestyle. If precautions are taken against the onset of these diseases, their impact on the body may be lessened or even avoided. Although every condition affected by lifestyle cannot be described, those that frequently occur and those on which lifestyle has the greatest impact are discussed, including diabetes, arthritis, osteoporosis, asthma, the common cold, influenza, and headaches.

Diabetes Mellitus

Diabetes mellitus is a group of diseases resulting from one of the following situations: The body doesn't make insulin, the body doesn't make enough insulin, or the body doesn't use insulin properly.[1] Diabetes is a metabolic disorder involving the pancreas. People with diabetes experience an abnormality in the way their bodies use glucose (blood sugar); this results from the deficient production of insulin by the pancreas or from resistance of the body's tissues to the action of insulin.[2] The blood may contain ample glucose (blood sugar), but without enough insulin available for use, the glucose cannot move from the bloodstream into the cells, where it is needed for fuel. As a result, people with diabetes cannot use the energy they consume, and high glucose levels build up in the blood and urine, leading to a condition known as *hyperglycemia* (high blood sugar). Large amounts of sugar in the urine require additional water, so that the sugar can be diluted for elimination. The body's increased need for water leads to a depletion of the body's water stores, causing excessive thirst and frequent urination. When the body becomes unable to completely break down glucose as a source of energy, fat must be used. Fat is metabolized differently than glucose, and its breakdown is incomplete when glucose is not available. Incomplete metabolism causes an excess amount of chemicals called *ketone bodies* to build up in the body. The buildup of ketones is used to perform the functions that glucose would perform under normal conditions (supplying energy), but the excess amounts of ketone bodies disrupt the body's chemical balance, altering the blood's chemistry and making it more acidic. Acidic conditions in the body are extremely hazardous.

Diabetes can be a serious disorder. The symptoms include excessive thirst; increased urination; hunger; a tendency to tire easily; wounds that heal slowly; blurred vision; and frequent skin, vaginal, and urinary tract infections. Dehydration and the buildup of ketones can cause ketoacidosis (the accumulation of ketones) and nausea, vomiting, abdominal pain, lethargy, and drowsiness. Ketoacidosis often leads to severe sickness, coma,

and even death. Of equal significance is that prolonged periods of elevated glucose levels disrupt normal enzyme and membrane functions.[3] Chronic complications that may result are eye disease, kidney disorders, painful nerve and muscle symptoms, and decreased circulation. Diabetes is a leading cause of foot and leg amputations. Diabetes can also produce impotence in men and increased risk for heart disease and heart attacks in both genders.

The prevalence of diabetes in the United States is 18.2 million people or 6.3 percent of the population. Of this number, 5.2 million people are unaware that they have diabetes. Approximately 1 in every 400 to 500 children and adolescents has Type 1 diabetes. Although nationally representative data for Type 2 diabetes are unavailable for youth, several studies indicate that Type 2 is becoming more common among children and adolescents.[4] Prevalence is becoming more common in American Indians, African Americans, and Hispanics. Rates are also increasing in white adolescents, but not at the same rate as that of the previously mentioned groups. Most researchers are attributing these alarming increases to sedentary lifestyles and the poor nutritional habits of adolescents.

Type 1 Diabetes

Diabetes consists of two diagnostic categories. *Type 1 diabetes* occurs most commonly in children and young adults, although it may develop at any age. Type 1 is an autoimmune disease in which the body produces antibodies that attack and damage its own cells—in this case, the insulin-producing cells of the pancreas.[2] The symptoms may be sudden and sometimes progress rapidly, requiring quick intervention to prevent death. People with Type 1 diabetes produce little or no insulin and require insulin injections to function. Before insulin was discovered, the average life span for a person with Type 1 diabetes was two years after diagnosis. Properly treated, these people now live almost as long as the general population.

Type 2 Diabetes

Type 2 diabetes is the most common type and is found primarily in people over the age of 40 (see Just the Facts: Type 2 Diabetes in Youth). Scientists believe that it is strongly linked to genetic factors. If an identical twin develops Type 2 diabetes, the other most likely will as well. People with Type 2 either develop a resistance to insulin activity or experience insufficient insulin action. Their bodies are usually capable of producing adequate amounts of insulin—something a person with Type 1 diabetes cannot do. The difficulty in Type 2 diabetes is that body cells become resistant to insulin at the receptor sites (the place where insulin attaches to the cell). There are several types of tests to diagnose diabetes. The

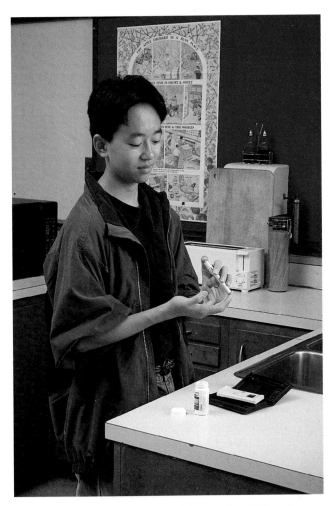

To manage their condition successfully, people with Type 1 diabetes must periodically test their blood glucose level.

most common test is the fasting glucose test. An individual is considered to have Type 2 diabetes if his or her fasting glucose value is above 125 mg/dL on at least two tests.[5] Type 2 is linked strongly to obesity. Almost 80 percent of diabetics with Type 2 are overweight at the time of diagnosis.[2]

Causes

Type 1 diabetes is an autoimmune disease. This means the body's immune system attacks a part of the body that is well. In Type 1 diabetes, the body produces antibodies that attack and damage the area of the pancreas that produces insulin. Initially, the ability to produce insulin is impaired, but eventually, usually in less than a year, little or no insulin is produced. The onset is usually before age 35 and often in childhood. Type 1 diabetes is sometimes associated with a viral infection within the insulin-producing cells, resulting in the inability to produce insulin.[1]

∿ Just the Facts ∿

Type 2 Diabetes in Youth

A growing number of children and adolescents are developing Type 2 diabetes. Typically, Type 2 diabetes occurs in youngsters who are overweight, are older than 10 years of age, are in middle to late puberty, and have a family history of Type 2 diabetes. Researchers expect that, as the American population becomes even more overweight, the frequency of Type 2 diabetes will increase in younger, prepubescent children. Since the development of Type 2 diabetes in children and adolescents is relatively new, accurate statistics regarding the number of Type 2 cases have not been reported, but it is estimated that between 8 and 45 percent of children with newly diagnosed cases of diabetes will have Type 2 diabetes.[5]

Heredity plays a role in Type 2 diabetes. In a study of 218 people with Type 2 diabetes, 66 percent reported at least one relative with diabetes, and 46 percent reported at least two relatives with diabetes. Patients whose mothers had diabetes were twice as likely to develop the disease than were those whose fathers had diabetes.[1]

Obesity also is an important factor (see Just the Facts: Preventing and Controlling the Effects of Diabetes). Not all people who are obese develop diabetes, but 90 percent of people with diabetes are overweight. Tumors of certain endocrine organs, such as the pituitary gland, adrenal glands, and pancreas, can all interfere

∿ Just the Facts ∿

Preventing and Controlling the Effects of Diabetes

Several lifestyle behaviors can significantly reduce the likelihood of developing Type 2 diabetes:

- Maintaining normal weight
- Exercising regularly
- Not smoking
- Maintaining blood pressure levels or treating high blood pressure
- Maintaining normal blood lipid levels
- Eating a low-fat, high-fiber diet

with or destroy insulin production. Taking cortico-steroids, used to treat asthma or arthritis, may result in latent diabetes.[1]

Treatment

Although there is no cure for diabetes, the disease can be controlled by diet, exercise, and/or insulin. People with Type 1 have to have insulin injections, usually several a day, and they must manipulate dosage levels according to dietary and activity levels (see Just the Facts: American Diabetes Association (ADA) Guidelines for Diabetes Screening). Self-administered blood glucose tests help them monitor blood sugar levels and determine the appropriate insulin dose. Good blood sugar control reduces the risk for the complications associated with Type 1 diabetes.

Many people with Type 2 diabetes can control their blood glucose by following a careful diet, exercising, losing weight, and taking oral medication. People with Type 2 may find it necessary to take medication to control their cholesterol and blood pressure. Of adults with diagnosed diabetes, 12 percent take both insulin and oral medication, 19 percent take insulin only, 53 percent take oral medication only, and 15 percent take neither insulin nor oral medication.[5] Losing weight helps lower insulin resistance, enabling the body to make more efficient use of the insulin available. Nutrition guidelines developed by the American Diabetes Association (ADA) dispel the notion of a diabetic diet that is good for everyone with the disease. For example, the previous emphasis on sugar consumption has given way to an emphasis on carbohydrate consumption.[6] The total amount of carbohydrate, regardless of its source, is what affects blood sugar levels.[6] Another example is that diabetics are now encouraged to consume monounsaturated fats. Type 2 studies at four medical centers showed better control of blood glucose levels when 45 percent of the calories came from fat, with highly monounsaturated olive oil as the predominant fat, and 40 percent from carbohydrate than when 55 percent came from carbohydrate and 30 percent came from fat.[7]

Evidence that links exercise to a decreased incidence of Type 2 diabetes is increasing. A study of 5,990 men showed that incidence rates declined as energy expenditure increased. For each 500-calorie increment in physical activity, the risk for Type 2 diabetes decreased by 6 percent. Men who increased their energy expenditure by 2,000 calories decreased their risk by 24 percent.[8,9] In a study of more than 21,000 male physicians, men who exercised just once a week had 23 percent less chance of developing Type 2 diabetes than did men who did not exercise.

Exercise lowers blood sugar levels by reducing the body's resistance to insulin. Cells become more sensitive

to insulin and more capable of absorbing glucose. The effect is lower levels of circulating blood sugar. This benefit of exercise, however, lasts for only 24 hours, which means exercise must be done every day. Regular activity doesn't seem to have the same dramatic effect on Type 1 diabetes, but it does lower the amount of insulin needed and the risk for cardiovascular disease.[1] (See Just the Facts: Advances in Treating Diabetes.)

Many of the complications associated with diabetes are preventable or treatable, but diagnosis and proper treatment are necessary (see Wellness for a Lifetime: Are

〜〜 Just the Facts 〜〜

Advances in Treating Diabetes[4]

Medications

There are new classes of blood glucose–lowering drugs. Those drugs are sulfonylureas, meglitinides, biguanides, alpha-glucosidase inhibitors, and thiazolidinediones. Each class of drugs increases insulin, slows absorption of blood sugar, or makes the body more sensitive to the effects of insulin.

New Types of Insulin

Newer types of insulin more closely mimic natural insulin. Newer types of insulin are absorbed more quickly and prevent glucose levels from rising too high after meals. One type is long-acting and requires only one injection a day. Researchers are hopeful that the long-acting varieties will enable more consistent blood sugar control over an entire day.

Methods of Delivering Insulin

The most common method of delivering insulin is with either a syringe or an insulin pen. Now available are insulin pumps, which provide a continuous supply through a tiny needle implanted under the skin, eliminating the need for shots. Other delivery systems being experimented with include skin patches, nasal sprays, and oral inhalers.

More Efficient Methods of Monitoring Glucose

The FDA has approved the first device that combines a glucose meter, insulin pump, and a dosing calculator. There also are new devices that use lasers and electrical currents to monitor blood glucose levels without having to prick a finger to obtain a blood sample.

Islet Cell Transplant

Islet cells are found in the pancreas and produce insulin. In Type 1 diabetes, when these cells are destroyed, diabetes develops. Researchers have developed a method to implant new islet cells in the liver. Although still experimental, this procedure is showing promise and may eventually lead to a cure for Type 1 diabetes. Better drugs to prevent rejection and new surgical techniques are eliminating many of the past problems with such transplants.

Pancreas Transplants

This procedure is usually reserved for people under age 45 and with Type 1 diabetes. Unfortunately, not all transplants are successful; however, when a successful transplant occurs, the need to take insulin is eliminated, but there is a need to take immune-suppressing drugs, which may lead to serious side effects.

Wellness for a Lifetime

Are Illness and Chronic Disease Inevitable as We Age?

As the population of the United States continues to age, chronic conditions are becoming increasingly common. The largest group of maturing adults, known as *baby boomers*, were born after World War II, between 1946 and 1964. Are they doomed to develop age-related conditions? Will you or someone close to you inevitably have to face a chronic condition or disease associated with aging?

The answer for all age groups is a resounding NO. We may have genetic predispositions of which we should be aware; however, we can embrace the concepts of wellness, including maintaining an active lifestyle, eating properly, not smoking, and controlling stress. By doing so, we may be able to delay the onset of many chronic conditions, diminish their severity, or prevent the factors that cause them. The earlier we begin to practice positive behaviors, the greater the likelihood of healthy outcomes.

All people can make health-related choices that enhance their well-being and that of their families and communities. It is imperative that we accept responsibility for improving our lives. Regardless of age, we are empowered through our attitudes and actions to create a high quality of life. Wellness is a journey, not a destination, filled with opportunities for joy, happiness, learning, and making the most of each day.

Illness and Chronic Disease Inevitable as We Age?). Neglect of diabetes and its complications may result in early death (see Just the Facts: Major Complications of Diabetes on page 442).

Prediabetes

In the past few years, physicians have identified a condition referred to as prediabetes. This condition exists when blood glucose levels are higher than normal but are not high enough for a diagnosis of diabetes. Prediabetes is sometimes referred to as impaired fasting glucose (IFG) or impaired glucose tolerance (IGT), depending on the test used to identify the condition. Individuals with

～～Just the Facts～～

Major Complications of Diabetes

Several serious complications can result from diabetes. Most of the following complications are caused by blood vessel damage:

- *Coronary heart disease (CHD):* People with diabetes have two to four times more risk of dying from CHD than do people without diabetes.

- *Nerve damage:* Between 60 and 70 percent of people with diabetes have some form of nerve damage.

- *Foot problems:* Because of peripheral nerve damage, foot problems can go unnoticed. Proper treatment for conditions such as athlete's foot, blisters, and calluses is extremely important. Any sign of infection should be treated immediately to avert the need for amputation.

- *Kidney damage:* Thirty to 40 percent of people with Type 1 diabetes and 20 percent of those with Type 2 diabetes eventually develop kidney disease, which can lead to kidney failure.

- *Peripheral vascular disease (PVD):* Diabetes and smoking can double or triple the risk for PVD (atherosclerosis) in the arteries of the legs, which increases the risk for foot and leg problems, including the possibility of amputation.

- *Skin problems:* People with diabetes are at increased risk for skin infections.

- *Stroke:* People with diabetes have a two to four times greater risk for stroke.

- *Vision loss:* Diabetic retinopathy (retina disease) is the leading cause of blindness. People with diabetes are also at increased risk for glaucoma and cataracts.

prediabetes are at a higher risk of developing Type 2 diabetes, heart disease, and stroke. An important point is that the progression from prediabetes to Type 2 diabetes is not inevitable. Research has indicated that, with weight loss and increased exercise, the progression to Type 2 can be delayed or prevented and that blood glucose levels may return to normal.[5] It is estimated that as many as 16 million people may have prediabetes.

Gestational Diabetes

Gestational diabetes is Type 2 diabetes that occurs in some women during pregnancy. It is more common among obese women and those with a family history of the disease. The condition must be normalized to prevent complications in the infant. After pregnancy, 5 to

10 percent are found to have Type 2 diabetes and those who have had gestational diabetes have a 20 to 50 percent chance of developing Type 2 diabetes in the next 10 years.[5]

Exercise and Diabetes

The need for exercise for the individual with diabetes is the same as that for anyone without the condition. The American Diabetes Association recommends a total of 30 minutes a day at least five days a week. The exercise routine for a diabetic should incorporate the same components as for a nondiabetic. It should include an aerobic component, strength training, and flexibility exercises.

There are several precautions a diabetic must take when engaging in an exercise program. A physician should be consulted to ensure that there are no exercise activities that would be contraindicated. An exercise stress test may be recommended to determine how the heart reacts to exercise. It is essential that the exerciser learn how his or her blood glucose responds to exercise. Checking the glucose level before and after exercise can demonstrate the benefits of exercise. If the blood glucose is above 300, exercise can elevate it even higher; thus, caution should be used when engaging in exercise. For those with Type 1 diabetes when the glucose level is above 250 and ketones are present in the urine, exercise should be avoided.

For the diabetic exerciser, avoiding low blood glucose (hypoglycemia) also is important. Sometimes eating a snack before exercising or adjusting medications will alleviate any problems with hypoglycemia. Blood glucose should be checked during exercise if symptoms, such as nervousness or shakiness, are noticed. If the blood glucose is 70 or below, fruit juice, a soft drink, or glucose tablets can be used to raise the glucose level.[10] There should always be snacks and water available during exercise. Lastly, it is imperative that a medical ID tag be worn, in case an emergency does occur.

Arthritis

Arthritis is an inflammatory disease of the joints. The more than 100 varieties of arthritis include gout, ankylosing spondylitis, systemic lupus erythematosis, osteoarthritis, and rheumatoid arthritis. Osteoarthritis and rheumatoid arthritis occur most often. Both result in pain and deformed joints.

Osteoarthritis, also known as *degenerative joint disease,* is the most common form of arthritis, affecting more than 20 million Americans. By age 40, about 90 percent of people have X-ray evidence of osteoarthritis in the weight-bearing joints, such as the hips and knees, although symptoms generally do not appear until later in life.[11] Men typically develop symptoms before age 45, whereas women usually have them after age 55. Men more often have osteoarthritis in the hips, knees, and spine, and women are more likely to have it in the hands and knees.[11] It is the most limiting chronic condition affecting women in the United States.[11]

Osteoarthritis is characterized by the gradual breakdown of cartilage, which comes with age. The first signs are microscopic pits and fissures on the cartilage surface that cause the cartilage to crack and lose its resilience.[13] Tiny pieces of cartilage may break off into the joint cavity. The result is a change in the contours of the articular surfaces. Finally, patches of exposed bone appear, causing mechanical-type friction and irritation. The bone responds by trying to repair itself, but the repair is disorderly. As a result, joint surfaces thicken and bone spurs (osteophytes) form.

The deterioration associated with osteoarthritis seems related to the wear and tear of daily living, age, and injury. Other factors may include heredity, diet, abnormal use of joints (for example, throwing a curve ball every day year after year), excessive weight, stress, and impaired blood supply to affected joints.

Treatment for osteoarthritis includes aspirin and cortisone drugs to relieve pain. Mild exercise, heat, cold, or a combination of heat and cold application accompanied by massage can be used. Exercise is used for therapeutic purposes to help maintain range of motion and to strengthen the muscles that can help alleviate joint problems. Research has shown that physical activity decreases joint pain, improves function, and delays disability. A special exercise program called PACE (People with Arthritis Can Exercise) teaches people how to safely increase their exercise activity.[13]

An eight-week walking study[14] involving patients with osteoarthritis of the knee (one of the most common arthritic problems) provides a reason for optimism regarding exercise. Patients who walked 30 minutes three times a week reported a 27 percent decrease in pain and an improved ability to walk longer distances, compared with a nonwalking control group. The researchers concluded that supervised walking can be helpful for people with significant arthritis of the knee. Stretching exercises also help relieve arthritis pain by lengthening tendons, which reduces muscle spasms, the source of much of the pain in osteoarthritis. However, the results of other studies have shown that exercise may not contribute to relief of pain. In addition, exercise of an arthritic joint may cause pain that can be relieved only by rest.

Rheumatoid arthritis is one of the most crippling forms of arthritis. It affects about 1 percent of the adult population worldwide. More than 2.5 million Americans have this condition, and more than 60 percent of those affected are women.[12] The onset of rheumatoid arthritis is usually between the ages of 20 and 45. Although the

exact causes are unknown, this form of arthritis may be an autoimmune disease. The most obvious damage occurs in joints, but the disease affects the whole body. The symptoms of rheumatoid arthritis include joint swelling, redness, stiffness, pain, muscle atrophy, joint deformity, and limited mobility. The condition is unpredictable because it can suddenly flare up and just as suddenly go into remission. Emotional stress is often associated with an attack. The disease frequently results in disability.

Treatment includes a mixture of rest periods, gentle exercise, physical therapy, and medication. The emphasis is on relieving pain, reducing inflammation, maintaining function of the joints, and preventing deformities (see Nurturing Your Spirituality: Living Well with a Chronic Condition on page 444).

Osteoporosis

Osteoporosis is a chronic disease in which the mineral content of the bones progressively decreases, so that the bones become brittle and are easily broken. It is linked to more than 1 million fractures of the hip, spine, and other bones each year. Vertebral bones in the spine shrink and fracture, causing a deformed spine. Bones in the wrist are also common fracture sites. Some 44 million Americans, 68 percent of whom are women,[15] are affected by osteoporosis. Although postmenopausal white and Asian women are at highest risk, men and women of all ages and ethnicities can be affected.[15]

Though bones may seem hard, they are made of living cells that require calcium and vitamin D (necessary for the optimum absorption of calcium) to grow and stay strong. Almost all of the body's calcium stores are located in bone.[15] During growth and development, bones typically receive more calcium than they give up. By age 25, when bone density peaks, calcium absorption levels off; at age 30, the bone-building process is over. This is when bone-mass maintenance and calcium are especially important.[15] If blood levels of calcium drop, the body withdraws what it needs from its bones. With adequate dietary intake of calcium, bones are spared the effects of calcium depletion that may accelerate osteoporosis.

Calcium is not the only factor associated with bone loss. Estrogen depletion during menopause triggers bone loss of up to 1 percent a year. By the time a woman is 80, she may have lost 30 to 40 percent of her bone mass. When bone-mass loss becomes excessive, a fall may not be needed to fracture bones. Bending over and lifting 25 pounds—a heavy bag of groceries—could cause injury.

Because nicotine is thought to decrease blood levels of estrogen, smoking also contributes to bone loss. Smokers go through menopause on average at least two years earlier than nonsmokers.[15] Genetics may also play a role in osteoporosis. Researchers have identified an osteoporosis gene that determines how well vitamin D

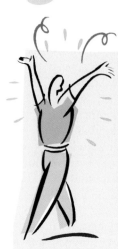

Nurturing Your Spirituality

Living Well with a Chronic Condition

Many people have potentially debilitating or even life-threatening conditions, such as asthma, diabetes, and high blood pressure. Proper management of these conditions makes it possible for these people to live long lives. A person with a chronic condition may even have a quality of life as high as that of someone who does not have a chronic condition. If you have a chronic disease, you can learn to manage it effectively.

First, you need to know as much as you can about your condition. Knowledge is power. The more you know, the better you will be able to understand the condition and its treatment. More important, great strides are being made every day in the treatment of many diseases, and a cure may be possible in your lifetime. A trusted physician who takes the time to listen to you and to explain your options can be helpful. You should explore your alternatives and participate in making decisions. Taking an active role helps

physically, because no one knows your body like you do, and it empowers you to avoid feeling like a victim.

Second, having a support system, such as your family or a group of people who have the same condition you do, can foster your emotional well-being in many ways. Having someone to whom you can express your frustrations or fears and from whom you can receive unconditional support provides security. Knowing others who share your feelings can make you feel less alone. Often, those who have the same condition as you can offer solutions you hadn't considered. You can also find ways to laugh together about those moments of utter distress when you feel different from everyone else. The bonds people create when they share their problems can be lifelong, making the difficult times easier to bear.

Life lessons can be learned in many situations. Everyone has his or her share of problems. Sometimes having a chronic condition may seem unfair, but we are all less lucky than some and better off than others. All people struggle to find ways to be grateful for life every day and to jump life's hurdles. Take care of yourself, make friends, find inner peace, and share with others. Then your life will be full no matter what challenges life hands you.

---

facilitates the absorption of calcium. People who have the gene are more resistant to absorbing available calcium. Caffeine and alcohol have also been implicated in bone loss. A recent study found that women who drank two or more cups of caffeinated coffee a day and drank no milk experienced significant loss of bone density after menopause. The effects of caffeine can be negated with consumption of milk. In the same study, coffee drinkers who drank at least one glass of milk per day had 6.5 percent higher bone density than the coffee-only group.[16]

The National Osteoporosis Foundation recommends several steps to reduce the risk of contracting this disease. First, consume adequate amounts of calcium, preferably from food. If this doesn't work, calcium supplements are recommended. The foundation suggests 1,500 mg, almost double the amount given in the RDA.[17] Second, consume enough vitamin D (400 IU) to permit absorption of the calcium. Third, consider hormone replacement therapy (estrogen) and discuss its use with your medical doctor, especially if you have a family history of osteoporosis. And fourth, participate in weight-bearing activities, such as walking, running, and weight training, to prevent bone loss. In one study, women who participated in a year-long exercise program and received daily doses of estrogen experienced a 7 percent increase in bone density and fared better than women on estrogen alone.[16] Physical exercise forces bones to adapt to the stresses imposed on them, and they hypertrophy in response. Bones atrophy when they are unstressed.

The Food and Drug Administration currently approves of three drugs for the prevention and treatment of postmenopausal osteoporosis. These drugs are alendronate, raloxifene, and resedronate. Another drug, teriparatide, is approved for postmenopausal women and for men at high risk for fracture. Estrogen hormone therapy is still utilized for treatment; however, because of the findings of The Women's Health Initiative (WHI) (see Chapter 13) estrogen replacement therapy should be considered carefully and only after a serious discussion with a physician. Even if accepted as a treatment, estrogen replacement therapy should be used on a short-term basis. Based on the results of the WHI study, the nonestrogen medications should be used instead.[15]

People with osteoporosis can and should exercise, but the type of physical activity and the intensity of exercise must be carefully selected. Forceful contractions of muscles and high-impact activities should be avoided because they may stress the bones beyond their breaking point. Swimming, water aerobics, stationary cycling, walking, and light weight training are good starting activities for those with osteoporosis.

Asthma

Asthma is a chronic respiratory condition characterized by attacks of wheezing and difficulty in breathing. The cause of asthma attacks is partial obstruction of bronchi and bronchioles resulting from the contraction or spasm of the muscles in the bronchial walls. Researchers have discovered that asthma results from immune malfunction.[23] Although the underlying cause of asthma is not known, there are three key features:

1. *Hyper-irritability.* Bronchi are very sensitive to **allergens,** such as cold air, cigarette smoke, fumes, and animal dander.
2. *Muscle spasm.* When the bronchial walls are exposed to an irritant, the walls constrict and narrow the bronchial passages. This is referred to as *reversible airway obstruction,* because bronchial muscles can still relax but the spasm causes wheezing. Some individuals who wheeze can breathe fairly efficiently while seriously impaired.
3. *Inflammation.* Most individuals with asthma have some chronic bronchial inflammation, which causes excess mucus production and swelling. The inflammation is probably caused by exposure to an irritant. It is bronchial inflammation that causes the coughing associated with asthma.

Attacks may be mild or severe and may last anywhere from a few minutes to a few days. Asthma may develop at any age, although many children with asthma outgrow the condition as they get older and the bronchial passages widen. Asthma may be hereditary.

The two major types of asthma are extrinsic and intrinsic. Extrinsic asthma is the most common type and is typically triggered by a hypersensitivity to irritants or allergens, such as dust, pollen, feathers, animal dander, molds, smoke, extremely cold or dry air, and air pollutants. For some asthmatics, drugs, food allergies, and exercise induce an attack.

Intrinsic asthma is caused by factors such as stress or frequent respiratory tract infections. This form of asthma is less common than extrinsic asthma, but its symptoms are similar.

There is no cure for asthma, but there are preventive measures and treatments that help reduce the severity and length of an attack. One form of prevention is immunotherapy, in which the asthmatic is desensitized through injections of weakened allergens. Medications, such as corticosteroid drugs, reduce inflammation and serve as a primary intervention for many asthmatics.

Bronchodilator drugs (medicines that open the bronchioles) are used routinely by asthmatics when an asthma attack occurs. These drugs are breathed in through an inhaler and usually restore normal breathing in several minutes. (See Wellness on the Web: Breathing Easier: Getting the Facts on Asthma.)

One way to anticipate an impending attack or to determine the severity of an actual attack is to use a peak-flow meter, a small, hand-held device (available at drugstores) that measures airflow. Peak airflow will go down hours and sometimes even a day or two

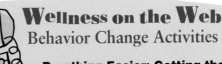

before an attack, so the meter can serve as an early warning system. During an attack, it provides an objective way to determine how much the air passages in the lungs narrow.

Exercise-induced asthma is common among asthmatics. The symptoms include a coughing attack and tightness in the chest during or shortly after exercise. It appears to be most common when the asthmatic exercises in cold, dry air. Still, physical activity remains an integral part of wellness for people with exercise-induced asthma. Improvements in fitness and health status occur in asthmatics who exercise. An added benefit is that, for many asthmatics, exercise is accompanied by a decrease in the frequency and severity of exercise-induced attacks (Figure 14-1, page 446). See Assessment Activity 14-2.

The Common Cold

More than 200 viruses, known as *rhinoviruses,* can cause the common cold.[18] A person may develop a temporary immunity to one or two viruses and still be infected by another. Anytime people are together, viruses that cause the common cold are present. Adults average 2 or 3 colds each year, and children experience 6 to 10. Most colds occur during the fall and winter. Their incidence begins in late August to early September, increasing slowly for a few weeks thereafter, and remains high until March/April. Seasonal changes in humidity seem to affect the

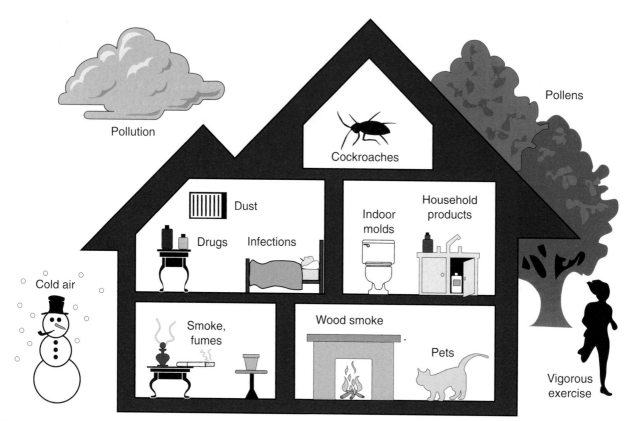

Figure 14-1 Common Asthma Triggers

If you have asthma, do you know which triggers are troublesome for you?

prevalence of colds, since the most common cold-causing viruses survive better in low humidity in the colder months of the year. The cold weather also tends to make the nasal passages drier and thus more vulnerable to viral infections. Colds can be spread by shaking hands, sneezing, and breathing. Evidence indicates that hand-to-hand contact is the most common way a cold is spread. When infected people blow or touch their noses, the virus is transferred to their hands. When an uninfected person touches the infected person's hands, the virus is again transferred. Touching the face with hands that carry the virus leads directly to developing a cold. Frequent hand washing may prevent the spread of the virus.

The signs and symptoms of a cold are easily recognized. They include a feeling of listlessness, general aches and pains, watery eyes, and runny nasal passages. As the cold progresses, the nasal membranes swell, resulting in a stuffy nose. Infections affecting the throat can lead to sore throats and coughing. These symptoms tend to last 7 to 10 days. As an old axiom points out, if a cold is treated, it will go away in 7 days and, if left alone, it will last a week. A cold may occasionally persist for several weeks, but complications are infrequent in adults and older children. When they do occur, they most often are middle ear or sinus infections.

Antibiotics do not cure the common cold because they fight only bacterial infections. Over-the-counter decongestants—in spray or pill form—constrict blood vessels to shrink nasal swelling and open air passages, providing temporary relief of cold symptoms. Nasal sprays are more effective because they deliver a greater concentration of medicine to the nasal passages and give immediate relief.[19] But their overuse can cause a rebound effect, making congestion even worse. Nasal sprays should not be used for more than three consecutive days. Antihistamines are not effective for cold symptoms and may lead to drowsiness. Cough suppressants, which may offer relief from nagging coughing episodes, should be used with caution. On the positive side, the cough reflex is nature's way of clearing the lungs; on the negative side, persistent coughing may irritate the airway. A pharmacist or medical doctor should be consulted for help matching the appropriate cough medicine with the type of cough (dry or loose mucus).

The best advice for treating a cold is to take aspirin, ibuprofen, or acetaminophen (young children shouldn't take aspirin with cold symptoms because it may cause Reye's syndrome); drink plenty of fluids; eat a nutritious diet; and get plenty of rest.

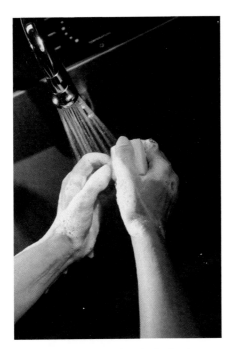

Washing your hands often is the best way to prevent the common cold.

Influenza

Influenza, or flu, is caused by a virus. There are three primary strains of the influenza virus: A, B, and C. Most influenza develops from the A and B strains. These strains can change genetically, reappearing in an altered form every few years. The symptoms of all types of flu include chills, fever, weakness, headache, sore throat, dry cough, nausea, vomiting, and muscular aches and pains. All symptoms may not be present, and the severity varies greatly among people. Treatment for flu is the same as for the common cold. Aspirin should not be taken by children or teenagers because the potentially fatal Reye's syndrome can develop.

Vaccines can prevent particular types of influenza. Current recommendations are that priority in vaccination should be given to children and adults with chronic cardiovascular and lung disorders; residents of nursing homes; medical personnel who may transmit the virus to high-risk patients; everyone over 65; and anyone with conditions such as diabetes, kidney disease, hereditary anemias, and impaired natural immunity.

Headaches

One of the conditions that causes great discomfort is the headache. Some **headaches** are the result of injury or brain disease, but most are caused by distress, tension, anxiety, and environmental factors. Tension headaches are the most common. Caused by involuntary contractions of the scalp, head, and neck muscles, tension headaches may be precipitated by anxiety, stress, and allergic reactions. Tension headaches can often be relieved by massaging the scalp and muscles in the neck. Aspirin, acetaminophen, or ibuprofen pain relievers usually alleviate tension headaches.

Migraine headaches are characterized by throbbing pain that can last for hours or even days. Nausea and vomiting occasionally occur. Migraines, which seem to be initiated by stress, range from mild to severe. Migraines are considered a neurological disease with a hereditary link.[20] An abnormal drop in serotonin (a brain chemical that regulates blood vessel changes and controls pain) causes blood vessels near the surface of the brain to dilate, prompting nerve sensations perceived as pain. People who experience migraines may experience what is called an "aura"—flicker or jagged points of light that distort vision. Other symptoms include a throbbing pain, usually on one side of the head and accompanied by nausea or vomiting.

There are two types of treatment for a migraine. The first treatment plan is to relieve the pain as quickly as possible. Treatment is begun immediately when a migraine is perceived to be starting. The second approach to treatment is to prevent migraines before they occur. Several drugs for prevention are available, including the serotonin antagonists, with the main drug for migraine called somatriptan (Imitrex). Other brand-name drugs include Zomig, Amerge, Maxait, Axert, and Frova. Also available is a nasal spray named Stadol. This spray is a narcotic and thus is habit-forming. Obviously, this medicine should be used cautiously.[20]

Cluster headaches usually cause a knifelike pain behind the eye that quickly spreads to the forehead. The pain can spread to the neck, to the back of the head, and even into the teeth. The nose often runs, and the involved eye tears. The pain is often described as one of the worst pains a person can endure. Cluster headaches get their name because they occur in clusters, at least one each day and sometimes several times a day. The attacks begin suddenly and may last from several minutes to several hours. In extreme cases, they last a few weeks or several months. Affected people may be symptom-free for weeks or months. The cause of cluster headaches is unknown, but these headaches appear to be related to arterial constriction and dilation.

A wide range of environmental factors may trigger headache pain. Exposure to smoke (including secondhand smoke), carbon monoxide (automobile exhaust, defective furnaces), alcohol, caffeine, and certain foods causes headaches in many people. Alcohol causes blood vessels to dilate, adding blood flow to irritated nerve endings. Caffeine in small amounts may help relieve headache pain by constricting blood vessels; in larger quantities (more than 2 cups), blood vessels dilate, which may lead to rebound headaches. Heavy coffee drinkers may experience withdrawal headaches if they try to cut out caffeine cold turkey. A progressive reduction in caffeine over the course of a week or two should provide an appropriate acclimatization. Food triggers are most likely to be those containing amines. Amines cause blood vessels to constrict and dilate. Common dietary sources are aged cheeses, red wine, citrus fruits, and chocolates. Food additives, such as nitrates in hot dogs, smoked foods, and cold cuts, and flavor enhancers, such as monosodium glutamate (MSG), are often accused of provoking headaches.[21]

Many illnesses can cause a headache. Sinusitis, teeth and gum problems, high blood pressure, hypothyroidism, acute anemia, Cushing's disease, and Addison's disease are common offenders.[21] A complete physical exam can help identify specific medical causes. A headache should be evaluated by a physician if it is chronic, associated with a fever, accompanied by numbness or paralysis, associated with a stiff neck, interfering with thinking or memory, and/or continuing to get worse.

Treatment of headache pain includes a full gamut of interventions. Techniques such as deep breathing, progressive relaxation, biofeedback, meditation, and visualization seem to help relieve the pain in some sufferers. New drugs that block headache pain without negatively

Real-World Wellness

Dealing with Headaches

I've heard about many remedies for headaches. What are the best ways to deal with the various types of headaches?

The following are some methods[22] for managing headaches:

• Migraine	Sumatriptan, an injectable, oral, or nasal application constricts the arteries of head; can be used alone or in combination with the drugs ergotamine, tartrate, cafergot, or belladonna
• Tension	Over-the-counter analgesics; if chronic, antidepressants
• Cluster	For acute attacks, sumatriptan or inhaled oxygen; preventive drugs, such as methysergide, steroids, or lithium
• Sinus	Decongestants; antibiotics if needed

affecting other parts of the body are in the final stages of testing and could become available in the near future (see Real-World Wellness: Dealing with Headaches).

Summary

- Diabetes mellitus is a group of diseases with one of the following symptoms: The body doesn't make insulin, it doesn't make enough insulin, or it doesn't use insulin properly.
- The two major categories of diabetes are Type 1 and Type 2.
- Type 1 diabetes usually occurs early in life and requires insulin injections because the pancreas loses its ability to produce insulin.
- Type 2 diabetes occurs most often in people over 40 years of age who do not exercise and are obese.
- Arthritis is an inflammatory disease of the joints. The most common form of arthritis is osteoarthritis, characterized by deterioration of the cartilage covering the surfaces of the bones in certain joints.
- It is believed that rheumatoid arthritis is a disease of the immune system that results in joint swelling, pain, deformity, and decreased mobility.
- Asthma may be caused by extrinsic factors, such as pollen or dust, or intrinsic factors, such as stress.

- The common cold is caused by rhinoviruses, of which there are more than 200 varieties. Antibiotics do not cure colds.
- Influenza is caused by only three strains of virus, but these agents have the ability to change and reappear in different forms. Because influenza can range widely in severity, certain high-risk groups are encouraged to have an annual flu vaccine.
- Osteoporosis is a chronic disease characterized by a loss of mineral content of the bones, which makes them brittle and vulnerable to breakage.
- Mild to moderate exercises are effective in promoting bone strength in the elderly.
- Headaches are divided into three categories—tension, cluster, and migraine. People who experience migraines can use techniques such as deep breathing and meditation to alleviate pain or prevent the onset of a headache.

Review Questions

1. Explain the difference between Type 1 and Type 2 diabetes.
2. Describe the main symptoms of diabetes.
3. What are the most serious potential complications of uncontrolled diabetes?
4. What steps can be taken to prevent the development of Type 2 diabetes?
5. Explain the differences between the two most common forms of arthritis, their causes, and their possible treatments.

6. Discuss the relationship among calcium, estrogen, exercise, and osteoporosis.
7. What are some measures and treatments that help reduce the severity and length of an asthma attack or prevent it altogether?
8. What behaviors may help prevent and treat the common cold?
9. Explain how the influenza viruses differ from the common cold viruses.
10. Explain the differences between tension headaches and migraine headaches. How do the causes, symptoms, and treatments differ?
11. What environmental factors can trigger headache pain?
12. What role does physical activity play in the various conditions discussed in this chapter?

References

1. Mayo Clinic. 1998. Diabetes-weight control and exercise may keep you off the road to high blood sugar. *Mayo Clinic Health Letter* 16(2).
2. Margolis, S., and C. D. Saudek. 2003. *The Johns Hopkins White Papers: Diabetes Mellitus—2003.* Baltimore, MD: The Johns Hopkins Medical Institution.
3. Margolis, S. 2001. *The Johns Hopkins consumer guide to medical tests.* New York: Rebus.
4. Mayo Clinic. 2004. Diabetes-taking action to prevent or control this condition. Medical Essay-Supplement to *Mayo Clinic Health Letter.* February.
5. National Diabetes Information Clearinghouse. 2004. National diabetes status (http://diabetes.niddk.nih.gov/dm/pubs/statistics/index.htm).
6. American Diabetes Association. 2004. Making healthy food choices (http://www.diabetes.org).
7. Editors. 1997. Dealing with diabetes: Diet and exercise hold key to control. *Environmental Nutrition—The Newsletter of Food, Nutrition and Health* 20(12).
8. Editors. 1994. Diabetic diet shifts emphasis from carbs toward "mono" fats. *Environmental Nutrition—The Newsletter of Food, Nutrition and Health* 17(10).
9. Helmrich, S. P., D. R. Ragland, and R. S. Paffenbarger. 1994. Prevention of noninsulin-dependent diabetes mellitus with physical activity. *Medicine and Science in Sports and Exercise* 26:824.
10. American Diabetes Association. 2004. Getting Started. Available online at http://www.diabetes.org.
11. Margolis, S., and J. A. Flynn. 1998. *Arthritis.* Baltimore, MD: The Johns Hopkins Medical Institution.
12. Margolis, S. 2002. *The Johns Hopkins medical guide to health after 50.* New York: Medical Letter.
13. American Osteopathic Association. 2004. Arthritis. Available online at http://www.osteopathic.org.
14. Lamb, L. 1992. Exercise helps osteoarthritis. *Health Letter* 39(11):4.
15. National Institutes of Health. 2004. Osteoporosis (http://www.osteo.org).
16. Alberts, N. 1995. Osteoporosis. *American Health* 14(9):70.
17. Liebman, B. 1994. Calcium: After the craze. *Nutrition Action Health Letter* 21(5):1.
18. National Institutes of Allergy and Infectious Disease. 2004. The common cold. Available online at http://www.naid.nih.gov/factsheets/cold.htm.
19. Consumers Union. 1996. Finding the right cold medicine. *Consumer Reports* 61–62.
20. Family Doctor. 2004. Migraine headache: Ways to deal with the pain (http://www.familydoctor.org).
21. Halpern, G. M. 1994. Headache can be a pain in the neck. *Healthline* 13(7):9.
22. Harvard University. 1998. Migraine—more than a headache. *Harvard Health Letter* 23(3):4.
23. American Academy of Allergy, Asthma, and Immunology. Patient's Guide to Asthma (http://www.aaaai.org).

Suggested Readings

Fanta, C., L. Cristian, and K. Haver. 2003. *Taking control of asthma.* New York: Tree Press.

This is a comprehensive, authoritative presentation of asthma written in layman's terms. It contains extensive coverage of current therapies, as well as the pros and cons of the various medications. Stress is singled out as an asthma trigger. Other allergens are identified and suggestions given for avoiding or alleviating asthma.

Ruderman, N., J. Devlin, and S. Schneider. 2002. *Handbook of exercise in diabetes.* Alexandria, VA: American Diabetes Association.

This book provides a comprehensive exercise program for the prevention and treatment of diabetes. It contains data on the effects of exercise on blood glucose and metabolism, treatment plans, and information on how exercise affects the many conditions associated with diabetes.

Tyrell, D., and M. Fielder. 2003. *Cold wars: The fight against the common cold.* New York: Oxford University Press.

This book traces the history of the common cold and the many remedies used to "help" sufferers. The progress in understanding the psychological aspects of colds and the latest research on prevention and cures are presented.

Name _____ Date _____ Section _____

Assessment Activity 14-2

Managing Your Asthma

Directions: If you have asthma, there are many things you can do to help manage your condition effectively. To assess your personal health management, place a check mark next to each statement that applies to you.

Reducing or Avoiding Asthma Triggers

_____ I have identified my asthma triggers.

_____ I do not smoke and I avoid environmental tobacco smoke.

_____ I use and properly maintain an air filter and an air conditioner to keep my home cleaner and more comfortable.

_____ I avoid vacuuming or I use a dust mask when vacuuming.

_____ I avoid mowing the lawn or I use a dust mask when mowing.

_____ I avoid woodstoves and fireplaces.

_____ I use dust-proof encasings on my pillows, mattress, and box spring.

_____ I use a dehumidifier as necessary in my home to reduce indoor mold.

_____ I use window shades or curtains made of plastic or other washable material for easy cleaning.

_____ My closets contain only needed clothing. Anything I do not currently wear is stored in plastic garment bags.

_____ I do not sleep or lie down on upholstered furniture.

_____ If I have a pet, it does not sleep in or go into my bedroom.

_____ I avoid perfume and cologne, cleaning chemicals, paint, and talcum powder as much as possible.

Preventing and Managing Asthma Attacks

_____ I have learned everything I can about asthma.

_____ I take my medications as prescribed by my physician.

_____ I carry my inhaler with me at all times.

_____ I have a crisis plan for managing a severe asthma attack.

_____ I keep emergency numbers by the phone and with me at all times.

_____ I know how quickly my asthma medications should work.

_____ I use a peak-flow meter to anticipate and respond quickly to asthma attacks.

Interpretation

17 or more items checked: You are doing a great job avoiding asthma triggers and preventing and managing asthma attacks.

14–16 items checked: In many ways, you are doing a good job of managing your asthma. However, you may be unnecessarily exposing yourself to common asthma triggers, or your plan for preventing and managing attacks may need some work.

13 or fewer items checked: You need to manage your asthma much more effectively. Remember that an asthma attack can be fatal.

Discuss this assessment with other members of your family or your roommates. Ask them to help you with your asthma prevention and management program.

15

Becoming a Responsible Health Care Consumer

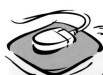

Online Learning Center

Log on to our Online Learning Center (OLC) for access to these additional resources:

- Chapter key term flashcards
- Learning objectives
- Additional goals for behavior change
- Concentration game
- Self-scoring chapter quizzes

- Additional lab activities

The OLC also offers Web links for study and exploration of wellness topics. Access these links through **www.mhhe.com/ anspaugh6e**, click on Student Center, click on Chapter 15, and then click on Web Activities.

Goals for Behavior Change

- Apply criteria for determining whether health information is valid, reliable, and based on scientifically controlled studies.
- Identify specific strategies for enhancing communication with your physician.
- Determine the diagnostic tests and immunizations appropriate for your age, gender, and health status.
- Find a specific online newsgroup or patient support group that might be helpful to you.

Key Terms

absolute risks
alternative medicine
contraindications
defensive medicine
diagnostic laboratory tests
direct access testing (DAT)
double-blind study
epidemiologic studies
false negative
false positive
health insurance
health maintenance
  organization (HMO)
iatrogenic condition
immunizations
implied consent
informed consent

periodic examinations
placebo
point of service (POS)
polypharmacy
preferred provider
  organization (PPO)
primary-care physician
relative risks
reliability
risk factor
scientifically controlled
  studies
selective health examinations
self-care
statistical relationship
statistical significance
validity

Objectives

After completing this chapter, you will be able to do the following:

- Explain how to evaluate the accuracy, validity, and reliability of health information.
- Discuss the criteria for determining when, where, and how to choose health care.
- Describe the functions and purposes of the major components of a physical examination.

raditionally, Americans have had a rather passive attitude toward health care. Whether taking medicine, purchasing health care products, undergoing surgery, or having a diagnostic test administered, people have operated as if following orders. Fortunately, this attitude is changing. People are viewing themselves as active participants in their health care. They are asking questions, placing demands on *health care providers* (people and/or facilities that provide health care services), getting second opinions, and sometimes even refusing treatments. People realize that they must assume more responsibility for safeguarding their health. With this responsibility, however, comes the challenge of knowing what one can and should ...lf. The purpose of this chapter is to lay the ... you to become an informed, active participant in ...re marketplace.

... ...th

Informa...

The first and perhaps m... sumers is to make sense of th... plosion. Many popular magaz... articles, newspapers often ... icine, the publications of hea... evision programs feature numerous heal... ... thousands of scientific, health-related studies are published daily. Interest in health information appears to have reached an all-time high.

The availability of so much health information has drawbacks; the major drawback is that so much of the information is confusing, sometimes even contradictory. Even medical experts have trouble separating fact from fiction. It is not unusual for a new finding to be headlined one day and completely refuted the next. For some people, the seemingly endless contradictions and medical flip-flops lead to an attitude that, carried to the extreme, completely disregards new developments and information, even those with life-saving potential. Two examples illustrate this point. For years eggs have been on everyone's list of foods to be avoided because they are high in cholesterol and increase the heart disease risk of many Americans. The assumption was that dietary cholesterol from egg yolks caused high blood cholesterol. The American Heart Association recently changed its position on this issue and no longer sets a limit on the number of eggs a healthy person can eat, as long as the total amount of dietary cholesterol averages no more than 300 milligrams a day (one egg contains 213 milligrams cholesterol).[1] Why the change? Now we know that saturated fat in the diet has more of an effect on blood cholesterol than dietary cholesterol. This was not known several years ago.

Another nutrition example is soy. For several years, experts have promoted the health benefits of soy products. Chapter 6 of this text identifies soy protein as a good nonmeat source of protein. Consumers have gotten the message and soy products are staple items in the grocery store. However, recently the power of soy consumption to lower heart disease risk was downgraded— in other words, another flip-flop. What are we to believe? Like many health claims, the truth is not clearly black or white. In the case of soy products, a consistent, high intake of soy foods every single day is required to produce heart health benefits. Experts caution people against relying on "casual" soy consumption to improve blood cholesterol levels.[2]

Countless other examples could be cited that explain the skepticism, even distrust, of many people toward medical information. The challenge for most people is to keep an open mind and realize that health information is constantly evolving. Cholesterol is a good example. At one time, cholesterol was thought to be the major risk factor for heart disease. Nothing else seemed to matter. Then it was learned that some people with high choles-... ...l... sign of atherosclerosis; conversely, ... for in-depth discussion of this risk factor). Now we know it is the cholesterol carriers in the form of low-density lipoproteins (LDLs) and high-density lipoproteins (HDLs) that earn our attention. Today's emphasis on LDLs and HDLs doesn't mean that the early messages about cholesterol were completely wrong. They were the first steps in understanding a complex issue. Without the early interest in cholesterol, it is unlikely that we would have learned what we know today about cholesterol carriers. Will today's knowledge about LDLs and HDLs be obsolete tomorrow? Possibly. But if that is the case, it is likely that it will have served as an important building block for the medical truths of tomorrow. Much of what is known about health and medicine is like this. The editor of a highly respected health newsletter states the dilemma clearly: "Science proceeds by one good article or study at a time. There's never a direct, final answer because our information keeps increasing. So consumers and doctors often need to make tough decisions amid incomplete, changing, and contradictory information."[3]

Given the mixed messages about health, it is perhaps a good idea to adopt a somewhat skeptical attitude, especially toward extreme and sensational health claims. The First Amendment to the U.S. Constitution, which guarantees freedom of the press, also guarantees Americans the right to publish health-related nonsense. The

Just the Facts

The Making of a Medical Flip-Flop[4]

Many of the health contradictions, or medical flip-flops, can be explained by the differences in motives between journalists and researchers. Journalists often highlight unusual findings to grab your attention. The goal is to sell newspapers, magazines, or, in the case of television, time. Researchers, on the other hand, typically view each new study as a steppingstone to the truth, well aware that the latest finding may not stand the test of time. It is the body of evidence—confirmed and reconfirmed—not the latest headlines, that should influence decisions.

Often, what seems like a flip-flop is a shift in emphasis for scientists. To the casual reader, it may appear as a contradiction. For example, it is common knowledge that dietary fat, especially saturated fat, is bad for health. But now it appears that an extremely low-fat diet may be worse for some people than a moderately fat diet, especially if much of it consists of monounsaturated and omega-3 fatty acids. To the layperson, the fat message appears to be flip-flopping; in reality, it isn't. It became more complex, requiring researchers to refine the message.

SOURCE: Forman, A. 2001. Why nutrition advice flip-flops all the time . . . or does it? *Environmental Nutrition* 24(3):1, 6.

more you read, generally the more contradictions you will uncover (see Just the Facts: The Making of a Medical Flip-Flop). This should not make you feel uncomfortable but, to the contrary, make you realize that medicine is still as much art as science.

Guidelines for Evaluating Health Information

Adhering to the guidelines that follow should help your search for correct health information.

Avoid Jumping to Conclusions

Most health misinformation is based on facts, not lies. The problem is that facts get exaggerated and sometimes lead people to wrong conclusions.

A good example involves potato chips, which have long been considered a junk food. Actually, the quick cooking process of potato chips preserves nutrients better than mashing, boiling, or baking potatoes. Ounce per ounce, potato chips provide more nutrients than do other forms of potatoes. This information alone might convince people to begin consuming large quantities of potato chips. However, because potato chips are cooked in oil, they are high in fat and calories and are not recommended for people trying to lose weight. This extra bit of information gives a completely different angle to the perspective on potato chips. By being aware that the truth of most health issues is not simple, the tendency to oversimplify and overgeneralize health information can be thwarted.

Remember That Health Discoveries Take Time

Health discoveries often make their way into media headlines, but a cardinal rule of science is that findings must be replicable. Health information based on a dramatic discovery is not usually considered valid unless it is confirmed in several follow-up studies or experiments.

Beware of Headline Reading

Newspaper, magazine, and television headlines are intended to arouse your curiosity primarily for one purpose: to make you buy or watch. A headline might cleverly capture the essence of a story or it might present a partial truth that leads to wrong conclusions. A common media strategy is to sensationalize a story by crafting a headline that contradicts conventional wisdom. Consider some recent examples: "Snacking Cuts Cholesterol," "Live Longer, Drink Wine," "Calcium Linked to Prostate Cancer." These headlines are fraught with possible deceptions. They may represent the results of isolated studies that run against mainstream medical thought. They may serve as punchlines for stories based on studies with many shortcomings. Or they may actually represent new trends in thinking supported by a medical consensus. The only way to know for sure is to become a well-informed, discriminating consumer of information the way you are a consumer of products, goods, and services. The challenge is to avoid the tendency toward headline reading and to apply the criteria for determining if health information is both valid and reliable.

Apply the Criteria for Determining Validity and Reliability of Health Information

Health information that can be trusted is based on studies that are valid, reliable, and reported in a way that includes research and statistics in their proper context. When assessing validity and reliability, know the type of study that serves as the basis for new information. Knowing the meanings of the following terms will help put new information in a proper context.

Validity

In health research, **validity** means *truthfulness*. If a study is designed and conducted properly, its findings are likely to be valid. For example, it was found that adding vitamin E to human cells in the laboratory stimulated cell division and growth. This was used to support the erroneous conclusion that vitamin E would delay the aging process. This was not a proper generalization because a simple laboratory experiment is not a valid procedure for demonstrating something as complex as aging.

Reliability

Reliability is another key criterion for evaluating health information. It is the extent to which health claims can be consistently verified. If a claim is reliable, it can be demonstrated to occur consistently in study after study. The test of time is perhaps the ultimate criterion for evaluating the trustworthiness of new information.

Statistical significance

Researchers and reporters often use the term **statistical significance** to give meaning and credibility to findings. For example, in one study a group of college students who ate breakfast every morning before going to class did better in school than a comparison group who skipped breakfast. The differences were reported to be statistically significant. Does this mean that the differences between the two groups were large, maybe equivalent to a full letter grade? Does this mean that breakfast is the key to academic success? Statistical significance does not necessarily imply largeness, but it does imply probability. *Statistical significance* means that the probability that a findings are due to chance alone is less than 5 percent. 95 of 100 times similarly designed studies or results. If the differences between statistically significant, they may be and might not show up again if a many studies are performed, statistically significant results Consequently, it takes hundreds of conflicting, to create a consensus. Any health claim worth considering numerous studies or experiments.

Statistical relationship

Statistical relationship more variables or events. Much health literature is based on statistical relationships or associations. For example, it is well known that a statistical relationship exists between the consumption of salt and blood pressure for some people. In other words, an increase in salt intake is accompanied by an increase in blood pressure. Conversely, a drop in salt intake is associated with a decrease in blood pressure. This is helpful information, but does it mean that high salt intake causes high blood pressure? No. If this were true, then all Americans who eat too much salt would have high blood pressure. The mistake many people make is to conclude that one event in a statistical relationship causes the other. Relationships are important and helpful clues to health and they provide a basis for better understanding health risks. However, they cannot and do not establish cause and effect.

Risk factor

The term **risk factor** refers to health habits and/or practices that increase the risk of getting certain diseases. The emphasis in Chapter 2, for example, is on those risk factors related to heart disease. Risk factors may be reported in terms of absolute risks or relative risks. **Absolute risks** indicate the actual number or percentage of people affected by a risk factor. **Relative risks** indicate the number or percentage of people affected by a risk factor in relation to or comparison with something else. Relative risks are often cited in the media because they are more impressive and make better headlines than absolute risks. But relative risks are also more misleading than absolute risks. For example, consider the following headline: "Bicycle Deaths Quadruple Auto Deaths on College Campus." The basis for the headline was a study that reported that the risk for death from bicycling to school increased 100 percent over the previous year, whereas deaths caused by driving to school increased by only 25 percent. The reporter incorrectly concluded that bicycling is four times more risky (relative risk) than driving. What is missing is information about baseline risk. If the baseline risk of deaths from bicycling is 1 in 1,000, a 100 percent increase raises it to 2 in 1,000. If the baseline risk for driving to school is 400 in 1,000, then a 25 percent increase boosts the risk for death by 100 to 500 in 1,000. Driving to school then turns out to be 250 times more risky (absolute risk) than bicycling to school, a complete reversal of the meaning of the headline. Although this example is hypothetical, it serves as a reminder of the importance of inquiring about the chances of getting a disease in the first place before drawing conclusions regarding risk factors, diseases, and death.

Risk factors are also often reported out of context. If they are reported fairly and accurately, they still are interpret. For example, how is a woman a diagnosis that indicates she has a 1 in 77 chance of developing breast cancer in the next five years? Does this imply a high risk, a low risk, or average risk? Is the risk sufficient to consider aggressive and sometimes dangerous treatments? She and her family may be alarmed by these odds until they learn that these are the same odds of dying in an automobile accident after 50 years of driving.[5] When confronted with a statistical assessment of risks, it is helpful and sometimes reassuring to ask for comparison benchmarks.

Ask Questions About Information

Answers to four questions about the nature and type of study will help you sort through the contradictory findings and claims reported in the popular press.

What type of study was used?

There are several types of studies and each has certain advantages and limitations. **Epidemiologic studies** are population studies (rather than scientifically controlled experimental studies) that observe the health habits and lifestyles of thousands of people for a period of time. The Framingham Study in Framingham, Massachusetts, is perhaps the longest-running and most famous epidemiologic study in the United States. It has yielded information that has been invaluable to our understanding of the risk factors associated with many diseases, especially heart disease. Epidemiologic studies may be *prospective* or *retrospective*. In a prospective study, researchers follow a group of people at a specific point in time and identify relationships between lifestyle and diseases. In a retrospective study, researchers look back in time to identify possible disease relationships. Retrospective studies are generally considered less reliable than prospective studies. An advantage of epidemiologic studies is that they tend to be more generalizable to the population at large. A disadvantage is that they do not prove cause and effect.

Scientifically controlled studies are experiments conducted in controlled settings. The classic study is a **double-blind study** that includes at least two groups, one that is an experimental group and receives some form of experimental treatment and another that is a control group and receives no treatment. The double-blind feature of a study ensures that neither the researcher nor the subjects know who is receiving an experimental treatment and, therefore, will not influence the outcome with that knowledge. If a researcher wanted to prove, for example, that a particular brand of soap prevents athlete's foot, one group of subjects would use the experimental soap and the other would use a **placebo,** or soap substitute. Researchers administering the soap treatment would not know which soap each subject was using, nor would the subjects in the experimental and control groups know. If the experimental group had significantly fewer cases of athlete's foot, the results could then be attributed to the treatment.

The experimental-control, double-blind requirement of scientific research is a difficult standard to meet. Such studies are costly and require considerable resources and manpower. Typically, they are referred to in the press as *clinical trials* or *population intervention studies*. The advantage of scientifically controlled studies is that they control the variables, so that it is often possible to establish cause-and-effect relationships. The disadvantage is that results usually apply to a narrowly defined population group and lack generalizability to the general population.

What were the characteristics of the people included in the study?

Scientific studies require random sampling of subjects to represent the diverse racial, religious, gender, and cultural characteristics of the population at large. Medical breakthroughs should not be based on a small number of homogeneous, or similar, subjects. Broadly designed human clinical trials that are randomized (a systematic sorting of subjects according to the laws of chance), that are placebo controlled, and that include a double blind offer the strongest proof of reliable information.[6] If a study is limited to one gender or ethnic group, its findings will not apply to anyone of a different gender or ethnicity. If the study involves animals, avoid drawing conclusions until subsequent human studies are conducted.

If you are at low risk for a condition being studied, the results probably do not apply to you. The consumption of alcohol illustrates the point. A number of studies report that one drink per day for a woman and up to two drinks a day for a man may reduce the risks associated with heart disease. These studies affect only people who have heart disease and consume alcoholic beverages. If you do not have heart disease and if you do not drink beverages that contain alcohol, the study findings are not relevant to you.

Remember, true breakthroughs in medical research are the exception rather than the rule.

How many people were in the study?

In general, the more people included in a study, the better. If a study reports findings that are based on a small number of subjects or patients, be cautious about drawing conclusions. Small-scale studies are seriously limited in their ability to generalize to the public, regardless of how tightly controlled they are. It is not unusual for the media, in their quest to be first to get the word out, to blow medical findings out of proportion. Sometimes small research projects give reason to be hopeful; sometimes they just lead to false hope. Large-scale studies involving many people and repeated over time lead to findings that are reliable and generalizable.

Who funded the study?

Businesses stand to gain or lose substantial sums of money (and reputation) from headline stories featuring their products. Consider the huge upswing in profits experienced by businesses in the pharmaceutical industry when several studies reported the weight-loss benefits of new diet drugs. Profits were staggering; so were the losses when the drugs were later pulled off the market. Before jumping to conclusions, inquire about the funding source.

Consider the Sources of Information

Valid and reliable health information comes from respected journals, magazines, and newsletters. Such publications have experienced health or medical editors who subject their articles to peer review and criticism by other scientists. Because little or no space is devoted to advertising, they are less inclined to be influenced by the need to protect the reputation or promote the product of a sponsor or an advertiser. Several of these newsletters are available free online (see Just the Facts: Health Help You Can Trust on the Internet).

Health information and the Internet

People who have access to a computer and an Internet service provider can obtain health and medical information that once was available only to those in the medical

Just the Facts

Health Help You Can Trust on the Internet

The Internet has grown so rapidly that it would take volumes to list all of the available Web sites that offer health information. Even if that were feasible, there would be little assurance that the information could be trusted. Fortunately, several respected health organizations have reviewed selected Web sites and identified the ones that are useful and reliable. A few of these sites are listed here. Remember that many more excellent sites are available. (A $$ sign indicates that the Web site may charge a fee for use.)

Newsletters

- Harvard Medical School publications at **www.harvardhealth.org**
- HealthNews at **www.webmd.com**
- Johns Hopkins InteliHealth Newsletter at **www.intelihealth.com**
- Mayo Health Oasis at **www.mayoclinic.org**
- Nutrition Action Health Letter at **www.cspinet.org**
- Tufts University Health and Nutrition Newsletter at **http://healthletter.tufts.edu**

Medical Database, Links, and/or Search Engines

- Achoo at **www.achoo.com**
- Centers for Disease Control and Prevention at **www.cdc.gov**
- Hardin Meta Directory of Internet Health Sources at **www.lib.uiowa.edu/hardin/md/pharm.html**
- Health-Resource at **www.thehealthresource.com** ($$)
- HealthAtoZ at **www.Healthatoz.com**
- Healthtouch at **www.healthtouch.com**
- HealthWeb at **www.healthweb.org**
- Medical Matrix at **www.medmarix.org**
- MedicineNet at **www.medicinenet.com**

- MEDLINE (also National Library of Medicine) at **www.medlineplus.gov**
- Medscape at **www.medscape.com**
- MedSearch at **www.medsearch.com** ($$)

Other Health Sites

- American Cancer Society at **www.cancer.org**
- American Dental Association at **www.ada.org**
- American Heart Association at **www.americanheart.org**
- American Medical Association at **www.ama-assn.org**
- American Psychiatric Association at **www.apa.org**
- Clinical trials at **www.clinicaltrials.gov**
- Institute for Safe Medication Practices at **www.ismp.org**
- Nutrition information at **www.navigator.tufts.edu**
- OncoLink cancer information at **www.oncolink.upenn.edu**
- U.S. Food and Drug Administration at **www.fda.gov**
- U.S. Pharmacopeia (pharmaceutical information) at **www.usp.org**

Other Health Sites

- Alternative medicine at **www.wholehealthmd.com**
- Children's health at **www.kidshealth.org**
- Department of Health and Human Services at **www.healthfinder.gov**
- Noncommercial health sites at **www.healthweb.org**
- Ratings of physicians at **www.healthgrades.com**
- The Merck Manual at **www.merck.com**
- The Merck Manual Home Edition at **www.merckhomeedition.com**

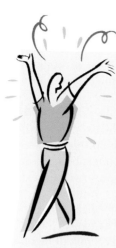

Nurturing Your Spirituality

Support Is Just a Click Away

Online patient support groups can be useful, especially for people with chronic illness. With the click of a mouse it is possible to interact with others who share health problems. One of the most direct methods of communicating with others on the Internet is through newsgroups. Newsgroups are locations where electronic messages (e-mail) related to a medical topic are posted. These are usually plain text messages rather than sophisticated, color-graphic presentations. Newsgroups are not a collection of news items. Essentially, they are virtual bulletin boards open to anyone who wants to participate. Newsgroups make it possible to locate other people experiencing the same health concerns you are and to hear about their experiences, as well as tell about yours.

There are more than 15,000 newsgroups available on the Internet.[5] To locate the name of a specific newsgroup that might be helpful to you, visit one of the following Web sites:

- Deja News at **www.dejanews.com**
- Dictionary.com at **www.dictionary.com**
- Self-Help Sourcebook at **www.mentalhelp.net/selfhelp/**
- Healthfinder at **www.healthfinder.gov**

Following are some popular newsgroups devoted to specific health issues:

- AIDS at **http://sdmc.cpcra.org/links.usenet.html**
- Arthritis at **misc.health.arthritis**
- Asthma at **alt.support.asthma**
- Cancer at **sci.med.diseases.cancer**
- Depression at **alt.support.depression**
- Diabetes mellitus at **misc.health.diabetes**
- Eating disorders at **alt.support.eating-disord**
- Headaches at **alt.support.headaches.migraine**
- Infertility at **misc.health.infertility**
- Stop smoking at **alt.support.stop-smoking**

A newsgroup may receive dozens and even hundreds of new postings each day. You can read all of them or select those that seem to be most relevant. Messages on a related topic often are grouped together in a *thread*, making it easier to follow a conversation. Often, participants share practical tips for daily living. Sometimes, experts offer medical advice. Some groups are managed by administrators who screen submissions. However, most groups are uncontrolled, which means that they may contain inaccurate information.

---

profession who had user privileges at major medical libraries and research centers. Web sites provide information regarding most diseases and health conditions. Some sites provide access to news groups, chat rooms, bulletin boards, support groups, and even medical specialists (see Nurturing Your Spirituality: Support Is Just a Click Away). Perhaps more than any other development of recent times, the Internet has been the best means of empowerment for people who want and need information so that they can be actively involved in their health care. Armed with the latest information, people can be better prepared to ask questions and become partners with their physicians when serious health issues occur.

According to a recent study in which medical consultants reviewed selected Web pages, much of the information available online is "as good as any you'll find in a good medical library—and in some cases more complete than the information your own physician could provide."[7] But the same study called the Internet a "wild frontier" mixed with all sorts of information—good and bad, true and false, complete and dangerously incomplete. Some information may be outdated and some may be presented in Web sites that are not managed by knowl-

edgeable sources or have not been subjected to peer review. How can you tell if the information on the Internet can be trusted? The following guidelines will help:

1. Check the date of Internet postings. Reputable Web sites provide dates of entry of its content. If dates are not included, it's probably because the Web site sponsor doesn't want you to know.
2. Identify the source or owner of the Web site. Established health and medical institutions usually provide valid and reliable information. Institutions that have earned a good reputation for the quality of programs and services they deliver to customers and patients can usually be counted on to go the extra mile to ensure quality Web sites. Web sites ending in "gov" and "edu" are managed by governmental and educational institutions, respectively, and can usually be trusted.
3. Determine if the Web site promotes products or procedures. Be skeptical if the Web site overwhelms you with ads. Also exercise caution if the Web site relies on testimonials and anecdotes to promote its products and services.

Managing Health Care

A major theme throughout this text is that you can control many factors that influence your health. An outgrowth of this attitude is the **self-care** movement, the trend toward becoming an active partner in the management of one's health rather than a passive recipient of medical treatment. Armed with correct information, you can manage many aspects of your health care that were once thought to be solely within the realm of a physician. An added bonus of becoming actively involved in self-care is a shift from feelings of helplessness and despair to feelings of control, responsibility, and involvement (see Assessment Activity 15-3).

Answers to the following questions guide the use of health care services, providers, and products and facilitate the self-care approach to wellness:

- When should you seek health care?
- What can you expect from a stay in the hospital?
- How can you select a health care professional?

When to Seek Health Care

Many people tend to fall into two extreme groups regarding health care: those who seek health care for every ache and pain and those who avoid health care unless experiencing extreme pain. Both groups unwisely use the health care establishment. Those in the first group fail to understand that too much health care can be ineffective or even harmful. They also fail to recognize the powerful recuperative powers of the body. The reality is that the majority of people who seek medical care are unaffected by the treatment. Most of the time the body is capable of healing itself. Of course, sometimes medical treatment is essential, but for every person who gets better from treatment another person experiences an **iatrogenic condition.** An iatrogenic condition is a health problem or condition caused by medical treatment. Several examples include drug reactions, medical mistakes, and infection. Sometimes the iatrogenic condition is worse than the presenting symptom. This does not mean that symptoms should be disregarded on the assumption the body will heal itself or if treatment is sought there is a 50:50 chance of an unnecessary complication. People who avoid health care at all costs fail to recognize the value of early diagnosis and detection of disease. The challenge, therefore, is to know when to seek health care and when to allow for the natural course of events that occurs in the healing process.

Perhaps the best way to find a balance between too much and too little health care is to establish a physician-patient relationship with a general practitioner. The general practitioner may be a family practice physician or an internist who specializes in internal medicine.

Visit your doctor while you are in good health. This permits your doctor to serve as a facilitator of wellness and provides him or her with a benchmark for interpreting symptoms when they occur.

A second important way to balance health care is to trust your instincts. Nobody knows when something is wrong with your body better than you do. Health and illness are subject to a wide variation in interpretation. If you are attuned to your body, you are your own best expert for recognizing signs and symptoms of illness.

Several signs and symptoms warrant medical attention without question.[8] Internal bleeding, as shown by blood in the urine, bowel movement, sputum, or vomit, or blood from any of the body's openings requires immediate attention. Abdominal pain, especially when it is associated with nausea, may indicate a wide range of problems from appendicitis to pelvic inflammatory disease and requires the diagnostic expertise of a physician. A stiff neck when accompanied by a fever may suggest meningitis and justifies immediate medical intervention. Injuries, many first-aid emergencies, and severe disabling symptoms require prompt medical care (see Just the Facts: When a Cut or Scrape Requires a Doctor at **www.mhhe.com/anspaugh6e** Student Center, Chapter 15, Just the Facts). Headaches that last longer than 24 hours, are severe and sudden, occur most mornings, are accompanied by nausea, or are more painful than you've had before may indicate a range of problems, including a severely inflamed artery, a stroke, an aneurysm, sleep apnea, a migraine, or hypertension and require medical intervention.[9] Back pain that is accompanied by leg weakness or pain radiating down the leg suggests the possibility of a herniated disk and demands the attention of a medical doctor.[9] A rash that spreads quickly, appears as red streaks on a leg or an arm, is painful and limited to one side of the body, accompanies fever, or is on or near the genitals may be difficult to diagnose and suggests hives, infection of the lymph vessels, shingles, Rocky Mountain spotted fever, or sexually transmitted diseases.[9]

There is debate about when medical care is needed in the case of fever. *Fever* means a reading over 99° F.[10] An elevated temperature may be a sign that the body's immune system is responding to an infection and working to destroy pathogens or disease-producing organisms. In other words, a fever is the body's own adaptive response that helps fight disease. However, if left untreated for an extended time, a fever may cause harm to sensitive tissues in the body, such as connective tissue found in joints and tissues in the valves of the heart. Body temperature is generally about 98.6° F. Body temperature varies with exercise, at rest, by climate, and by gender. It is not usually necessary for an adult to seek medical care for a fever. Home treatment in the form of aspirin, acetaminophen, and sponge baths usually lowers fever. You should consult your physician if fever remains above

102° F despite your actions or, in the case of a low-grade fever (99° F to 101° F), if there is no improvement in 72 hours.[11] Some ailments, such as sore throat, ear pain, diarrhea, urinary problems, and skin rash, may be the cause of a fever and should be treated. Fever in young children should be discussed with a physician. (See Real-World Wellness: When to Seek Treatment for a Fever.)

Unintended weight loss may trigger a doctor's visit. Some people's weight loss fluctuates more than others. But if you haven't been trying to lose weight and you lose weight outside your normal fluctuations, consult your physician. It might signify any number of problems, such as thyroid problems, diabetes, cancer, or depression.[11]

Persistent heartburn may suggest something more serious than the occasional bout of indigestion. If you take antacids frequently, ulcers, acid reflux, or stomach cancer may be implicated. Seek medical advice.

Headaches are difficult to diagnose and suggest a wide range of conditions ranging from muscle tension to a brain tumor. If you haven't been prone to headaches before—or if you're experiencing a new type of headache—consult with your physician. Seek medical attention without delay if headache pain follows a head injury, occurs only on one side of your head, is made worse by lying down, or occurs together with weakness or numbness. All of these may indicate a significant underlying problem from a brain tumor to a blot clot.[11]

Dizziness may suggest one or more of 64 different conditions ranging from drug reactions to inner ear infection.[11] If dizziness is particularly severe or if it interferes with your daily activities, it should be checked by a medical doctor.

Entering a Hospital

Hospitals are driven by the goal of saving lives. They range in size and service from small units that provide general care and low-risk treatments to large, specialized centers offering dramatic and experimental therapies. You may be limited in your choice of a hospital by factors beyond your control, including insurance coverage, your physician's hospital affiliation, and the type of care accessible in your location.

The large majority of Americans benefit from the care and services provided by hospitals. More than 42 million procedures are performed on hospital inpatients and include everything from elective cosmetic surgery to leading-edge transplant surgery. The five most common health problems that require inpatient hospitalization are heart disease, childbirth delivery, psychoses, pneumonia, and malignant neoplasms (see Figure 15-1, page 464).[12] People usually check in, receive treatment, and leave better off than they were when they were admitted. The length of stay varies according to

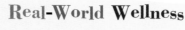

Real-World Wellness

When to Seek Treatment for a Fever[10]

If a fever is the body's way of making it an unfriendly host to viruses and bacteria, should I try to stop a fever with medications? When should I let a fever run its natural course and when should I seek treatment?

The body's immune system responds to infections with a sequence of reactions that leads to an increase in body temperature (fever). The elevated temperature helps destroy the pathogens that cause us to become sick. In this sense, a fever is a natural response and serves a useful purpose. It's the body's built-in defense system. Some experts suggest that our efforts to reduce fever may be counterproductive. In animals with severe infections, those with a high fever have a higher survival rate. Those who receive treatments to reduce the fever have a higher mortality rate. Evidence in humans is similar: Fever boosts the body's resistance to infections and shortens the duration of illness.

Even though a fever helps the body rid itself of infection-producing viruses and bacteria, it may also increase the risk for injury to sensitive tissues in the body, such as connective tissues in the joints and valves in the heart. A sustained low-grade fever may signal serious underlying conditions that require medical care, while a high fever of short duration may cause conditions ranging from heart palpitations to convulsions.

Some guidelines for fever treatment are as follows:

1. If you have a low-grade fever for a couple of days and are tolerating it well, let it run its course. If, on the other hand, you are uncomfortable, unable to rest or work, take a fever-reducing medicine.
2. If you have a high fever, 102° F or higher, consult with your physician.
   a. High fever during the first three months of pregnancy can cause birth defects.
   b. High fever in children can cause convulsions.
   c. High fever in heart patients may cause irregular heartbeats.
3. If any fever lasts longer than 72 hours, regardless of temperature reading, consult a physician to rule out underlying infections that may spell danger and require aggressive medical treatment.

many factors, such as the health and age of patients, the seriousness of the health problem, the presence of multiple risk factors, and insurance coverage. Figure 15-2 on page 464 presents the average length of hospital stay for seven common conditions.

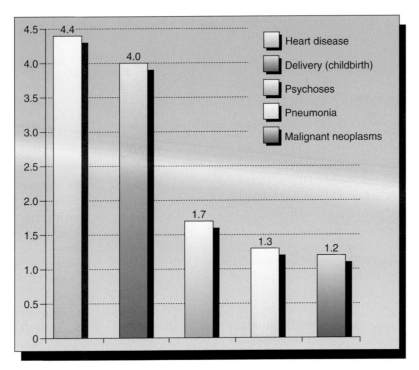

Figure 15-1 Inpatient Hospitalizations (Millions)

SOURCE: DeFrances, C. J., and M. J. Hall. 2004. *2002 National hospital discharge survey*. Hyattsville, MD: National Center for Health Statistics.

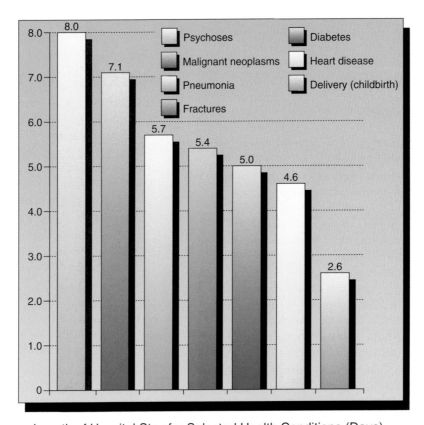

Figure 15-2 Average Length of Hospital Stay for Selected Health Conditions (Days)

SOURCE: DeFrances, C. J., and M. J. Hall. 2004. *2002 National hospital discharge survey*. Hyattsville, MD: National Center for Health Statistics.

∿ Just the Facts ∿

Grading Hospitals[15]

The following Web sites provide ranking and rating scores of U.S. hospitals.

1. *U.S. News and World Report*
   a. Lists the top 50 hospitals in 17 specialties
   b. Web site: **www.usnews.com**

2. Leapfrog Group
   a. Develops a safety score based on survey results of 30 safety practices
   b. Web site: **www.leapfroggroup.org**

3. Consumer Checkbook
   a. Lists hospital ratings based on surveys of physicians, mortality rates, and adverse outcome rates for surgery
   b. Web site: **www.checkbook.org**

4. Health Grades, Inc.
   a. Grades hospitals on a five-star rating system that is based on mortality data from Medicare
   b. Web site: **www.healthgrades.com**

While Americans enjoy the benefit of some of the world's best hospitals, you should still be aware of possible dangers. Well-known hospital hazards are unnecessary operations, unexpected drug reactions, harmful or even fatal blunders, and hospital-borne infections. An estimated 44,000–98,000 people die each year in the United States as a result of medical errors, the eighth-leading cause of death.[13] The greatest danger that a hospital presents is infection, largely preventable by the most basic of infection-control health practices: hand washing.[14]

What can laypeople do to ensure proper and safe care while in the hospital? The following guidelines should be considered:

- If you have a choice of hospitals, inquire about their accreditation status, reputation, and ratings from consumer groups (see Just the Facts: Grading Hospitals). Hospitals are subject to inspection to make sure they are in compliance with federal standards.

- Before checking into a hospital, you need to decide on your accommodations. Do you want to pay extra for a single room? Do you need a special diet? Do you need a place to store refrigerated medicine? If someone will be staying with you, will he or she need a cot? You should try to avoid going in on a weekend when few procedures are done. When you get to your room, speak up immediately if it is unacceptable.

- You need to be familiar with your rights as a patient (see Just the Facts: Do You Know Your Medical Rights?). Hospitals should provide an information booklet that includes a Patient's Bill of Rights. The booklet will inform you that you have the right to considerate and respectful care; information about tests, drugs, and procedures; dignity; courtesy; respect; and the opportunity to make decisions, including about when to leave the hospital.

- You should make informed decisions. Before authorizing any procedure, you must be informed about your medical condition, treatment options, expected risks, and prognosis and the name of the person in

∿ Just the Facts ∿

Do You Know Your Medical Rights?

The following is a short list of some of your rights as a patient in the health care system:

- You have the right as a parent to stay with your children during tests and treatments, provided you don't interfere with medical treatment or are not suspected of child abuse.

- You have the right to request that a relative or friend accompany you during a test, treatment, hospitalization unless you're in a semiprivate room.

- You have the right to see your medical records if your state law permits it. Some states allow you to copy parts of your record under certain conditions[16] (see Just the Facts: Are Your Medical Records Yours? at **www.mhhe.com/anspaugh6e** Student Center, Chapter 15, Just the Facts).

- You have the right to emergency care, whether you have insurance or not.

- You have the right to refuse to sign any form. The health care provider can also refuse to provide treatment in the absence of your signed authorization.

- You have the right to a second opinion, but your doctor can also stop treating you for challenging him or her.

- You have the right to leave the hospital at any time, even against medical advice or without paying the bill.

- You have the right to refuse or stop any treatment, whether or not it is experimental.

- You have the right to an itemized, detailed bill for all medical services.

- You have the right to know the results of all tests unless the doctor has reason to believe that the information will be harmful (for example, cause you to commit suicide).

charge of treatment. Your agreement to a procedure based on your having been informed of these matters is called **informed consent**. The only instances in which hospitals are not required to obtain informed consent are life-threatening emergencies, cases involving unconscious patients when no relatives are present, and compliance with the law or a court order, such as those regulating sexually transmitted diseases. If you are asked to sign a consent form, you should read it first. If you want more information, you should ask before signing. If you are skeptical, you have the right to postpone a procedure and discuss it with your doctor.

- Authorization of a medical procedure may be given nonverbally, such as through your appearance at a doctor's office for treatment, your cooperation during the administration of tests, or your failure to object when you could easily refuse consent. Your agreement to a procedure in such situations is called **implied consent**.

- You need to weigh the risks of drug therapy (see Just the Facts: "Brown Bag" Solution to Polypharmacy Problems), X-ray examinations, and laboratory tests against their expected beneficial results. When tests or treatments are ordered, you should ask about their purpose, possible risks, and possible actions if a test finds that something is wrong. Finally, you should inquire about prescribed drugs. Avoid taking drugs, including pain and sleeping medication, unless you feel confident of their benefits and are aware of their hazards. This is particularly true for antibiotics, which in general have been overprescribed to the point that some bacteria no longer respond to their use. Your chances of harboring drug-resistant bacteria are greater if you have taken many antibiotics or have not taken them as prescribed. Even if you have never had an antibiotic, you can still acquire drug-resistant bacteria. It's important to remember that people don't become resistant to antibiotics; bacteria do.[18] If you contract a bacterial infection, the strain of bacteria present in your body will determine how your body responds to antibiotic treatment, not your history with antibiotics.

- When scheduled for surgery, prepare for anesthesia. In rare cases, general anesthesia can cause brain damage and death. One cause of such catastrophes is vomiting while unconscious. To reduce the risk, avoid eating or drinking anything after midnight the night before surgery. However, it is usually acceptable to take medications with a sip of water up to two hours before surgery.[19] First check with your physician or surgeon.

- You need to know who is in charge of your care, record his or her office number, and note when you can expect a visit. If your doctor is transferring your

care to someone else, you need to know who it is. If your doctor is not available and you do not know what is happening, you can ask for the nurse in charge of your case.

- You should keep a daily log of procedures, medicines, and doctor visits. When you get your bill, compare each item with your written record. Insist on an itemized bill.

- You should stay active within the limits of your medical problem. Many body functions begin to suffer from just a few days' inactivity. Moving about, walking, bending, and contracting muscles help clear body fluids, reduce the risk for infections (especially in the lungs), and minimize the stress of hospital procedures, which can add to the depression and malaise of hospitalization.

- Eating habits change for many people following surgery, and it is not uncommon to experience a deficiency in nutrients. This is particularly true if

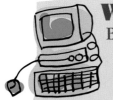

Wellness on the Web
Behavior Change Activities

How Can You Choose Quality Health Care?

If you're like most people, you want the best health care available—but you may not know how to evaluate the quality of care you're receiving. The Agency for Health Care Policy and Research (AHCPR), a part of the U.S. Department of Health and Human Services, is the lead agency charged with supporting research designed to improve the quality of health care, reduce its cost, and broaden access to essential services. AHCPR's research programs bring practical, science-based information to medical practitioners as well as consumers and other health care purchasers. The agency has published "Your Guide to Choosing Quality Health Care," which shows how you can rate the quality of health care services you and your family receive. It describes quality measures, including consumer ratings, clinical performance measures, and accreditation—what they are, where to find them, and how to use them. The guide has checklists, questions, charts, and other tools to help you make the health care decisions that are right for you. Take a moment to read about this information, which you'll find online at **www.mhhe.com/anspaugh6e**, Student Center, Chapter 15, Wellness on the Web, Activity 1.

Choosing a Physician Who's Right for You

The most important factor in the quality of health care you receive is your personal physician, or primary-care provider.

At certain times in your life, you may need to choose a physician. You may have moved recently or perhaps have a new health care plan that doesn't work with your provider. You may have become dissatisfied with your current physician and want to make a switch. Whatever the reason, selecting a new physician can be a daunting task if you're unsure where to begin. How do you know who's right for you or your family if all you have to go on is a list of names? You could just call a doctor's office at random and make an appointment, but chances are you'll make a better choice if you do a little homework up front. Go to the Web site listed previously and click on Activity 2 to learn more about choosing a physician who's right for you.

What Insurance Coverage Meets Your Needs?

The search for quality medical care can be challenging—and so can the search for comprehensive yet affordable health insurance. The cost of health care in the United States is high and continues to escalate. Few Americans can afford the cost of medicines, physicians' fees, or hospitalization without some form of health insurance. Health insurance is a contract between an insurance company and an individual or a group for the payment of medical care costs. Choosing health coverage can be a complex and confusing task, because health plans differ greatly in services performed, choice of providers, and out-of-pocket costs. The more you know, the easier it will be for you to decide what insurance plan best fits your personal needs and budget. Go to the Web site listed previously and click on Activity 3 to learn more about choosing a plan that meets your needs.

---

you are on a sodium-restricted or calorie-restricted diet. Some medical experts recommend a complete multivitamin/mineral supplement when hospitalized, whether it is added to your IV fluids or it is taken as a pill.[20]

- Ask questions until you know all you need to know. Know the three Ps: Be polite, be pleasant, and most of all be persistent. According to some experts, the best way to avert hospital errors can be summarized in two words: "Speak up!"[21] The more you assert yourself and the more questions you ask, the fewer mistakes that will result.

- Insist that hospital workers who enter your room wash their hands for at least 15 seconds with soap or alcohol-treated wipes in your presence. Infectious disease–control experts suggest that this is one of the most important things a patient can do to prevent the spread of infection. Concern for this basic hygiene measure takes on added importance when patients are subjected to invasive diagnostic procedures and/or surgery.

Selecting a Health Care Professional

Choosing a physician for your general health care is an important and necessary duty. Only physicians are discussed here, but this information applies to the selection of all health care practitioners. You must select one who will listen carefully to your problems and diagnose them accurately. At the same time, you need a physician who can move you through the modern medical maze of technology and specialists (see Just the Facts: Selected Health Care Specialists on page 468).

For most people, good health care means having a **primary-care physician,** a professional who assists you as you assume responsibility for your overall health and directs you when specialized care is necessary. Your primary-care physician should be familiar with your complete medical history as well as your home, work, and other environments. You will be better understood in periods of sickness if your physician has also seen you during periods of wellness.

Just the Facts

Selected Health Care Specialists

The following lists show the fields of specialty of selected health care specialists.

Name of Specialist	Field of Specialty
Medical Specialists	
Allergist	Allergic conditions
Anesthesiologist	Administration of anesthesia (such as during surgery)
Cardiologist	Coronary artery disease, heart disease
Dermatologist	Skin conditions
Endocrinologist	Diseases of the endocrine system
Epidemiologist	Study of the causes and sources of disease
Family practice physician	General-care physician
Gastroenterologist	Stomach, intestines, digestive system
Geriatrician	Diseases and conditions of the aged
Gynecologist	Female reproductive system
Hematologist	Study of blood
Immunologist	Diseases of the immune system
Internist	Diseases in adults
Neonatologist	Newborns
Nephrologist	Kidney disease
Neurologist	Nervous system
Neurosurgeon	Surgery of the brain and nervous system
Obstetrician	Pregnancy, labor, childbirth
Oncologist	Cancer, tumors
Ophthalmologist	Eyes
Orthopedist	Skeletal system
Otolaryngologist	Head, neck, ears, nose, throat
Otologist	Ears
Pathologist	Study of tissues and the essential nature of disease
Pediatrician	Childhood diseases and conditions
Plastic surgeon	Use of material to alter or rebuild tissues
Primary-care physician	General health and medical care
Proctologist	Disorders of the rectum and anus
Psychiatrist	Mental illnesses
Radiologist	Use of X rays
Rheumatologist	Diseases of connective tissues, joints, muscles, tendons
Rhinologist	Nose
Surgeon	Surgery
Urologist	Urinary tracts of men and women and reproductive organs of men
Dental Specialists	
Dentist	General care of teeth and oral cavity
Endodontist	Diseases of teeth below the gum line (root canal therapy)
Orthodontist	Teeth alignment, malocclusion
Pedodontist	Dental care of children
Periodontist	Diseases of supporting structures
Prosthodontist	Construction of artificial appliances for the mouth

For adults, primary-care physicians are usually family practitioners, once called "general practitioners," and internists, specialists in internal medicine. Pediatricians often serve as primary-care physicians for children. Obstetricians and gynecologists, who specialize in pregnancy, childbirth, and diseases of the female reproductive system, often serve as primary-care physicians to women. General surgeons may offer primary care in addition to the surgery they perform. In some states, osteopathic physicians also practice family medicine. (Doctors of osteopathic medicine are licensed medical physicians whose approach to health care emphasizes the treatment of the whole person, not just signs and symptoms of disease.)

There are several sources of information about physicians in your area:

- Local and state medical societies can identify doctors by specialty and tell you a doctor's basic credentials. You should check on the doctor's hospital affiliation and make sure the hospital is accredited. Another sign of standing is the type of societies in which the doctor has membership. The qualifications of a surgeon, for example, are enhanced by a fellowship in the American College of Surgeons (abbreviated as FACS after the surgeon's name). An internist fellowship in the American College of Physicians is abbreviated FACP. Membership in academies indicates physicians' special interests.
- All physicians board certified in the United States are listed in the *American Medical Directory* published by the American Medical Association and available in larger libraries.
- The American Board of Medical Specialists (ABMS) publishes the *Compendium of Certified Medical Specialties* (www.ama-assn.org), which lists physicians by name, specialty, and location.
- Pharmacists can be asked to recommend names.
- Hospitals can give you names of staff physicians who also practice in the community.
- Local medical schools can identify faculty members who also practice privately.
- The American College of Surgeons (www.facs.org) can identify doctors who are a fellow of the college. This suggests that the surgeon has passed a peer-reviewed evaluation and is staying current with the latest developments in his or her field.
- Many colleges and universities have health centers that keep lists of physicians for student referral.
- Friends may have recommendations, but you should allow for the possibility that your opinion of a doctor may differ from theirs.
- Detailed reports on doctors, including credentials, degrees, and possible disciplinary actions and malpractice judgments, are available online (www.consumerinfocentral.com) for a fee. You can also

check your state department of health Web site for information on licensure for all health professionals.

Once you have identified a leading candidate, you can make an appointment. You need to check with the office staff about office hours, availability of emergency care at night or on weekends, backup doctors, procedures when you call for advice, hospital affiliation, and payment and insurance procedures. You should schedule your first visit while in good health. Once you have seen your doctor, reflect on the following: Did the doctor seem to be listening to you? Were your questions answered? Was a medical history taken? Were you informed of possible side effects of drugs or tests? Was respect shown for your need of privacy? Was the doctor open to the suggestion of a second opinion?

Patient-physician communication

Most doctors are not disinterested in you, but they are busy—so busy that many patients complain that their doctors cannot or will not listen to them. There isn't much time to state your problem: Doctor visits last 18 minutes on average.[21,22] This is a problem because, according to the American Society of Internal Medicine, correct diagnoses depend largely on what you tell your doctor. Patients who do not speak up and who do not insist on being heard may get plenty of medical advice and prescription drugs, but they do not necessarily get the best results. Studies have shown that patients trained to ask questions, interrupt when necessary, and explain how their symptoms affect their lives have better health outcomes than those who are passive. Research also shows that better communication between patients and doctors can lead to a more accurate diagnosis, fewer tests, increased adherence to treatment, and greater satisfaction with care. Patients who report that their doctors communicate well are more likely to say their conditions improved than those who feel their doctors communicate poorly.[21] (See Assessment Activity 15-1.)

Patients can do much to facilitate the development of a physician-patient partnership. Understanding the meaning of commonly used medical words, abbreviations, suffixes, and prefixes can enhance this communication (see Just the Facts: Communicating with Health Care Professionals on page 470). The following are some tips to ensure good communication:

- Take along a family member or close friend. According to one highly respected health newsletter, this is the single most important piece of advice anyone can give.[23] It is not unusual for a patient who is unaccompanied at the doctor's office to return home unable to explain what was said, done, or recommended. The patient benefits from a second pair of eyes and ears, and the physician benefits because

Just the Facts

Communicating with Health Care Professionals

Following are some words, abbreviations, suffixes, and prefixes often used in health and medical care.

Term	Meaning
A (prefix)	Without
Aberration	Different from normal action
Acute	A condition that occurs suddenly
Adult	Developed fully
Affinity	Attraction
-algia (suffix)	Pain in
Angio- (prefix)	Vessels (veins or arteries)
Arrest	Stopping, restraining
Arthr- (prefix)	Joint-related
Asymptomatic	Without symptoms
Bowel	Intestine
BP	Blood pressure
Cardiac (cardio-)	Relating to the heart
Carpo- (prefix)	Wrist
CAT	Computer-assisted X ray
CCU	Coronary care unit
Chronic	A condition that occurs for a long time
Coma	Complete loss of consciousness
Congenital	Existing at or before birth
Contraindication	A reason for not prescribing a drug, procedure, or treatment
Coronary	Relating to the heart
CVA	Cerebrovascular accident (stroke)
Degenerative	Deterioration of a part of the body
Diagnosis	Determining of a disease
Dilation	Stretching, increase in size
Distention	Widening or enlargement
DO	Doctor of osteopathy
Dose	Amount of medication to be given at one time
Dys- (prefix)	Bad, difficult
Dysfunction	Impairment of function
Edema	Swelling from accumulation of fluid
EEG	Electroencephalogram
EKG, ECG	Electrocardiogram
Embolus	Blood clot floating free in the bloodstream
Emia- (prefix)	In the blood
Endemic	Disease prevalent in a particular area
Entero- (prefix)	Intestine
Epidemic	Disease prevalence that is higher than normal
ER/ED	Emergency room/emergency department
Etiology	Reference to the cause of a disease
Extra- (prefix)	Outside of
Gastr- (prefix)	Stomach
GP	General practitioner
Hem- (prefix)	Blood
Hemorrhage	Bleeding
Hyper- (prefix)	Excessive
Hypo- (prefix)	Insufficient

continued

Just the Facts

continued

Term	Meaning
Indication	Condition that leads to a prescribed drug, procedure, or treatment
ICU	Intensive care unit
Innate	Hereditary, congenital
Innocuous	Harmless
Insidious	Refers to a disease that does not show early symptoms of its advent
-ism (suffix)	Condition, theory, method
-itis (suffix)	Inflammation
IV	Intravenous (within a vein)
Jaundiced	Yellow
Macro	Large
Mal- (prefix)	Bad, deficient
Malady	Illness
Malaise	Uneasiness
MD	Medical doctor
MI	Myocardial infarction
Micro- (prefix)	Small
MRI	Magnetic resonance imaging
Myo- (prefix)	Muscle
Nephro- (prefix)	Kidney
-opothy (suffix)	Cause unknown
Pandemic	Disease that is prevalent over a large region
Pernicious	Severe, fatal
Phag- (prefix)	To eat
-philia (suffix)	Attraction, affinity
Presby- (prefix)	Old
Primary	Principal, most important
Prognosis	Medical outlook of a disease
Pulmo- (prefix)	Lung
Renal	Kidney
Sepsis	Infection
Sign	Something tangible that can be observed
Stenosis	Constricted, decreasing in size
Symptom	Intangible evidence of a disease
Symptomatic	Relating to symptoms
Syndrome	Set of symptoms that occur together for unknown causes
Systemic	Affecting all systems of the body
Thrombus	Solid blood clot
TIA	Transient ischemic attack
TPR	Temperature, pulse, respiration
Trauma	Injury from external force
Tumor	Growth
-uria (suffix)	Urine, urination

patients are usually calmer and the family member or close friend can provide insight into the patient.

- When you see your physician about a problem, you should state the most important problem first. Doctors tend to believe that the first thing a patient says is most important.

- You should be specific. If you have a headache, where does it hurt? How long does it last? How often does it occur?

- You should know your family history. Because many illnesses run in families, you may be at higher risk for certain diseases. Before your first visit, you should

Wellness for a Lifetime

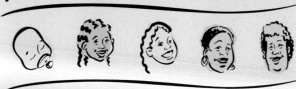

Older Adults Can Go Too Far with Self-Care

In an effort to assume responsibility for their own health care, people sometimes go too far. This is especially true for older people—those over 65 years of age—who are taking medications, both over-the-counter and prescription drugs. Common mistakes include the following: (1) taking larger doses of over-the-counter medicines than called for on the label; (2) mixing different types of medicines, both over-the-counter and prescription, without understanding the potential impact of taking two different drugs at the same time (such as analgesics and alcohol); and (3) taking someone else's medicine.

The risks and potential dangers for self-medication mistakes increase for the elderly. Drug companies typically set dosages for new drugs high enough to be effective for 90 percent of the intended population. Many times this dosage is too high even for people under age 65, and for those over 65, the risk for harmful side effects increases significantly.[24] Three characteristics are used to determine dosages by drug companies: (1) how much of the drug is absorbed into the bloodstream from the intestine; (2) how much of the drug is broken down in the body; and (3) how quickly the drug is eliminated from the body. The tests used to determine these characteristics are usually completed on healthy, young volunteers with healthy, young intestines, livers, and kidneys.

Unfortunately, as humans age, their organs tend to decline in function and the processes responsible for eliminating drugs decrease, thus allowing an "overloading" effect on the user. This problem is made worse when an elderly person is taking more than one type of drug, as many elderly people do. The more drugs ingested, the greater the possibility of drug interactions. Drug interactions can increase the potency of a drug, render it ineffective, or cause other side effects that might be life-threatening. Older people in particular seem to be highly sensitive to drugs that affect the central nervous system, such as tranquilizers, antidepressants, and sleeping pills. Generally, older people are at increased risk for side effects if they are taking antidepressants, arthritis medications, blood thinners, dementia drugs, diabetes drugs, muscle relaxants, pain relievers, or sedatives or tranquilizers.[24]

To avoid potential overdoses, elderly patients should make both the physician and the pharmacist aware of all medications being taken, so that more appropriate dosages can be prescribed and closer monitoring of effects can occur.

---

contact your parents and close relatives to learn of their health problems, especially heart disease, cancer, stroke, arthritis, diabetes, alcoholism, and tuberculosis.

- You need to list medications and treatments you are receiving, including over-the-counter drugs. The possibility of overdosing on either prescription or over-the-counter drugs is a growing problem, especially for older people—those over 65 years of age (see Wellness for a Lifetime: Older Adults Can Go Too Far with Self-Care).[24] You will also need to identify any allergies and drug reactions. Remember the "brown bag" approach to polypharmacy.

- You should tell about dietary supplements, including herbs, vitamins, and minerals. Just because supplements are advertised as "natural" doesn't mean they're safe. Like drugs, supplements can have side effects and interact with each other and medicines.

- You should ask questions. You can take a written list of questions but try to make them brief and specific. You should ask about anything that is unclear and repeat the answers in your own words.

- Before leaving the doctor's office, you need to make certain you know the diagnosis or how to follow the recommended treatment. If drugs are prescribed, you should inquire about the possible **contraindications** (reasons for not using a drug), side effects, and generic substitutions.

- When appropriate, ask your physician to write down instructions or recommend reading material for more information on a particular subject. Inquire about the next steps in the treatment, if and when a return visit is required, and danger signs to look for and report to your physician.

- Ask your doctor if he or she communicates with patients by e-mail. There is a trend toward e-mail communication between doctors and patients and in some states insurers pay doctors for online consultations. If your doctor encourages e-mail communication, inquire about confidentiality and security issues. Ask if anyone else reads messages directed to the doctor. Also ask about the turnaround time for responding to messages. If you are impatient by nature and can't wait the required time for a response, don't write. Your impatience will likely lead to subsequent e-mails, possible telephone calls, and then a visit for the same problem. This is overkill and, except in emergency situations, is wasteful of both your time and your doctor's. Some guidelines for facilitating e-mail communication include the following:[25,26]

- Keep messages brief. If this isn't possible, you need to see the doctor face-to-face.
- Write a subject line that is descriptive, such as "surgery question."
- E-mail messages may not accurately describe who you are. In the body of your message, indicate your full name, birth date, and address.
- Edit your message before sending it. A good suggestion is to print your message, let it sit for a couple of hours, check it again for errors, revise it as needed, and then send it. Ask about the turnaround time.
- If a follow-up visit to the doctor's office is required, take a copy of your message(s) and the doctor's responses with you.
- Don't expect a doctor to respond to your questions if he or she hasn't seen you or doesn't have a medical file on you.
- E-mail, like any other form of communication, can be misused and abused. It is ideal and efficient for many circumstances. Still, it is no substitute for periodic office visits.

Second opinions

Chronic pain, recurring illnesses, and conditions involving elective surgery often benefit from a second opinion. A second opinion is often appropriate, and peace of mind is a sufficient reason for seeking it.

In some cases, such as elective surgery, your health insurer may require a second or third opinion before authorizing payment for certain treatments. (See Real-World Wellness: How to Get a Second Opinion for advice on getting a second opinion.)

If you decide to ask for a second opinion, common courtesy dictates that you discuss it with your physician. Your physician may suggest bringing in a consultant to assess your situation and discuss it with you and your physician. You can also ask your physician for the name of someone to see separately.

A physician may feel that a second opinion is a waste of time or money. Regardless, your wish for more information should be respected. Reputable physicians do not feel threatened by another opinion; to the contrary, they welcome another perspective on a difficult case. If your physician expresses displeasure for or resists your wish to have a second opinion, you may want to consider looking for another doctor.

Another good resource for a second opinion is your pharmacist. Pharmacists are experts on drugs, drug

Real-World Wellness

How to Get a Second Opinion

I am considering elective surgery and want a second opinion. What are some good sources for referral?

Following are some options for finding second opinions:

- Ask your primary-care physician for the names of two or three experts in the field.
- Call a medical center or hospital and ask to talk to the chief of surgery for a surgical opinion or to the chief of medicine for a nonsurgical question.
- Call the county medical society.
- Call the Second Surgical Opinion Hotline (800-638-6833) for medical organizations, which provides referrals on surgical questions.
- Call the Health Benefits Research Corporation, which offers a Second Opinion Hotline (800-522-0036, 800-631-1220 in New York) and referral service. Consultation with a board-certified specialist is available for a fee.
- Call the American Board of Medical Specialists to determine if the opinion you're getting is from a board-certified physician. The number is 800-776-CERT.

interactions, contraindications, and side effects. Pharmacists are a crucial part of the health care team, whether it's in the drug store, hospital, clinic, or long-term health care facility. In 2006, pharmacists will be officially recognized as health care providers, allowing them to counsel older adults about changing medications and assessing possible interactions of various medications. Medicare will pay for the service. The physician will still have to approve any recommended changes the pharmacist makes.[27]

Alternative Medicine

Alternative medicine, also called *complementary medicine* or *integrative medicine,* is the body of therapies not taught in U.S. medical schools and generally unavailable from doctors or hospitals.[28] Almost two-thirds of the public have tried alternative medical therapy, despite the skepticism of many providers of traditional medical care (also called *allopathic* medicine, which refers to the treatment of diseases using scientifically proven and established measures).[28] These therapies vary considerably in their approach and include prayer, meditation, natural products, deep breathing exercises, chiropractic care, yoga, massage, and diet-based therapies (see Table 15-1, page 474).

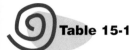

Table 15-1 Ten Most Commonly Used Alternative Medicine Therapies

Rank	Therapy	Percentage of Adults
1	Use of prayer for one's own health	43.0
2	Prayer by others for one's own health	24.4
3	Natural products	18.9
4	Deep breathing exercises	11.6
5	Participation in prayer group for one's own health	9.6
6	Meditation	7.6
7	Chiropractic care	7.5
8	Yoga	5.1
9	Massage	5.0
10	Diet-based therapies	3.5

SOURCE: Barnes, P. M., E. Powell-Griner, K. McFann, and R. L. Nahin. 2004. *Complementary and alternative medicine use among adults: United States, 2002.* Hyattsville, MD: National Center for Health Statistics.

Proponents of alternative medicine acknowledge that allopathic medicine is superb when it comes to surgery, emergency, and trauma. But they claim that alternative approaches work better for almost everything else, especially chronic degenerative diseases, because they focus on prevention and target causes rather than symptoms. Many alternative methods are thought to work by helping the body heal itself instead of by introducing strong drugs often to compensate for the side effects of other drugs.[29]

Skeptics of alternative medicine claim that its effectiveness has not been proven and worry about the indiscriminate use of some therapies. They offer numerous reasons for their concerns:[30]

- Patients often delay starting conventional medical treatment that has a proven track record to try an alternative approach touted as a miracle cure.
- There is the false perception that "natural" remedies are risk-free. Many herbal medicines may negate the effects of important medicines. St. John's wort, for example, affects the action of drugs such as warfarin (Coumadin), the anticlotting drug, and indinavir (Crixivan), an AIDS drug. Ginkgo biloba and ginseng interact with warfarin; kava interacts with sedatives. These interactions aren't monitored closely because the FDA has little authority over alternative medicines.[31]
- There is a lack of evidence from scientifically controlled studies that demonstrate a therapy's effectiveness to make good on its promise.
- Proponents tend to rely on anecdotal records (isolated incidents) and testimonials to promote therapies.

- Because herbs and vitamins are processed and excreted primarily by the liver and kidneys, as are most drugs, they can cause serious drug interactions with prescription and over-the-counter medications.

Many health problems, such as chronic pain, lower-back problems, and stress-related problems (such as anxiety and insomnia), don't respond well to conventional medical approaches. If at first conventional treatments aren't effective, alternative therapies may offer some benefit. If you consider using a form of alternative medicine, experts recommend you do the following:[32]

- Keep a diary to track symptoms. Writing down when symptoms begin and when they abate is a good way to determine if there is an association between treatment and relief.
- Add one therapy at a time. It is hard to know which therapy may be helping and which may be causing side effects when multiple therapies are used. Use the diary to track one treatment at a time.
- Discuss alternative therapies with your conventional physician. Potential interactions between conventional and alternative therapies can cause serious health problems.
- Discuss conventional therapies with your alternative physician. If an alternative physician suggests discontinuing a drug, check with your conventional physician first.

Assessing Your Health

Many tests, procedures, gadgets, and machines assess various aspects of health and wellness. They range from the hands-on physical examination to the use of sophisticated diagnostic tests.

The Physical Examination

Until recently, the annual physical examination was viewed as a normal and necessary part of health care. Now, considerable debate exists among medical experts as to who needs a physical examination, how often it is needed, and what it should include. The emphasis today is on the use of selective health examinations and periodic examinations. **Selective health examinations** are specific tests used for specific problems. The assumption of this approach is that tests are more useful if they are matched to specific complaints. **Periodic examinations** are assessments given according to age, health habits, predisposition for certain conditions, and/or risk factors.

The periodic exam includes only those tests warranted by the information coming from a thorough medical history and discussion of those lifestyle factors related to diseases. The assumption is that behavior and habits are the best criteria for predicting disease risk.

Criticisms of the comprehensive annual physical examination for a healthy adult are not meant to undermine the doctor-patient relationship. They simply cast doubt about the efficacy of the physical examination. However, this does not nullify the value of regular visits to the doctor. To the contrary, seeing a physician for a limited examination at regular intervals can be good preventive medicine.

How often?

The need for a complete physical exam depends on a person's age, health, and lifestyle. People over the age of 65 benefit from a checkup every year. People in good health and between 40 and 65 should see their physicians for routine tests at least every 1 to 5 years.[33] Healthy people between the ages of 18 and 39 should have two complete physical exams in their twenties.[33] During the first exam, ask to have your blood profile checked (cholesterol, LDLs, HDLs). Height, weight, body mass index, and blood pressure should also be checked.

Regardless of their age, people with family histories of heart disease, stroke, high blood pressure, cancer, and diabetes can benefit from periodic checkups, even if they are in good health. The same is true for people whose health habits or occupations put them at higher than normal risk for chronic diseases and disabling conditions. Even in these cases, good judgment and discretion should rule the choice of tests to be included in the physical examination.

Components

The three basic tools for completing a physical examination are medical history, hands-on examination, and diagnostic/laboratory tests. A medical history is the most important part of the physical examination, especially during the first visit with your physician.[34] This includes information about health habits, lifestyle, family history, and symptoms. Many physicians use health-risk appraisals, detailed questionnaires that provide information about health habits. This is one area of the physical examination for which a patient can prepare. By following the guidelines for communicating with your physician presented earlier in this chapter, you can help your physician obtain an accurate health profile.

The hands-on examination is the second part of the physical examination. It consists of touching, looking, and listening. Physicians can feel, or palpate, for enlarged glands, growths, and tumors with procedures such as the breast examination, pelvic examination, rectal examination, and hernia examination. Thumping the back and chest lets the physician know whether any fluid has built up in or around the lungs. Tapping a knee for reflexes may reveal nervous system damage. A stethoscope is used to listen to the heart, lungs, abdomen, and glands located near the surface of the skin. Possible problems that can be detected with the stethoscope range from a heart murmur to poor circulation, a lung infection, intestinal blockage, and an overactive thyroid gland.

Physicians have access to a number of instruments to inspect visually for problems. An ophthalmoscope is used to view the brain through the eye. The first sign of some brain diseases is an unhealthy-looking optic nerve. Leakage in the blood vessels of the eye may be a sign of diabetes or hypertension. An otoscope is used to inspect the ear, particularly the tympanic membrane. The proctoscope and sigmoidoscope are used to examine the rectum and colon. The laryngoscope and bronchoscope provide a look at the larynx and bronchial tubes.

The last part of the physical examination includes **diagnostic laboratory tests,** which vary from a simple urinalysis to invasive dye tests. The effectiveness of these tests is being debated. Tests conducted for specific symptoms may be invaluable in pinpointing disabling conditions. They may be just as valuable for what they do not reveal as they are for what they do reveal. This can be reassuring to the patient and physician. On the negative side, many physicians rely too heavily on laboratory tests. Patients often demand or acquiesce to more tests than are necessary and sometimes than are good for them.

Many times tests are recommended more for the purpose of protecting the doctor against medical malpractice suits than for their diagnostic value. This practice, called **defensive medicine,** paints a sobering picture of the difficulty in making medical decisions for doctors and patients. A doctor may know with 99 percent certainty a particular diagnosis but order a test or procedure, anyway, as protection against liability, should he or she be sued later. Malpractice suits are a reality; over 1 million hospital patients will suffer an injury as a result of a medical mistake. More than 10 percent of these patients will die, partly as the result of the mistake.[35] To avoid the threat of a malpractice lawsuit, it is not unusual for physicians to order a battery of extra tests. Of course, patients always have the right to decline prescribed tests. The decision must be made by patient and doctor and should be based on the test's potential for contributing to an effective medical intervention.

Thus, when you go for a physical examination, you can determine which tests you are willing to be subjected to by asking the right questions:

- *What do you expect to find?* You should start by asking why you need the test. How will it help facilitate a diagnosis? You need to ask about alternatives and the disadvantage of waiting and not testing. Sometimes the best test is the test of time. Agreeing to a test because it is routine procedure is not a satisfactory explanation.

- *What risks are associated with the test?* No test is risk-free; you should compare potential benefits and risks.

One problem with tests is that they are not 100 percent accurate. An inaccurate result can lead to a wrong diagnosis. A **false positive,** in which a test incorrectly reveals an abnormality, may occur. False positives provoke needless anxiety, causing some people to feel and even act sick. Conversely, normal results do not necessarily indicate good health. A **false negative,** in which a test indicates normality even though a person is sick, may occur. These results may lead to a false sense of health and may delay much needed treatment at critical stages of a disease. Statistically, test results are accurate for about 95 percent of the population. Thus, 5 percent of patients can be expected to have false positives or false negatives on any laboratory tests. Other factors that may cause test errors are the taking of certain medications, exercise, stress, diet, time of day, and mistakes in handling or processing specimens.

Another problem with tests is that they may involve physical risks. Some of the more common risks are infection; bleeding; damage to vital structures; and reactions to anesthetics, drugs, and dye-contrast materials. Again, it is important to ask questions.

- *What are the options after the test?* If a test is positive, then what? If none of the options is plausible to you, why have the test administered? If it is impossible to treat a disease that a test reveals, the test is not justified. The diagnosis of a treatable disease, on the other hand, usually justifies the test.
- *What is the value of the test?* This question need not be perceived as confrontational. If approached with sincerity and courtesy, discussions about the physical examination in general and laboratory tests in particular can serve as a basis for forming an active partnership with your physician in making decisions about your health care.

Common Diagnostic Laboratory Tests

Americans are having many diagnostic tests performed. Home medical tests, available from most pharmacies, allow you to monitor a growing list of medical conditions including high blood pressure, high body temperature, asthma, allergies, urinary tract infections, pregnancy, diabetes mellitus, colon cancer, high cholesterol, and HIV infection. The tests should not be viewed as substitutes for your doctor. The accuracy rates and reliability of over-the-counter medical kits vary considerably, and their instructions do not always explain how to interpret the results. These test procedures are also

ᨑᨑ Just the Facts ᨑᨑ

Essentials for Your Medicine Cabinet

With the exception of personal items and prescription medicines, what should you keep in your medicine cabinet? The following are the essentials, according to experts:

1. A *thermometer* to assess body temperature (oral, rectal, ear, and electronic models available)
2. *Ipecac* to induce vomiting in case of poisoning
3. *Acetaminophen* to reduce fever and pain (in liquid form for children; aspirin should not be given to children under 15 years of age because of its link to Reye's syndrome)
4. An *antiseptic*, such as hydrogen peroxide, for cleaning open wounds
5. *Gauze* and *tape* to treat minor wounds
6. An *ice bag* to reduce swelling
7. *Ace bandages* to wrap pulled muscles or twisted ankles or to bind a splint
8. *Benadryl* or a similar antihistamine to reduce allergic reactions
9. An *antibiotic ointment* or *cream* to prevent infections from cuts
10. *Antidiarrheal medication* to treat diarrhea

subject to human error, but they provide a useful way to get involved in your health care.

Some other inexpensive items should be included in your medicine cabinet (see Just the Facts: Essentials for Your Medicine Cabinet). These items should help you cope with most common minor aches and pains.

Depending on your health status, gender, age, symptoms, and risk for a disease, some of the more common tests may be recommended when you go to your physician for a checkup. *Multiple blood screening tests* check for high blood sugar, which indicates diabetes; blood urea nitrogen, an indicator of kidney function; an overactive parathyroid gland; blood count, a screen for anemia; and much more (see Assessment Activity 15-2).

A *complete blood lipid profile* checks for high LDL cholesterol, low HDL cholesterol, and triglyceride levels. (See Chapter 2 for a thorough discussion of cholesterol and lipoproteins—HDLs and LDLs.) This assessment is recommended every five years, starting at age 20.[36]

A *thyroid stimulating hormone (TSH) blood test* checks for an overactive or underactive thyroid gland or thyroid disease. This test is recommended every five years, starting at age 35.[36]

Fecal occult-blood tests, also called *hemoccult tests,* are used to detect hidden blood in bowel movements. If a test is positive, it may indicate signs of an early cancer of the colon. People over 50 should either test themselves (home screening kits are available in most pharmacies) or have their stools tested for blood every year.[36] (See Just the Facts: Fecal Occult-Blood Tests: Reducing False Positives at www.mhhe.com/anspaugh6e Student Center, Chapter 15, Just the Facts.) Two more options, both of which are invasive, are recommended in combination with or in place of the fecal occult-blood test. One option is a *sigmoidoscopy,* a procedure that involves the insertion of a flexible viewing scope into the lower third of the colon, where about one-half of colorectal cancers occur.[37] It is more accurate than a fecal occult-blood test, but it cannot detect tumors in the upper part of the colon. Another option is a *colonoscopy,* which is similar to sigmoidoscopy in that it involves the insertion of a flexible viewing scope, but it is different in that it examines the entire colon. It is the only procedure that permits the removal of polyps during the test. The colon should be checked at age 50 and repeated every 10 years if a colonoscopy is used or every 5 years if a sigmoidoscopy is used in combination with an annual fecal occult-blood test.[36] A noninvasive option is the use of a CT scanner that produces 3-D images of the colon. However, this option is not widely available and may not be covered by health insurance; if it yields suspicious results, it is followed by a colonoscopy.

Pulse rate may be an indicator of a health problem. The normal resting heart rate is between 60 and 80 beats a minute. Resting heart rates above 80 beats per minute put a person in a higher risk category for heart attacks and sudden death. The high heart rate does not increase the risk but is an indicator of basic problems, such as cigarette smoking, too much caffeine, stress, anxiety, hyperthyroidism, and most commonly a poor level of physical fitness. Slow heart rates are normally found in physically fit people; in them, slow heart rates are a sign of good health. Very slow rates below 50 beats per minute can occur in people who are not fit and who have heart problems. These people should seek medical advice.

Blood pressure measurements should be monitored regularly, especially for people who have had previously high readings or have family histories of hypertension (high blood pressure). Inexpensive, accurate home blood pressure kits can be purchased at most drugstores. Because all kits are not equally reliable, you should ask your pharmacist for a recommendation. People who have measurements higher than 140 over 90 mmHg or lower than 100 over 60 mmHg should keep records of their blood pressure and present them to their physicians during periodic checkups.

Mammography, an X-ray examination of the breast, detects early signs of breast cancer. Women should be screened every one to two years, starting at age 40.[36] High-risk women may be advised to have mammograms more often and at an earlier age.

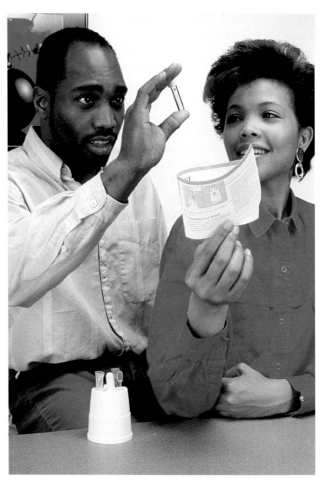

Self-care medical kits, such as home pregnancy tests, allow you to become more involved with your health care.

Pelvic examinations and *Pap smears* detect abnormalities of the ovaries, uterus, and cervix. Pap smears should be performed annually for three years beginning at age 21 or three years after the age of first intercourse. If they are normal, they may be performed every two to three years thereafter.[36] Pap smears should not be done during the menstrual period. The test is more accurate during the first half of the cycle if oral contraceptives are taken. Midcycle is preferred in most other menstruating women. No Pap smear is recommended for women over 65 if no abnormal results occurred in the previous decade or after hysterectomy unless the cervix remains or the hysterectomy was performed to treat cervical cancer.[36,37]

A complete *eye examination* includes a test for visual acuity; *tonometry,* a painless test for glaucoma; and a cataract (a clouding over the lens) check. To check for glaucoma, macular degeneration, and other vision problems, such as cataracts, an eye exam is recommended every 3 to 5 years before age 45 and every 1 to 3 years after that.[36]

Electrocardiograms (ECGs) are used to detect irregularities of the heart. Although there is some debate about the use of ECGs as routine screening procedures for *asymptomatic* (without symptoms), low-risk people, periodic ECG readings starting at age 40 are recommended.[36] Chest pain, hypertension, and symptoms of cardiovascular disease justify earlier ECGs. *Stress tests* use ECGs to assess how the heart functions under the stress of exercise. They are routine when symptoms are present.

Chest X-ray examinations are valuable diagnostic tools for people with chest symptoms, respiratory diseases, and heart problems. For people without symptoms, their routine use is questionable. Several groups of experts, including those associated with the Food and Drug Administration, recommend the discontinuation of routine chest X-ray examinations.[38] However, if you go to a hospital or often visit a doctor's office, you can anticipate a chest X-ray study more out of the need to comply with business policy than for diagnostic potential. Avoid a chest X-ray test if you may be pregnant.

Prostate cancer tests detect prostate cancer, a leading cause of cancer among men. The blood test that looks for prostate-specific antigens (PSAs) should be performed in combination with a digital rectal examination on men every one to two years, starting at age 50 in white men and age 40 in African-American men.[36] Because not all experts endorse this procedure, discuss the advantages and disadvantages of PSAs with your physician.

An *HIV test* is recommended for people who think they may have been infected with the HIV virus. This includes people who have had unprotected sex or a blood transfusion, have used IV drugs, or have participated in high-risk behaviors. After the blood test, these people should avoid high-risk behavior for six months to a year and then retest.

A *visual skin test* for skin cancer is recommended every three years for people 20 to 39 and annually for people over 40. An annual skin examination performed by a dermatologist is important for anyone with a history of many moles, pale skin, and a family history of melanoma.

A fasting *blood glucose test* is recommended to detect diabetes mellitus. The test requires a small blood sample following a 12-hour fast. It is recommended for people with symptoms of diabetes, including excessive thirst and frequent urination, people who are overweight, and those who have strong family histories of the disease.

A *bone density test* detects bone thinning and/or loss and is recommended for women soon after menopause and every two to three years after 65.[36] It is also recommended for women at high risk for osteoporosis regardless of age. The test involves the use of an X-ray-type machine at two sites: spine and hip. Test results are reported in terms of a T-Score, which describes how much

∼∽Just the Facts∼∽

Interpreting Your T-Score[39]

A bone density test for possible signs of bone thinning and/or loss may signal the development of osteoporosis. Test results are presented as T-Scores and can be interpreted as follows:

- T-Scores ranging from −1 to +1 or higher mean that bone density is "normal" and suggest low risk for bone fractures due to osteoporosis.
- T-Scores ranging from −1 to −2.5 indicate low bone mass (*osteopenia*) and a greater risk for bone fractures.
- T-Scores of −2.5 and lower indicate the presence of osteoporosis.

the bone density varies from what's considered normal. "Normal" is based on the typical bone mass of people in their thirties, when bone mass is at its peak.[39] (See Just the Facts: Interpreting Your T-Score.)

Ultrasound, also known as sonography, is a reliable, radiation-free imaging technique that can detect blood clots, assess heart valve and muscle function (*echocardiogram*), and determine the size and development of a developing fetus. Although ultrasound is useful in detecting fetal abnormalities, the American College of Obstetricians and Gynecologists has advised against its routine use in pregnancy.[39]

Direct-Access Testing (DAT)

Direct-access testing, or **DAT,** is an emerging trend in medical testing that offers patients convenience, privacy, and a sense of control. Patients simply order a particular test, go to a commercial or hospital lab affiliated with the DAT vendor, and submit a blood test; within a couple of days, test results are mailed or made available online. This is done without a visit to the physician's office or a prescription. Convenience is the number one reason patients seek DAT; "no need to see a physician" is the number two reason.[40]

DAT providers offer medical tests for chronic conditions, such as diabetes and heart disease, and acute conditions, such as infections. Some tests are modestly priced (e.g., less than $25), while others cost several hundred dollars or more. DAT is not available in some states and it is not usually covered by health insurance.

The American College of American Pathology, the professional group that oversees medical testing, warns against the indiscriminate use of DAT. However, it does not restrict its members from offering DAT. Criticisms of DAT include

- A "positive" will require a follow-up appointment with a doctor and probably a repeat of the same test.
- DAT may raise patients' anxiety levels and ultimately result in more tests, more visits to health care providers, and ultimately higher costs. This is particularly true for false positives.
- If doctors are not in the loop during the testing phase, neither are they in the loop to interpret test results and plan follow-up treatment options.
- Some test results will be false negative and therefore lead to a false sense of well-being.
- Patients who think they have a little knowledge about a particular health issue may use the results of DAT to mistakenly self-diagnose and actually exacerbate their condition.

Regardless of these criticisms, DAT is an option for patients who demand privacy and convenience and have the financial resources to pay for it. Advice for DAT users include[40]

- Use DAT discriminately; it is not intended to be a substitute for your physical or your physician. To quote the editors of the highly respected *Tufts University Health and Nutrition Letter,* "testing should never be an entirely do-it-yourself project."[41]
- Investigate and ask questions about the test just as you do for those administered in the doctor's office.
- If DAT yields abnormal results, consult with your doctor.

Immunizations for Adults

Many people believe that **immunizations** (administrations of preparations or vaccines, usually in the form of injections, for providing immunity or preventing a disease) are only for children. Consequently, many thousands of adults die every year of diseases they would not have acquired if they had received standard vaccines. Adult immunization is recommended to prevent or ameliorate influenza, pneumonia, some forms of hepatitis, measles, rubella (German measles), tetanus, diphtheria, and chicken pox.

People born after 1956 may need to be reimmunized for measles, mumps, and rubella (MMR) because the earlier vaccine may not have provided complete coverage.[42] A booster is not suggested for those born before 1957 because of the likelihood that they have natural immunity.

Booster shots should be given for tetanus and diphtheria every 10 years (tetanus and diphtheria vaccines are usually combined). A booster shot is required annually for protection against common strains of influenza, whereas a pneumonia vaccine is usually good for life if administered after age 65. Some experts recommend the initial pneumonia vaccine at age 50.[43] If administered before the age of 65, a booster shot is recommended at least 5 years after the first shot.[42]

Vaccines against hepatitis A, hepatitis B, and chicken pox are recommended for adults at risk because of their jobs, travel, or exposure to susceptible children or infected people. Hepatitis A vaccine lasts for several years. No booster shots are required for hepatitis B or chicken pox. If you are not sure whether you've had the disease, a blood test can check for antibodies.

Paying for Health Care

The cost of health care in the United States is expensive and is escalating. A majority of Americans cannot afford the cost of medicines, physicians' fees, or the cost of hospitalization without some form of health insurance. **Health insurance** is a contract between an insurance company and a person or group for the payment of medical care costs. After the person or group pays a premium to an insurance company, the insurance company pays for part or all of the medical costs, depending on the type of insurance and benefits provided. The type of insurance policy purchased greatly influences where a person goes for health care, who provides the health care, and what medical procedures can be performed.

Preferred Provider Organization (PPO)

A **preferred provider organization** (PPO) is a network of independent physicians, hospitals, and other health care providers who contract with an insurance company to provide medical care at discount rates. Subscribers are given incentives (reduced costs) if they use PPO-approved providers. This plan usually includes a *deductible,* an amount paid by the patient before being eligible for benefits from the insurance company. For example, if your expenses are $1,000, you may have to pay $200 before the insurance company will pay the other $800. After the deductible is met, the insurance provider pays a percentage of the remaining balance. PPO subscribers can use out-of-network providers, but they then usually pay more because the care is not discounted. The advantages of this plan are that a patient usually has more options in choosing health care providers and is not required to obtain a referral from a primary-care physician to seek the services of a specialist. Several disadvantages of this insurance option are that substantial costs may be incurred if unexpected illnesses or injuries occur and patients may not routinely receive comprehensive, preventive health care.

Point of Service (POS)

A **point of service** (**POS**) is an insurance plan in which subscribers use approved providers who have agreed to accept fixed copayments. The delivery of health care starts with and is coordinated by the primary-care physician. Before going to a specialist, a patient must first be referred by the primary-care physician. Out-of-plan providers can be seen but at a higher cost. Medical charges above the maximum allowed by the insurance company are the responsibility of the patient. Advantages of this insurance option are comprehensive health care coordinated by the primary-care physician, lower costs in the case of unexpected illnesses or accidents, and no deductibles. A disadvantage is the loss of accessibility to specialists without first obtaining referral approval.

Health Maintenance Organization (HMO)

A **health maintenance organization** (**HMO**) is a managed health care plan that provides a full range of medical services for a prepaid amount of money. For a fixed monthly fee, usually paid through pay-roll deductions by an employer, and often a small copayment, subscribers receive care from physicians, specialists, allied health professionals, and educators hired or contractually retained by the HMO.

HMOs offer an advantage in that they provide comprehensive care, including preventive care, at a lower cost than private insurance over a long period of coverage. One drawback is that patients are limited in their choice of providers to those who belong to the HMO.

Indemnity Plan

An indemnity plan is one in which a person pays a premium, which ensures health care on a fee-for-service basis. In addition to the premium, subscribers pay part of the cost for medical care. Typically, the insurance company pays 80 percent after the deductible has been met, and the subscriber pays 20 percent. Usually, there are fixed indemnity benefits, specified amounts paid for particular procedures. If your policy pays $500 for a tonsillectomy and the actual cost is $1,000, you owe the health care provider $500. There are often exclusions, certain services not covered by the policy. Common examples of exclusions are elective surgery, dental care, vision care, and preexisting illnesses and injuries. An advantage of an indemnity plan is that there are no limits on the providers you can use or on how often you see them. A disadvantage is that this type of insurance usually costs more than PPOs, POSs, and HMOs.

Government Insurance

In a government insurance plan, the government at the federal, state, or local level pays for health care costs of eligible participants. Two prominent examples of this plan are Medicare and Medicaid. Medicare is financed by Social Security taxes and is designed to provide health care for people 65 years of age and older, the blind, the severely disabled, and those requiring certain treatments, such as kidney dialysis. Medicare Part A covers hospital, skilled nursing, and home health care costs. People who qualify for Social Security also qualify for Part A. Medicare Part B is optional for an extra premium and covers physician fees and costs of outpatient care and physical therapy. Medicaid is subsidized by federal and state taxes. It provides limited health care, generally for people eligible for benefits and assistance from two programs: Aid to Families with Dependent Children and Supplementary Security Income.

Summary

- Health information that can be trusted is based on scientifically controlled studies that yield consistent results over time.
- A study is considered reliable if its findings can be confirmed in repeated studies conducted over the course of many years.
- Scientifically controlled studies involve experimental and control groups, use randomly selected participants, and feature double-blind procedures.
- *Statistical significance* is a term health journalists and researchers use to indicate probability. If a finding is statistically significant, 95 of 100 times similar studies yield similar findings.
- *Statistical relationship* is a term used to indicate the degree of association between two or more variables (e.g., dietary fat and heart disease). Statistical relationships do not demonstrate cause and effect.
- In the health literature the term *absolute risk* refers to the actual number of people affected by a risk factor. *Relative risk* refers to the percentage of people affected by a risk factor in comparison with some benchmark. Relative risks are often used in the news media because they tend to produce more sensational headlines but they are more prone to deception than absolute risks.
- Epidemiologic studies are population studies that observe the health habits and lifestyles of many people over time. They may be prospective or retrospective.

- The discriminating use of the Internet can yield helpful information for most health conditions.
- Signs and symptoms that warrant immediate medical attention are signs of internal bleeding; abdominal pain associated with nausea; a stiff neck accompanied by fever; headaches that last longer than 24 hours or are severe and sudden; back pain that is accompanied by leg weakness or pain radiating down the leg; a rash that spreads quickly; and serious first-aid emergencies and injuries.
- People can help ensure proper and safe care while in a hospital by checking on the hospital's accreditation status, deciding on accommodations before admission, knowing their patient rights, discussing treatments and procedures with their physicians, asking questions, and staying active.
- Good health care means establishing a doctor-patient relationship while in good health.
- The doctor who manages the general care of patients and directs patients to specialized services is the primary-care physician.
- Alternative medicine is the use of therapies not taught in U.S. medical schools and generally unavailable from doctors or hospitals.
- When telling a physician about a problem, you can enhance good communication by presenting the most important problem first, being as specific as possible, being familiar with your family medical history, knowing the names of medicines you are taking, and asking questions. If possible, take a friend or close relative when seeking medical care or treatment.

- The three major components of a physical examination are the medical history, the hands-on examination, and diagnostic laboratory tests.
- A medical history is the most important part of the physical examination, especially during the initial visit to a doctor.
- A selective health examination involves the use of specific tests for specific problems. A periodic exam involves the use of tests and procedures after a complete medical history and a discussion of personal lifestyle factors and risk factors.
- Defensive medicine is the practice of prescribing tests and procedures for the purpose of protecting doctors from medical-malpractice lawsuits.
- Direct-access testing (DAT) empowers patients with the ability to purchase medical testing without a prescription or a trip to the doctor's office. DAT may be more convenient than scheduling an appointment with a doctor, but it is also expensive (not usually covered by insurance) and if the test results are not favorable the doctor is left out when he or she is needed the most.
- The eight diseases for which adults need to maintain immunization are influenza, pneumonia, hepatitis, measles, rubella, tetanus, diphtheria, and chicken pox.
- Health insurance options include the preferred provider organization (PPO), the point of service (POS), the health maintenance organization (HMO), the indemnity plan, and government insurance.

Review Questions

1. How does health fatalism negatively influence understanding of health information?
2. What are some examples of health information contradictions?
3. What criteria must a research study satisfy before its claims can be trusted?
4. What are some techniques and strategies that manufacturers and producers of health products use to mislead and deceive the public?
5. Explain the meaning and significance of scientifically controlled, double-blind studies. Cite an example.
6. What do the terms *statistical significance* and *statistical relationship* mean in reference to health studies?
7. Differentiate between the terms *absolute risk* and *relative risk*. Which of these two terms tends to be misleading? Why?
8. How do epidemiologic studies differ from scientifically controlled studies?
9. How can you tell if health information on the Internet can be trusted? Identify three criteria or guidelines.
10. Identify four signs or symptoms that require immediate medical attention.
11. A high body temperature, a fever, is described in the chapter as "an adaptive response." What does this mean?

12. Why is it important to see a physician while in good health?
13. What can laypeople do while in a hospital to ensure that they receive safe and proper care?
14. Define the term *polypharmacy*. What can people do to prevent health complications caused by polypharmacy?
15. Identify the five health conditions that are responsible for the greatest number of inpatient hospitalizations.
16. What is the major role and function of a primary-care physician?
17. Define *alternative medicine*. What reasons do conventional medical doctors give for being concerned about the indiscriminate use of alternative medicine?
18. List four sources of information for researching physicians and specialists in your geographical area.
19. Identify four techniques that facilitate communication between patient and physician.
20. List four guidelines for facilitating e-mail communication between you and your health care provider.
21. Identify six rights patients have when in a hospital.
22. Differentiate among selective health exam, periodic exam, and comprehensive physical examination.
23. Identify five items that should be included in the home medicine cabinet. What is the purpose of each?

24. In reference to medical tests, differentiate among the terms *positive, negative, false positive,* and *false negative.*
25. Define *defensive medicine.* Discuss its impact on both the quantity and the quality of health care provided to patients.
26. Identify 5 of the 10 most commonly used alternative medical therapies.
27. What does the acronym DAT mean? What are the pros and cons of DAT?
28. Identify immunizations for adults.
29. Compare and contrast the basic plans of health insurance.

References

1. Klausner, A. 2003. The sunny side ups (and downs) of egg substitutes. *Environmental Nutrition* 26(10):2.
2. Tufts Media. 2003. Soy's power to lower cholesterol downgraded. *Tufts University Health and Nutrition Letter* 21(2):1.
3. Sandroff, S. 2000. Frustrations of science. *Consumer Reports on Health* 12(8):2.
4. Forman, A. 2001. Why nutrition advice flip-flops all the time . . . or does it? *Environmental Nutrition* 24(3):1, 6.
5. *New England Journal of Medicine.* 2003. Assessing your health risks. *HealthNews* 9(12):3.
6. Harvard Medical Information Publications Group. 1999. Health information: Turn of the news. *Harvard Health Letter,* 24(11):1–2.
7. Consumers Union. 1997. Finding medical help online. *Consumer Reports* 62(2):27–31.
8. Mayo Foundation for Medical Education and Research. 1997. Health info on the Internet. *Mayo Clinic Health Letter* 15(4):6.
9. Consumers Union. 2004. Doctoring yourself: When is it wise? *Consumer Reports on Health* 16(1):1, 4–6.
10. Consumers Union. 2002. When to treat a fever. *Consumer Reports on Health* 14(9):10.
11. Tufts University. 2000. When nagging symptoms should trigger a doctor's visit. *Tufts University Health and Nutrition Letter* 18(5):4–5.
12. DeFrances, C. J., and M. J. Hall. 2004. *2002 National hospital discharge survey.* Hyattsville, MD: National Center for Health Statistics.
13. Bernstein, A. B., E. Hing, A. J. Moss, K. F. Allen, A. B. Siller, and R. B. Tiggle. 2003. *Health care in America: Trends in utilization.* Hyattsville, MD: National Center for Health Statistics.
14. Associated Press. 2002. Hospital infections killed 103,000 in 2000, study says. *The Commercial Appeal,* 21 July, A2.

15. Harvard Medical Information Publications Group. 2004. Hospital report cards: Making the grade. *Harvard Health Letter* 29(8):1–2.
16. Sandroff, R. 1997. AHAdvocate. *American Health* 16(6):41–43.
17. Consumers Union. 2001. Medication errors—Yours and theirs. *Consumer Reports on Health* 13(11):1, 4–6.
18. *Environmental Nutrition.* 2002. Antibiotic use in animals leaves people vulnerable to "superbugs." *Environmental Nutrition* 25(8):1, 6.
19. Mayo Foundation for Medical Education and Research. 2004. Surgery: What to expect and how to prepare. *Mayo Clinic Health Letter* 22(6):1–8.
20. *Environmental Nutrition.* 2004. Hospitalized? Insist on getting a multi. *Environmental Nutrition* 27(8):3.
21. Consumers Union. 2001. Doctor, can we talk? *Consumer Reports on Health* 13(7):7–8.
22. Consumers Union. 2001. Rushed doctor visits. *Consumer Reports on Health* 13(9):3.
23. Harvard Medical Information Publications Group. 2004. Nine tips for patients. *Harvard Health Letter* 29(9):1–2.
24. Consumers Union. 1998. Special report on health guide to medication. *Consumer Reports* 63(4):1–8.
25. Lipman, M. 2004. E-mailing your doctor. *Consumer Reports on Health* 16(4):11.
26. Consumers Union. 2002. Take two aspirins and e-mail me in the morning. *Consumer Reports* 67(1):59, 61.
27. *New England Journal of Medicine.* 2004. Advice from the pharmacy. *HealthNews* 11(9):14.
28. Barnes, P. M., E. Powell-Griner, K. McFann, and R. L. Nahin. 2004. *Complementary and alternative medicine use among adults: United States, 2002.* Hyattsville, MD: National Center for Health Statistics.
29. The Burton Goldberg Group. 1998. *Alternative medicine, the definitive guide.* Puyallup, WA: Future Medicine.

30. Atkinson, H. 1997. Discussing alternative medicine. *HealthNews* 3(10):4–5.
31. Harvard Medical Information Publications Group. 2000. Alternative medicine. *Harvard Health Letter* 25(11):1–3.
32. Harvard Medical Information Publications Group. 1997. Alternative medicine, time for a second opinion. *Harvard Health Letter* 23(1):1–3.
33. MedlinePlus. 2004. Physical exam frequency (www.nlm.nih.gov/medlineplus/ency/article/002125.htm).
34. Harvard Medical Information Publications Group. 1999. The physical exam: Close encounter of a medical kind. *Harvard Health Letter* 24(10):1–3.
35. Medical Malpractice Victims Organization. 2001. Some startling facts about medical malpractice (www.a-r-m.org).
36. Consumers Union. 2004. Which tests do you really need? *Consumer Reports on Health* 16(2):1, 4–5.
37. Consumers Union. 2002. To screen or not to screen. *Consumer Reports on Health* 14(6):1, 4–6.
38. Lipman, M. 2001. Imaging tests: Are more always better? *Consumer Reports on Health* 13(2):11.
39. Mayo Foundation for Medical Education and Research. 1999. Understanding your T-Score. *Mayo Clinic Health Letter* 17(11):3.
40. *New England Journal of Medicine.* 2003. What's DAT? *HealthNews* 9(7):5.
41. Tufts University. 2003. Putting home tests to the test. *Tufts University Health and Nutrition Letter* 21(8):1–4.
42. Tufts University. 2002. Vaccines? Yes, you. *Tufts University Health and Nutrition Letter* 20(9):3.
43. Harvard Medical School. 2003. Boomers, not just babies, need to get their shots. *Harvard Health Letter* 28(11):7.

Suggested Readings

Gallin, P. F. 2003. *How to survive your doctor's care: Get the right diagnosis, the right treatment, and the right experts for you.* St. Louis, MO: Lifeline Press.

This guide is a roadmap for navigating the medical system. The importance of choosing a hospital before choosing a doctor is emphasized, along with the value of second opinions. Real-world examples are used to explain the inner workings of the medical world. After reading this book, patients can improve their chances for getting good health care, selecting the right doctor, evaluating the doctor, and knowing what to do when receiving medical care.

Medical Economics Co. 2003. *The PDR pocket guide to prescription drugs.* 6th ed. St. Louis, MO: Pocket Books.

This pocket-sized book provides FDA-approved information on drugs according to brand name and generic cross-reference, along with benefits, risks, and side effects. Possible food/drug interactions and overdose information are included. Drug profiles are based on information from the trusted *Physicians' Desk Reference.*

Soden, K. J. 2003. *The art of medicine: What every doctor and patient should know.* St. Louis, MO: Mosby.

This book reinforces the age-old advice that medicine is part science and part art. Topics ranging from death and dying to sexuality, spirituality, and wellness are discussed using stories, anecdotes, and even cartoons. While it was designed originally to teach medical students how to interact with patients and deal with difficult medical situations, it is equally applicable to patients who expect their doctors to serve as both physician and partner.

Name _____ Date _____ Section _____

Assessment Activity 15-2

Assessing the Results of Diagnostic Tests

Directions: Use this assessment to record the dates and results of commonly administered diagnostic medical tests. Refer to information in this chapter to review the purposes of these tests.

Test Name	Typical Reference Range	What's Being Tested	Your Results	Date
1. Alanine aminotransferase (ALT)	10–40 U/L	Heart, liver, muscle damage		
2. Albumin	3.5–5.2 g/dL	Kidneys		
3. Alkaline phosphate	35–128 mg/dL	Liver, parathyroid glands, bone disease		
4. Aspartate aminotransferase (AST)	10–59 U/L	Liver, heart, muscle damage		
5. Bilirubin	0.3–1.5 mg/dL	Liver, kidneys		
6. Blood urea nitrogen (BUN)	8–22 mg/dL	Kidneys		
7. Calcium	8.6–10.0 mg/dL	Parathyroid glands, cancer, bone disease		
8. Carbon dioxide	22–28 mEq/L	Lungs and heart		
9. Chloride	98–107 mEq/L	Dehydration		
10. Cholesterol (total)	< 200 mg/dL	Heart and artery disease		
11. Creatinine	0.7–1.3 mg/dL	Kidneys		
12. Free T4 hormone	1.0–4.3 mg/dL	Thyroid gland		
13. Globulin	1.5–3.8 g/dL	Infections		
14. Glucose	< 120 mg/dL	Diabetes mellitus		
15. Hematocrit	42–52%	Anemia		
16. High-density lipoprotein (HDL)	> 40 mg/dL	Heart and artery disease		
17. Iron (total)	50–175 mg/dL	Anemia		
18. Lactic dehydrogenase	100–190 U/L	Liver		
19. Low-density lipoprotein (LDL)	< 130 mg/dL	Heart and artery disease		
20. Lymphocyte	20–40%	Immune deficiency disorder		
21. Phosphorous	2.3–4.6 mg/dL	Kidneys		
22. Potassium	3.4–4.4 mEq/L	Kidneys		
23. Protein	6.4–8.3 g/dL	Kidneys, nutrition		
24. Red blood cells (RBC)	4.2–6.1 m/mL	Anemia		
25. Sedimentation rate	(< 50) 15–20 mm/h	Infections		

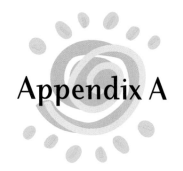

Appendix A

Food Composition Table

Nutritional Content of Common Foods

For this Food Composition Table, foods are listed within the following groups:

1. Breads, cereals, rice, and pasta
2. Vegetables
3. Fruit
4. Milk, yogurt, and cheese
5. Meat, poultry, fish, dry beans, eggs, and nuts
6. Fats, oils, sweets, and alcoholic beverages

SOURCE: U.S. Department of Agriculture, Agricultural Research Service. 2004. *USDA Nutrient Database for Standard Reference, Release 17* (**www.nal.usda.gov/fnic/foodcomp**).

Breads, Cereals, Rice, and Pasta

Name	Amount	Weight (g)	Energy (Calories)	Protein (g)	Carbohydrate (g)	Fiber (g)	Total Fat (g)	Saturated Fat (g)	Cholesterol (mg)	Sodium (mg)	Vitamin A (RE)	Vitamin C (mg)	Calcium (mg)	Iron (mg)
Bagel, plain	1 bagel, 4″ diameter	89	245	9.3	47.5	2.0	1.4	0.2	0	475	0	0	16	3.2
Barley, pearled, cooked	½ cup	79	97	1.8	22.2	3.0	0.3	0.1	0	2	1	0	9	1.0
Bulgur, cooked	½ cup	83	110	3.0	23.5	4.5	0.1	0	0	4	0	0	11	0.5
Biscuit	1 biscuit, 2½″ diameter	27	93	1.8	12.8	0.4	4.0	1.0	0	325	0	0	5	0.7
Bread, corn	1 piece	60	188	4.3	28.9	1.4	6.0	1.6	37	467	26	0	44	1.1
Bread, french	1 slice	64	175	5.6	33.2	1.9	1.9	0.4	0	390	0	0	48	1.6
Bread, oatmeal	1 slice	27	73	2.3	13.1	1.1	1.2	0.2	0	162	1	0	18	0.7
Bread, pita, white	1 pita, 6½″ diameter	60	165	5.5	33.4	1.3	0.7	0.1	0	322	0	0	52	1.6
Bread, pita, whole-wheat	1 pita, 6½″ diameter	64	170	6.3	35.2	4.7	1.7	0.3	0	340	0	0	10	2.0
Bread, pumpernickel	1 slice	26	65	2.3	12.3	1.7	0.8	0.1	0	174	0	0	18	0.7
Bread, raisin	1 slice	32	88	2.5	16.7	1.4	1.4	0.3	0	125	0	0	21	0.9
Bread, rye	1 slice	32	83	2.7	15.5	1.9	1.1	0.2	0	211	0	0.1	23	0.9
Bread sticks	2 sticks, 7⅝″× ⅝″	20	82	2.4	13.6	0.6	1.9	0.3	0	131	0	0	4	0.8
Bread stuffing	½ cup	100	178	3.2	21.7	2.9	8.6	1.7	0	543	81	0	32	1.1
Bread, white	1 slice	30	80	2.5	14.9	0.7	1.1	0.2	0	161	0	0	32	0.9
Bread, whole-grain	1 slice	32	80	3.2	14.8	2.0	1.2	0.3	0	156	0	0.1	29	1.1
Bread, whole-wheat	1 slice	28	69	2.7	12.9	1.9	1.2	0.3	0	148	0	0	20	0.9
Buckwheat groats, cooked	½ cup	84	77	2.8	16.8	2.3	0.5	0.1	0	3	0	0	6	0.7
Bun, hamburger/hot dog	1 roll	43	123	3.7	21.6	1.2	2.2	0.5	0	241	0	0	60	1.4
Cake, angelfood	1/12 of 10″ cake	50	129	3.1	29.4	0.1	0.2	0	0	255	0	0	42	0.1
Cake, chocolate w/frosting	⅛ of 18 oz cake	64	235	2.6	34.9	1.8	10.5	3.1	27	214	16	0.1	28	1.4
Cake, yellow w/icing	⅛ of 18 oz cake	64	243	2.4	35.5	1.2	11.1	3.0	35	216	21	0	23	1.3
Cereal, All-Bran	½ cup	30	53	3.7	22.7	15.3	0.9	0.2	0	127	260	17.3	116	5.2
Cereal, Bran Chex	⅗ cup	28	90	2.9	22.6	4.6	0.8	0.1	0	200	6	15.0	17	8.1
Cereal, Cheerios	1 cup	30	110	3.1	22.9	2.6	1.8	0.4	0	284	375	15.0	55	8.1
Cereal, cornflakes	1 cup	28	102	1.8	24.2	0.8	0.2	0.1	0	298	210	14.0	1	8.7
Cereal, Cream of Wheat	½ cup	126	67	1.9	13.8	0.9	0.3	0	0	168	0	0	25	5.1
Cereal, frosted flakes	¾ cup	31	119	1.2	28.3	0.6	0.2	0.1	0	200	225	15.0	1	4.5
Cereal, granola	½ cup	31	135	3.0	22.4	1.9	4.2	0.6	0	8	0	0.1	24	1.3
Cereal, raisin bran	1 cup	61	186	5.6	47.1	8.2	1.5	0	0	354	250	0	35	5.0
Cereal, Total	¾ cup	30	105	3.0	23.9	2.6	0.7	0.2	0	199	375	60.0	258	18.0
Cereal, Wheaties	1 cup	30	110	3.2	0.9	2.1	0.9	0.2	0	222	225	15.0	55	8.1
Coffee cake w/topping	1 piece	63	263	4.3	29.4	1.3	14.7	3.7	20	221	21	0.2	34	1.2
Cookie, chocolate chip	1 medium cookie	16	78	0.9	9.3	0.4	4.5	1.3	5	58	26	0	6	0.4
Cookie, fig bar	1 cookie	16	56	0.6	11.3	0.7	1.2	0.2	0	56	1	0	10	0.5
Cookie, fortune	1 cookie	8	30	0.3	6.7	0.1	0.2	0.1	0	22	0	0	1	0.1
Cookie, oatmeal	1 large cookie	18	81	1.1	12.4	0.5	3.3	0.8	0	69	0	0.1	7	0.5
Cookie, sandwich	1 cookie	10	47	0.5	7.0	0.3	0.3	0.4	0	60	0	0	3	0.4
Corn grits, cooked	½ cup	121	73	1.7	15.7	0.2	0.2	0	0	0	7	0	0	0.8
Cornmeal, dry	¼ cup	35	126	2.9	26.8	2.6	0.6	0.1	0	1	14	0	2	1.4
Couscous, cooked	½ cup	79	88	3.0	18.2	1.1	0.1	0	0	4	0	0	6	0.3
Cracker, Crispbread, rye	3 crispbreads	30	110	2.4	24.7	5.0	0.4	0	0	79	0	0	9	0.7
Cracker, Goldfish	24 goldfish	12	70	1.0	8.0	1.0	4.0	0	0	100	0	0	8	0.4
Cracker, graham	3 squares	28	119	2.0	21.3	1.0	2.8	0.4	0	185	0	0	22	1.2
Cracker, matzo	1 matzo	28	112	2.8	23.7	0.9	0.4	0.1	0	1	0	0	4	0.9
Cracker, melba toast	6 pieces	30	117	3.6	23.0	1.9	1.0	0.1	0	249	0	0	28	1.1
Cracker, Ritz	5 crackers	16	79	1.2	10.3	0.3	3.7	0.6	0	124	0	0	24	0.6
Cracker, saltine	10 squares	30	130	2.8	21.5	0.9	3.5	0.9	0	390	0	0	36	1.6
Cracker, whole-wheat	6 crackers	24	106	2.1	16.5	2.5	4.1	0.8	0	158	0	0	24	0.7
Croissant, butter	1 medium	57	231	4.7	26.1	1.5	12.0	6.6	38	424	106	0.1	21	1.2

Name	Amount	Weight (g)	Energy (Calories)	Protein (g)	Carbohydrate (g)	Fiber (g)	Total Fat (g)	Saturated Fat (g)	Cholesterol (mg)	Sodium (mg)	Vitamin A (RE)	Vitamin C (mg)	Calcium (mg)	Iron (mg)
Danish pastry, cheese	1 pastry	71	266	5.7	26.4	0.7	15.5	4.8	11	320	32	0	25	1.1
Doughnut, glazed	1 medium	45	192	2.3	22.9	0.7	10.3	2.7	14	181	1	0	27	0.5
English muffin, plain	½ muffin	29	67	2.2	13.1	0.8	0.5	0.1	0	132	0	0	50	0.7
French toast	1 slice	65	149	5.0	16.3	0	7.0	1.8	75	311	86	0.2	65	1.1
Macaroni, cooked	½ cup	70	99	3.3	19.8	0.9	0.5	0.1	0	1	0	0	5	1.0
Muffin, blueberry	2″ by 2¾″	57	158	3.1	27.4	1.5	3.7	0.8	17	255	5	0.6	32	0.9
Muffin, oat bran	2¼″ by 2½″	57	154	4.0	27.5	2.6	4.2	0.6	0	224	0	0	36	2.4
Noodles, chow mein	½ cup	23	119	1.9	12.9	0.9	6.9	1.0	0	99	2	0	5	1.1
Noodles, egg, cooked	½ cup	80	106	3.8	19.9	0.9	1.2	0.2	53	6	5	0	10	1.3
Noodles, Japanese soba	½ cup	57	56	2.9	12.2	0	0.1	0	0	34	0	0	2	0.3
Oatmeal, instant	1 packet	155	153	4.1	31.4	2.6	1.8	0.4	0	234	302	0	105	3.9
Oats, uncooked	¼ cup	20	78	3.2	27.1	2.1	1.3	0.2	0	1	2	0	11	0.9
Pancake	4″ pancake	38	74	2.0	13.9	0.5	1.0	0.2	5	239	12	0.1	48	0.6
Pasta, cooked	½ cup	57	75	2.9	14.2	0	0.6	0.1	19	3	3	0	3	0.7
Popcorn, air-popped	2 cups	16	61	1.9	12.5	2.4	0.7	0.1	0	1	3	0	2	0.4
Popcorn, oil-popped	2 cups	22	110	1.9	12.6	2.2	6.2	1.0	0	194	3	0	2	0.6
Pretzels	10 twists	60	229	5.5	47.5	1.9	2.1	0.5	0	1,029	0	0	22	2.6
Quinoa, uncooked	¼ cup	43	159	5.6	29.3	2.5	2.5	0.3	0	9	0	0	26	3.9
Rice, brown, cooked	½ cup	71	109	2.3	22.9	1.8	0.8	0.3	0	1	0	0	10	0.5
Rice cake	1 cake	9	35	0.7	7.3	0.4	0.3	0	0	29	0	0	1	0.1
Rice, white, cooked	½ cup	93	121	2.2	26.6	0.3	0.2	0.1	0	0	0	0	3	1.4
Rice, wild, cooked	½ cup	82	83	3.3	17.5	1.5	0.3	0	0	3	0	0	2	0.5
Roll, dinner	1 roll, 2″ square	28	84	2.4	14.1	0.8	2.0	0.5	0	146	0	0	33	0.9
Spaghetti, cooked	½ cup	70	99	3.3	19.8	1.2	0.5	0.1	0	70	0	0	5	1.0
Taco shell	1 medium	13	62	1.0	8.3	1.0	3.0	0.4	0	49	0	0	21	0.3
Tortilla chips	1 oz	28	142	2.0	17.8	1.8	7.4	1.4	0	150	6	0	44	0.4
Tortilla, corn	1 medium	26	58	1.5	12.1	1.4	0.7	0.1	0	42	0	0	46	0.4
Tortilla, flour	1 medium	49	159	4.3	27.2	1.6	3.5	0.9	0	234	0	0	61	1.6
Wheat germ, toasted	¼ cup	28	108	8.3	14.1	3.7	3.0	0.5	0	1	0	1.7	13	2.6

Vegetables

Name	Amount	Weight (g)	Energy (Calories)	Protein (g)	Carbohydrate (g)	Fiber (g)	Total Fat (g)	Saturated Fat (g)	Cholesterol (mg)	Sodium (mg)	Vitamin A (RE)	Vitamin C (mg)	Calcium (mg)	Iron (mg)
Artichoke, cooked	1 medium	120	60	4.2	13.4	6.5	0.2	0	0	114	22	12.0	54	1.5
Arugula, raw	1 cup	20	5	0.5	0.7	0.3	0.1	0	0	3	24	3.0	16	0.1
Asparagus, cooked	6 spears	90	22	2.3	3.8	1.4	0.3	0	0	10	49	9.7	18	0.7
Bamboo shoots, canned	½ cup	66	13	1.1	2.1	0.9	0.3	0.1	0	5	1	0.7	5	0.2
Bean sprouts, raw	½ cup	35	43	4.6	3.3	0.4	2.3	0.3	0	5	0	5.4	23	0.7
*Beans, baked (plain)	½ cup	127	118	6.1	26.0	6.4	0.6	0.1	0	504	22	3.9	64	0.4
*Beans, black, cooked	½ cup	86	114	7.6	20.4	7.5	0.5	0.1	0	1	1	0	23	1.8
*Beans, fava, cooked	½ cup	85	94	6.5	16.7	4.6	0.3	0.1	0	4	2	0.3	31	1.3
Beans, green snap, cooked	½ cup	63	22	1.2	4.9	2.0	0.2	0	0	2	42	6.1	29	0.8
*Beans, kidney, cooked	½ cup	89	112	7.7	20.2	6.5	0.4	0.1	0	2	0	1.1	25	2.6
*Beans, lentils, cooked	½ cup	99	115	8.9	19.9	7.8	0.4	0.1	0	2	1	1.5	19	3.3
*Beans, lima, cooked	½ cup	94	108	7.3	19.6	6.6	0.4	0.1	0	2	0	0	16	2.2
*Beans, navy, cooked	½ cup	91	129	7.9	23.9	5.8	0.5	0.1	0	1	0	0.8	64	2.3
*Beans, pinto, cooked	½ cup	86	117	7.0	21.9	7.4	0.4	0.1	0	2	0	1.8	41	2.2
*Beans, refried	½ cup	126	118	6.9	19.6	6.7	1.6	0.6	10	377	0	7.6	44	2.1

*Dry beans and peas (legumes), which can be counted as servings of vegetables or as servings from the meat, poultry, fish, dry beans, eggs, and nuts group.

Name	Amount	Weight (g)	Energy (Calories)	Protein (g)	Carbohydrate (g)	Fiber (g)	Total Fat (g)	Saturated Fat (g)	Cholesterol (mg)	Sodium (mg)	Vitamin A (RE)	Vitamin C (mg)	Calcium (mg)	Iron (mg)
Beans, yellow snap, cooked	½ cup	63	22	1.2	4.9	2.1	0.2	0	0	2	5	6.1	29	0.8
Beet greens, cooked	½ cup	144	39	3.7	7.9	4.2	0.3	0	0	347	734	35.9	164	2.7
Beets, cooked	½ cup	74	37	1.4	8.5	1.7	0.2	0	0	65	3	3.1	14	0.7
Broccoli spears, cooked	2 spears	78	22	2.3	3.9	2.3	0.3	0	0	20	108	58.2	36	0.7
Brussels sprouts, cooked	4 sprouts	84	33	2.1	7.3	2.2	0.4	0.1	0	18	60	52.1	30	1.0
Cabbage, cooked	½ cup	75	17	0.8	3.3	1.7	0.3	0	0	6	10	15.1	23	0.1
Cabbage, raw	½ cup	45	11	0.6	2.4	1.0	0.1	0	0	8	6	14.3	21	0.3
Carrot juice	¾ cup	177	71	1.7	16.4	1.4	0.3	0	0	51	1,938	15.0	42	0.8
Carrots, cooked	½ cup	78	35	0.9	8.2	2.6	0.1	0	0	51	1,915	1.8	24	0.5
Carrots, raw	1 medium	61	26	0.6	6.2	1.8	0.1	0	0	21	1,716	5.6	16	0.3
Cauliflower, cooked	½ cup	62	14	1.1	2.5	1.7	0.3	0	0	9	1	27.4	10	0.2
Celery, raw	8 sticks	32	5	0.2	1.2	0.5	0	0	0	28	4	2.2	13	0.1
Chard, cooked	½ cup	88	18	1.6	3.6	1.8	0.1	0	0	156	275	15.8	51	2.0
Coleslaw, homemade	½ cup	60	41	0.8	7.4	0.9	1.6	0.2	5	14	49	19.6	27	0.4
Collards, cooked	½ cup	95	25	2.0	4.7	2.7	0.3	0	0	9	297	17.3	113	0.4
Corn, yellow, cooked	½ cup	82	89	2.7	20.6	2.3	1.1	0.2	0	14	18	5.1	2	0.5
Cucumber, raw	½ cup	52	7	0.4	1.4	0.4	0.1	0	0	1	11	2.8	7	0.1
Eggplant, cooked	½ cup	50	14	0.4	3.3	1.2	0.1	0	0	1	3	0.6	3	0.2
Endive, raw	½ cup	25	4	0.3	0.8	0.8	0.1	0	0	6	51	1.6	13	0.2
Hominy, canned	½ cup	83	94	1.2	11.8	2.1	0.7	0.1	0	173	0	0	8	0.5
Kale, cooked	½ cup	65	18	1.2	3.6	1.3	0.3	0	0	15	481	26.7	47	0.6
Lettuce, iceberg	1 cup	55	7	0.6	1.1	0.8	0.1	0	0	5	18	2.1	10	0.3
Lettuce, looseleaf	1 cup	56	10	0.7	2.0	1.1	0.2	0	0	5	106	10.1	38	0.8
Lettuce, romaine	1 cup	56	8	0.9	1.3	1.0	0.1	0	0	4	152	13.4	20	0.6
Mushrooms, cooked	½ cup	78	21	1.7	4.0	1.7	0.3	0	0	2	0	3.1	5	1.4
Mushrooms, raw	½ cup	35	9	1.0	1.4	0.4	0.1	0	0	1	0	0.8	2	0.4
Mustard greens, cooked	½ cup	70	11	1.6	1.5	1.4	0.2	0	0	11	212	17.7	52	0.5
Okra, cooked	½ cup	92	26	1.9	5.3	2.6	0.3	0.1	0	3	47	11.2	88	0.6
Onion, raw	½ cup	80	30	0.9	6.9	1.4	0.1	0	0	2	0	5.1	16	0.2
Parsnip, raw	½ cup	67	50	0.8	12.0	3.2	0.2	0	0	7	0	11.3	24	0.4
*Peas, blackeye, cooked	½ cup	86	100	6.6	17.9	5.6	0.5	0.1	0	3	1	0.3	21	2.2
*Peas, chickpeas (garbanzos)	½ cup	82	134	7.3	22.5	6.2	2.1	0.2	0	6	2	1.1	40	2.4
Peas, edible podded	10 peapods	34	14	1.0	2.6	0.9	0.1	0	0	1	5	20.4	15	0.7
Peas, green	½ cup	80	62	4.1	11.4	4.4	0.2	0	0	70	54	7.9	19	1.2
*Peas, split, cooked	½ cup	98	116	8.2	20.6	8.1	0.4	0.1	0	2	1	0.4	14	1.3
Pepper, green chili, canned	½ cup	70	15	0.5	3.2	1.2	0.2	0	0	276	9	23.8	25	0.9
Pepper, sweet green, raw	1 small	74	20	0.7	4.8	1.3	0.1	0	0	1	47	66.1	7	0.3
Pepper, sweet red, raw	1 small	74	20	0.7	4.8	1.5	0.1	0	0	1	422	140.6	7	0.3
Pickle, dill	1 medium	65	12	0.4	2.7	0.8	0.1	0	0	21	833	1.2	6	0.3
Potato, baked w/skin	1 medium	173	188	4.0	43.5	4.1	0.2	0	0	14	0	22.3	17	2.3
Potato, boiled	1 potato, 2½″ diameter	136	118	2.5	27.4	2.4	0.1	0	0	5	0	17.7	7	0.4
Potato, french fries	10 fries	50	109	1.7	17.0	1.6	4.1	1.9	0	141	0	4.8	5	0.7
Potato, mashed w/milk	½ cup	105	81	2.0	18.4	2.1	0.6	0.3	2	318	6	7.0	27	0.3
Potato salad	½ cup	125	179	3.4	14.0	1.6	10.3	1.8	85	661	41	12.5	24	0.8
Pumpkin, canned	½ cup	123	42	1.3	9.9	3.6	0.3	0.2	0	6	2,702	5.1	32	1.7
Radish	13 medium	58	12	0.3	2.1	0.9	0.3	0	0	13.9	1	13.2	12	0.2
Rutabaga, mashed	½ cup	120	47	1.5	10.5	2.2	0.3	0	0	24	67	22.6	58	0.6
Sauerkraut, drained	½ cup	121	13	0.6	3.0	1.8	0.1	0	0	469	1	10.5	21	1.0
Soybeans, green, boiled	½ cup	90	127	11.1	9.9	3.8	5.8	0.7	0	13	14	15.3	131	2.3

*Dry beans can be counted as servings from this group or the vegetables group; data on dry beans is listed under vegetables (see items marked with an asterisk).

Name	Amount	Weight (g)	Energy (Calories)	Protein (g)	Carbohydrate (g)	Fiber (g)	Total Fat (g)	Saturated Fat (g)	Cholesterol (mg)	Sodium (mg)	Vitamin A (RE)	Vitamin C (mg)	Calcium (mg)	Iron (mg)
Spinach, cooked	½ cup	95	27	3.0	5.1	2.9	0.2	0	0	82	739	11.7	139	1.4
Spinach, raw	1 cup	30	7	0.9	1.1	0.8	0.1	0	0	24	202	8.4	30	0.8
Squash, summer, cooked	½ cup	90	18	0.8	3.9	1.3	0.3	0	0	1	26	5.0	24	0.3
Squash, summer, raw	½ small squash	59	12	0.7	2.6	1.1	0.1	0	0	1	12	8.7	12	0.3
Squash, winter	½ cup	100	39	0.9	8.8	2.8	0.6	0.1	0	1	356	9.6	14	0.3
Sweet potato, baked	½ cup	100	103	1.7	24.3	3.0	0.1	0	0	10	2,182	24.6	28	0.5
Sweet potato, canned w/syrup	½ cup	100	108	1.3	25.4	3.0	0.3	0.1	0	39	716	10.8	17	1.0
Tomato juice	¾ cup	182	31	1.4	7.7	1.5	1.4	0	0	18	102	33.3	16	1.1
Tomato, raw	1 medium	123	26	1.0	5.7	1.4	0.4	0.1	0	11	76	23.5	6	0.6
Tomato sauce	½ cup	123	37	1.6	1.7	1.7	0.2	0	0	741	120	16.0	17	0.9
Turnip, cooked, mashed	½ cup	115	24	0.8	5.6	2.3	0.1	0	0	108	0	13.3	25	0.3
Vegetable juice	¾ cup	182	35	1.1	8.3	1.5	0.2	0	0	491	213	50.4	20	0.8
Vegetables, mixed	½ cup	91	54	2.6	11.9	4.0	0.1	0	0	32	389	2.9	23	0.7
Vegetable soup	1 cup	241	72	2.1	12.0	0.5	1.9	0.3	0	822	301	1.4	22	1.1
Water chestnuts	½ cup	70	35	0.6	8.7	1.8	0	0	0	6	0	0.9	3	0.6

Fruit

Name	Amount	Weight (g)	Energy (Calories)	Protein (g)	Carbohydrate (g)	Fiber (g)	Total Fat (g)	Saturated Fat (g)	Cholesterol (mg)	Sodium (mg)	Vitamin A (RE)	Vitamin C (mg)	Calcium (mg)	Iron (mg)
Apple	1 medium	138	81	0.3	21.0	3.7	0.5	0.1	0	0	7	7.9	10	0.2
Apple juice	¾ cup	179	84	0.3	20.7	0.2	0.2	0	0	13	0	44.8	11	0.5
Applesauce, unsweetened	½ cup	122	52	0.2	13.8	1.5	0.1	0	0	2	4	25.9	4	0.1
Apricots	2 medium	70	34	1.0	7.8	1.7	0.3	0	0	1	183	7.0	10	0.4
Apricots, dried	9 halves	32	75	1.2	19.4	2.8	0.1	0	0	3	228	0.8	14	1.5
Avocado	1 medium	173	306	3.7	12.0	8.5	30.0	4.5	0	21	105	13.7	19	2.0
Banana	1 medium	118	109	1.2	27.6	2.8	0.6	0.2	0	1	9	10.7	7	0.4
Blackberries	½ cup	72	37	0.5	9.2	3.8	0.3	0	0	0	12	15.1	23	0.4
Blueberries	½ cup	73	41	0.5	10.2	2.0	0.3	0	0	4	7	9.4	4	0.1
Cantaloupe	¼ melon, 5″ diameter	138	48	1.2	11.5	1.1	0.4	0.1	0	12	444	58.2	15	0.3
Carambola (starfruit)	1 small	70	23	0.4	5.5	1.9	0.2	0	0	1	34	14.8	3	0.2
Cherries, canned in syrup	½ cup	128	116	0.9	29.8	1.4	0.1	0	0	9	91	2.6	13	1.7
Cherries, sweet, raw	11 cherries	75	54	0.9	2.3	1.7	0.7	0.2	0	0	16	5.2	11	0.3
Cranberries, raw	½ cup	48	23	0.2	6.0	2.0	0.1	0	0	1	2	6.4	3	0.1
Cranberry juice cocktail	¾ cup	190	108	0	27.3	0.2	0.2	0	0	4	0	67.1	6	0.3
Cranberry sauce	¼ cup	139	105	0.1	26.9	0.7	0.1	0	0	20	1	1.4	3	0.2
Currants, dried	¼ cup	36	109	1.5	26.7	2.4	0.1	0	0	3	3	1.7	31	1.2
Dates, dried	¼ cup	45	122	0.9	32.7	3.3	0.2	0.1	0	1	2	0	14	0.5
Figs, raw	2 medium	100	74	0.8	19.2	3.3	0.3	0.1	0	1	14	2.0	35	0.4
Fruit cocktail, heavy syrup	½ cup	124	91	0.5	23.4	1.2	0.1	0	0	7	25	2.4	7	0.4
Fruit cocktail, light syrup	½ cup	121	69	0.5	18.1	1.2	0.1	0	0	7	25	2.3	7	0.4
Fruit cocktail, juice	½ cup	119	55	0.5	14.1	1.2	0	0	0	5	37	3.2	9	0.3
Grapefruit	½ medium	128	41	0.8	10.3	1.4	0.1	0	0	0	15	44.0	15	0.1
Grapefruit juice	¾ cup	185	70	1.0	16.6	0.2	0.2	0	0	2	2	54.1	13	0.4
Grapes	12 grapes	60	43	0.4	10.7	0.6	0.3	0	0	1	4	6.5	7	0.2
Guava	1 fruit	90	46	0.7	10.7	4.9	0.5	0.2	0	3	71	165.2	18	0.3
Honeydew	⅛ melon, 5½″ diameter	125	44	0.6	11.5	0.8	0.1	0	0	13	5	31.0	8	0.1
Kiwifruit	1 large	91	56	0.9	13.5	3.1	0.4	0	0	5	16	68.3	24	0.4
Kumquats	5 fruits	100	63	0.9	16.4	6.6	0.1	0	0	6	30	37.4	44	0.4
Lemon, with peel	1 fruit	108	22	1.3	11.6	5.1	0.3	0	0	3	3	83.2	66	0.8

Name	Amount	Weight (g)	Energy (Calories)	Protein (g)	Carbohydrate (g)	Fiber (g)	Total Fat (g)	Saturated Fat (g)	Cholesterol (mg)	Sodium (mg)	Vitamin A (RE)	Vitamin C (mg)	Calcium (mg)	Iron (mg)
Lemon juice	2 tablespoons	31	6	0.1	2.0	0.1	0.1	0	0	6	1	7.6	3	0
Mango	½ medium	103	65	0.5	17.0	1.8	0.3	0.1	0	2	389	27.7	10	0.1
Nectarine	1 fruit	136	67	1.3	16.0	2.2	0.6	0.1	0	0	101	7.3	7	0.2
Orange	1 medium	131	62	1.2	15.4	3.1	0.2	0	0	0	28	69.7	52	0.1
Orange juice	¾ cup	187	82	1.5	18.8	0.4	0.5	0.1	0	2	15	61.6	19	0.3
Papaya	½ medium	152	59	0.9	14.9	2.7	0.2	0.1	0	5	43	93.9	36	0.2
Passion fruit	½ cup	118	114	2.6	27.6	12.3	0.8	0.1	0	33	83	35.4	14	1.9
Peach, canned in juice	½ cup	124	55	0.8	14.3	1.6	0	0	0	5	47	4.4	7	0.3
Peach, raw	1 medium	98	42	0.7	10.9	2.0	0.1	0	0	0	53	6.5	5	0.1
Pear, canned	½ cup	124	62	0.4	16.0	2.0	0.1	0	0	5	1	2.0	11	0.4
Pear, raw	1 medium	166	98	0.6	25.1	4.0	0.7	0	0	0	3	6.6	18	0.4
Pineapple, canned in juice	½ cup	125	75	0.5	19.5	1.0	0.1	0	0	1	5	11.8	17	0.3
Pineapple, raw	1 slice, 3½″ × 3¼″	84	41	0.3	10.4	1.0	0.4	0	0	1	2	12.9	6	0.3
Plantain, raw	1 medium	179	218	2.3	57.1	4.1	0.7	0.3	0	7	6	2.3	5	1.1
Plums	1½ medium	99	55	0.8	13.0	1.5	0.6	0	0	0	32	9.5	4	0.1
Prune juice	¾ cup	192	136	1.2	33.5	1.9	0.1	0	0	8	0	7.9	23	2.3
Prunes, dried	5 prunes	42	80	1.1	26.3	3.0	0.2	0	0	2	84	1.4	21	1.0
Raisins	¼ cup	43	129	1.4	34.0	1.7	0.2	0.1	0	5	0	1.4	21	0.9
Raspberries	½ cup	62	30	0.6	7.1	4.2	0.3	0	0	0	8	15.4	14	0.4
Rhubarb, raw	1 stalk	51	11	0.5	2.3	0.9	0.1	0	0	2	5	4.1	44	0.1
Strawberries	5 large	90	27	0.6	6.3	2.1	0.3	0	0	1	3	51.0	13	0.3
Tangerine	1 medium	84	40	0.5	9.4	1.9	0.2	0	0	1	77	25.9	12	0.1
Watermelon	1⁄16 melon	286	92	1.8	20.5	1.4	1.2	0.1	0	6	106	27.5	23	0.5

Milk, Yogurt, and Cheese

Name	Amount	Weight (g)	Energy (Calories)	Protein (g)	Carbohydrate (g)	Fiber (g)	Total Fat (g)	Saturated Fat (g)	Cholesterol (mg)	Sodium (mg)	Vitamin A (RE)	Vitamin C (mg)	Calcium (mg)	Iron (mg)
Buttermilk, low-fat	1 cup	245	98	8.1	11.7	0	2.2	1.3	10	257	20	2.5	284	0.1
Cheese, American	2 oz	57	186	11.1	4.1	0	13.9	8.8	36	905	124	0	325	0.5
Cheese, blue	1½ oz	43	150	9.1	1.0	0	12.2	7.9	32	593	97	0	225	0.1
Cheese, cheddar	1½ oz	43	171	10.6	0.5	0	14.1	9.0	45	264	118	0	307	0.3
Cheese, cottage, creamed	1 cup	210	216	26.2	5.6	0	9.5	6.0	32	850	101	0	126	0.3
Cheese, cottage, low-fat (1%)	1 cup	226	163	28.0	6.1	0	2.3	1.5	9	918	25	0	138	0.3
Cheese, cottage, fat-free	1 cup	145	123	25.0	2.7	0	0.6	0.4	10	19	12	0	46	0.3
Cheese, cream	2 oz	57	198	4.3	1.5	0	19.8	12.5	62	168	216	0	45	0.7
Cheese, cream, fat-free	2 oz	57	55	8.2	3.3	0	0.8	0.5	5	311	159	0	105	0.1
Cheese, feta	1½ oz	43	112	6.0	1.7	0	9.0	6.4	38	475	54	0	210	0.3
Cheese, Mexican	1½ oz	43	151	9.6	1.2	0	12.0	7.6	45	279	27	0	281	0.2
Cheese, monterey	1½ oz	43	159	10.4	0.3	0	12.9	8.1	38	228	108	0	317	0.3
Cheese, mozzarella, part-skim	1½ oz	43	108	10.3	1.2	0	6.8	4.3	25	198	75	0	275	0.1
Cheese, parmesan, grated	2 tablespoons	10	46	4.2	0.4	0	3.0	1.9	8	186	17	0	138	0.1
Cheese, process spread	2 oz	56	170	9.1	5.5	0	12.3	8.1	45	839	100	0.1	261	0.1
Cheese, provolone	1½ oz	43	149	10.9	0.9	0	11.3	7.3	29	373	112	0	321	0.2
Cheese, ricotta, part skim	½ cup	124	171	14.1	6.4	0	9.8	6.1	38	155	140	0	337	0.5
Cheese, Swiss	1½ oz	43	160	12.1	1.4	0	11.7	7.6	39	111	19	0	409	0.1
Ice cream, chocolate	1 cup	132	285	5.0	37.2	1.6	14.2	9.0	45	100	151	0.9	144	1.2
Ice cream, vanilla, rich	1 cup	148	357	5.2	33.2	0	24.0	14.8	90	83	272	1.0	173	0.1
Ice cream, vanilla, light	1 cup	132	183	5.0	30.0	0	5.7	3.5	18	112	62	1.1	183	0.1
Ice cream, vanilla, soft serve	1 cup	172	370	7.1	38.2	0	22.4	12.9	157	105	265	1.4	225	0.4
Milk, chocolate	1 cup	250	208	7.9	25.9	2.0	8.5	5.3	30	150	73	2.3	280	0.6
Milk, fat-free (nonfat)	1 cup	245	86	8.4	11.9	0	0.4	0.3	5	127	149	2.5	301	0.1

Name	Amount	Weight (g)	Energy (Calories)	Protein (g)	Carbohydrate (g)	Fiber (g)	Total Fat (g)	Saturated Fat (g)	Cholesterol (mg)	Sodium (mg)	Vitamin A (RE)	Vitamin C (mg)	Calcium (mg)	Iron (mg)
Milk, low-fat (1%)	1 cup	244	102	8.0	11.7	0	2.6	1.6	10	124	144	2.4	300	0.1
Milk, reduced fat (2%)	1 cup	244	122	8.1	11.7	0	4.7	2.9	20	122	139	2.4	298	0.1
Milk, whole	1 cup	244	149	8.0	11.4	0	8.2	5.1	34	120	76	2.2	290	0.1
Pudding, made with milk	½ cup	142	158	4.5	25.6	1.4	4.8	3.0	17	146	37	1.0	158	0.5
Yogurt, frozen, vanilla	1 cup	144	229	5.8	34.8	0	8.1	4.9	3	125	82	1.2	206	0.4
Yogurt, low-fat, plain	8 oz container	227	143	11.9	16.0	0	3.5	2.3	14	159	36	1.8	415	0.2
Yogurt, low-fat, with fruit	8 oz container	227	238	11.0	42.2	0	3.2	2.1	14	148	136	1.6	384	0.2
Yogurt, nonfat, plain	8 oz container	227	127	13.0	17.4	0	0.4	0.3	5	175	5	2.0	452	0.2

Meat, Poultry, Fish, Dry Beans, Eggs, and Nuts

Name	Amount	Weight (g)	Energy (Calories)	Protein (g)	Carbohydrate (g)	Fiber (g)	Total Fat (g)	Saturated Fat (g)	Cholesterol (mg)	Sodium (mg)	Vitamin A (RE)	Vitamin C (mg)	Calcium (mg)	Iron (mg)
Bacon	3 slices	19	109	5.7	0.1	0	9.4	3.3	19	303	0	0	2	0.3
Bacon, Canadian	2 slices	47	86	11.3	0.6	0	3.9	1.3	27	719	0	0	5	0.4
Beef, ½" fat	3 oz	85	344	19.9	0	0	28.7	11.9	78	48	0	0	9	2.1
Beef, corned beef	3 oz	85	213	23.0	0	0	12.7	5.3	73	856	0	0	10	1.8
Beef, ground, extra lean, broiled	3 oz	85	218	21.6	0	0	13.9	5.5	71	60	0	0	6	2.0
Beef, ground, lean, broiled	3 oz	85	231	21.0	0	0	15.7	6.2	74	65	0	0	9	1.8
Beef, ground, regular, broiled	3 oz	85	246	20.5	0	0	17.6	6.9	77	71	0	0	9	2.1
Beef, lean, fat trimmed	3 oz	85	179	25.4	0	0	7.9	3.0	73	56	0	0	7	2.5
Beef liver, braised	3 oz	85	137	20.7	2.9	0	4.2	1.6	331	60	9,011	19.6	6	5.8
Beef ribs, broiled	3 oz	85	306	18.7	0	0	25.1	10.2	70	53	0	0	10	1.8
Chicken breast, w/skin, roasted	½ breast	98	193	29.2	0	0	7.6	2.1	82	70	26	0	14	1.0
Chicken, dark meat, w/skin, roasted	3 oz	85	215	22.1	0	0	13.4	3.7	77	74	49	0	13	1.2
Chicken, dark meat, w/o skin, roasted	3 oz	85	168	22.2	0	0	7.9	2.2	76	76	18	0	12	1.1
Chicken, dark meat, w/skin, fried	3 oz	85	253	18.6	8.0	0	15.8	4.2	76	251	26	0	18	1.2
Chicken, drumstick, w/skin, roasted	1 drumstick	52	112	14.1	0	0	5.8	1.6	47	47	16	0	6	0.7
Chicken, light meat, w/skin, roasted	3 oz	85	189	24.7	0	0	9.2	2.6	71	64	27	0	13	1.0
Chicken, light meat, w/o skin, roasted	3 oz	85	147	26.3	0	0	3.8	1.1	72	65	8	0	13	0.9
Chicken, light meat, w/skin, fried	3 oz	85	235	20.0	8.1	0	13.1	3.5	71	243	20	0	17	1.1
Chicken liver, chopped	½ cup	70	110	17.1	0.8	0	3.8	1.3	442	36	3,439	11.1	10	5.9
Chicken, thigh, w/skin, roasted	1 thigh	62	153	15.5	0	0	9.6	2.7	58	52	30	0	7	0.8
Chicken, wing, w/skin, roasted	1 wing	34	99	9.1	0	0	6.6	1.9	29	28	16	0	5	0.4
Egg white, large	1 egg white	33	17	3.5	0.3	0	0	0	0	55	0	0	2	0
Egg, whole, large	1 egg	50	75	6.2	0.6	0	5.1	1.6	213	63	97	0	25	0.7
Egg yolk, large	1 yolk	17	59	2.8	0.3	0	5.1	1.6	213	7	97	0	23	0.6

Name	Amount	Weight (g)	Energy (Calories)	Protein (g)	Carbohydrate (g)	Fiber (g)	Total Fat (g)	Saturated Fat (g)	Cholesterol (mg)	Sodium (mg)	Vitamin A (RE)	Vitamin C (mg)	Calcium (mg)	Iron (mg)
Fish, catfish, baked/broiled	3 oz	85	129	15.9	0	0	6.8	1.5	54	68	13	0.7	8	0.7
Fish, cod, baked/broiled	3 oz	85	89	19.5	0	0	0.7	0.1	40	77	9	2.6	7	0.3
Fish, halibut, baked/broiled	3 oz	85	119	22.7	0	0	2.5	0.4	35	59	46	0	51	0.9
Fish, salmon, baked/broiled	3 oz	85	175	18.8	0	0	10.5	2.1	54	52	13	3.1	13	0.3
Fish, salmon, canned	3 oz	85	130	17.4	0	0	6.2	1.4	37	457	45	0	203	0.9
Fish, salmon, smoked	3 oz	85	99	15.5	0	0	3.7	0.8	20	1,700	22	0	9	0.7
Fish, sardine, canned in oil	1 can (3.75 oz)	92	191	22.7	0	0	10.5	1.4	131	465	62	0	351	2.7
Fish, snapper, baked/broiled	3 oz	85	109	22.3	0	0	1.5	0.3	40	48	30	1.4	34	0.2
Fish sticks	3 sticks	84	228	13.1	19.9	0	10.3	2.6	94	489	26	0	17	0.6
Fish, swordfish, baked/broiled	3 oz	85	132	21.6	0	0	4.4	1.2	43	98	35	0.9	5	0.9
Fish, trout, baked/broiled	3 oz	85	162	22.6	0	0	7.2	1.3	63	57	16	0.4	47	1.6
Fish, tuna, canned in oil	3 oz	85	158	22.6	0	0	6.9	1.4	26	337	20	0	3	0.6
Fish, tuna, canned in water	3 oz	85	109	20.1	0	0	2.5	0.7	36	320	5	0	12	0.8
Ham, extra lean	3 oz	85	116	18.0	0.4	0	4.1	1.4	26	965	0	0	5	0.8
Ham, regular	3 oz	85	192	17.5	0.4	0	12.9	4.3	53	800	0	11.9	7	1.2
Lamb, trimmed	3 oz	85	218	20.8	0	0	14.3	6.7	74	65	0	0	14	1.6
Lunch meat, beef pastrami	3 oz	85	297	14.7	2.6	0	24.8	8.9	79	1,043	0	0	8	1.6
Lunch meat, beef, sliced	3 oz	85	151	23.9	4.9	0	3.3	1.4	35	1,224	0	0	9	0.8
Lunch meat, bologna (beef)	3 slices	85	265	10.4	0.7	0	24.2	10.3	49	834	0	0	10	1.4
Lunch meat, bologna (turkey)	3 slices	85	169	11.7	0.8	0	12.9	4.3	84	747	0	0	71	1.3
Lunch meat, chicken breast	3 oz	85	108	14.3	1.9	0	4.7	1.2	50	1,005	0	0	14	1.3
Lunch meat, franks (beef)	1 frank	57	180	6.8	1.0	0	16.2	6.9	35	585	0	0	11	0.8
Lunch meat, franks (chicken)	1 frank	45	116	5.8	3.1	0	8.8	2.5	45	617	17	0	43	0.9
Lunch meat, ham, lean, sliced	3 slices	85	111	16.5	0.8	0	4.2	1.4	40	1,215	0	0	6	0.6
Lunch meat, liverwurst	3 oz	85	277	12.0	1.9	0	24.2	9.0	134	731	7,059	0	22	5.4
Lunch meat, salami, dry	8 slices	80	334	18.3	2.1	0	27.5	9.8	63	1,488	0	0	6	1.2
Lunch meat, turkey breast	3 oz	85	94	19.1	0	0	1.3	0.4	35	1,216	0	0	6	0.3
Nuts, almonds	⅓ cup	47	274	10.1	9.3	5.6	24.0	1.8	0	0	0	0	117	2.0
Nuts, cashews, dry roasted	⅓ cup	46	262	7.0	14.9	1.4	21.2	4.2	0	7	0	0	21	2.7
Nuts, chestnuts, dry roasted	⅓ cup	48	117	1.5	25.2	2.4	1.0	0.2	0	1	1	12.4	14	0.4
Nuts, macadamia, dry roasted	⅓ cup	45	321	3.5	6.0	3.6	34.0	5.3	0	2	0	0.3	31	0.3
Nuts, pecans	⅓ cup	36	249	3.3	5.0	3.5	25.9	2.2	0	0	3	0.4	25	0.9
Nuts, pine	⅓ cup	45	257	10.9	6.4	2.0	23.0	3.5	0	2	1	0.8	12	4.2
Nuts, pistachios, dry roasted	⅓ cup	43	244	9.1	11.8	4.4	19.6	2.4	0	4	23	1.0	47	1.8
Nuts, walnuts	⅓ cup	40	262	6.1	5.5	2.7	26.1	2.5	0	1	2	0.5	39	1.2
Peanut butter, chunky	2 tablespoons	32	188	7.7	6.9	2.1	16.0	3.1	0	156	0	0	13	0.7
Peanut butter, smooth	2 tablespoons	32	190	8.1	6.2	1.9	16.3	3.3	0	149	0	0	12	0.6
Peanuts, dry roasted	⅓ cup	49	285	11.5	10.5	3.9	24.2	3.4	0	3	0	0	26	1.1
Pork chop, pan fried	3 oz	85	190	23.5	0	0	10.0	3.7	60	44	2	0.3	4	0.7
Pork ribs, braised	3 oz	85	337	24.7	0	0	25.8	9.5	103	79	3	0	40	1.6
Pork roast	3 oz	85	214	22.9	0	0	12.9	4.5	69	41	3	0	5	0.8
Pumpkin seeds, roasted	¼ cup	57	296	18.7	7.6	2.2	23.9	4.5	0	10	22	1.0	24	8.5
Sausage, beef	1 sausage	43	134	6.1	1.0	0	11.6	4.9	29	486	0	0	3	0.8
Sausage, pork	1 sausage	67	216	13.4	1.0	0	17.2	6.1	52	618	0	1.3	16	1.0
Sausage, smoked links	32″ links	48	161	6.4	0.7	0	14.6	5.1	34	454	0	0	5	0.7
Shellfish, clams, canned	3 oz	85	126	21.7	4.4	0	1.7	0.2	57	95	145	18.8	78	23.8
Shellfish, clams, steamed	10 clams	95	140	24.3	4.9	0	1.9	0.2	64	106	542	21.0	87	26.6
Shellfish, crab, steamed	3 oz	85	82	16.4	0	0	1.3	0.1	45	911	8	6.5	50	0.6
Shellfish, oysters, fried	6 medium	88	173	7.7	10.2	0	11.1	2.8	71	367	79	3.3	55	6.1
Shellfish, shrimp, canned	3 oz	85	102	19.6	0.9	0	1.7	0.3	147	144	15	2.0	50	2.3
Shellfish, shrimp, fried	4 large	30	73	6.4	3.4	0.1	3.7	0.6	53	103	17	0.5	20	0.4

Name	Amount	Weight (g)	Energy (Calories)	Protein (g)	Carbohydrate (g)	Fiber (g)	Total Fat (g)	Saturated Fat (g)	Cholesterol (mg)	Sodium (mg)	Vitamin A (RE)	Vitamin C (mg)	Calcium (mg)	Iron (mg)
Sunflower seeds, dry roasted	¼ cup	32	186	6.2	7.7	3.6	15.9	1.7	0	1	0	0.4	22	1.2
Tempeh	½ cup	83	160	15.4	7.8	0	9.0	1.8	0	7	0	0	92	2.2
Tofu, firm	½ cup	126	183	19.9	5.4	2.9	11.0	1.6	0	18	21	0.3	861	13.2
Turkey, dark meat, w/o skin, roasted	3 oz	85	138	24.5	0	0	3.7	1.2	95	67	0	0	22	2.0
Turkey, dark meat, w/skin, roasted	3 oz	85	155	23.5	0	0	6.0	1.8	99	65	0	0	23	2.0
Turkey, light meat, w/o skin, roasted	3 oz	85	119	25.7	0	0	1.0	0.3	73	48	0	0	13	1.3
Turkey, light meat, w/skin, roasted	3 oz	85	139	24.5	0	0	3.9	1.1	81	48	0	0	15	1.4
Veal, sirloin, roasted	3 oz	85	172	21.4	0	0	8.9	3.8	87	71	0	0	11	0.8
Vegetarian bacon, cooked	1 oz	16	50	1.7	1.0	0.4	4.7	0.7	0	234	1	0	4	0.4
Vegetarian franks	1 frank	51	118	12.1	1.5	1.5	7.1	0.8	0	224	0	0	10	1.0
Vegetarian patties	1 patty	67	119	11.2	10.2	4.0	3.8	0.5	0	382	76	0	48	1.2
Vegetarian sausage	1 patty	38	97	7.0	3.7	1.1	6.9	1.1	0	337	24	0	24	1.4

Fats, Oils, Sweets, and Alcoholic Beverages

Name	Amount	Weight (g)	Energy (Calories)	Protein (g)	Carbohydrate (g)	Fiber (g)	Total Fat (g)	Saturated Fat (g)	Cholesterol (mg)	Sodium (mg)	Vitamin A (RE)	Vitamin C (mg)	Calcium (mg)	Iron (mg)
Alcoholic beverage, beer	1 can or bottle	356	146	1.1	13.2	0.7	0	0	0	18	0	0	18	0.1
Alcoholic beverage, liquor	1.5 oz	42	97	0	0	0	0	0	0	0	0	0	0	0
Alcoholic beverage, wine	5 oz	148	103	0	2.1	0	0	0	0	12	0	0	12	0.5
Beverage, cola	1 can	370	152	0	38.5	0	0	0	0	15	0	0	11	0.1
Beverage, fruit punch	1 cup	247	114	0	28.9	0.2	0	0	0	10	2	108.4	10	0.2
Beverage, kiwi strawberry drink	1 cup	236	113	0.2	27.8	0	0	0	0	10	0	0	0	0
Beverage, lemon-lime soda	1 can	368	147	0	38.3	0	0	0	0	40	0	0	7	0.3
Beverage, tea, bottled, sweetened	1 bottle	480	178	0	40.8	0	0	0	0	0	0	0	0	0
Butter	1 tablespoon	14	102	0.1	0	0	11.5	7.1	31	117	107	0	3	0
Candy, caramels	1 piece	10	39	0.5	7.8	0.1	0.8	0.7	1	25	1	0.1	14	0
Candy, fudge	1 piece	17	65	0.3	13.5	0.1	1.4	0.9	2	11	8	0	7	0.1
Candy, jelly beans	10 large	28	104	0	26.4	0	0.1	0	0	7	0	0	1	0.3
Candy, milk chocolate	1 bar	44	226	3.0	26.0	1.5	13.5	8.1	10	36	24	0.2	84	0.6
Chocolate syrup	2 tablespoons	38	105	0.8	24.4	0.7	0.4	0.2	0	27	1	0.1	5	0.8
Cream, half and half	2 tablespoons	30	39	0.9	1.3	0	3.5	2.2	11	12	32	0.3	32	0
Cream, heavy, whipped	½ cup	60	206	1.2	1.7	0	22.1	13.8	82	23	252	0.4	39	0
Cream, sour	1 tablespoon	12	26	0.4	0.5	0	2.5	1.6	5	6	23	0.1	14	0
Frosting, chocolate	1⁄12 package	38	151	0.4	24.0	0.2	6.7	2.1	0	70	75	0	3	0.5
Honey	1 tablespoon	21	64	0.1	17.3	0	0	0	0	1	0	0.1	1	0.1
Jam/preserves	1 tablespoon	20	56	0.1	13.8	0.2	0	0	0	6	0	1.8	4	0.1
Lard	1 tablespoon	13	115	0	0	0	12.8	5.0	12	0	0	0	0	0
Marmalade	1 tablespoon	20	49	0.1	13.3	0	0	0	0	11	1	1.0	8	0
Margarine, hard	1 tablespoon	14	101	0.1	0.1	0	11.4	2.1	0	133	113	0	4	0
Margarine, liquid	1 tablespoon	14	102	0.3	0	0	11.4	1.9	0	111	113	0	9	0
Margarine, soft	1 tablespoon	14	101	0.1	0	0	11.3	2.0	0	152	113	0	4	0
Margarine-like spread	1 tablespoon	14	50	0.1	0.1	0	5.6	1.1	0	138	115	0	3	0
Mayonnaise, fat-free	1 tablespoon	16	11	0	2.0	0.3	0.4	0.1	2	120	1	0	1	0
Mayonnaise, regular	1 tablespoon	15	57	0.1	3.5	0	4.9	0.7	4	105	12	0	2	0

Name	Amount	Weight (g)	Energy (Calories)	Protein (g)	Carbohydrate (g)	Fiber (g)	Total Fat (g)	Saturated Fat (g)	Cholesterol (mg)	Sodium (mg)	Vitamin A (RE)	Vitamin C (mg)	Calcium (mg)	Iron (mg)
Oil, canola	1 tablespoon	14	124	0	0	0	14.0	1.0	0	0	0	0	0	0
Oil, corn	1 tablespoon	14	120	0	0	0	13.6	1.7	0	0	0	0	0	0
Oil, olive	1 tablespoon	14	119	0	0	0	13.5	1.8	0	0	0	0	0	0.1
Popsicle	1 single stick	88	63	0	16.6	0	0	0	0	11	0	9.4	0	0
Salad dressing, blue cheese	2 tablespoons	31	154	1.5	2.3	0	16.0	3.0	5	335	20	0.6	25	0.1
Salad dressing, French	2 tablespoons	31	134	0.2	5.5	0	12.8	3.0	0	427	40	0	3	0.1
Salad dressing, Italian	2 tablespoons	29	137	0.2	3.0	0	14.2	2.1	0	231	7	0	3	0
Salad dressing, Italian light	2 tablespoons	30	32	0	1.5	0	2.9	0.4	2	236	0	0	1	0.1
Sherbet	½ cup	74	102	0.8	22.5	0	1.5	0.9	0	34	10	2.3	40	0.1
Shortening, vegetable	1 tablespoon	13	113	0	0	0	12.8	3.2	0	0	0	0	0	0
Sugar, brown	1 tablespoon	14	52	0	13.4	0	0	0	0	5	0	0	12	0.3
Sugar, white	1 tablespoon	13	49	0	12.6	0	0	0	0	0	0	0	0	0
Syrup, corn	1 tablespoon	20	56	0	15.3	0	0	0	0	24	0	0	1	0
Syrup, maple	¼ cup	79	206	0	52.9	0	0.2	0	0	7	0	0	53	0.9

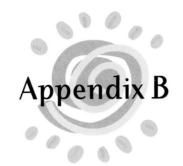

Appendix B

Nutritional Content of Popular Items from Fast-Food Restaurants

Arby's

	Serving Size (g)	Calories	Protein (g)	Total Fat (g)	Saturated Fat (g)	Total Carbohydrate (g)	Sugars (g)	Fiber (g)	Cholesterol (mg)	Sodium (mg)	Vitamin A	Vitamin C	Calcium	Iron	Calories from Fat
Regular roast beef	154	320	21	13	6	34	5	2	45	950	0	0	6	20	110
Giant roast beef	224	450	32	19	9	41	6	2	75	1,440	0	0	6	30	170
Beef 'n cheddar	195	440	22	21	7	44	8	2	50	1,270	2	2	8	20	180
Chicken breast fillet	233	500	25	25	4	48	8	3	55	1,220	10	15	8	15	220
Market fresh roast turkey, ranch and bacon	379	830	49	38	10	75	16	5	110	2,260	10	6	35	30	38
Southwest chicken wrap	259	550	35	30	9	45	1	30	75	1,690	10	10	40	10	270
Chicken club salad	284	140	18	1	0	15	11	3	40	360	130	60	6	10	10
Curly fries—small	106	340	4	18	3	39	N/A	4	0	790	8	8	4	10	160
Homestyle fries—small	113	300	3	13	2	44	1	3	0	550	0	10	2	6	110
Bacon 'n egg croissant	125	410	13	26	12	31	4	< 1	190	670	10	0	4	15	230
Jamocha shake—regular	397	500	13	13	8	81	78	0	35	390	8	10	50	4	120
Tangy southwest sauce	57	330	1	35	5	5	4	0	30	370	2	2	0	0	310

SOURCE: Arby's® 2005 Nutrition, Ingredient & Allergen Information (U.S.), **www.arbysrestaurant.com**.

N/A: not available.

Burger King

	Serving Size (g)	Calories	Protein (g)	Total Fat (g)	Saturated Fat (g)	Total Carbohydrate (g)	Sugars (g)	Fiber (g)	Cholesterol (mg)	Sodium (mg)	Vitamin A	Vitamin C	Calcium	Iron	Calories from Fat
Whopper® with cheese	316	800	35	49	18	53	9	4	110	1,450	25	15	25	30	440
Whopper® Jr. with cheese	160	430	19	26	9	32	5	2	55	770	10	6	15	15	230
Bacon double cheeseburger	196	570	35	34	17	32	6	2	110	1,250	10	2	25	25	310
Chicken Whopper®	272	570	38	25	4.5	48	5	4	75	1,410	15	10	6	40	230
Chicken Tenders® 4-pc.	62	170	11	9	2.5	10	0	0	25	420	0	0	0	2	90
French fries—small	74	230	3	11	3	29	0	2	0	410	0	8	2	2	100
Onion rings—small	51	180	2	9	2	22	3	2	0	260	0	0	6	0	80
Ranch dipping sauce	28	140	1	15	2.5	1	1	N/A	5	95	0	0	0	0	130
TenderCrisp™ garden salad	383	410	25	22	5	28	5	5	40	1,170	140	45	20	15	200
Croissan'wich® sausage, egg, cheese	163	500	18	36	12	26	7	1	220	1,060	10	0	15	15	330
French toast sticks	112	390	6	20	4.5	46	11	2	0	440	0	0	6	10	180

SOURCE: Burger King Corporation, 2005, www.bk.com.

N/A: not available.

Kentucky Fried Chicken

	Serving Size (g)	Calories	Protein (g)	Total Fat (g)	Saturated Fat (g)	Total Carbohydrate (g)	Sugars (g)	Fiber (g)	Cholesterol (mg)	Sodium (mg)	Vitamin A	Vitamin C	Calcium	Iron	Calories from Fat
Original Recipe® chicken—breast	161	380	40	19	6	11	0	0	145	1,150	0	0	0	6	170
Original Recipe® chicken—thigh	126	360	22	25	7	12	0	0	165	1,060	0	0	0	6	230
Extra crispy chicken—breast	162	460	34	28	8	19	0	0	135	1,230	0	0	0	8	250
Extra crispy chicken—thigh	114	370	21	26	7	12	0	0	120	710	0	0	0	6	230
Honey BBQ sandwich	147	300	21	6	1.5	41	18	4	50	640	2	4	6	15	50
Biscuit w/savory	57	190	2	10	2	23	1	0	1.5	580	0	0	0	4	90
Mashed potatoes w/gravy	108	110	2	4	1	18	0	1	0	260	2	4	0	2	35
Potato wedges—small	102	240	4	12	3	30	0	3	0	830	0	6	2	10	110
Corn on the cob (3")	82	70	2	1.5	0.5	13	5	3	0	5	0	6	4	4	15
BBQ beans	136	230	8	1	1	48	22	7	0	720	8	6	15	30	10
Coleslaw	130	190	1	11	2	22	13	3	5	300	25	40	4	0	100
Double choc. chip cake	76	400	4	29	5	31	27	2	45	230	0	0	4	8	260

SOURCE: KFC Corporation, 2005, www.kfc.com.

N/A: not available.

Taco Bell

	Serving Size (g)	Calories	Protein (g)	Total Fat (g)	Saturated Fat (g)	Total Carbohydrate (g)	Sugars (g)	Fiber (g)	Cholesterol (mg)	Sodium (mg)	Vitamin A	Vitamin C	Calcium	Iron	Calories from Fat
Crunchy taco	78	170	8	10	4	13	< 1	< 1	25	350	4	0	6	6	90
Crunchy Taco Supreme®	113	220	9	14	7	14	2	1	35	360	8	6	8	6	120
Soft taco—beef	99	210	10	10	4	21	2	< 1	25	620	4	0	10	8	90
Soft Taco Supreme®	135	260	11	14	7	23	3	1	35	640	8	6	15	8	130
Ranchero chicken soft taco	135	270	14	14	4	21	3	2	35	710	6	8	10	6	130
Bean burrito	198	370	14	10	3.5	55	4	8	10	1,200	10	8	20	15	90
Burrito Supreme®—chicken	248	410	21	14	6	50	5	5	45	1,270	15	15	20	15	130
Gordita Supreme®—beef	153	310	14	16	7	30	7	2	35	600	8	6	15	15	140
Chalupa Supreme®—chicken	153	370	17	20	8	30	4	1	45	530	6	8	10	6	180
Tostada	170	250	11	10	4	29	2	7	15	710	10	8	15	8	90
Mexican pizza	216	550	21	31	11	47	3	5	45	1,040	15	8	35	20	280
Fiesta Taco Salad™	548	870	31	47	16	80	10	12	65	1,780	20	20	40	35	430
Chicken quesadilla	184	540	28	30	13	40	4	3	80	1,380	15	4	50	10	270
Nachos BellGrande®	380	780	20	43	13	80	5	11	35	1,300	8	8	20	15	380

SOURCE: Taco Bell Corporation, 2005, www.tacobell.com.

N/A: not available.

Visit the following Web sites for complete nutritional information:

Arby's www.arbys.com
Back Yard Burgers www.backyardburgers.com
Boston Market www.bostonmarket.com
Burger King www.bk.com
Dairy Queen www.dairyqueen.com
Domino's Pizza www.dominos.com
Hardees www.hardees.com
Jack in the Box www.jackinthebox.com
Kentucky Fried Chicken www.kfc.com
McDonald's www.mcdonalds.com
Papa John's www.papajohns.com
Pizza Hut www.pizzahut.com
Quizno's Subs www.quiznos.com
Rally's/Checkers Drive-In www.checkers.com
Sonic www.sonicdrivein.com
Subway www.subway.com
Taco Bell www.tacobell.com
Taco John's www.tacojohns.com
Wendy's www.wendys.com
White Castle www.whitecastle.com

Appendix C

A Self-Care Guide for Common Medical Problems

This self-care guide will help you manage some of the most common symptoms and medical problems:

- Fever
- Sore throat
- Cough
- Nasal congestion
- Ear problems
- Nausea, vomiting, or diarrhea
- Heartburn and indigestion
- Headache
- Low-back pain
- Strains and sprains
- Cuts and scrapes

Each symptom is described here in terms of what is going on in your body. Most symptoms are part of the body's natural healing response and reflect your body's wisdom in attempting to correct disease. Self-care advice is also given, along with some guidelines about when to seek professional advice. In most cases, the symptoms are self-limiting; that is, they will resolve on their own with time and simple self-care strategies.

No medical advice is perfect. You will always have to make the decision about whether to self-treat or get professional help. This guide is intended to provide you with more information, so you can make better, more informed decisions. If the advice here differs from that of your physician, discuss the differences with him or her. In most cases, your physician will be able to customize the advice to your individual medical situation.

The guidelines given here apply to *generally healthy adults*. If you are pregnant or nursing, or if you have a chronic disease, particularly one that requires medication, check with your physician for appropriate self-care advice. Additionally, if you have an allergy or a suspected allergy to any recommended medication, check with your physician before using it.

If you have several symptoms, read about your primary symptom first and then proceed to secondary symptoms. Use your common sense when determining self-care. If you are particularly concerned about a symptom or confused about how to manage it, call your physician to get more information.

Fever

Body temperature is generally about 98.6° F. Body temperature varies with exercise, at rest, by climate, and by gender. Fever means a reading over 99° F. It is most commonly a sign that your body is fighting an infection. Fever may also be due to an inflammation, an injury, or a drug reaction. Chemicals released into your bloodstream during an infection reset the thermostat in the hypothalamus of your brain. The message goes out to your body to turn up the heat. The blood vessels in your skin constrict, and you curl up and throw on extra blankets to reduce heat loss. Meanwhile, your muscles begin to shiver to generate additional body heat. The resulting rise in body temperature is a fever. Later, when your brain senses that the temperature is too high, the signal goes out to increase sweating. As the sweat evaporates, it carries heat away from the body surface.

A fever may not be all bad; it may even help you fight infections by making the body less hospitable to bacteria and viruses. A high body temperature appears to bolster the immune system and may inhibit the growth of infectious microorganisms.

Most generally healthy people can tolerate a fever as high as 103° to 104° F (39.5° to 40° C) without problems. Therefore, if you are essentially healthy, there is little need to reduce a fever unless you are very uncomfortable. Older adults and those with chronic health problems, such as heart disease, may not tolerate the increased metabolic demand of a high fever, and fever reduction may be advised.

Most problems with fevers are due to the excessive loss of fluids from evaporation and sweating, which may cause dehydration.

Self-Assessment

1. If you are sick, take your temperature several times throughout the day. Oral temperatures should not be measured for at least 10 minutes after smoking, eating, or drinking a hot or cold liquid. When using an oral glass thermometer, first clean it with rubbing alcohol or cool soapy water (hot water may break it). Then shake it down until it reads 95° F or lower. Place the thermometer under your tongue and leave it in place for a *full 3 minutes*. (If you leave it in for only 2 minutes, the temperature reading will be off by at least half a degree.) To read the thermometer, notice where the colored column ends and compare it with the degrees marked in lines on the thermometer. If you are using an electronic digital thermometer, follow the directions that came with it.

   "Normal" temperature varies from person to person, so it is important to know what is normal for you. Your normal temperature will also vary throughout the day, being lowest in the early evening. If you exercise or if it is a hot day, your temperature may normally rise. Women's body temperature typically varies by a degree or more through the menstrual cycle, peaking around the time of ovulation. Rectal temperatures normally run about 0.5° to 1.0° F higher than oral temperatures. If your recorded temperature is more than 1.0° to 1.5° F above your normal baseline temperature, you have a fever.

2. Watch for signs of dehydration: excessive thirst; very dry mouth; infrequent urination with dark, concentrated urine; and light-headedness.

Self-Care

1. Drink plenty of fluids to prevent dehydration—at least 8 ounces of water, juice, or broth every 2 hours.
2. Take a sponge bath using lukewarm water; this will increase evaporation and help reduce body temperature naturally.
3. Don't bundle up. This decreases the body's ability to lose excess heat.
4. Take an aspirin substitute (acetaminophen, ibuprofen, or naproxen sodium). For adults, two standard-size tablets every 4 to 6 hours can be used to reduce the fever and the associated headache and achiness. Do not use aspirin in anyone younger than age 20, because some younger people with chicken pox, influenza, or other viral infections have developed a life-threatening complication, Reye's syndrome, after taking aspirin.

When to Call the Physician

1. Fever over 101° F despite self-care actions
2. Low-grade fever (99° to 100° F) if there is no improvement in 72 hours
3. If fever last more than 5 days, regardless of improvement
4. Recurrent, unexplained fevers
5. Fever accompanied by a rash, stiff neck, severe headache, difficulty breathing, cough with brown sputum, severe pain in the side or abdomen, painful urination, convulsions, or mental confusion
6. Fever with signs of dehydration
7. Fever after starting a new medication

Sore Throat

A sore throat is caused by inflammation of the throat lining resulting from an infection, allergy, or irritation (especially from cigarette smoke). If you have an infection, you may also notice some hoarseness from swelling of the vocal cords and "swollen glands," which are enlarged lymph nodes that produce white blood cells to help fight the infection. The lymph nodes, part of your body's defense system, may remain swollen for weeks after the infection subsides.

Most throat infections are caused by viruses, so antibiotics are not effective against them. However, about 20 to 30 percent of throat infections are due to streptococcal bacteria. This type of microbe can cause complications, such as rheumatic fever and rheumatic heart disease, and therefore should be diagnosed by a physician and treated with antibiotics. Strep throat is usually characterized by very sore throat, high fever, swollen lymph nodes, a whitish discharge at the back of the throat, and the absence of other cold symptoms, such as a cough and runny nose (which suggest a viral infection). Allergy-related sore throats are usually accompanied by a runny nose, sneezing, and watery, itchy eyes.

Self-Assessment

1. Take your temperature.
2. Look at the back of your throat in a mirror. Is there a whitish, puslike discharge on the tonsils or in the back of the throat?
3. Feel the front and back of your neck. Do you feel enlarged, tender lymph nodes?

Self-Care

1. If you smoke, stop smoking to avoid further irritation of your throat.
2. Drink plenty of liquids to soothe your inflamed throat.
3. Gargle with warm salt water (¼ tsp salt in 4 oz water) every 1 to 2 hours to help reduce swelling and discomfort.
4. Suck on throat lozenges, cough drops, or hard candies to keep your throat moist.
5. Use throat lozenges, sprays, or gargles that contain an anesthetic to numb your throat temporarily and make swallowing less painful.

6. Try an aspirin substitute to ease throat pain.
7. For an allergy-related sore throat, try an antihistamine, such as chlorpheniramine.

When to Call the Physician

1. Great difficulty swallowing saliva or breathing
2. Sore throat with fever over 101° F (38.3° C), especially if you do not have other cold symptoms, such as nasal congestion or a cough
3. Sore throat with a skin rash
4. Sore throat with whitish pus on the tonsils
5. Sore throat and recent contact with a person who has had a positive throat culture for strep
6. Enlarged lymph nodes lasting longer than 3 weeks
7. Hoarseness lasting longer than 3 weeks

Cough

A cough is a protective mechanism of the body to help keep the airways clear. There are two types of cough: a dry cough (without mucus) and a productive cough (with mucus). Common causes of cough include infection (viral or bacterial), allergies, and irritation from smoking and pollutants. If you have a cold, the cough may be the last symptom to improve, because the airways may remain irritated for several weeks after the infection has resolved.

Your airways are lined with hairlike projections called cilia, which move back and forth to help clear the airways of mucus, germs, and dust. Infections and cigarette smoking paralyze and damage this vital defensive mechanism.

Self-Assessment

1. Take your temperature.
2. Observe your mucus. Thick brown or bloody mucus suggests a bacterial infection.

Self-Care

1. If you are a smoker, stop smoking. Smoking irritates the airways and undermines your body's immune defenses, leading to more serious infections and longer-lasting symptoms. Most people do not feel like smoking when they have a cold with a cough. If you want to quit, a cold may provide an excellent opportunity to do so.
2. Drink plenty of liquids (at least six 8-ounce glasses a day) to help thin mucus and loosen chest congestion.
3. Use moist heat from a hot shower or vaporizer to help loosen chest congestion.
4. Suck on cough drops, throat lozenges, or hard candy to keep your throat moist and help relieve a dry, tickling cough.
5. If you have a dry, nonproductive cough or the cough keeps you from sleeping, you can use a cough

syrup or lozenge that contains the nonprescription cough suppressant dextromethorphan. Because a cough that produces mucus is protective, it is generally not advisable to suppress a productive cough.

When to Call the Physician

1. Cough with thick brown or bloody sputum
2. Cough with high fever—above 102° F (38.8° C)—and shaking chills
3. Severe chest pains, wheezing, or shortness of breath
4. Cough that lasts longer than 4 weeks

Nasal Congestion

Nasal congestion is most commonly caused by infection or allergies. With infection, the nasal passages become congested because of increased blood flow and mucus production. This congestion is actually part of the body's defense to fight infection. The increased blood flow raises the temperature of the nasal passages, making them less hospitable to germs. The nasal secretions are rich in white blood cells and antibodies to help fight and neutralize the invading organisms and flush them away. Nasal congestion associated with sore throat, cough, and fever usually indicates a viral infection. Green nasal discharge is common with viral infections; it does not mean you need an antibiotic.

Nasal congestion caused by allergies is often accompanied by a thin, watery discharge; sneezing; and itchy eyes; it is sometimes associated with a seasonal pattern. In an allergic reaction, the offending allergen (such as pollen, dust, mold, or dander) triggers the release of histamine and other chemicals from the cells lining the nose, throat, and eyes. These chemicals cause swelling, discharge, and itching. Antihistamine drugs block the release of these irritating chemicals.

Self-Assessment

1. Take your temperature.
2. Observe the color and consistency of your nasal secretions. A thick brown or bloody discharge suggests a bacterial sinus infection.
3. Tap with your fingers over the sinus cavities above and below the eyes. If the tapping causes increased pain, you may have a bacterial sinus infection.

Self-Care

1. If you smoke, stop smoking to prevent continuing irritation of the nasal passages.
2. Use moist heat from a hot shower or vaporizer to help liquefy congested mucus.
3. Use a decongestant nasal spray or drops to relieve congestion temporarily. However, if these decongestants are used for more than 3 days, they can cause

"rebound congestion," which actually creates more nasal congestion. As an alternative, use saltwater nose drops (¼ tsp salt in ½ cup of boiled water, cooled before using).

4. Try an oral decongestant, such as pseudoephedrine (60 mg every 6 hours), to help shrink swollen mucous membranes and open nasal passages. In some people, these medications can cause nervousness, sleeplessness, or heart palpitations. If you have uncontrolled high blood pressure, heart disease, or diabetes, check with your physician before using decongestants.

When to Call the Physician

1. Nasal congestion with severe pain and tenderness in the forehead, cheeks, or upper teeth and a high fever (above 102° F or 38.8° C)
2. Thick brown or bloody nasal discharge
3. Nasal congestion and discharge unresponsive to self-care treatment and lasting longer than 3 weeks

Ear Problems

Ear symptoms include earache, discharge, itching, stuffiness, and hearing loss. They may be caused by problems in the external ear canal, eardrum, middle ear, or eustachian tube (the passageway that connects the middle ear space to the back of the throat). The ear canal can become blocked by excess wax, producing hearing loss and a sense that the ear is plugged. An infection of the external ear canal due to excessive moisture and trauma is often referred to as "swimmer's ear." It can cause pain, a sense of fullness, discharge, and itching. Congestion and blockage of the eustachian tube by a cold or allergy can result in pain, a sense of fullness, and hearing loss. A middle ear infection often produces severe pain, hearing loss, and fever.

Self-Assessment

1. Take your temperature. A fever may be a sign of infection.
2. Have someone look into the ear canal with a flashlight or an otoscope. Look for wax blockage or a red, swollen canal indicating an external ear infection.
3. Wiggle the outer part of the ear. If this increases the pain, an infection or inflammation of the external canal is the likely cause.

Self-Care

1. If blockage of the ear canal with wax is the problem, first try a hot shower to liquefy the wax, and use a wash cloth to wipe out the ear canal. You can also use a few drops of an over-the-counter wax softener and then flush the canal gently with warm

water in a bulb syringe. Do not use sharp objects or cotton swabs; they can scratch the canal or push the wax in deeper.

2. To treat mild infections of the external ear canal, you must thoroughly dry the ear canal. A few drops of a drying agent (Burrow's solution) on a piece of cotton gently inserted into the canal can act as a wick to dry the canal.
3. To relieve congestion and blockage of the eustachian tube, try a decongestant, such as pseudoephedrine; a nasal spray (but for no longer than 3 days); or an antihistamine. Hot showers or a vaporizer may help loosen secretions, and yawning or swallowing may help open the eustachian tube. For a mild plugging sensation without fever or pain, pinch your nostrils and blow gently to force air up the eustachian tube and "pop" your ears.

When to Call the Physician

1. Severe earache with fever
2. Puslike or bloody discharge from the ear
3. Sudden hearing loss, especially if accompanied by ear pain or recent trauma to the ear
4. Ringing in the ears or dizziness
5. Any ear symptom lasting longer than 2 weeks

Nausea, Vomiting, or Diarrhea

Nausea, vomiting, and diarrhea usually are defensive reactions of your body to rapidly clear your digestive tract of irritants. These symptoms may be caused by a viral infection, foodborne illness, medications, or other types of infection. Vomiting dramatically ejects irritants from your stomach, and nausea discourages eating to allow the stomach to rest. With diarrhea, overstimulated intestines flush out the offending irritants.

The major complications of vomiting and diarrhea are dehydration from fluid losses and decreased fluid intake and a risk of bleeding from irritation of the digestive tract.

Self-Assessment

1. Take your temperature. A fever is often a clue that an infection is causing the symptoms.
2. Note the color and frequency of vomiting and diarrhea. This will help you estimate the severity of fluid losses and check for bleeding (red, black, or "coffee grounds" material in the stool or vomit; iron tablets and Pepto-Bismol can also cause black stools).
3. Watch for signs of dehydration: very dry mouth; excessive thirst; infrequent urination with dark, concentrated urine; and light-headedness.
4. Look for signs of hepatitis, an infection of the liver: a yellow color in the skin and the white parts of the eyes.

Self-Care

1. To replace fluids, take frequent, small sips of clear liquids, such as water, noncitrus juice, broths, flat ginger ale, or ice chips.
2. When the vomiting and diarrhea have subsided, try nonirritating, constipating foods, such as the BRAT diet: bananas, rice, applesauce, and toast.
3. For several days, avoid alcohol, milk products, fatty foods, and aspirin and other medications that might irritate the stomach. Do not stop taking regularly prescribed medications without discussing this change with your physician.
4. Medications are not usually advised for vomiting. For diarrhea, over-the-counter medications containing kaolin, pectin, or attapulgite may help thicken the stool. Loperamide, now available without a prescription, can be used to ease diarrhea.

When to Call the Physician

1. Inability to retain any fluids for 12 hours or signs of dehydration
2. Severe abdominal pains not relieved by the vomiting or diarrhea
3. Blood in the vomit (red or "coffee grounds" material) or in the stool (red or black, tarlike material)
4. Vomiting or diarrhea with a high fever (above 102° F or 38.8° C)
5. Yellow color in skin or white parts of the eyes
6. Vomiting with severe headache and a history of a recent head injury
7. Vomiting or diarrhea that lasts 3 days without improvement
8. If you are pregnant or have diabetes
9. Recurrent vomiting and/or diarrhea

Heartburn and Indigestion

Indigestion and heartburn are usually a result of irritation of the stomach or the esophagus, the tube that connects the mouth to the stomach. The stomach lining is usually protected from stomach acids, but the esophagus is not. Therefore, if stomach acids "reflux," or back up into the esophagus, the result is usually a burning discomfort beneath the breastbone. The esophagus is normally protected by a muscular valve that allows food to enter the stomach but prevents stomach contents from flowing upward into the esophagus. Certain foods (such as chocolate), medications, and smoking can loosen and open this protective sphincter valve. Overeating, lying down, or bending over can also cause the stomach acids to gain access to the sensitive lining of the esophagus.

Recurrent or persistent abdominal pain may be a symptom of an ulcer, a raw area in the lining of the stomach or duodenum (the first part of the small intestine).

About 1 in 5 men and 1 in 10 women develop an ulcer at some time in their lives. Most ulcers are linked to infection with the bacterium *Helicobacter pylori*; people who regularly take nonsteroidal anti-inflammatory drugs, such as aspirin or ibuprofen, are also at risk for ulcers, because these drugs irritate the lining of the stomach. *H. pylori* infection is relatively easy to diagnose and treat, and other medications are available to treat ulcers linked to other causes. Many of the self-care measures described here are also frequently recommended for people with ulcers.

Self-Assessment

1. Look for a pattern in the symptoms. Do they occur after eating certain foods, after taking certain medications, or when you bend over or lie down? Do certain foods or an antacid relieve the symptoms?
2. Observe your bowel movements. Black, tarlike stools may indicate bleeding in the stomach (iron tablets and Pepto-Bismol can also cause black stools).

Self-Care

1. Avoid irritants, such as smoking, aspirin, ibuprofen, naproxen sodium, alcohol, caffeine (coffee, tea, cola), chocolate, onions, carbonated beverages, spicy or fatty foods, acidic foods (vinegar, citrus fruits, tomatoes), or any other foods that seem to make your symptoms worse.
2. Take nonabsorbable antacids, such as Maalox, Mylanta, or Gelusil, every 1 to 2 hours and especially before bedtime, or try an acid reducer available without a prescription (Pepcid, Tagamet, or Zantac).
3. Avoid tight clothing.
4. Avoid overeating; eat smaller, more frequent meals.
5. Don't lie down for 1 to 2 hours after a meal. Elevate the head of your bed with 4- to 6-inch blocks of wood or bricks. Adding extra pillows usually makes things worse by creating a posture that increases pressure on the stomach. Using a waterbed also usually makes reflux worse. Try sleeping on your left side, which may reduce reflux, compared with sleeping on your back or right side.
6. If you are overweight in the abdominal area, weight loss may help. Abdominal obesity can increase pressure on the stomach when you are lying down.

When to Call the Physician

1. Stools that are black and tarlike or vomit that is bloody or contains material that looks like coffee grounds
2. Severe abdominal or chest pain
3. Pain that goes through to the back
4. No relief from antacids
5. Symptoms lasting longer than 3 days

Headache

Headache is one of the most common symptoms. There are four major types of headache: tension, migraine, cluster, and sinus. Tension headaches, migraines, and cluster headaches are described in Chapter 14. Sinus headaches are caused by blockage of the sinus cavities, with resulting pressure and pain in the cheeks, forehead, and upper teeth. Headache caused by elevated blood pressure is very uncommon and occurs only with very high pressures.

Self-Assessment

1. Take your temperature. The presence of fever may indicate a sinus infection. Fever, severe headache, and a very stiff neck suggest meningitis, a rare but serious infection around the brain and spinal cord.
2. Tap with your fingers over the sinus cavities in your cheeks and forehead. If this causes increased pain, it may indicate a sinus infection.
3. For recurrent headaches, keep a headache journal. Record how often and when your headaches occur, associated symptoms, activities that precede the headache, and your food and beverage intake. Look for patterns that may provide clues to the cause(s) of your headaches.

Self-Care

1. Try applying ice packs or heat on your neck and head.
2. Gently massage the muscles of your neck and scalp.
3. Try deep relaxation or breathing exercises.
4. Take aspirin or an aspirin substitute for pain relief. Over-the-counter products containing a combination of aspirin, acetaminophen, and caffeine are approved by the FDA for treating migraines.
5. If pain is associated with nasal congestion, try a decongestant medication, such as pseudoephedrine.
6. Try to avoid emotional and physical stressors (such as poor posture and eyestrain).
7. Try avoiding foods that may trigger headaches, such as aged cheeses, chocolate, nuts, red wine, alcohol, avocados, figs, raisins, and any fermented or pickled foods.

When to Call the Physician

1. Unusually severe headache
2. Headache accompanied by fever and a very stiff neck
3. Headache with sinus pain, tenderness, and fever
4. Severe headache following a recent head injury
5. Headache associated with slurred speech, visual disturbance, or numbness or weakness in the face, arms, or legs
6. Headache persisting longer than 3 days
7. Recurrent unexplained headaches
8. Increasing severity or frequency of headaches
9. Severe migraine headaches; in recent years, many new prescription medications have been approved for the prevention and treatment of migraines

Low-Back Pain

Pain in the lower back is a very common condition; it is most often due to a strain of the muscles and ligaments along the spine, often triggered by bending, lifting, or other activity. Low-back pain can also result from bone growths (spurs) irritating the nerves along the spine or pressure from ruptured or protruding discs, the "shock absorbers" between the vertebrae. Sometimes back pain is caused by an infection or stones in the kidney. Fortunately, however, simple muscular strain is the most common cause of low-back pain and can usually be effectively self-treated.

Self-Assessment

1. Take your temperature. Back pain with high fever may indicate a kidney or other infection.
2. Check for blood in your urine or frequent, painful urination, which may also indicate a kidney problem.
3. Observe for tingling or pain traveling down one or both legs *below* the knee with bending, coughing, or sneezing. These symptoms suggest a disc problem.

Self-Care

1. Lie on your back or in any comfortable position on the floor or a firm mattress, with knees slightly bent and supported by a pillow. Rest for 1 to 3 days if the pain persists.
2. Use ice packs on the painful area for the first 3 days, and then continue with cold or change to heat, whichever gives more relief.
3. Take aspirin or an aspirin substitute for pain relief as needed.
4. After the acute pain has subsided, begin gentle back and stomach exercises. Practice good posture and lifting techniques to protect your back. Try to resume gentle, everyday activities, such as walking, as soon as possible. Bed rest beyond 3 days is not advised. To learn more about proper back exercises and use of your back, consult a physical therapist or your physician.

When to Call the Physician

1. Back pain following a severe injury, such as a car crash or a fall
2. Back pain radiating down the leg *below* the knee on one or both sides

3. Persistent numbness, tingling, or weakness in the legs or feet
4. Loss of bladder or bowel control
5. Back pain associated with high fever (above 101° F or 38.3° C), frequent or painful urination, blood in the urine, or severe abdominal pain
6. Back pain that does not improve after 2 weeks of self-care

Strains and Sprains

Missteps, slips, falls, and athletic misadventures can result in a variety of strains, sprains, and fractures. A strain occurs when you overstretch a muscle or tendon (the connective tissue that attaches muscle to bone). Sprains are caused by overstretching or tearing ligaments (the tough, fibrous bands that connect bone to bone). Depending on the severity and location, a sprain may actually be more serious than a fracture, because bones generally heal very strongly, while ligaments may remain stretched and lax after healing. After a sprain, it may take 6 weeks for the ligament to heal.

After most injuries, you can expect pain and swelling. This is the body's way of immobilizing and protecting the injured part, so that healing can take place. The goal of self-assessment is to determine whether you have a minor injury that you can safely self-treat or a more serious injury to an artery, a nerve, or bone that should be treated by your physician.

Self-Assessment

1. Watch for coldness, blue color, or numbness in the limb beyond the injury. These may be signs of damage to an artery or a nerve.
2. Look for signs of a possible fracture, which include a misshapen limb, reduced length of the limb on the injured side compared with the uninjured side, an inability to move or bear weight, a grating sound with movement of the injured area, extreme tenderness at one point along the injured bone as you press with your fingers, or a sensation of snapping at the time of the injury.
3. Gently move the injured area through its full range of motion. Immobility or instability suggests a more serious injury.

Self-Care

1. Immediately immobilize, protect, and rest the injured area until you can bear weight on it or move it without pain. Remember: If it hurts, don't do it.
2. To decrease pain and swelling, immediately apply ice (a cold pack or ice wrapped in a cloth) for 15 minutes every hour for the first 24 to 48 hours. Then apply ice or heat as needed for comfort.

3. Immediately elevate the injured limb above the level of your heart for the first 24 hours to decrease swelling.
4. Immobilize and support the injured area with an elastic wrap or a splint. Be careful not to wrap so tightly as to cause blueness, coldness, or numbness.
5. Take aspirin or an aspirin substitute for pain as needed.

When to Call the Physician

1. An injury that occurred with great force, such as a high fall or motor vehicle crash
2. A snap heard or felt at the time of the injury
3. A limb that is blue, cold, or numb
4. A limb that is bent, twisted, or crooked
5. Tenderness at specific points along a bone
6. Inability to move the injured area
7. A wobbly, unstable joint
8. Marked swelling of the injured area
9. Inability to bear weight after 24 hours
10. Pain that increases or lasts longer than 4 days

Cuts and Scrapes

Cuts and scrapes are common disruptions of the body's skin. Fortunately, the vast majority of these wounds are minor and don't require stitches, antibiotics, or a physician's care. An abrasion involves a scraping away of the superficial layers of skin. Abrasions, though less serious, are often more painful than cuts, because they disrupt more skin nerves. There are two types of cuts: lacerations (narrow slices of the skin) and puncture wounds (stabs into deeper tissues).

Normal healing of a cut or an abrasion is a remarkable process. After the bleeding stops, small amounts of serum—a clear, yellowish fluid—may leak from the wound. This fluid is rich in antibodies to help prevent an infection. Redness and swelling may normally occur as more blood is shunted to the area, bringing white blood cells and nutrients to speed healing. There may also be some swelling of nearby lymph nodes, which are another part of your body's defense against infection. Finally, a scab forms. This is "nature's bandage," which protects the area while it heals.

The main concerns about cuts are the possibilities of damage to deeper tissues and the risk for infection. Damage to underlying blood vessels may lead to severe bleeding, as well as blueness and coldness in areas beyond the wound. Injured nerves may produce numbness and a loss of the ability to move parts of the body beyond the injured area. Damaged muscles, tendons, and ligaments can also result in an inability to move areas beyond the cut.

Wound infection usually does not take place until 24 to 48 hours after an injury. Signs of infection include increasing redness, swelling, pain, pus, and fever. One of the most serious, though fortunately uncommon, complications of puncture wounds is tetanus ("lockjaw"). This bacterial infection thrives in areas not exposed to oxygen, so it is more likely to develop in deep puncture wounds or dirty wounds. Tetanus is not likely to develop in minor cuts or wounds caused by clean objects, such as knives. You need a tetanus immunization shot following a cut under the following conditions:

- If you have never had the basic series of three tetanus immunization injections
- If you have a dirty or contaminated wound and it has been longer than 5 years since your last injection
- If you have a clean, minor wound and it has been longer than 10 years since your last injection

Self-Assessment

1. Look for warning signs of complications: persistent bleeding, numbness, an inability to move the injured area, or the later development of pus, increasing redness, and fever.
2. Measure the size of the cut. If your cut is shallow (less than ¼ inch deep), less than an inch long, and not in a high-stress area (such as a joint, which bends) and you can easily hold the edges of the wound closed, it probably won't need stitches.

Self-Care

1. Apply direct pressure over the wound until the bleeding stops. The only exception is puncture wounds, which should be encouraged to bleed freely (unless spurting a large amount of blood) for a few minutes to flush out bacteria and debris.

2. Try to remove any dirt, gravel, glass, or foreign material from the wound with tweezers or by gentle scrubbing.
3. Wash the wound vigorously with soap and water, followed by an application of hydrogen peroxide solution as an antiseptic.
4. If it is an abrasion, cover the area with a sterile adhesive bandage until a scab forms. For minor lacerations, close the cut with a butterfly bandage or a sterile adhesive tape, drawing the edges close together but not overlapping. If there is an extra flap of clean skin, leave it in place for extra protection. Do not attempt to close a puncture wound. Instead, soak the wound in warm water for 15 minutes several times a day for several days. Soaking helps keep the wound open and thus prevents infection.

When to Call the Physician

1. Bleeding that can't be controlled with direct pressure
2. Numbness, weakness, or an inability to move the injured area
3. Any large, deep wound
4. A cut in an area that bends and with edges that cannot easily be held together
5. Cuts on the hands or face unless clean and shallow
6. A contaminated wound from which you cannot remove the foreign material
7. Any human or animal bite
8. If you need a tetanus immunization (see indications noted earlier)
9. Development of increasing redness, swelling, pain, pus, or fever 24 hours or more after the injury
10. If the wound is not healing well after 3 weeks

Appendix D

Resources for Self-Care

Books and Audiotapes

American College of Obstetricians and Gynecologists. 2000. *Encyclopedia of women's health and wellness.* Washington, DC: American College of Obstetricians and Gynecologists. *A comprehensive look at women's health that includes checklists, questionnaires, and many other helpful tools.*

American Medical Women Association. 2001. *Complete family health book.* New York: Golden Books. *A comprehensive guide to family health.*

Ammer, C. 2000. *The new A to Z of women's health: A concise encyclopedia.* 4th ed. New York: Facts on File. *An easy-to-use reference covering a wide variety of women's health topics.*

Brubaker, M., et al. 1999. *Surgery: A patient's guide from diagnosis to recovery.* San Francisco: UCSF Nursing Press. *A comprehensive look at surgery from diagnosis to the postsurgery recovery process at home.*

Griffith, H. W. 2000. *Complete guide to prescription and nonprescription drugs, 2001 edition.* New York: Perigee. *A comprehensive guide to side effects, warnings, and precautions for the safe use of over 4,000 brand-name and generic drugs.*

Griffith, H. W. 2000. *The complete guide to symptoms, illness, and surgery.* 4th rev. ed. New York: Perigee. *An up-to-date reference covering signs and symptoms, illnesses and disorders, and surgeries.*

Hogan, R. W. 2000. *The PDR pocket guide to prescription drugs.* 4th ed. New York: Pocket Books. *An easy-to-use reference to over 1,000 prescription drugs.*

Inlander, C. B., K. Morales, and the People's Medical Society. 2000. *Family health for dummies.* Foster City, CA: IDG Books. *Addresses a wide range of health topics.*

Kemper, D. W. 1999. *Healthwise handbook: A self-care manual for you.* Boise, ID: Healthwise. *Practical guidelines for home care of common medical problems in adults and children.*

Komaroff, A. L., ed. 1999. *Harvard Medical School family health guide.* New York: Simon & Schuster. *A comprehensive, easy-to-use guide to symptoms, disorders, treatments, medical emergencies, and the health care system.*

Lerner, P., and J. Lerner. 2000. *Lerner's consumer guide to health care.* Seattle, WA: Lerner Communications. *Presents advice on how to obtain quality medical care and to negotiate the bureaucracy of the health care system.*

Lorig, K., et al. 2000. *Living a healthy life with chronic conditions.* Palo Alto, CA: Bull. *A helpful guide to dealing with chronic illness.*

Medical Economics Staff, ed. 2001. *PDR family guide to prescription drugs.* 8th ed. New York: Three Rivers Press. *A comprehensive guide to prescription drugs.*

Medical Economics Staff, ed. 2001. *PDR for nonprescription drugs and dietary supplements.* 22d ed. Montvale, NJ: Medical Economics. *A clinical reference covering food and drug interactions, side effects, contraindications, costs, and other information on over-the-counter drugs and supplements.*

Men's Health Books, ed. 2000. *The complete book of men's health.* Emmaus, PA: Rodale Press. *An illustrated guide to men's health, with an emphasis on prevention.*

Muth, A. S. 2001. *Surgery sourcebook: Basic consumer health information about major surgery and outpatient surgeries.* Detroit: Omnigraphics. *A comprehensive, consumer-oriented look at surgery.*

Naparastek, B. *Health journeys.* Akron, OH: Image Paths (800-800-8661; www.healthjourneys.com). *A selection of high-quality audiotapes for imagery for relaxation, mental health, illness management, and preparation for surgery.*

Pryor, J. L., and S. Glass. 2000. *It's in the male: Everyone's guide to men's health.* Minnetonka, MN: Appladay Press. *A concise guide to key men's health concerns.*

Rothenberg, M. A., and C. F. Chapman. 2000. *Dictionary of medical terms: For the nonmedical person.*

4th ed. Hauppauge, NY: Barrons Educational Series. *Includes basic definitions of many medical terms.*

Rybacki, J. J., and J. W. Long. 2001. *The essential guide to prescription drugs.* New York: HarperResource. *A comprehensive drug reference that includes descriptions of how each drug works, possible side effects, and other precautions.*

Self-care advisor: The essential home health guide for you and your family. 2000. Alexandria, VA: Time-Life. *Provides advice on more than 300 common health problems, including symptoms, suggestions for home care, advice on when to call the doctor, and tips for prevention.*

Shannon, J. B., ed. 1999. *Medical tests sourcebook.* Detroit: Omnigraphics. *Provides basic consumer information on a wide variety of medical tests.*

Silverman, H., ed. 2000. *The pill book.* 9th rev. ed. New York: Bantam. *Provides descriptions and illustrations of more than 1,500 of the most commonly prescribed drugs.*

Sobel, D., and R. Ornstein. 1998. *Mind and body health handbook.* Los Altos, CA: DRx. *Presents step-by-step instructions for how to use your mind to relieve stress, boost immunity, improve mood, and manage illness.*

See Chapter 1 for a list of general health-related newsletters and magazines.

Health Information Centers

Consumer Information Center (Pueblo, CO 81009, 888-8PUEBLO; www.pueblo.gsa.gov).

National Health Information Center (P.O. Box 1133, Washington, DC 20013, 800-336-4797; www.health.gov/nhic).

Office of Minority Health Resource Center (P.O. Box 37337, Washington, DC 20013, 800-444-6472; www.omhrc.gov).

Self-Help and Mutual Aid Groups

Self-help groups provide information and peer support for nearly every conceivable medical condition or problem. Look in the telephone book for a local chapter, or contact one of the following self-help clearinghouses for the names of self-help groups in your community.

American Self-Help Clearinghouse (St. Clare's Health Services, 25 Pocono Road, Denville, NJ 07834, 973-326-8853; www.mentalhelp.net/selfhelp).

National Self-Help Clearinghouse (365 5th Avenue, Suite 3300, New York, NY 10016, 212-817-1822; www.selfhelpweb.org).

Telephone Hot Lines

For hot lines relating to the main topics of this text, see the For More Information sections at the end of each chapter. Additional hot lines are listed here. Extensive lists of health-related hot lines and clearinghouses are available from the National Health Information Center (800-336-4797; www.health.gov/nhic), the American Self-Help Clearinghouse (973-326-8853, www.mentalhelp.net/selfhelp/fonenums/helpline.htm), and Johns Hopkins InfoNet (http://www.hopkinsmedicine.org).

Blindness: American Foundation for the Blind, 800-232-5463; National Library Service for the Blind and Physically Handicapped, 800-424-8567; Recording for the Blind and Dyslexic, 800-221-4792.

Chronic fatigue syndrome: CFIDS Association, 800-442-3437.

Consumer products: U.S. Consumer Product Safety Commission, 800-638-2772: FDA National Hotline, 888-463-6332.

Deafness/hearing problems: American Speech Language and Hearing Association, 800-638-8255; Dial-a-Hearing Screening Test, 800-222-EARS: National Institute on Deafness and Other Communication Disorders, 800-241-1044, 800-241-1055 (TTY).

Disabling conditions: Americans with Disabilities Act Hotline, 800-949-4232 (Voice/TTY); Job Accommodation Network, 800-232-9675 (Voice/TDD).

Down syndrome: National Down Syndrome Society, 800-221-4602.

Endometriosis: Endometriosis Association, 800-992-3636.

Epilepsy: Epilepsy Foundation of America, 800-EFA-1000; Epilepsy Information Service, 800-642-0500.

Gambling: National Council on Compulsive Gambling, 800-522-4700.

Headache: National Headache Foundation, 800-843-2256; American Council for Headache Education, 800-255-ACHE.

Hemophilia: National Hemophilia Foundation, 888-463-6643.

Irritable bowel syndrome: International Foundation for Functional Gastrointestinal Disorders, 888-964-2001.

Kidney disease: American Kidney Fund, 800-638-8299; National Kidney Foundation, 800-622-9010.

Lung disease/respiratory disorders: Lung Line, sponsored by the National Jewish Medical and Research Center, 800-222-LUNG, 800-552-LUNG (recorded information, 24 hours); American Lung Association, 800-LUNG-USA.

Lupus: Lupus Foundation of America, 800-558-0121.

Multiple sclerosis: Multiple Sclerosis Foundation, 800-441-7055.

Parkinson's disease: American Parkinson's Disease Association, 800-223-2732; National Parkinson Foundation, 800-327-4545.

Rare disorders: National Organization for Rare Disorders, 800-999-6673.

Self-abuse and self-mutilation: SAFE (Self-Abuse Finally Ends), 800-DONT-CUT.

Sickle cell disease: Sickle Cell Disease Association of America, 800-421-8453.

Spina bifida: Spina Bifida Association of America, 800-621-3141.

Spinal cord injury: Christopher Reeve Paralysis Association, 800-225-0292.

Sports and sports injures: Women's Sports Foundation, 800-227-3988.

Sudden infant death: American SIDS Institute, 800-232-SIDS.

The Internet

The Internet is a global network of computers that links together commercial online communication services, such as America Online and CompuServe, with tens of thousands of university, government, and corporate networks. The Internet is composed of many parts, including World Wide Web documents, e-mail, newsgroups, mailing lists, and chat rooms. With access to the Internet, you can obtain in-depth information about hundreds of wellness topics and keep up with the latest research; you can also connect with people worldwide who share a medical problem or another challenge to wellness.

To reach the Internet, you need a computer, a modem, access to the network through a provider, and browser software, which allows you to navigate. Internet access is often available to students at little or no cost through college computer centers. If you have to obtain access through a commercial Internet service provider, choose one that suits your needs and your budget. Bare-bones access is available at low cost, but you may need to obtain additional software, including a browser, such as Netscape Navigator or Microsoft Internet Explorer. Online services, such as America Online, CompuServe, and Microsoft Network, are often more expensive, but they provide all the necessary software and offer many features, including e-mail, newsgroups, and Web browsers.

The World Wide Web   The World Wide Web is made up of computer files, called Web pages or Web sites, that have been created by individuals, companies, and organizations. The Web is considered a user-friendly part of the Internet because it offers easy access and navigation and has media capabilities, such as audio, video, and animation.

Each Web site is identified by an address or uniform resource locator (URL), such as www.healthfinder.gov. To access a site, you can type the URL into the appropriate screen of your browser or you can click on a *hyperlink,* a shortcut to another Web page or to a different part of the current page. When you view a Web page, hyperlinks may appear as images or as text that is a different color and/or is underlined. By clicking on links, you can jump quickly from one Web site to related sites, even if they are located on the other side of the world.

To search out information on a particular topic, you need to use a search engine or directory, such as one of the following:

AltaVista	www.altavista.com
Ask Jeeves	www.ask.com
Excite	www.excite.com
Fast Search	www.alltheweb.com
Go	www.go.com
Google	www.google.com
Hotbot	www.hotbot.com
Lycos	www.lycos.com
Northern Light	www.northernlight.com
Yahoo!	www.yahoo.com

These search engines search a unique database of Web pages, so you will obtain different results from different search engines. A meta–search engine such as the following ones simultaneously submits your search to multiple search engines:

Dogpile	www.dogpile.com
MetaCrawler	www.go2net.com/search.html

To use a search engine, you may need to enter key words or navigate through a series of increasingly more specific directories; some search engines offer both key word and directory searches. Within seconds, the search engine will generate a list of sites (with hyperlinks) that match your search parameters, often with a brief description of each site.

When you are searching, it's best to make your searches as specific as possible. Searching for key words, such as *AIDS* or *cancer,* will yield thousands or even millions of matches. Use more specific phrases, such as "HIV vaccine" or "cervical cancer treatment." If the search engine has a help section, take a look at it. Different engines have different rules for how best to enter key words. For example, you may need to enclose phrases in quotation marks or put plus or minus signs between words to obtain an appropriate result. If you don't find the information you are looking for using one search engine, try another. In addition, there are search engines and directories that specialize in health and medicine:

eHealth	www.hon.ch
Health A to Z	www.healthatoz.com
HealthWeb	healthweb.org

Karolinska Institutet — micf.mic.ki.se/Diseases
Medical Matrix — www.medmatrix.org
MedWeb — www.medweb.emory.edu/MedWeb
MedWorld: Medbot — www-med.stanford.edu/medworld/medbot
WebMD® — www.webmd.com

Listed next is a sampling of Web sites that contain information on a variety of wellness topics and/or links to many other appropriate sites. For Web sites dealing with a specific wellness topic, refer to the *Wellness: Concepts and Applications* Online Learning Center (www.mhhe.com/anspaugh6e).

American Academy of Family Physicians
    aafp.org
    www.familydoctor.org
CDC Health Information A to Z
    www.cdc.gov/health/diseases.htm
Dr. Koop's Community
    www.drkoop.com
Duke University Healthy Devil On-Line
    http://gilligan.mc.duke.edu/h-devil
FirstGov for Consumers
    www.consumer.gov/health.htm
Go Ask Alice
    www.goaskalice.columbia.edu
Healthfinder
    www.healthfinder.gov
HealthTouch Online
    www.healthtouch.com
InteliHealth
    www.intelihealth.com
MayoClinic.com
    www.mayoclinic.com
Medem
    www.medem.com
MedicineNet
    www.medicinenet.com
National Center for Health Statistics
    www.cdc.gov/nchs
National Women's Health Resource Center
    www.healthywomen.org
NetWellness
    www.netwellness.org
New York Online Access to Health
    www.noah-health.org
NIH Health Information Index
    http://health.nih.gov
Seek Wellness
    www.seekwellness.com
WebMD
    webmd.com

Usenet Newsgroups Newsgroups consist of archived messages, articles, and postings about a particular topic; they are similar to bulletin boards. Commercial online services maintain members-only newsgroups, but many more are available on the Internet. To locate a newsgroup on a particular topic, use a search engine or visit a site devoted to newsgroups, such as Deja.com (www.deja.com).

You are free to browse any newsgroup's articles. Postings on related topics are often grouped together in a "thread," consisting of an original message that began a discussion and all the replies to that message. A busy newsgroup can receive thousands of postings a day, and older articles are deleted to make room for new ones. If you find an article of interest, print it or save it to your computer—it may be deleted from the newsgroup by your next visit.

In addition to browsing, reading, and saving newsgroup postings, you can also be an active participant. You can reply to a message, either to the person who posted it or to the entire newsgroup, or you can post a new message that starts a new thread of discussion. To ensure that your postings are appropriate, it's often a good idea to observe a newsgroup for a while or look at its "frequently asked questions" page prior to becoming an active member.

Listserv Mailing Lists Listservs are similar to newsgroups, except that messages are delivered by e-mail to all subscribers to the mailing list rather than posted at a public site. Once you subscribe to a mailing list, you receive messages posted by other subscribers and you can post your own messages. As with newsgroups, it's a good idea to read messages for a while before joining the discussion. You can stop subscribing to a mailing list at any time.

To locate listservs for a particular topic, do a key word search using a search engine by entering the topic and the word *listserv*. Or try the extensive mailing list directory at Topica (www.topica.com).

Real-Time Communication: Chat Rooms With access to the Internet, you may also have the opportunity to participate in real-time communication with people from around the world. You can sign on to a particular chat group and communicate with others who are signed on to the same group at that time. You can have a "public" conversation, in which everyone in the chat room is included, or a "private" conversation between you and one other person. Many chat groups have a moderator, who can kick people off and/or refuse them further access if they don't behave appropriately. For reasons of privacy and security, many people suggest that chat room participants avoid divulging too much personal information.

Evaluating Information from the Internet Anyone can post information and advice on the Internet—true or false, good or bad. When evaluating information from the Internet, ask the following questions:

- *What is the source of the information? Who is the author or sponsor of the Web page?* Web sites maintained by government agencies, professional organizations, or established academic or medical institutions are likely to present trustworthy information. Many other groups and individuals post accurate information, but it is important to watch your sources carefully. Many sites will describe their sponsor on the home page; alternatively, they may have an "about us" or "who we are" link that provides this information. Take a look at the backgrounds, qualifications, and credentials of the people who are behind the information at the site. Beware of sites that don't indicate the sources of the information they post; if you don't know where it comes from, you can't assess its validity.

  As you click on links and move from page to page, also pay attention to where you are. Even if you start out at a trustworthy site, the click of a button can catapult you into a completely different site. Learn how to read your current Web address, so that you know when you've left one site and entered another. Look at the abbreviation in the server name in the URL, which will change according to the sponsor's purpose—for example, "org" for organizational, "gov" for governmental, "edu" for educational, and "com" for commercial.

- *How often is the site updated?* Most Web pages will indicate the date of their most recent modifications. Major organizations may update their Web sites on a daily or weekly basis. Look for sites that are updated frequently.

- *What is the purpose of the page? Does the site promote particular products or procedures? Are there obvious reasons for bias?* The same common sense you'd use to evaluate any factual claim applies to the Internet. Be wary of sites that sell specific products, use testimonials as evidence, appear to have a social or political agenda, or ask for money. Many sites sponsored by commercial companies and lay organizations do provide sound, useful information; however, it's a good idea to consider possible sources of bias in the information they present.

- *What do other sources say about a topic?* To get a broad perspective on a piece of information, check out other online sources or ask a professional. You are more likely to obtain and recognize quality information if you use several different sources. Be wary of claims that appear at only one site.

- *Does the site conform to any set of guidelines or criteria for quality and accuracy?* A number of organizations have developed codes of conduct or ethical standards for health-related sites; these codes include criteria such as use of information from respected sources and disclosure of the site's sponsors. These organizations include the following:

American Accreditation HealthCare Commission
www.urac.org

American Medical Association
www.ama-assn.org

Health Internet Ethics
www.hiethics.com

Health on the Net Foundation
www.hon.ch

Internet Healthcare Coalition
www.ihealthcoalition.org

Look for sites that identify themselves as conforming to some code or set of principles.

- *Is the site easy to use? Does it have links to other sites?* In addition to having strong content, good Web pages should be easy to use, be clearly organized, and have a good search capability. For more on finding and evaluating online wellness-related information, check out the following Web sites:

California Medical Association (select Health Care Links)
www.cmanet.org

CDC: Internet Health Related Hoaxes and Rumors
www.cdc.gov/hoax_rumors.htm

Oncolink Source Reliability Information
www.oncolink.upenn.edu

Science Panel on Interactive Communication and Health
www.scipich.org

Search Engine Watch
www.searchenginewatch.com

Glossary

absolute risk the actual number or percentage of people affected by a risk factor.

abstinence to refrain completely from engaging in a particular behavior.

acesulfame a nonnutritive sweetener that is 200 times sweeter than sucrose and marketed as "sunette" in many food products.

acquaintance rape forced sexual intercourse between people who know one another well.

acquired immunodeficiency syndrome (AIDS) viral destruction of the immune system, causing loss of ability to fight infections.

acute illness an illness that occurs suddenly, often has no identifiable cause, is usually treatable, and often disappears in a short time.

addiction a pathological need for a substance that has life-damaging potential.

addictive behavior behavior that is excessive, compulsive, and psychologically and physically destructive.

adipose cells fat cells.

adrenocorticotropic hormone (ACTH) a hormone released by the hypothalamus during periods of stress that initiates various physiological responses.

aerobic literally "with oxygen"; when applied to exercise, activities in which oxygen demand can be supplied continuously by individuals during performance.

aerobic capacity maximum oxygen consumption.

alcohol a socially acceptable drug.

alcoholism the disease in which an individual loses control over drinking; an inability to refrain from drinking.

allergens substances that cause allergic reactions.

alternative medicine the body of therapies that are not taught in U.S. medical schools and are generally unavailable from doctors or hospitals.

amenorrheic the cessation of menstruation.

amino acids chemical structures that form protein.

anabolic steroids drugs closely related to testosterone that increase muscle mass in humans.

anaerobic literally "without oxygen"; when applied to exercise, high-intensity physical activities in which oxygen demand is greater than the amount that can be supplied during performance.

android the deposition of fat that is characteristic of men; fat tends to accumulate in the abdomen and upper body.

aneurysm a weak spot in an artery that forms a balloonlike pouch that can rupture.

angina chest pain that is the result of ischemia (see *ischemia*).

angioplasty a procedure in which narrowed arteries are dilated through the use of a catheter.

anorexia nervosa a serious illness of deliberate self-starvation with profound psychiatric and physical components.

antioxidants compounds that block the oxidation of substances in food or the body (vitamins C and E and beta-carotene are examples).

arthritis inflammatory disease of the joints.

asthma a chronic respiratory condition characterized by difficulty breathing.

asymptomatic without symptoms.

atherosclerosis a slow, progressive disease of the arteries characterized by the deposition of plaque on the inner lining of arterial walls.

ATP adenosine triphosphate, the unit of energy used for muscular contraction.

atrophy a decrease in the size of organ, muscle, and body tissues from disease or disuse.

autogenics the form of suggestion that precipitates relaxation.

autoimmune disease a disease in which the immune system fails to recognize the body's own parts and produces antibodies against them to the point of causing injury.

autonomic nervous system the part of the nervous system that is concerned with control of involuntary body functions.

avoidance a behavioral strategy that emphasizes eliminating circumstances associated with undesirable behavior.

ballistic stretching repetitive contractions of agonist muscles to produce rapid stretches of antagonist muscles.

balloon angioplasty a surgical procedure that involves the insertion of a catheter with a balloon at the tip used to compress fatty deposits and plaque against the walls of the artery.

bariatric surgery surgery to reduce weight.

basal cell carcinoma the most common type of skin cancer; it grows slowly and usually does not metastasize (spread).

basal metabolic rate (BMR) the number of calories needed to sustain life.

behavioral contract a written agreement in a lifestyle-change program.

behavior assessment the process of counting, recording, observing, measuring, and describing behavior.

behavior substitution a lifestyle change technique in which an incompatible behavior is substituted for a behavior being altered.

benign noncancerous; refers to a growth that is unable to spread.

binge drinking consuming five or more drinks in a single session at least once during the previous two weeks, with the intent to become intoxicated.

binge-eating disorder the practice of eating large amounts of food in a short period of time.

biofeedback an educational tool used to provide information about an individual's physiological actions.

blood alcohol concentration (BAC) the percentage of alcohol content in the blood.

body composition the amount of lean versus fat tissue in the body.

body dysmorphic disorder (BDD) a psychiatric disorder characterized by a preoccupation with perceived imperfections in physical appearance that cause the person to withdraw from social activities.

body image the perception of and about the body.

body mass index (BMI) the ratio of body weight in kilograms to height in meters squared.

botanicals plants that are thought to have medicinal properties (also called *herbs* and *phytomedicinals*).

bulimia nervosa an eating disorder characterized by episodes of secretive binge eating and purging.

caesarean section delivery the surgical removal of the fetus through the abdominal wall.

caffeine a stimulant that increases the heart rate.

caloric deficit a deficit that occurs when the number of calories burned exceeds the number of calories consumed.

caloric expenditure calories expended by physical activity and metabolism.

caloric intake calories supplied by food.

calorie short for *kilocalorie*, which is the unit of measurement for food energy; a calorie is the amount of heat required to raise the temperature of 1 gram of water 1 degree Centigrade.

cancer a group of diseases characterized by uncontrolled, disorderly cell growth.

capillaries the smallest vessels transporting blood from the heart to the tissues.

carbohydrate loading the practice of increasing carbohydrate intake for six days before an event, while decreasing exercise duration.

carbon monoxide a colorless, tasteless, odorless gas that is the product of incomplete combustion of carbon-containing fuels.

carcinogens substances that cause cancer or enable the growth of cancer cells; cancer-causing agents.

carcinoma cancer of a body surface or body cavity, such as cancer of the breast, lung, skin, stomach, testis, or uterus.

cardiac output the amount of blood ejected by the heart in 1 minute.

cardia dysrhythmia an irregular heart rate that is sometimes intractable.

cardiorespiratory endurance the ability to take in, deliver, and extract oxygen for physical work.

cariogenic promoting of dental caries, or cavities.

catheterization the process of examining the heart by introducing a catheter into a vein or an artery and passing it into the heart.

cause and effect in medical research, the type of a relationship in which one variable is scientifically proved to cause a certain effect.

cerebral hemorrhage the bursting of a blood vessel in the brain.

chemoprevention nutritional intervention to prevent diseases, such as cancer, by bolstering the immune system.

chemotherapy the use of drugs and hormones to treat various cancers.

child abuse the physical, emotional, or sexual mistreatment of a child.

chlamydia one of the most common sexually transmitted diseases.

cholesterol a steroid that is an essential structural component of neural tissue and cell walls and is required for the manufacture of hormones and bile.

chronic disease a disease that usually begins gradually and persists for an indefinite period of time, usually months or years.

chronic effects of exercise the physiological changes that result from cardiorespiratory training.

circuit resistance training a total of 8 to 15 exercises are usually used in a circuit; the exerciser goes through the circuit three times, with minimum rest between exercise stations.

cocaine a stimulant used in powdered form.

cognitive dissonance an internal conflict that occurs when a person's behaviors are inconsistent with his or her beliefs, values, or knowledge.

colonoscopy   a procedure involving the insertion of a flexible viewing scope that examines the entire colon.

communicable diseases   diseases that can be transmitted from one person to another.

complete protein   a protein that contains all the essential amino acids.

complex carbohydrates   polysaccharides, including starch and fiber.

concentric contraction   the shortening of a muscle as it develops the tension to overcome an external resistance.

condyloma   warts on the genitalia.

contracting   a behavior change strategy that involves a written statement of health goals, target dates for completion of each goal, intervention strategies, rewards, and incentives.

contraindication   a reason for not prescribing a drug or treatment.

control group   in health research, the group receiving no treatment.

coping   effort(s) made to manage or deal with stress.

coronary artery bypass surgery   a procedure involving the removal of a leg vein, which is used as a shunt around the blocked area in the coronary artery.

countering   substituting a new behavior for an undesirable one.

crack   a smokable form of cocaine that is extremely dangerous and very addictive.

Crohn's disease   a type of inflammatory bowel disease whose cause is unknown; Crohn's disease is characterized by frequent and intense diarrhea, abdominal pain, gas, fever, and rectal bleeding.

cross-training   the attainment of physical fitness by participating in a variety of activities regularly.

crude fiber   residue of plant food following chemical treatment in the laboratory.

cunnilingus   oral sex performed on the female genitalia.

daily values (DVs)   nutritional guidelines for the ingestion of carbohydrate, fat, saturated fat, cholesterol, sodium, potassium, and dietary fiber.

date rape   forced sexual intercourse between people who are in a dating situation.

deceptive advertising   advertising that misleads consumers by overstating or exaggerating the performance of a product.

deductible   the amount paid by a patient before being eligible for benefits from an insurance company.

defensive medicine   the practice of prescribing medical tests to protect doctors against malpractice lawsuits.

dehydration   the excessive loss of body water.

delta-9-tetrahydrocannabinol (THC)   a major psychoactive drug found in marijuana.

depressants   sedatives and tranquilizers; these agents slow the central nervous system.

designer drugs   illegally manufactured drugs that mimic controlled substances.

diabetes mellitus   a metabolic disorder involving the pancreas and the failure to produce insulin; a risk factor for cardiovascular disease.

diagnostic laboratory tests   tests conducted for specific symptoms during a physical examination.

dietary fiber   the residue of plant food after digestion in the human body; 1 gram of crude fiber equals 2 to 3 grams of dietary fiber.

Dietary Reference Intakes (DRIs)   the replacement for the Recommended Dietary Allowance as the standards for presenting nutrient recommendations.

diet resistance   the inability to lose weight by dieting.

direct-access testing (DAT)   testing in which a patient purchases a particular test online or at a participating lab, submits blood, and receives results without visiting a physician.

disability insurance   insurance that pays for income lost because of the inability to work due to an illness or injury.

disordered eating   sporadic eating, poor nutrition, unnecessary dieting, or occasional bingeing and purging, but not classified as full-blown problem areas by the American Psychiatric Association.

distress   the form of stress that results in negative responses.

diuretics   substances that increase water output and the body's need for water.

diverticulitis   an infection of the diverticula of the intestines.

diverticulosis   the condition of having saclike swellings (diverticula) in the walls of the intestines.

domestic violence   violence that occurs when an individual is in some way hurt by a person whom he or she knows.

double-blind study   the type of health research in which neither the researcher nor the subjects know who is receiving an experimental treatment.

drug   a chemical substance that has the potential to alter the structure and functioning of a living organism.

eating disorders   eating disorders that meet specific criteria established by the American Psychiatric Association.

eccentric contraction   the lengthening of a muscle as the weight or resistance is returned to the starting position.

echocardiography   a noninvasive technique that uses sound waves to determine the shape, texture, and movement of the valves of the heart.

ectomorph   the body shape characterized by a thin body frame.

elderly abuse   physical, emotional, sexual, or medical abuse of an elderly person; most often the abuser is an adult child of the victim.

electrocardiograph (ECG) a device for recording electrical variations in action of the heart muscle.

embolus a mass of undissolved matter in the blood or lymphatic vessels that detaches from the vessel walls.

endomorph the body shape characterized by rounded physical features and large body frame.

endorphins mood-elevating, pain-killing substances produced by the brain.

energy nutrients nutrients, such as carbohydrates, fat, and protein, that provide a source of energy for the body.

enhanced food food that has been modified and/or supplemented for the purpose of achieving or facilitating a health benefit.

environmental dimension of wellness aspects of wellness that improve quality of life in the community, including laws and agencies that safeguard the physical environment.

epidemiologic studies population studies that observe the health habits and diseases of large numbers of people.

epinephrine a hormone produced by the adrenal medulla that speeds up body processes.

essential fat fat that is indispensable for individuals to function biologically and necessary to support life.

essential hypertension high blood pressure caused by unknown reasons.

essential nutrients nutrients that cannot be made by the body and must be supplied in the diet.

ethyl alcohol the intoxicating agent in alcoholic drinks; a colorless liquid with a sharp, burning taste.

eustress stress judged as "good," positive stress or stress that contributes to positive outcomes.

exclusion a medical service that is not covered by an insurance policy.

experimental group in health research, the group receiving some form of experimental treatment.

false negative a test result that incorrectly shows a person is healthy when an abnormality actually exists.

false positive a test result that incorrectly shows an abnormality when a person is actually healthy.

family practitioner a medical doctor who serves as a general practitioner for an individual or a family.

fasting complete starvation; avoidance of food consumption.

fat a mixture of triglycerides.

fellatio oral sex performed on the male genitalia.

female athletic triad a condition characterized by disordered eating, lack of menstrual periods, and low age-adjusted bone density.

fiber substances in food that resist digestion; formerly called *roughage*.

fight or flight syndrome the initial phase of the general adaptation syndrome (GAS); when a stressor is encountered, the body responds by preparing to stand and fight or run away, depending on the situation; also called the *alarm phase* of the GAS.

fixed indemnity benefits specified amounts that are paid by an insurance company for particular medical procedures.

flexibility range of motion at a joint.

folate a vitamin B nutrient found primarily in leafy vegetables.

foodborne illness illness caused by ingestion of foods containing toxic substances produced by microorganisms.

fraternal twins twins who emanate from separate eggs and do not have identical genes.

freebasing smoking liquefied cocaine.

free radicals naturally produced chemicals that arise from cell activity.

fructose fruit sugar.

functional foods foods that provide a specific health benefit above and beyond their inherent nutritional value.

gastroplasty bariatric surgery performed to limit the size of the stomach.

general adaptation syndrome (GAS) a series of physiological changes that occur when a stressor is encountered; the GAS is conceived of as having three phases: alarm, resistance, and exhaustion.

genital warts warts on the genitalia.

glucose the primary source of energy used by the body; blood sugar.

Glycemic Index (GI) an assessment of food in terms of its ability to increase blood sugar in the two to three hours after eating.

glyceride fat compound, including triglyceride, monoglyceride, and diglyceride.

Golgi tendon organ a proprioceptor that responds to muscle stretch and tension.

goniometer a protractor-like instrument used to measure the flexibility of various joints.

gonorrhea a bacterial disease that is sexually transmitted and can lead to serious complications if left untreated, including sterility and scarring of the heart valves.

gynoid a fat deposition characteristic of females, in whom fat tends to accumulate on the hips and thighs.

hardiness the label used in describing the type of personality that tends to remain healthy even under extreme stress; the three components of hardiness are challenge, commitment, and control.

hate crimes crimes directed at individuals or groups solely because of their racial, ethnic, or religious background, sexual orientation, or other differences from the perpetrator.

headache a common discomfort that is often caused by distress, tension, and anxiety; may be the result of injury or brain disease.

health the balancing of the physical, emotional, social, and spiritual components of personality in a manner that is conducive to optimal well-being and a higher quality of existence.

health behavior gap a discrepancy between what people know and what they actually do regarding their health.

health care providers people and facilities, such as physicians and hospitals, that provide health care services.

health disparities the disproportionate prevalence of diseases and health problems among certain population groups.

health fatalism in health information, the view that new information cannot be believed or trusted because it will inevitably be refuted.

health insurance a contract between an insurance company and an individual or a group for the payment of medical care costs.

health maintenance organization (HMO) a prepaid group insurance program that provides a full range of medical services.

health-promoting behaviors things done to maintain and improve one's level of wellness.

health promotion the art and science of helping people change their lifestyle to move toward a higher state of wellness.

health-related fitness the components of fitness that include cardiorespiratory endurance, muscular strength, muscular endurance, flexibility, and body composition.

health risk appraisals questionnaires used to provide information about health habits, lifestyle, and medical history.

heat exhaustion a serious heat-related condition characterized by dizziness, fainting, rapid pulse, and cool skin.

heat stroke a heat-related medical emergency characterized by high temperature (106° F or higher) and dry skin and accompanied by some or all of the following: delirium, convulsions, and loss of consciousness.

hemoglobin the substance in blood that carries oxygen.

hepatitis B one of five types of viral hepatitis; hepatitis B is the most serious type and can be transmitted sexually.

herbs see *botanicals.*

herpes simplex virus (HSV) the virus responsible for herpes genitalis, a sexually transmitted disease.

highly polyunsaturated fat a fatty acid composed of triglycerides in which the carbon chain has room for many hydrogen atoms.

homeostasis a state of balance or constancy; the body is continually attempting to maintain homeostasis.

homicide the intentional taking of another person's life; murder.

homocysteine an amino acid that is thought to increase the risk for heart disease.

homogeneous group a group of subjects with similar characteristics.

human immunodeficiency virus (HIV) the virus that is the source of AIDS.

human papilloma virus (HPV) the causative agent of condyloma (genital warts).

hydrogenation the process of adding hydrogen to unsaturated fatty acid to make it more saturated.

hyperglycemia high blood sugar.

hyperplasia an increase in the number of cells.

hypertension high blood pressure.

hyperthermia an excessive buildup of heat in the body.

hyperthyroidism a disease caused by an overactive thyroid gland.

hypertrophy an increase in the size of organs and muscle tissue.

hypokinesis physical inactivity.

hypothalamus the part of the limbic system that contains the center for many body functions; in stressful situations, the hypothalamus releases specific hormones to elicit appropriate body responses.

hypothermia a cold weather–related condition that results in abnormally low body temperature.

hypothyroidism a disease caused by an underactive thyroid gland.

iatrogenic condition a condition caused by receiving medical care.

identical twins twins who emanate from the same egg.

immunization a vaccine or another preparation administered to prevent disease.

immunotherapy in relation to cancer, a technique for stimulating the body's immune system to destroy cancer cells.

implied consent the nonverbal authorization of a medical procedure, such as cooperation during the administration of tests.

incomplete protein protein that does not contain all the essential amino acids in the proportions needed by the body.

infarction the death of heart muscle tissue.

inflammatory bowel disease (IBD) a variety of diseases that cause inflammation of the intestines; the two most common types are Crohn's disease and ulcerative colitis.

influenza an illness commonly called *flu;* caused by a virus.

informed consent a legal provision requiring a patient's authorization of any medical procedure, therapy, or treatment.

inhalants substances that cause druglike effects when inhaled.

insoluble fiber fiber that does not dissolve in water; comes from wheat bran and vegetables.

insulin a hormone, secreted by the pancreas, that increases the use of glucose by the tissues of the body.

intensity the degree of vigorousness of a single bout of exercise.

internist a medical doctor specializing in internal medicine and sometimes serving as a primary care physician.

ischemia a diminished supply of blood to the heart muscle.

isoflavones the phytoestrogens in soybeans that are thought to help prevent breast cancer by blocking natural estrogens.

isokinetic a method for developing muscular strength that involves a constant rate of speed and changes in the amount of weight resistance.

isometric the use of static contractions to develop strength.

isotonic a method for developing muscular strength that involves a variable rate of speed and a constant weight resistance.

lactic acid a metabolite formed in muscles as a result of incomplete breakdown of sugar.

lactose a simple sugar; milk sugar.

lactovegetarian a person who eats plant foods and dairy products but excludes eggs, fish, poultry, and meat from the diet.

Leading Health Indicators (LHIs) healthy lifestyle issues identified in the document *Healthy People 2010* as health priorities for Americans.

legumes foods that come from plants with seed pods that split on two sides when ripe.

leptin a protein made in fat cells that controls weight gain and loss.

leukemia cancer of the blood-forming tissues, including the bone marrow and spleen.

life insurance insurance that pays a death benefit.

lifestyle diseases diseases and/or health conditions largely caused by health habits and practices under the control of the individual.

limbic system a large, C-shaped area in the brain that contains the centers for emotions, memory storage, learning relay, and hormone production (the pituitary gland, thalamus, and hypothalamus).

lipid the class of nutrients more commonly referred to as *fat*.

lipoprotein fat-carrying protein.

liposuction the surgical removal of fat tissue.

locus of control the perspective from which an individual views life; individuals with an *internal* locus of control believe that their decisions make a difference and that they have control over their lives; people with an *external* locus of control see themselves as "victims" and consider other people, situations, and conditions as being the controlling factors in their lives.

low-calorie diet a diet that limits intake to 800 to 1,000 calories a day; results in atrophy of heart muscle.

low-carb diet a diet that limits carbohydrate intake to below the recommended 45 to 65 percent of calories in daily intake.

lymphoma cancer that develops in the lymphatic system, including the neck, armpits, groin, and chest.

macronutrients nutrients required by the body in large amounts; usually refers to the energy nutrients: protein, fat, and carbohydrates.

mainstream smoke smoke that is inhaled and exhaled by the smoker.

major minerals minerals required in large amounts (more than 5 grams a day).

malignant cancerous; refers to a growth that has the ability to spread to other areas of the body.

mammography X-ray examination of the breast to detect cancer.

marijuana cannabis; a plant that produces mild effects similar to both a stimulant and a depressant; also labeled as a mild hallucinogen.

megadose a large dose, usually in the form of supplements.

melanoma a dangerous form of skin cancer that has a strong tendency to spread to other areas of the body.

mesomorph a body shape characterized by a muscular, athletic body build.

metabolism all chemical reactions that occur within the cells of the body.

metastasis the process by which cancerous cells spread from their original location to another location in the body.

micronutrients nutrients required by the body in small amounts; usually refers to vitamins and minerals.

migraine headaches headaches characterized by throbbing pain that can last for hours or days, sometimes accompanied by nausea and vomiting; migraines are thought to be the result of dilation of blood vessels in the head.

minerals inorganic compounds in food necessary for good health.

mitochondria the cell's "powerhouse."

moderate-calorie diet a diet that limits caloric intake to 1,300 to 1,600 calories a day.

monocytes white blood cells that grow into macrophages, which protect the body by ingesting foreign material.

monounsaturated fat fatty acid composed of triglycerides in which the carbon chain has room for two hydrogen atoms.

morbidity the incidence of disease and/or sickness.

mortality the incidence of death.

muscular endurance the application of repeated muscular force developed by many repetitions against resistances considerably less than maximum.

muscular strength the maximal force that a muscle or muscle group can exert in a single contraction.

myocardial infarction a heart attack; the death of heart muscle tissue.

narcotics powerful painkillers.

negative reinforcers avoidance of something unpleasant.

neoplasm an abnormal mass of cells; also called a *tumor;* can be benign or malignant.

net carbs the total grams of carbohydrate per serving after subtracting grams of fiber and sugar alcohols.

neutraceuticals natural ingredients intended to promote and maintain health.

newsgroup a location on the Internet where electronic messages related to a medical topic are posted.

nicotine the addictive substance and alkaloid poison found in tobacco.

novelty diets fad diets often based on gimmicks that typically promote certain nutrients or foods as having unique weight-loss qualities.

nucleoside analogs a combination of drugs (AZT & ddI) that seems to prevent the development of opportunistic infections associated with AIDS.

nutrient a substance found in food that is required by the body.

nutrient density the ratio of nutrients to calories; also called the *index of nutritional quality.*

nutrition the science that deals with the study of nutrients and the way the body ingests, digests, absorbs, transports, metabolizes, and excretes these nutrients.

obesity an excessive amount of storage fat.

ob gene a gene found in fat cells that produces leptin; also called the *fat gene.*

occupational dimension of wellness aspects of wellness that help achieve a balance between work and leisure in a way that promotes health and a sense of personal satisfaction.

Olestra a synthetic fat that has the flavor and taste of real fat but yields no calories.

omega-3 fatty acids the type of fatty acid found in cold-water seafood and thought to lower the risks for heart disease.

oncogene a cancer-causing gene.

osteoarthritis the most common form of arthritis, characterized by the deterioration of the articular cartilage that covers the gliding surfaces of the bones in certain joints.

osteophyte a bone spur.

osteoporosis a progressive decrease in the mineral content of bone, making bones brittle.

overcompensatory eating an eating pattern characterized by overconsumption of low-fat foods, which causes an increase in total caloric intake.

overfat may or may not be within normal guidelines for weight but with an excessive ratio of fat, compared with lean tissue.

overweight excessive weight for one's height without regard for body composition.

ovolactovegetarian a person who eats plant foods, eggs, and dairy products but excludes fish, poultry, and meat from the diet.

partner abuse physical or emotional abuse committed by an adult against his or her partner.

passive smoking the inhalation of environmental cigarette smoke by a nonsmoker.

pathogen a disease-producing organism.

pelvic inflammatory disease (PID) a chronic infection in the uterus, fallopian tubes, and upper reproductive areas; the leading cause of infertility in women.

performance-related fitness sports fitness; composed of speed, power, balance, coordination, agility, and reaction time.

periodic examination a physical exam in which tests and assessments are prescribed according to risk factors.

pescovegetarian a person who eats plant foods, eggs, dairy products, and fish but excludes red meat from the diet.

phytochemicals plant chemicals that exist naturally in foods.

phytoestrogen the plant hormone (estrogen) that exists naturally in foods.

phytomedicinals see *botanicals.*

placebo an inactive substance, such as a fake drug.

point of service (POS) a type of health insurance plan in which subscribers use approved providers who have agreed to accept fixed co-payments.

pollovegetarian a person who eats plant foods, eggs, dairy products, fish, and poultry but excludes red meat.

polypharmacy the administration of many drugs at the same time.

polyunsaturated fat fatty acid composed of triglycerides in which the carbon chain has room for four or more hydrogen atoms.

positive reinforcers rewards earned for achieving goals in a lifestyle-change program.

preferred provider organization (PPO) a group of private practitioners who sell their services at reduced rates to insurance companies.

preventive health behaviors health practices associated with the promotion of wellness and the prevention of sickness and death.

primary-care physician a medical doctor who is responsible for an individual's overall health.

primary site in reference to cancer, the original site of cancer cell formation.

proprioceptive neuromuscular facilitation (PNF) several stretching techniques that involve a combination of contraction and static stretching and holding agonist and antagonist muscle groups.

prospective study an epidemiologic study in which researchers predict possible disease relationships and patterns among groups of people.

protease inhibitor inhibits the enzyme protease, which allows HIV to develop.

protein complementing combining plant protein with cereal/grain protein to provide complete protein.

psychoactives drugs that can alter feelings, moods, and/or perceptions.

psychoneuroimmunology (PNI) the medical discipline whose philosophy rests on the connections among brain function, the nervous system, and the body's response to infection and abnormal cell division.

psychosomatic disease a disease (physical symptom) caused by psychological and emotional stressors.

radiotherapy the use of radiation to either destroy cancer cells or destroy their reproductive mechanism so they cannot replicate.

rape trauma syndrome psychological reactions following a rape; characterized by fear, nightmares, fatigue, crying spells, digestive upset, and perhaps impaired sexual desire/functioning.

reactance motivation a behavioral response to force or coersion in which the behavior is the opposite of that intended (e.g., a child refuses to eat a particular food because of parental force).

recidivism the tendency to revert to original behaviors/conditions after completing a behavior change program.

Recommended Dietary Allowances (RDAs) daily recommended intakes of nutrients for normal, healthy people in the United States.

Reference Daily Intakes (RDIs) minimum standards for essential nutrients; replaces the U.S. recommended daily allowance established in 1968.

relative risk the number or percentage of people affected by a risk factor in relation to or comparison with something else.

relaxation techniques techniques used in coping with and managing stress.

reliability the extent to which health studies yield consistent results.

reminders a behavioral strategy used to formulate action goals.

residual volume the amount of air remaining in the lungs after expiration.

retrospective study an epidemiologic study in which researchers review previously gathered data to identify possible disease relationships and patterns among groups of people.

reward deficiency syndrome a variety of disorders that have in common the traits of impulsiveness, addiction, and compulsiveness.

rheumatoid arthritis the most crippling form of arthritis, characterized by inflammation of the joints, pain, swelling, and deformity.

risk factors conditions that threaten wellness and increase the chances of contracting a disease.

road rage overly aggressive driving, which includes physical or verbal assault against another driver after a traffic dispute.

saccharides sugars.

safer sex a pattern of behavior in which steps are taken to protect oneself and one's partner from pregnancy and infection with HIV and sexually transmitted diseases; these steps can include using condoms or dental dams and having periodic medical tests and examinations.

sarcoma cancer of a connective tissue, such as bone and muscle.

saturated fat a fatty acid composed of triglycerides in which all the fatty acids contain the maximum number of hydrogen atoms.

scientifically controlled study a study conducted in a controlled setting that involves a treatment (experimental) group and a placebo (control) group.

secondary site in reference to cancer, the location of cancer cells after they have spread from the primary site.

sedentary physically inactive.

selective health examination a specific test used in response to specific symptoms or for diagnosing a specific problem.

self-care the movement toward individuals taking increased responsibility to prevent or manage certain health conditions.

self-efficacy people's belief in their ability to accomplish a specific task or behavior; that belief then affects the outcome of the task or behavior; the theory that individuals who expect to succeed tend to succeed and those who expect to fail tend to fail.

self-help the approach to lifestyle change that assumes individuals can plan and execute their own plans.

set point theory the theory that the body has a preference for maintaining a certain amount of weight and defends that weight quite vigorously.

sexually transmitted diseases (STDs) diseases spread through sexual contact, such as AIDS, chlamydia, gonorrhea, and herpes.

shaping up a behavioral strategy in which a person acclimates to desired behaviors in small increments.

sidestream smoke smoke given off by burning tobacco products.

sigmoidoscopy the insertion of a flexible viewing scope into the lower third of the colon.

skinfold measures the method for determining the amount of body fat by using skin calipers.

sleep apnea a condition characterized by loud snoring and brief periods during which breathing ceases.

soluble fiber fiber that dissolves in water; comes from fruit pectins and oat bran.

squamous cell carcinoma the second most common type of skin cancer; it rarely spreads to other areas, but it grows more quickly than basal cell carcinoma.

starch plant polysaccharides composed of glucose and digestible by humans.

static stretching the passive stretching of antagonist muscles by slowly stretching and holding a position for 15 to 30 seconds.

statistical relationship   an association between two or more variables or events.

statistical significance   the probability that a study's findings are reliable and are not due to chance.

stimulants   drugs that speed up the central nervous system.

stimulus control   the technique in lifestyle management involving the elimination and/or manipulation of stimuli related to a specific behavior.

stress   the body's nonspecific response to any demands made on it.

stressor   any physical, psychological, or environmental event or condition that initiates the stress response.

stretch reflex   the myotatic reflex.

stroke volume   the amount of blood that the heart can eject in one beat.

subliminal advertising   a technique in which messages, words, and symbols are embedded or hidden in advertisements.

sucrose   table sugar.

syndrome X   a combination of high blood pressure, high blood sugar, high blood lipids, and abdominal obesity.

syphilis   a sexually transmitted disease.

tar   a black, sticky, dark fluid composed of thousands of chemicals and found in tobacco.

tension headache   the most common kind of headache; caused by

involuntary contractions of the scalp, head, and neck muscles; may be precipitated by anxiety, stress, and allergic reactions.

thermic effect of food (TEF)   the amount of energy required by the body to digest, absorb, metabolize, and store nutrients.

thrombus   a stationary blood clot; can occlude an artery supplying the brain.

trace minerals   minerals required by the body in small amounts.

trans fatty acids   saturated fat found in processed food that has been hydrogenated.

transmit time   the time it takes food to move through the body.

transtheoretical model of behavior change   a self-help approach to lifestyle change consisting of six well-defined stages; it is based on the principles of the behavior change model developed by James Prochaska.

triglyceride   a compound composed of carbon, hydrogen, and oxygen with three fatty acids.

tropical oils   oils that come from the fruit of coconut and palm trees.

ulcerative colitis   chronic inflammation of the colon lining; the symptoms are the same as those of Crohn's disease, but the only area affected is the colon lining.

unintentional injury   any injury that occurs as a result of an accident or reckless behavior.

unsaturated fat   fatty acid composed of triglycerides in which the carbon chain has room for more hydrogen atoms.

validity   the extent to which the research design of a health study permits the assertion of certain health claims.

variable resistance   provides increasing resistance as a weight is lifted through the full range of motion.

vegan   a person whose diet is limited to plant foods; also called a *strict vegetarian.*

very low-calorie diet (VLCD)   a diet containing fewer than 800 calories a day.

viral hepatitis   an inflammation of the liver caused by one or more viruses.

visualization   a form of meditation that makes use of the imagination.

vital capacity   the amount of air that can be expired after a maximum inspiration.

vitamins   organic compounds in food necessary for good health.

vitamin supplements   natural and synthetic compounds taken orally to supplement the vitamins consumed in food.

water intoxication   the consumption of more water than the kidneys can excrete.

weight cycling   a potentially harmful pattern of repeated weight loss and weight gain.

weight maintenance   the consistent maintenance of weight within certain limits between any two points in time.

wellness   engaging in activities and behaviors that enhance quality of life and maximize personal potential.

Photo Credits

Index